W9-BAW-278

Praise for *The Art of Fermentation*

"*The Art of Fermentation* is much more than a cookbook. . . . Sure, it tells you how to do it, but much more important, it tells you what it means, and why an act as quotidian and practical as making your own sauerkraut represents nothing less than a way of engaging with the world. Or rather, with several different worlds, each nested inside the other: the invisible world of fungi and bacteria; the community in which you live; and the industrial food system that is undermining the health of our bodies and the land. This might seem like a large claim for a crock of sauerkraut, but Sandor Katz's signal achievement in this book is to convince you of its truth. To ferment your own food is to lodge an eloquent protest—of the senses—against the homogenization of flavors and food experiences now rolling like a great, undifferentiated lawn across the globe. It is also a declaration of independence from an economy that would much prefer we were all passive consumers of its commodities, rather than creators of unique products expressive of ourselves and the places where we live."

—MICHAEL POLLAN, from the Foreword

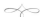

"*The Art of Fermentation* is an extraordinary book, and an impressive work of passion and scholarship. It lays the foundation for fermenting all kinds of foods, and whoever reads it will be able to negotiate any recipe for ferments (and conquer any lingering nervousness about fermentation) with impunity. I am so impressed—and ready to begin! Thank you, Sandor Katz."

—DEBORAH MADISON, author, *Vegetarian Cooking for Everyone* and *Local Flavors*

"Sandor Katz has proven himself to be the king of fermentation with this new book, an exhaustive yet very readable compendium of fermentation wisdom and techniques from around the world. A must-have in the libraries of anyone interested in food and nutrition."

—SALLY FALLON MORELL, President, The Weston A. Price Foundation

"Sandor Katz has already awakened more people to the diversity and deliciousness of fermented foods than any other single person has over the last century. Once you look at the world through the fresh eyes of such a genius, there is no going back to the tasteless world you had previously occupied. *The Art of Fermentation* is a wonder—so rich in its knowledge and so practical in its application. This book will be a classic for the next millennium."

—GARY PAUL NABHAN, author, *Renewing America's Food Traditions* and *Desert Terroir*

"*The Art of Fermentation* is a remarkable testimony to the astonishing passion that Sandor Katz has for all matters fermentative. History, science, and simple how-to wisdom are woven together in this extensive journey through the amazing diversity of foods and beverages that are founded upon fermentation."

—DR. CHARLIE BAMFORTH, Professor, Department of Food Science and Technology, University of California, Davis, and author, *Food, Fermentation and Micro-organisms*

"This is, quite simply, the finest book on fermentation available. It is comprehensive, erudite, and surprisingly profound. Sandor Katz is the guru of a large and growing tribe of fermentation enthusiasts, and this book will awaken you to the thrilling world of benign bacteria all around us. Not only do they provide us with pickles, cheese, bread, alcohol—but our existence depends on bacteria and they deserve our reverence and respect."

—KEN ALBALA, food historian and coauthor, *The Lost Arts of Hearth and Home: The Luddite's Guide to Domestic Self-Sufficiency*

"*The Art of Fermentation* appeals to our personal and fundamental well-being, with a thoroughly engaging account of wild, tamed, and unaccounted-for microorganisms. Based on theory, science, and practical observations, Sandor Katz casts thousands of dots onto the pages for us to connect with our own experiences and interests. There are things he writes in this book that are relevant to everyone. Whether we are at war or peace with the tiny creatures we call microorganisms, we can't help but conclude that they are the building blocks of the communities we observe as organisms. His obsession with ferment is contagious. With the flip of a page it's easy to find oneself discovering our own personal journey embedded in this thoroughly engaging book."

—CHARLIE PAPAZIAN, author, *The Complete Joy of Homebrewing*

"Sandor Katz has captured the essence of fermentation in this new book, which bubbles over with scientific, historical, and practical information about humankind's first biotechnology and earth's first energy source. The mystery and sensory allure of naturally fermented products ranging from fruit, honey, milk, all manner of starchy grain, tuber, and stalk—even fish and meat—are laid bare and enthusiastically and lucidly brought to life for both epicure and the do-at-homer."

—PATRICK E. MCGOVERN, Scientific Director, Biomolecular Archaeology Laboratory, University of Pennsylvania Museum, and author, *Ancient Wine* and *Uncorking the Past*

The ART of FERMENTATION

The ART of FERMENTATION

AN IN-DEPTH EXPLORATION OF ESSENTIAL CONCEPTS AND PROCESSES FROM AROUND THE WORLD

Sandor Ellix Katz

Foreword by Michael Pollan

Chelsea Green Publishing
White River Junction, Vermont

Project Manager: Patricia Stone
Developmental Editor: Makenna Goodman
Copy Editor: Laura Jorstad
Proofreader: Eileen M. Clawson
Indexer: Margaret Holloway
Bacteria Border Illustration: Caroline Paquita
Chapter Illustrations: Elara Tanguy
Designer: Maureen Forys, Happenstance Type-O-Rama

All photographs by Sandor Ellix Katz, unless otherwise credited.

DISCLAIMER: *Information offered in this book is based on years of experimentation, experience, and research. Parameters for safety and warnings of dangers are presented throughout the book and ought to be heeded. However, the author is not a trained professional in food science, food safety, health care, or any other field; neither he nor the publisher is responsible for the consequences of the application or misapplication of any information or ideas presented herein.*

Printed in the United States of America
First printing April 2012
13 12   17 18 19

Our Commitment to Green Publishing
Chelsea Green sees publishing as a tool for cultural change and ecological stewardship. We strive to align our book manufacturing practices with our editorial mission and to reduce the impact of our business enterprise in the environment. We print our books and catalogs on chlorine-free recycled paper, using vegetable-based inks whenever possible. This book may cost slightly more because it was printed on paper containing recycled fiber, and we hope you'll agree that it's worth it. Chelsea Green is a member of the Green Press Initiative (www.greenpressinitiative.org), a nonprofit coalition of publishers, manufacturers, and authors working to protect the world's endangered forests and conserve natural resources. *The Art of Fermentation* was printed on on FSC®-certified paper supplied by LSC Communications containing recycled fibers.

Library of Congress Cataloging-in-Publication Data
Katz, Sandor Ellix, 1962-
The art of fermentation : an in-depth exploration of essential concepts and processes from around the world/Sandor Ellix Katz ; foreword by Michael Pollan.
p. cm.
ISBN 978-1-60358-286-5 (hardcover)—ISBN 978-1-60358-364-0 (ebook)
1. Fermentation. 2. Fermented foods. I. Title.

TP371.44.K369 2012
664'.024—dc23

2011052014

Chelsea Green Publishing
85 North Main Street, Suite 120
White River Junction, VT 05001
(802) 295-6300
www.chelseagreen.com

For my father, Joe Katz, whose favorite thing to talk about is the vegetables coming out of his garden and all the things he and my stepmother Pattie do with them; the acorn doesn't fall far from the tree. I dedicate this book to him and to the many other teachers, mentors, and elders who have guided and inspired me throughout my life.

CONTENTS

FOREWORD

The Art of Fermentation is an inspiring book, and I mean that literally. The book has inspired me to do things I've never done before, and probably never would have done if I hadn't read it. In fact, Katz's book is the main reason that my kitchen counters and basement floor have lately sprouted an assortment of mason jars, ceramic crocks, jelly jars, bottles, and carboys, the clear ones glowing with unearthly colors. Since falling under the spell of Katz's fermentation evangelism, I have launched big crocks of sauerkraut and kimchi; mason jars of pickled cucumbers, carrots, beets, cauliflower, onions, peppers, and ramps; jelly jars of yogurt and kefir; and five-gallon carboys of beer and mead. All of them, I am regularly reminded, are alive. When it's late at night and quiet in the house, I can hear my ferments gurgling contentedly. It's become a deeply pleasing sound, because it means my microbes are happy.

I read cookbooks all the time and never make a thing from them, so why was *The Art of Fermentation* different? For one thing, Sandor Katz writes about the transformative power of fermentation with such infectious enthusiasm that he makes you want to try things *just to see what happens.* It's the same way I felt the day my elementary school teacher told us something miraculous would happen if we mixed up some vinegar with baking soda. These microbial transformations *are* miraculous and so, very often, are the results: striking new flavors and interesting new textures, wrought from the most ordinary ingredients, and not by us but by bacteria and fungi.

Another reason Katz inspires us to try recipes to make things you never even knew existed (kvass? *shrub*?!) is that he never intimidates. To the contrary. As a cookbook—and, as I will get to, it is so much more than a cookbook—*The Art of Fermentation* is empowering. Though the book traffics in many kinds of microbial mystery, Katz is by temperament a demystifier: it's not that complicated, he assures us, anyone can make sauerkraut; here's all you need to do. And if something goes wrong? If your kraut grows an alarming-looking beard of mold? No need to panic; just shave off the mold and enjoy the kraut beneath it.

But this attitude has something more behind it than Sandor Katz's easygoing temperament in the kitchen; there is a politics at work here as well. *The Art of Fermentation* is much more than a cookbook. Or rather, it is a cookbook in the same way that *Zen and the Art of Archery* is a how-to about bows and arrows. Sure, it tells you how to do it, but much more important, it tells you what it means, and why an act as quotidian and practical as making your own sauerkraut represents nothing less than a way of engaging with the world. Or rather, with several different worlds, each nested inside the other: the invisible world of fungi and bacteria; the community in which you live; and the industrial food system that is undermining the health of our bodies and the land.

This might seem like a large claim for a crock of sauerkraut, but Sandor Katz's signal achievement in this book is to convince you of its truth. To ferment your own food is to lodge an eloquent protest—of the senses—against the homogenization of flavors and food experiences now rolling like a great, undifferentiated lawn across the globe. It is also a declaration of independence from an economy that would much prefer we were all passive consumers of its commodities, rather than creators of unique products expressive of ourselves and the places where we live. Because your sauerkraut or homebrew will be nothing like mine or anyone else's.

The Koreans, who know a thing or two about fermentation, distinguish between the "tongue taste" of various foods and the "hand taste." Tongue taste is a simple matter of molecules making contact with taste buds—the kind of cheap and easy flavors any food scientist or food corporation can produce. "Hand taste" is the far more complex experience of a food that bears the indelible mark—the care and sometimes even the love—of the person who made it. The sauerkraut you make yourself will have hand taste.

And you will have plenty of it to give away, trust me. One of the best things about making your own ferments is sharing them with others, off the grid of the cash economy. I now swap bottles of beer and mead with other homebrewers and take part in a steady trade in mason jars, which leave my house brimming with sauerkraut only to return brimming with other people's kimchi or pickles. To delve into the world of fermented foods is to enter the community of fermentos, who happen to be a most interesting, eccentric, and generous bunch.

But of course there is another community to which *The Art of Fermentation* serves as a kind of passport or visa: the unseen community of fungi and bacteria all around us and within us. If this book has an underlying agenda (and it assuredly does) it is to help us reconceive our relationship with what biologist Lynn Margulis calls the "microcosmos." Since Louis Pasteur discovered the role of microbes in disease more than a century ago, most of us have found ourselves on a war footing with respect to bacteria. We dose our children with antibiotics, keep them as far away from microbes as possible, and generally strive to sanitize their world. We are living in the Age of Purell. And yet biologists have come to appreciate that the war on bacteria is not only futile—the bacteria, which can out-evolve us, will always win—but counterproductive.

The profligate use of antibiotics has produced resistant bacteria as lethal as any we managed to kill. Those drugs, along with a processed food diet lacking in both bacteria and food for bacteria (aka fiber), have disordered the microbial ecology in our gut in profound ways that we are just beginning to understand, and which may well explain many of our health problems.

Children protected from bacteria turn out to have higher rates of allergy and asthma. We are discovering that one of the keys to our well-being is the well-being of the microflora with whom we share these bodies, and with whom we co-evolved. And it looks like they really, really like sauerkraut.

In the war on bacteria, Sandor Katz is a confirmed pacifist. But he isn't just sitting out the war, or speechifying about it. He's doing something to end it. A Post-Pasteurian, Katz would have us renegotiate the terms of our relationship with the microcosmos, and *The Art of Fermentation* is an eloquent and practical manifesto showing us exactly how to do that, one crock of sauerkraut at a time. I fully expect that, like a particularly vibrant microbial culture, this book will spawn thousands of new fermentos, and not a moment too soon. Welcome to the party.

—MICHAEL POLLAN
December 22, 2011

ACKNOWLEDGMENTS

*A*lthough I am the lone author of this book, and any errors, misinterpretations, or omissions you may encounter are my sole responsibility, in many ways the process of writing it has been highly collaborative. My education in fermentation, although experiential and without any single central mentor figure, has been highly interactive, informed and guided by an uncountable number of communications, in person and via the Internet. I learned the things that made me decide it was time to write this book not only from the people who shared family recipes, or a microbiologist's perspective, or sent me interesting articles, but from all the people who have posed questions that forced me to reflect and research and further experiment, in order to understand fermentation more deeply, and learn to better explain it. I have no single teacher, but literally thousands of you reading this book have been my teachers. Thank you.

Many people, some quoted in the book, many more not, shared fermentation wisdom they have gleaned. With apologies in advance to anyone I have neglected to include in this list, I thank the following people who shared information, ideas, articles, books, images, and stories: Ken Albala, Dominic Anfiteatro, Nathan and Padgett Arnold, Erik Augustijns, David Bailey, Eva Bakkeslett, Sam Bett, Áron Boros, Jay Bost, Joost Brand, Brooke Budner, Justin Bullard, Jose Caraballo, Astrid Richard Cook, Crazy Crow, Ed Curran, Pamela Day, Razzle F. Dazzle, Michelle Dick, Lawrence Diggs, Vinson Doyle, Fuchsia Dunlap, Betsey Dexter Dyer, Orese Fahey, Ove Fosså, Brooke Gillon, Favero Greenforest, Alexandra Grigorieva, Brett Guadagnino, Eric Haas, Christy Hall, Annie Hauck-Lawson, Lisa Heldke, Sybil Heldke, Kim Hendrickson, Vic Hernandez, Julian Hockings, Bill Keener, Linda Kim, Joel Kimmons, Qilo Kinetichore, David LeBauer, Jessica Lee, Jessieca Leo, Maggie Levinger, Liz Lipski, Raphael Lyon, Lynn Margulis, E. Shig Matsukawa, Sarick Matzen, Patrick McGovern, April McGreger, Trae Moore, Jennifer Moragoda, Sally Fallon Morell, Merril Mushroom, Alan Muskat, Keith Nicholson, Lady Free Now, Sushe Nori, Rick Otten, Caroline Paquita, Jessica Porter, Elizabeth Povinelli, Lou Preston, Thea Prince, Nathan and Emily Pujol, Milo Pyne, Lynn Razaitis, Luke Regalbuto, Anthony Richter, Jimmy Rose, Bill Shurtleff, Josh Smotherman, Sterling, Betty Stechmeyer, Aylin Öney Tan, Mary Morgaine Thames, Turtle T. Turtlington, Alwyn de Wally, Pamela Warren, Rebekah Wilce, Marc Williams, and Valencia Wombone. I thank the Oxford Symposium on Food and Cookery for inviting me to present a paper at their 2010 conference, which had the theme "Cured, Fermented, and Smoked," and I thank the other presenters and participants there for the varied perspectives and stimulation I encountered.

I have had great helpers to assist me in experimentation, research, and organizing information. Special appreciations to Caeleb Grey, Spiky, MaxZine Weinstein, and Malory Foster. For invaluable long-distance research assistance, I thank Char Booth and my lifelong friend Laura Harrington. For providing me with a writer's retreat early in the process of writing this book, I thank Layard Thompson, Rya Kleinpeter, and Benjy Russell. For reading my manuscript as it evolved and providing me with feedback, I thank Spiky, Silverfang, MaxZine Weinstein, Betty Stechmeyer, Merril Mushroom, and Helga Thompson. I thank Michael Pollan for contributing the foreword to this book. I thank all the good people of Chelsea Green Publishing, with a special shout out to my wonderful editor Makenna Goodman. I thank my agent Valerie Borchardt.

I thank the creators of the food I so love to eat, experiment with, and write about: the plants and the animals, and the people who tend them. Specifically, I thank Simmer and Krista for milk; Branch, Sylvan, Daniel, Junebug, and Dashboard for eggs; Neal Appelbaum and Bill Keener (Sequatchie Cove Farm) for meat; Hush and Boxer for honey; Hector Black and Brinna for blueberries; and many people for vegetables, especially: Daz'l, Spiky, and the other garden faeries at Short Mountain; MaxZine and the ever-shifting IDA garden crew; Billy Kaufman, Stoney, John Whittemore, Jimmy Rose, and the Woofers at Little Short Mountain Farm; Mike Bondy and Rob Parker; Daniel; Jeff Poppen (the barefoot farmer of Long Hungry Creek Farm); and many more generous friends. I thank Angie Ott and Daz'l for providing so many of us with such varied and healthy starts; and Merril and Daz'l for always sharing their saved seeds. Being part of this network of food production and exchange is very inspiring and rewarding.

Most of all, I thank my beautiful friends and families, who have continued to indulge and encourage my obsession with fermentation. I thank my family of birth; I feel very lucky to have a family that I like so much, and in which I have received such steady support. While writing this book, I made the difficult decision to move out of the commune where I lived for 17 years, and into my own place down the road. I'm settling in to a new routine, and all is good. I thank everyone who lives at Short Mountain Sanctuary and IDA and our extended faeborhood community for your love and devotion, and for tasting all the experimental ferments I show up with. Among this group, and our regular visitors, are my dearest friends and intimates. You know who you are, and you know how much I love you.

INTRODUCTION

*L*ittle could I have imagined, as a New York City kid who loved pickles, that those delicious, crunchy, garlicky sour pickles would lead me on such an extraordinary journey of discovery and exploration. In fact, products of fermentation—not only pickles, but also bread, cheese, yogurt, sour cream, salami, vinegar, soy sauce, chocolate, and coffee, as well as beer and wine—were prominent in my family's diet (as they are in many, if not most, people's), though we never talked about them as such. Yet, as my path through life led me to various nutritional ideas and dietary experiments, I did learn about the digestive benefits of bacteria present in living fermented foods and began to experience their restorative powers. And when I found myself with a garden, faced with a surplus of cabbages and radishes, sauerkraut beckoned me. Our love affair endures.

The first time I taught a sauerkraut-making workshop, at the Sequatchie Valley Institute in 1999, I learned that there is a tremendous fear in our culture of aging food outside of refrigeration. In our time, most people are raised to view bacteria as dangerous enemies and refrigeration as a household necessity. The idea of leaving food outside of refrigeration in order to encourage bacterial growth triggers fears of danger, disease, and even death. "How will I know whether the right bacteria are growing?" is a common question. People largely assume that for microbial transformations to be safe, they require extensive knowledge and control and are therefore a specialized domain best left to experts.

Most food and beverage fermentation processes are ancient rituals that humans have been performing since before the dawn of history, yet we have largely relegated them to factory production. Fermentation has mostly disappeared from our households and communities. Techniques evolved by disparate human cultures over millennia, through observation of natural phenomena and manipulating conditions with trial and error, have become obscure and are in danger of being lost.

I have spent nearly two decades exploring the realm of fermentation. I do not have a background in microbiology or food science; I am just a food-loving back-to-the-land generalist who became obsessed with fermentation, spurred by a voracious appetite, a practical desire for food not to go to waste, and a willful desire to maintain good health. I have experimented widely, talked to many, many people about the subject, and done a lot of reading on it. The more

I experiment and the more I learn, the more I realize how little of an expert I remain. People grow up in households in which some of these traditional ferments are the daily context, and their knowledge is far more intimate. Others become commercial manufacturers and develop technical mastery in order to produce and market consistent and profitable products; countless such people know much more than I about brewing beer, making cheese, baking bread, curing salamis, or brewing *saké*. Microbiologists or other scientists who study very specific facets of the genetics, metabolism, kinetics, community dynamics, or other mechanisms of fermentations understand it all in terms I can only barely comprehend.

Nor do I possess anything approaching encyclopedic knowledge of fermentation. The infinite variation that exists in how people on every continent ferment all the various foods they eat is too vast for any individual to have comprehensive knowledge. However, I have had the privilege to hear a lot of wonderful stories, and taste many homemade and artisan-fermented concoctions. Many readers of my books, visitors to my website, and participants in my workshops have recounted tales of their grandparents' fermentation practices; immigrants have excitedly told me about ferments from the old country, often lost to them through migration; travelers have reported on ferments they have encountered; people have divulged their quirky family variations; and other experimentalists such as myself have shared their adventures. I have also fielded thousands of troubleshooting questions, causing me to research and think about many more aspects of the inevitable variations that occur in home fermentations.

This book is a compendium of the fermentation wisdom I have collected. I have included many other people's voices throughout. Though I have made an attempt to be thorough, this book is far from encyclopedic. My intention with it is to identify patterns and convey concepts to empower you with tools so you can explore and reclaim fermentation into your life. I am on a mission of sharing skills, resources, and information related to this important art, in the hope that these long-standing coevolutionary relationships, embedded in cultural practices, are not lost but rather spread, cross-pollinated, and adapted.

One word that repeatedly comes to the fore in my exploration and thinking about fermentation is *culture*. Fermentation relates to culture in many different ways, corresponding with the many layers of meaning embedded in this important word, from its literal and specific meanings in the context of microbiology to its broadest connotations. We call the starters that we add to milk to make yogurt, or to initiate any fermentation, cultures. Simultaneously, culture constitutes the totality of all that humans seek to pass from generation to generation, including language, music, art, literature, scientific knowledge, and belief systems, as well as agriculture and culinary techniques (in both of which fermentation occupies a central role).

In fact, the word *culture* comes from Latin *cultura*, a form of *colere*, "to cultivate." Our cultivation of the land and its creatures—plants, animals, fungi, and bacteria—is essential to culture. Reclaiming our food and our participation in cultivation is a means of cultural revival, taking action to break out of the confining and infantilizing dependency of the role of consumer (user), and taking back our dignity and power by becoming producers and creators.

This is not just about fermentation (even if, as a biological force upon our food, that is inevitable), but about food more broadly. Every living creature on this Earth interacts intimately with its environment via its food. Humans in our developed technological society, however, have largely severed this connection, and with disastrous results. Though affluent people have more food choices than people of the past could ever have dreamed of, and though one person's labor can produce more food today than ever before, the large-scale, commercial methods and systems that enable these phenomena are destroying our Earth, destroying our health, and depriving us of dignity. With respect to food, the vast majority of people are completely dependent for survival upon a fragile global infrastructure of monocultures, synthetic chemicals, biotechnology, and transportation.

Moving toward a more harmonious way of life and greater resilience requires our active participation. This means finding ways to become more aware of and connected to the other forms of life that are around us and that constitute our food—plants and animals, as well as bacteria and fungi—and to the resources, such as water, fuel, materials, tools, and transportation, upon which we depend. It means taking responsibility for our shit, both literally and figuratively. We can become creators of a better world, of better and more sustainable food choices, of greater awareness of resources, and of community based upon sharing. For culture to be strong and resilient, it must be a creative realm in which skills, information, and values are engaged and transmitted; culture cannot thrive as a consumer paradise or a spectator sport. Daily life offers constant opportunities for participatory action. Seize them.

Just as the microbial cultures exist only as communities, so too do our broader human cultures. Food is the greatest community builder there is. It invites people to sit and stay awhile, and families to gather together. It welcomes new neighbors and weary travelers and beloved old friends. And it takes a village to produce food. Many hands make light work, and food production often gives rise to specialization and exchange. And even more than food in general, fermented foods—especially beverages—play a significant role in community building. Not only are many feasts, rituals, and celebrations organized around products of fermentation (such as bread and wine), ferments are also among the oldest and most important of the foods that add both value and stability to the raw products of agriculture, essential to the economic underpinnings of all communities. The brewer and the baker are central participants in any grain-based economy; and wine transforms perishable grapes into a stable and coveted commodity, as does cheese for milk.

Reclaiming our food means reclaiming community, engaging its economic interconnectivity of specialization and divisions of labor, but at a *human* scale, promoting awareness of resources and local exchange. Transporting goods around the globe takes a huge amount of resources and wreaks environmental havoc. And while exotic foods can be thrilling treats, it's inappropriate and destructive to organize our lives primarily around them; most globalized food commodities are grown in vast monocultures, at the expense of forests and diverse subsistence crops. And by being totally dependent on an infrastructure of global trade, we make ourselves exceedingly vulnerable to disruptions for any number of reasons, from natural disasters (floods, earthquakes, tsunamis) and resource depletion (peak oil), to political violence (war, terrorism, organized crime).

Fermentation can be a centerpiece of economic revival. Relocalizing food means a renewal not only of agriculture but also of the processes used to transform and preserve the products of agriculture into the things that people eat and drink every day, including ferments such as bread, cheese, and beer. By participating in local food production—agriculture and beyond—we actually create important resources that can help fill our most basic daily needs. By supporting this local food revival, we recycle our dollars into our communities, where they may repeatedly circulate, supporting people in productive endeavors and creating incentives for people to acquire important skills, as well as feeding us fresher, healthier food with less fuel and pollution embedded in it. As our communities feed ourselves more and thereby reclaim power and dignity, we also decrease our collective dependency on the fragile infrastructure of global trade. Cultural revival means economic revival.

Everywhere I go I meet people who are making the choice to be part of this culture of revival. Perhaps this is exemplified best by the growing number of young people who are choosing to take up farming. The second half of the 20th century saw the near extinction of the tradition of regional food self-sufficiency in the United States and many other places. Today that tradition is in revival. Let us support and become part of it. Productive local food systems are better than globalized food for many reasons: They yield fresher and more nutritious food; local jobs and productivity; less dependence on fuel and infrastructure; and greater food security. We must become more closely connected to the land via our food, and we must have people willing to do the hard physical work of agriculture. Value and reward that work. And get involved with it.

I don't want to give the impression that this culture of revival is brand new. There always have been holdouts who resist new technologies, such as farmers who never adopted chemical methods, or never stopped using and saving the legacy of seed resources they inherited, or still use horses in lieu of tractors, or families who have unceasingly maintained fermentation practices. There have always been seekers looking to reconnect to old ways, or unwilling to accept the "conveniences" of modern culture. As much as culture is always reinventing itself in unprecedented ways, culture is continuity. There are always roots.

Cultural revival certainly does not require abandoning cities and suburbs for some remote rural ideal. We must create more harmonious ways of life where people and infrastructures are, and that is mostly cities and suburbs. "Sustainability" or "resilience" cannot be remote ideals you have to go somewhere else to fully realize. They are ethics we can and must build into our lives however we are able to and wherever we find ourselves.

Nearly 20 years ago, I moved from a lifetime in Manhattan to an off-the-grid rural commune in Tennessee, and I'm so glad I did. Sometimes a dramatic change is exactly what you need. I was 30 years old, had recently tested HIV+, and was searching for a big change I could not yet imagine, when a chance encounter led me to a communal homestead of queers in the woods. I can personally testify that rural resettlement can be a rewarding path. But rural living is certainly not intrinsically better or more sustainable than city life. In fact, rural dwelling, as most of us (myself included) are practicing it, involves driving frequently to get around. In the city I grew up in, most people do not have cars and get around using mass transit.

Cities are where most people are, and much incredibly creative and transformative work is being done in urban and suburban areas. Urban farming and homesteading are on the rise, flourishing especially in cities with large expanses of abandoned properties. The revival of artisan fermentation enterprises is centered around cities, mainly because they hold the major markets, no matter where production may occur.

The late, great urbanist Jane Jacobs put forth an intriguing theory that agriculture developed and spread from cities rather than rural outposts. In her book *The Economy of Cities*, Jacobs rejects the prevailing assumption that "cities are built upon a rural economic base," which she calls the "dogma of agricultural primacy."[1] Instead she argues that the inherent creativity of urbanism fostered the innovations that spawned (and continually reinvent) agriculture. "The first spread of the new grains and animals is from city to city. . . . The cultivation of plants and animals is, as yet, only city work."[2] Her basic idea is that a trading settlement that is a crossroads for people migrating from different areas provides a dynamic environment for incidental seed crossing and selective breeding, as well as greater opportunities for specialization and the development and spread of techniques.

If Jacobs's theory is correct, then fermentation practices must also have urban roots. Rural dwellers may frequently be guardians of inherited legacies such as seeds, cultures, and know-how; however, it is primarily urbanites who are spurring agricultural change in the countryside by creating demand— starting farmer's markets and providing the bulk of the community support for what is known as community supported agriculture (CSA). Urbanites can grow gardens and ferment, just as rural dwellers can. They can also tap into the deep currents of creativity that exist in cities, and the inevitable cross-pollination that occurs there, to foster change. That change can incorporate ancient wisdom that is in danger of disappearing, just as much as it can foster innovation. In any case, cultural revival is not exclusively or even primarily a rural endeavor.

Much of the 20th-century literature of fermentation promoted moving production away from small-scale community-based cottage industry into factories and replacing traditional starter cultures passed down from generation to generation with laboratory-bred improved strains, in the name of improved hygiene, safety, nutrition, and efficiency. "When an attempt was made to introduce Western-type beverages such as beer, Coca-Cola, and other soft drinks to the Bantu people, they were rejected," Clifford W. Hesseltine and Hwa L. Wang, of the US Department of Agriculture Fermentation Laboratory, reported in 1977, "so the Bantu beer process, as practiced in the native villages, was investigated. When the native process was understood and the yeast and bacteria occurring in the process had been isolated, an industrial fermentation process was developed using modern malting and fermentation equipment. The Bantu beer made in these modern fermentation plants was readily accepted. . . . The product, produced under sanitary conditions, is of uniform quality and sells at a low price."[3] A cheap and uniform product, mass-produced under sanitary conditions, is taken as unequivocally superior to the traditional village-produced product, regardless of the cultural and economic importance of the practice in the village context. Meanwhile, Paul Barker, from South Africa, writes: "Traditional fermentation along with many other practices are dying out in our African cultures and need to be recorded before lost to the likes of KFC, Coca Cola and Levi's."

My objective with this book is to encourage a reclaiming of fermentation in our homes and in our communities, as a means of reclaiming food, and with it a broad web of connections. Rather than fermenting just grapes, barley, and soybeans, let's ferment acorns, turnips, sorghum, or whatever food surpluses we can access or create. The great global monoculture ferments are wonderful, indeed, but the practical thrust of localism must be learning to make the most of surpluses that make themselves, such as acorns, or are so well adapted that they practically grow themselves with only a minimum of intervention, such as turnips or radishes in Tennessee gardens.

This book is organized around types of ferments, and specifically how to make them. The first three chapters are broad overviews, contextualizing fermentation in terms of evolution, practical benefits, and basic operational concepts. Most of the rest is organized by substrates—what foods are fermenting—and whether or not the products are primarily alcoholic. The end chapters address considerations for people thinking about turning their passion for fermentation into a commercial enterprise, non-food applications of fermentation, and finally a cultural revivalist manifesto.

In the processes-focused core of the book, I have abandoned the recipe format (aside from a few sidebars with recipes contributed by others). Rather than specific recipes, I wish to communicate concepts with broad applicability. I offer general proportions, or ranges of proportions, and process parameters, and sometimes even seasoning suggestions. I have attempted to explain what to do in each ferment, and why. Fermentation is more dynamic and variable than cooking, for we are collaborating with other living beings. The hows and whys of these sometimes complex relationships are more important than the specific quantities and combinations of ingredients, which inevitably vary among recipes and traditions. I want to help you understand the hows and whys of fermentation. With that understanding, recipes are everywhere, and you can creatively explore.

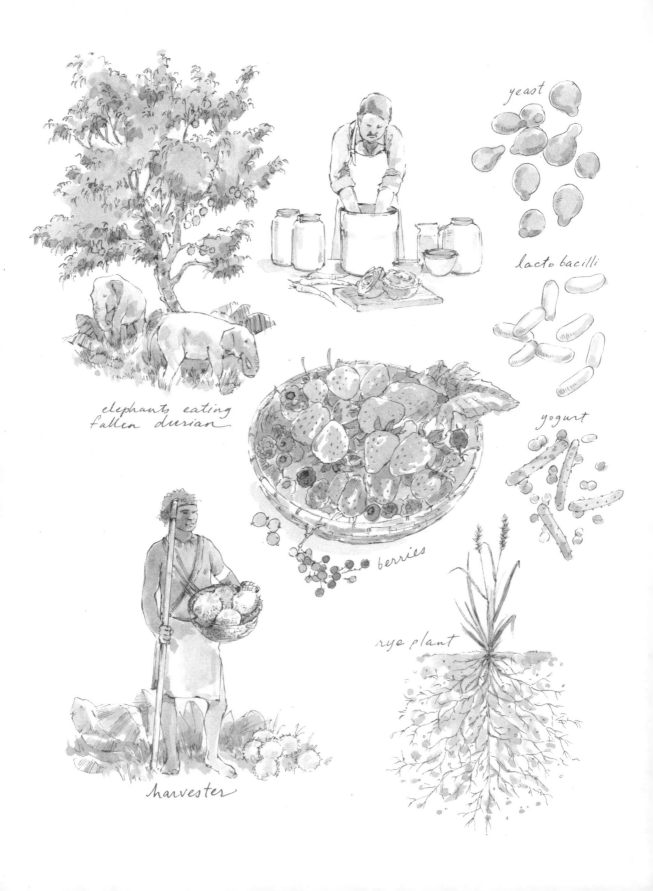

yeast

lacto bacilli

yogurt

elephants eating
fallen durian

berries

rye plant

harvester

CHAPTER 1

Fermentation as a Coevolutionary Force

*M*ost of the information you will find in this book pertains to techniques for fermenting delicious, nutritious foods and beverages for human consumption. In this context, fermentation is the transformation of food by various bacteria, fungi, and the enzymes they produce. People harness this transformative power in order to produce alcohol, to preserve food, and to make it more digestible, less toxic, and/or more delicious. By some estimates, as much as one-third of all food eaten by human beings worldwide is fermented,[1] and fermented food production, taken as a whole, constitutes one of the world's largest industries.[2] Fermentation has played an instrumental role in human cultural evolution, as we shall explore. It is important to recognize, however, that fermentation is a natural phenomenon much broader than human culinary practices; cells in our bodies are capable of fermentation. In other words, humans did not invent or create fermentation; it would be more accurate to state that fermentation created us.

 ## Bacteria: Our Ancestors and Coevolutionary Partners

Biologists use the term *fermentation* to describe *anaerobic* metabolism, the production of energy from nutrients without oxygen. Fermenting bacteria are thought to have emerged relatively early from the primordial prebiotic soup, before the atmosphere had a sufficient concentration of oxygen to support or evolve aerobic life-forms. "In the first two billion years of life on Earth, bacteria—the only inhabitants—continuously transformed the planet's surface and atmosphere and invented all of life's essential, miniaturized chemical systems," writes biologist Lynn Margulis.[3] The research of Margulis and others has convinced many biologists that symbiotic relationships between fermenting bacteria and other early single-cell life-forms became permanently embodied as the first *eukaryotic* cells that plants, animals, and fungi comprise.[4] As Margulis and Dorion Sagan explain in their book *Microcosmos*, the symbiosis may have begun as a predator-prey relationship:

> Eventually some of the prey evolved a tolerance for their aerobic predators, which then remained alive and well in the food-rich interior of the host. Two types of organisms used the products of each other's metabolisms. As they reproduced inside the invaded cells without causing harm, the predators gave up their independent ways and moved in for good.[5]

Evolution derived from such symbiosis is known as *symbiogenesis*. Microbiologists Sorin Sonea and Léo G. Mathieu elaborate on the concept: "*Symbiogenesis* with thousands of different bacterial genes has decisively enriched the limited metabolic potential of eukaryotic organisms, accelerating and facilitating their adaptation much more than would have been achieved by random mutation alone."[6]

Bacterial fermentation processes have been part of the context for all life. Fermentation plays such a broad and vital role in nutrient cycling that all beings coevolved with it, ourselves included. Through symbiosis and coevolution, bacteria fused into new forms, spawning all other life. "For the past [billion] years, members of the Bacteria superkingdom have functioned as a major selective force shaping eukaryotic evolution," state molecular biologists Jian Xu and Jeffrey I. Gordon. "Coevolved symbiotic relationships between bacteria and multicellular organisms are a prominent feature of life on Earth."[7] The importance of bacteria and our bacterial interactions cannot be overstated. We could not exist or function without our bacterial partners.

berries

Like all complex multicellular life-forms, the human body is host to an elaborate indigenous biota. Some geneticists argue that we are " a composite of many species," with a genetic landscape that encompasses not only the human genome but also those of our bacterial symbionts.[8] In our bodies, bacteria outnumber the cells containing our unique DNA by more than 10 to 1.[9] The vast majority of these bacteria—a mind-boggling 100 trillion (10^{14}) in number—are found in our intestines.[10] Bacteria break down nutrients we would not otherwise be able to digest[11] and play an important role, just beginning to be recognized, in regulating the balance between energy use and storage.[12] Intestinal bacteria produce certain necessary nutrients for us, including B and K vitamins.[13] They provide us with vital defense by "outcompeting invading pathogens for ecological niches and metabolic substrates."[14] In addition, intestinal bacteria are able to modulate "expression" of some of our genes, related to "diverse and fundamental physiological functions,"[15] including immune response. "Evidence of an active dialogue is rapidly unfolding" between intestinal bacteria and the immune cells of the intestine linings.[16]

That's just the bacteria in our intestines. On our bodies' surfaces, microbial communities exist in a great range of distinct niches. "For example, hairy, moist underarms lie a short distance from smooth dry forearms, but these two niches are likely as ecologically dissimilar as rainforests are to deserts," observed a 2009 study of the genetic diversity of skin bacteria.[17] Bacteria inhabit all our surfaces, particularly the warmer sweaty places that stay moist, as well as our eyes, upper respiratory tract, and orifices; more than 700 species have been detected in the healthy oral cavity.[18]

Even our reproduction requires fermentation. The human vagina has been found to secrete glycogen that supports an indigenous population of lactobacilli, which ferment the glycogen into lactic acid, thereby protecting the vagina from pathogenic bacteria, which cannot survive in an acid environment. "The presence of lactobacilli as a part of the normal vaginal flora is an important component of reproductive health."[19] Our indigenous bacteria protect us everywhere and enable us to function in myriad ways that are just beginning to be understood. From an evolutionary perspective, this extensive microbiota "endows us with functional features that we have not had to evolve ourselves."[20] This is a miracle of coevolution—the bacteria that coexist with us in our bodies enable us to exist. Microbiologist Michael Wilson notes that "each exposed surface of a human being is colonized by microbes exquisitely adapted to that particular environment."[21] Yet the dynamics of these microbial populations, and how they interact with our bodies, are still largely unknown. A 2008 comparative genomics analysis of lactic acid bacteria acknowledges that research is "just now beginning to scratch the surface of the complex relationship between humans and their microbiota."[22]

harvester

Bacteria are such effective coevolutionary partners because they are highly adaptable and mutable. "Bacteria continually monitor their external and internal environments and compute functional outputs based on information provided by their sensory apparatus," explains bacterial geneticist James Shapiro, who reports "multiple widespread bacterial systems for mobilizing and engineering DNA molecules."[23] In contrast with our eukaryotic cells, with fixed genetic material, prokaryotic bacteria have free-floating genes, which they frequently exchange. For this reason, some microbiologists consider it inappropriate to view bacteria as distinct species. "There are no species in prokaryotes," state Sorin Sonea and Léo G. Mathieu.[24] "Bacteria are much more of a continuum," explains Lynn Margulis. "They just pick up genes, they throw away genes, and they are very flexible about that."[25] Mathieu and Sonea describe a bacterial "genetic free market," in which "each bacterium can be compared to a two-way broadcasting station, using genes as information molecules." Genes "are carried by a bacterium only when needed . . . as a human may carry sophisticated tools."[26]

The emerging details of gene transfer are fascinating. In addition to exchanging genes directly with other bacteria, bacteria have receptors to receive genes from *prophages*, which Sonea and Mathieu call "a unique type of biological but inanimate construction: a micro-robot for gene exchanges . . . organized like an ultra-microscopic syringe with a hollow container ('head'), and an ultra-microscopic needle ('tail'). . . . This exclusively bacterial type of instrument for gene exchange among living beings may be carried across large distances by water, wind, animals, etc."

With so many mechanisms for genetic exchange, "all the world's bacteria essentially have access to a single gene pool and hence to the adaptive mechanisms of the entire bacteria kingdom," summarize Margulis and Sagan.[27] Beyond genetic flexibility, "bacteria utilise sophisticated mechanisms for inter-cellular communication and even have the ability to commandeer the basic cell biology of 'higher' plants and animals to meet their own needs," writes geneticist James Shapiro.[28] A new understanding of bacteria is emerging; far from being simplistic "lower forms" of life, they are becoming recognized as highly evolved, with elaborate systems for adaptability and resilience.

In any particular environment, some subset of the total bacterial gene pool is present. Interesting research recently identified a new class of enzymes, produced by a marine bacteria, *Zobellia galactanivorans*, that can digest a polysaccharide called *porphyran*, found in some seaweed (including nori), where the bacteria were found. Through genome analysis, investigators identified specific genes in the bacteria that produce the enzyme.

rye plant

Then, searching gene-sequencing databases, the investigators found the same genes in bacteria in the intestines of Japanese populations, but not North Americans. "This indicates that seaweeds with associated marine bacteria may have been the route by which these novel [enzymes] were acquired in human gut bacteria," conclude the researchers, elaborating that "contact with non-sterile food may be a general factor in [enzyme] diversity in human gut microbes."[29] What this means is that, to some degree, the microbes on the food we eat determine our metabolic capabilities.

This finding raises huge questions about both the past and the future. "It remains to be determined how, during human evolution, changes in food production and preparation such as agriculture and cooking have influenced the intestinal microbiota," notes a discussion in the journal *Nature*. "Consumption of hyper-hygienic, mass-produced, highly processed and calorie-dense foods is testing how rapidly the microbiota of individuals in industrialized countries can adapt while being deprived of the environmental reservoirs of microbial genes that allow adaptation by lateral transfer."[30]

We need not continue to deprive ourselves! If sterilized, processed food is starving our microbiota of genetic stimulation, live-culture foods that are rich depositories of bacterial genes are part of our human cultural legacy, everywhere. Through dietary change, we can indulge ourselves, and eat a variety of bacteria-rich living foods, precisely in order to build such genetic reservoirs inside our intestines, to enhance our metabolic capabilities, our immune function, and many other regulatory physiological functions.

Humans are not unique in having coevolved with bacterial symbionts. Plants also coevolved with and are dependent upon bacterial partners. A symbiotic relationship between photosynthesizing bacteria and other prokaryotes is thought by many to be the origin of the photosynthesizing chloroplasts in plant cells.[31] The soil around plant roots makes up what is known as the *rhizosphere*, where plants find sustenance through elaborate interaction with a multifaceted "soil food web." "We know more about the stars in the sky than about the soil under our feet," points out soil microbiologist Elaine Ingham.[32] Roots and their surfaces for soil interaction are actually far more elaborate than meets the eye. A single rye plant, growing but a season, has millions of rootlets, altogether running an estimated 680 miles/1,094 km, and each of the rootlets is covered with still smaller root hairs, numbering in the billions on each plant, altogether running 6,600 miles/10,600 km.[33] All these microscopic root hairs release *exudates* into the soil, highly regulated excretions including sugars, amino acids, enzymes, and many other nutrients and unique chemical compounds, creating a very selective environment in which they "literally call the proper bacteria to the area where [the plant] is growing," according to Stephen Harrod Buhner.[34] Like us, plants rely on bacteria for their survival and have evolved elaborate mechanisms for attracting and interacting with them.

Because we have evolved eating both plants and animals—and have coevolved with them—our coevolutionary histories encompass not only the plants and animals themselves but also their microbial associates. It is the ubiquitous presence of these life-forms, present from the very beginning but invisible until the past few centuries, which results in the ferments, nearly all prehistoric, that we love to eat and drink. The ferments, in spontaneously occurring forms, predate our consciousness of how to manipulate conditions so as to guide their development. But our consciousness did develop, and as part of that, so did the fermentation arts. The ferment itself, and our ability to

yogurt

produce it, is as much a product of coevolution as the person, plant, yeast, or bacterium. Thus coevolution encompasses even culture.

 ## Fermentation and Culture

What exactly is culture? In contrast with the realm of biological reproduction, where information is coded and copied as genes, in the cultural realm information is encoded as memes. Memes are transmitted through words, concepts, images, processes, abstractions—stories, pictures, books, films, photographs, computer programs, ledgers. Secret family recipes. Life lessons, like learning to identify edible plants, learning to garden, learning to cook, learning to fish, learning to procure, use, and preserve precious food resources. Fermenting.

It is largely our history of interacting with plants (and associated microbes) that gives rise to what we call "culture." After all, the word *culture* comes from Latin *cultura*, a form of the verb *colere*, to cultivate or till. The first definition of culture in the *Oxford English Dictionary* is simply: "The cultivation of land, and derived senses." Through these derived senses, and the many varied manifestations of cultivation, ideas of what could be cultivated grew. People culture pearls, we culture cells, and we culture milk. We practice aquaculture, viticulture, and horticulture, not to mention popular culture. Many people work hard to imbue their children with culture. Sometimes people decry cultural appropriation or defend cultural purity. Culture begins with cultivating the land, planting seeds, bringing intentionality to cycles that we act to perpetuate. Indeed, a more ancient origin of the word *culture* is the Indo-European root *kwel*, meaning "to revolve," from which *cycle*, *circle*, *chakra*, and many other words, along with *culture*, are derived.[35] Culture is cultivation, but it is not an isolated act; it is, by definition, part of a cyclical ongoing process, passed from generation to generation.

As my exploration of fermentation unfolds, I keep coming back to the profound significance of the fact that we use the same word—*culture*—to describe the community of bacteria that transform milk into yogurt, as well as the practice of subsistence itself, language, music, art, literature, science, spiritual practices, belief systems, and all that human beings seek to perpetuate in our varied and overlapping collective existences. As described earlier, successful coexistence with microbes in our midst is a biological imperative, and the fermentation arts are human cultural manifestations of this essential fact. If we are to enjoy surpluses of food, then we must have strategies for preserving them in the presence of the microbial ecology, such as it is. Clearly, as a group, fermented foods and beverages are more than incidental culinary novelties; they appear to be found in some form in every culinary tradition. I have searched—without success—for examples of cultures that do not incorporate any form of fermentation. Indeed, ferments are central features of many, perhaps even most, cuisines. Immigrants crossing continents and oceans—their only belongings the ones they could carry—have often brought their sourdoughs and other starters with them, or at the very least their fermentation knowledge and practices. The fermentation starters themselves, and the knowledge of how to use them, are tangible embodiments of culture, deeply embedded in our desires and cravings, not lightly abandoned.

How can we even imagine the cultural realm without alcoholic beverages? Though some religions and nations ban alcohol altogether, thus defining themselves in opposition to it, alcohol is known and used everywhere, and of widespread importance in ritual, ceremony, and celebration. "Their preeminence and universal allure—what might be called their biological, social, and religious imperatives—make them significant in understanding the development of our species and its cultures," states anthropologist Patrick E. McGovern, who has identified alcohol residues in 9,000-year-old pottery shards. "Our species' intimate relationship with fermented beverages over millions of years has, in large measure, made us what we are today."[36] Most people seem to enjoy manipulating our gift and burden of consciousness, and do so by whatever means available. Alcohol has been far and away the most widely available and widely used intoxicant.

lacto bacilli

We do not know the origins of alcohol. The alcohol that Professor McGovern identified from the Neolithic settlement of Jiahu in China was made from a mixture of rice, honey, and fruit.[37] It would appear that these early human alcohol makers were combining available carbohydrate and yeast sources, however they might have conceptualized the process. Is it possible that, rather than humans "discovering" alcohol and mastering its production, we evolved always already knowing it? Anthropologist Mikal John Aasved points out that "all vertebrate species are equipped with a hepatic enzyme system with which to metabolize alcohol."[38] Many animals have been documented consuming alcohol in their natural habitats. One of them, a daily consumer of alcohol in the Malaysian jungle, is the pentailed treeshrew (*Ptilocercus lowii*). Interestingly, this mammal is considered to be "the morphologically least-derived living descendant of early ancestors of primates," regarded as a "living model" for the ancestral lineage from which primates radiated.[39] The alcohol these treeshrews consume occurs naturally on the bertram palm (*Eugeissona tristis*), on "specialized flower buds that harbor a fermenting yeast community."[40] And the treeshrews are pollinators for the bertram palm. This tree, its pollinating shrews, and the fermenting yeast community all coevolved this arrangement together. It would be absurd to think of one species as the primary actor in this mutualistic community.

As the primate family diverged from the treeshrews, it lost such highly specialized alcohol-laced relationships. But our primate and humanoid ancestors presumably ate lots of fruit, which ferments when ripe, especially quickly in the warm and wet jungle climate. Biologist Robert Dudley theorizes that our precursors were routinely exposed to alcohol in fruit, and that "this exposure in turn elicited corresponding physiological adaptations and preferences over an evolutionary time scale that are retained in modern humans."[41]

While alcohol is present in fruits at low concentrations compared with alcoholic beverages, the fleeting availability of seasonal fruits encourages gorging. I know I respond to plentiful ripe berries that way. And I am not unique in this regard. Addiction researcher Ronald Siegel describes animals responding to fallen, split, fermenting durian fruits in Malaysia:

> A menagerie of jungle beasts, alerted by the ripening odor, parade to the fallen fruit. . . . Elephants that may have migrated from great distances sometimes gorge themselves on the fermented fruit remaining on the ground; they start swaying in a lethargic manner. The monkeys frequently lose motor coordination, have difficulty climbing, and start head-shaking. The flying foxes, which are the largest bats in the world and have the same tastes as humans, feed at night on mostly fermented and rotten fruit . . . [which] fouls the bat's sonar, thus causing navigational difficulties; the bats keep falling down and waddling on the ground.[42]

Alcohol "forms part of an intricate web of interrelationships between yeasts, plants, and animals as diverse as the fruit fly, elephant, and human, for their mutual benefit and propagation," summarizes Patrick McGovern.[43] Maybe our primate progenitors periodically participated in festivities similar to the Malaysian jungle feast described above and enjoyed the alterations alcohol provides. If this is the case, then our human lineage, rather than discovering alcohol, knew it all along, evolved with it, and applied our growing conceptual capabilities and tool-making skills to assure a steady supply. "By the time we became distinctly human 100,000 years ago, we would have known where there were certain fruits we could collect to make fermented beverages," argues McGovern. "We would have been very deliberate about going at the right time of the year to collect grains, fruits and tubers and making them into beverages at the beginning of the human race."[44]

Understanding how to manipulate conditions to make alcohol, and being able to share that information, are huge milestones in our cultural evolution. Even more important, or at least more necessary at a day-to-day level, is the cultural information required to effectively store food. At least a rudimentary knowledge of food storage strategies is required in order

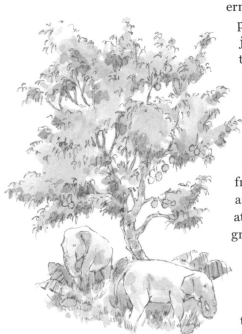

elephants eating fallen durian

to survive without daily hunting and gathering. The only way people could escape from a daily preoccupation with feeding themselves was by acquiring the ability to preserve food for the future.

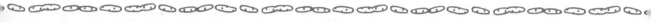

FERMENTATION RHYTHM

Blair Nosan, Detroit, Michigan

The rhythms of fermentation have become a part of my life in a way that is so deeply satisfying, I feel that they'll stay with me for a long time. Fermentation requires cycles of us, to return to, to inspect, to refresh and renew. Just as Shabbat comes once a week, so too do I renew my batch of yogurt every Saturday or Sunday, and check whatever else is brewing under my kitchen counter. I feel grateful for these rhythms because they help me feel rooted in a world without grounding, and they help me engage with a past where humans' daily lives were suffused with awareness of the cycles of our climate and our seasons. I just feel grateful for the opportunity to cultivate that awareness in an otherwise thoroughly modern (and ever modernizing) world.

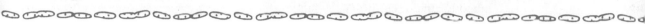

Anthropologist Sidney Mintz makes the point that squirrels and many other animals "instinctively collect and hide food for the future, when they can." What humans do is different, less instinct than "an invented, constructed, symbolically transmitted technology," he explains.[45] In emergent human societies, cultural information, transmitted via symbol and language, enhanced ancient coevolutionary relationships. In fact, "the development of agroecology cannot be separated from the human ability to symbol," argues theorist David Rindos.

> Language can be used to classify resources according to the amount and type of utility, both immediate and potential. Language in humans permits the preferential preservation of resources at times before their utility is apparent. . . . Such behaviors, modified though they may be by symbolic factors, will vastly increase the ability of people to affect coevolutionary relationships that already exist.[46]

Genes were supplemented by memes as vectors of coevolutionary change. Information about cultivation, storage, and processing could be communicated and taught. The challenges of fermentation and food storage led to creative solutions such as pottery vessels that constituted major technological advances. Food storage capabilities reinforced the logic of generating surplus food. And surpluses drove the need for more effective storage strategies. Specialization and elaboration ensued.

Food storage does not necessarily involve fermentation. In many cases it primarily consists of keeping foods dry but not too dry, cool but not too cold, and dark. But it is not easy, with limited technology, to create ideal conditions for storage. Learning the lessons it takes to dry and store food effectively involves errors and accidents: seeds and grains getting moist, resulting in germination and/or molds; fruits and vegetables fermenting and/or rotting; milk aging in various environments; meats and fish faring quite differently depending upon moisture and salt content. Learning to understand the dynamics of how foods aged under different storage conditions was a necessary aspect of coevolving with the more limited range of plants and animals that agricultural societies increasingly came to rely upon. Settling into a sedentary life primarily subsisting on agricultural crops and/or milk or meat animals requires such an understanding. Without it, agricultural societies could not have developed.

Distinctions between fresh and rotten food are fundamental, both as a life lesson for survival and as a narrative theme in mythology across human cultures.[47] Understanding what is and isn't appropriate to put in our mouths is some of the earliest cultural information we each acquire as babies. In the creative space between the binary opposites of fresh and rotten is the food that is effectively preserved: the cultured foods, the ferments so deeply embedded in our cultural particulars.

Fermentation and Coevolution

What is fascinating about the concept of coevolution is the recognition that the processes of becoming are infinitely interconnected. As a dynamic between two species, coevolution has been described as "an evolutionary change in a trait in the individuals of one population in response to a trait of the individuals of a second population, followed by an evolutionary response by the second population to the change in the first."[48] Life, however, is never so simple as to be limited to just two interrelated species; coevolution is a complex and multivariable process through which all life is linked.

All the plants our hunter-gatherer ancestors ate, like those our primate ancestors ate, consisted of unique chemical compounds, along with enzymes, bacteria, and other associated microbial forms, to which our ancestors and their microbiota adapted (or not, but they are not here to tell the tale). The plants' coevolutionary histories do not revolve exclusively around us. For instance, could certain large fruits have evolved to attract the attention and seed-spreading potential of extinct megafauna, to our enduring benefit?[49] Some plants we eventually coevolved with in ways we came to describe as domesticated. "We automatically think of domestication as something we do to other species," writes Michael Pollan in *The Botany of Desire*. "But it makes just as much sense to think of it as something certain plants and animals have done to us, a clever evolutionary strategy for advancing their own interests. The species that have spent the last ten thousand or so years figuring out how best to feed, heal, clothe, intoxicate, and otherwise delight us have made themselves some of nature's greatest success stories."[50]

The influence of coevolution changes all involved. To say that one species is the creation or the master of another is a self-serving oversimplification. What we call "domestication" is a process that exists along a continuum, which ethnobotanist Charles R. Clement describes as running from wild, to "incidentally coevolved," to "incipiently domesticated," to "semi-domesticated," to "landraces" and "modern cultivars," representing "a continuum of human investment in selection and environmental manipulation."[51] Like any coevolutionary process, domestication has repercussions for all parties. Coevolutionary success can lead to very specialized relationships. Treeshrews eating the fermenting nectar while pollinating the bertram palms, discussed already, is one vivid example. With the major human food crops, our great investment in selection and environmental manipulation makes us "obligate agents," meaning "sufficiently dependent upon certain plants so that [our] survival, at new densities, is dependent on the survival of the plants."[52]

In that dependence, in all our cultural particulars, we are manifestations of coevolutionary processes with the plants as much as they are manifestations of coevolutionary processes with us. Humans are not the only actors in these relationships. Nor are plants the only other life-forms to benefit from their close association with us. How about *Saccharomyces cerevisiae*, the primary yeast used to produce alcoholic beverages and bread? Yeasts are widespread in nature, but this particular one developed—through its long association with humans and our willingness to grow and process plants, in huge quantities, to its preferred specifications, to feed it generously and cultivate it continuously over the course of the millennia—into the coevolutionary partner we now know as *S. cerevisiae*. "Microorganisms are [our] most numerous servants," wrote Carl S. Pederson in a 1979 microbiology textbook, epitomizing a worldview of humans as the supreme creation of evolution, with all other life-forms ours to freely exploit.[53] To view ourselves as masters and microorganisms as our servants denies our mutual interdependence. Rather than *Saccharomyces cerevisiae* being the servant of humanity, it could be said that we are its doting fan and servant, much as we are to *Vitis vinifera* (grapes) or *Hordeum vulgare* (barley).

Although we rarely pay much attention to them, we have also consorted with many varied lactic acid bacteria (LAB). By 2007, geneticists could state emphatically: "Every person in the world has contact with lactic acid bacteria. From birth, we are exposed to these species through our food and environment."[54] The LAB's genetic diversity "allows them to inhabit a variety of ecological niches ranging from food matrices such as dairy products, meats, vegetables, sourdough bread, and wine to human mucosal surfaces such as the oral cavity, vagina, and gastrointestinal tract."[55] Comparative genome analysis suggests that in nutrient-rich niches, the LAB specialize efficiency by shedding genes for metabolic pathways they are not using. "The specialized adaptation to milk is particularly interesting," notes the analysis, "because this fermentation environment would not exist without human intervention. The selective pressure came not only from the natural environment, but also from anthropogenic environments created by humans."

Who exactly is the servant of whom? Are the acidifying bacteria in milk or the yeasts in grape juice *our* servants, or are we doing their bidding by creating the specialized environments in which they can proliferate so wildly? We must stop thinking in such hierarchical terms and recognize that we, like all creation, are participants in infinite interrelated biological feedback loops, simultaneously unfolding a vast multiplicity of interdependent evolutionary narratives.

 ## Fermentation as a Natural Phenomenon

Fermented foods were not exactly human inventions; they are natural phenomena that people observed and then learned how to cultivate. Depending on the place, varying natural phenomena were observed, because different foods were being produced in surplus, processed in distinctive ways, and stored under specific conditions in each environment. The distinctness of cultures arises out of the specificity of place: Different plants (and animals) grow abundantly and produce surpluses, and different microbial communities develop on them. In China, rice and millet were developed, and their complex carbohydrates came to be digested by molds into simple sugars for alcohol fermentation. "The discovery of the *mould ferment* in the Neolithic period is the result of the happy conjunction of three factors," writes H. T. Huang. "Firstly, the nature of the ancient cereals cultivated by the Chinese, that is, rice and millets, secondly, the development of steaming as a preferred method for cooking such cereals, and thirdly, the kinds of fungal spores that were present in the environment. . . . As far as we know, the convergence of these distinctive factors occurred only in China."[56] In the "Fertile Crescent" of the Middle East, it was barley and wheat instead that developed, and a very different method, germination (malting), that came to be used to digest them into sugars for fermentation.

Both available foods and spontaneous fermentation phenomena vary dramatically between the extremes of tropical heat and arctic cold. In cold climates, fermentation is absolutely essential for survival. In summer, when waterways are accessible, people catch fish, as well as birds, and bury them in pits, where they ferment for months, until winter food scarcity requires their use. People in tropical climates are not driven by such stark seasonal imperatives, yet fermentation is no less important there. Hamid Dirar documented more than 80 distinct ferments in the Sudan alone. In tropical heat, rapid microbial transformations of food are inevitable. Fermentation is a strategy used to guide that transformation to create delicacies rather than decomposition. "Sudan's foods are almost all fermented," notes Dirar.[57] Clifford W. Hesseltine and Hwa L. Wang, of the US Department of Agriculture Fermentation Laboratory,[58] state: "Fermented foods are essential parts of diets in all parts of the world."[59]

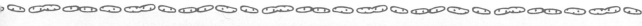

KRAUT PRAYER

Eli Brown, Oakland, California

Myriad beings beneath my sight, thank you for your transformations. May you nourish me as I nourish you. May you thrive in me as I thrive on the earth. In all the worlds may nourishment follow hunger as the echo follows the call.

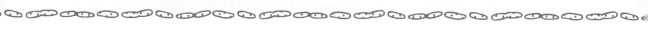

The War on Bacteria

The biological reality—that bacteria are our ancestors and the context for all life; that they perform many important physiological functions for us; and that they improve, preserve, and protect our food—contrasts sharply with the widespread perception of bacteria as our enemies. Because the earliest triumphs of microbiology involved identifying bacterial pathogens and developing effective weapons against them, our culture has embraced a project that I call the "War on Bacteria." We've heard for a decade about the War on Terror, and for two decades before that about the War on Drugs. Although it rarely gets named as such, the War on Bacteria is much older than either of these, and over the past few generations it has indoctrinated almost everyone. Beyond antibiotic drugs that individuals take, sometimes for important reasons (but typically overprescribed), we routinely feed antibiotics to livestock, chemically sterilize our water, and use antibacterial soaps marketed with the seductive promise of killing 99.9 percent of bacteria.

The problem with killing 99.9 percent of bacteria is that most of them protect us from the few that can make us sick. Continuous indiscriminate killing of bacteria in, on, and around our bodies makes us *more* vulnerable to infection rather than less vulnerable. Because of bacteria's genetic mutability, pathogenic bacteria are rapidly developing resistance to commonly used antibacterial compounds. "The use of common antimicrobials for which acquired resistance has been demonstrated in bacteria as ingredients in consumer products should be discontinued," states the American Medical Association.[60] The constant generalized assault of bacteria, and the ideology that fuels it, is misguided and dangerous. "Those who hate and want to kill bacteria indulge in self-hatred," notes Lynn Margulis.[61]

As a result of the War on Bacteria, our bacterial context is rapidly shifting. One bacterium formerly ubiquitous in humans, *Helicobacter pylori*, which resides in the stomach, is now found in fewer than 10 percent of American children and may be headed toward extinction.[62] *H. pylori* has been associated with humans for at least 60,000 years, and there is evidence that closely related bacteria have lived in the stomachs of mammals since their emergence 150 million years ago. Often people seek to categorize bacteria as either "good" or "bad." *H. pylori* has been correlated with health problems such as ulcers and stomach cancer, and these have decreased along with the bacteria's incidence in the population. But even though *H. pylori* may contribute to problems for us, it is part of us and we coevolved dependent upon it for certain regulatory functions. Among the roles this particular bacterium is thought to play (or have played) in our bodies is regulating stomach acid levels, certain immune responses, and the hormones that control appetite. The disappearance of *H. pylori* may be implicated in increased levels of obesity, asthma, acid reflux, and esophageal cancers.[63] "The accuracy of classifying commensal bacteria as 'detrimental' or 'beneficial' remains highly speculative," cautions epidemiologist Volker Mai, "because such classifications are based on examining their effects on only a few specific aspects of human health, and attempts have not been made to associate microflora composition with overall health."[64] Microbiologist and medical doctor Martin Blaser argues that "changing selection for our endogenous microbial populations is responsible for some of the emerging patterns in human health and disease," and suggests that "*H. pylori* might therefore be considered an 'indicator organism' for changing human microecology and disease risk."[65] We eradicate our evolutionary partners at great risk.

Cultivating a Biophilic Consciousness

As you read this book, and experiment with fermenting foods and beverages, I encourage you to cultivate not only the specific bacterial and fungal communities necessary for the ferments, but a consciousness of ourselves as coevolutionary beings, part of a greater web of life. Biologist Edward O. Wilson has dubbed such consciousness *biophilia*.[66] While this word may be new, such a consciousness has been part of humanity since the beginning. Unfortunately, we have become increasingly isolated from the natural world, lacking awareness of and conscious interaction with animals, plants, fungi, and bacteria in our midst. Rather than continuing to distance ourselves from interaction with the larger web of life, we must reclaim these relationships. Fermentation is a tangible way of cultivating this consciousness and these relationships.

As evolutionary beings, we must recognize in bacteria not only our cellular origins and mutualistic partners, but our best hope for biological pathways into the future. How else can we possibly adapt to all the toxic compounds and waste we are creating? Bacteria have already been found to decompose many pollutants, including rubber tires,[67] organophosphorus compounds used in pesticides, plasticizers, jet fuel, and chemical warfare,[68] and phthalates used in plastics and cosmetic products.[69] After the horrific months-long 2010 oil spill from the *Deepwater Horizon*, the journal *Science* reported that the spill stimulated deep-sea "proteobacteria" that helped biodegrade the spilled oil.[70] Fungi also offer promising detoxifying and adaptive potential.[71] If our evolutionary imperative is to adapt to shifting conditions, then we must embrace, encourage, and work with microorganisms rather than attempting, however futilely, to eradicate them; or imagining that we can engineer them to our will in precise and predictable ways. Coevolution affects all beings involved, too infinitely compounded to be predictable. We cannot control coevolutionary fate; we can only adapt to shifting conditions as best we can.

There is no generic formula for adapting to change. Yet we must. We can only transform by looking beyond the seductions of cultural innovation—the television, the computer, even the printed page before you—and reclaiming our cultural roots and biological inheritance. We must build community not only with people, but by restoring our broad web of coevolved relationships. The practice of fermentation gives us the opportunity to get to know and work with a range of microorganisms with which we have already coevolved. Into the future they go, with us or without us.

FERMENTING GROWTH
Shivani Arjuna, Wisconsin

Learning to ferment opens people's minds to the possibility that they can provide for themselves in other ways they haven't ventured into yet. It's empowering.

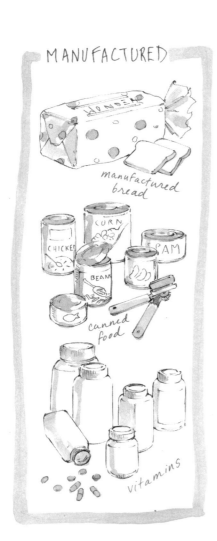

manufactured
bread

CORN
CHICKE
BEANS
PAM

canned
food

vitamins

HOME-GROWN / FERMENTED

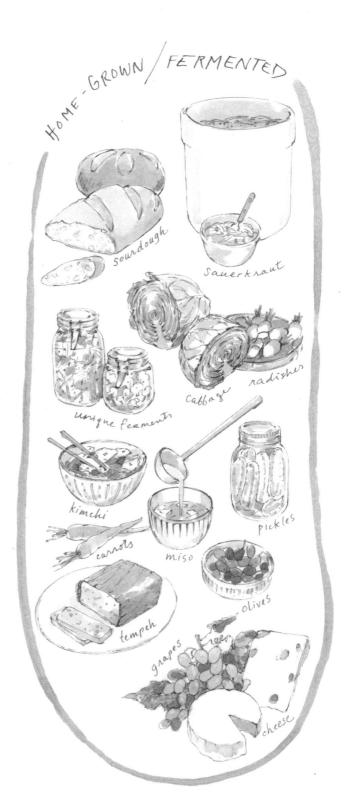

sourdough

sauerkraut

unique ferments

cabbage

radishes

kimchi

miso

pickles

carrots

tempeh

olives

grapes

cheese

CHAPTER 2

Practical Benefits of Fermentation

*B*eyond sacred alcohol, fermentation has been valued throughout history primarily for its usefulness in preserving food. Think about how stable cheddar cheese is compared with milk, for example. Although recent generations have seen fermentation eclipsed as a food preservation method by canning, freezing, chemical preservatives, and irradiation, this ancient food preservation wisdom is still applicable and may be a key to continued survival in a future filled with uncertainty. Many people are becoming interested in fermentation for its nutritional and health benefits, which are considerable and can be quite dramatic. Scientific investigation has been confirming the link between live-culture foods and good health intuitively understood by cultures around the world. Bacteria play crucial roles in many aspects of our physiological functioning, and fermented foods can support, replenish, and diversify our microbial ecology, which may also be key to adapting to shifting conditions. Fermentation has also been used as a strategy for saving fuel, since fermentation digests certain nutrients that otherwise would require long cooking, and enables foods to remain stable at ambient temperatures without refrigeration. This energy-saving aspect of fermentation also has increased relevance given all the uncertainty about future energy supplies. Yet ultimately more compelling (at least for me) than preservation, health, or energy efficiency benefits are the complex edgy flavors of fermentation, which got me interested in all this in the first place. Food is not strictly utilitarian, after all. It can and does bring us great pleasure. In this chapter, we will explore each of these four major benefits of fermentation: preservation, health, energy efficiency, and flavor.

The Preservation Benefits of Fermentation, and Their Limits

Try to imagine life without refrigeration, while still maintaining a supply of food to eat. Like most of the people I expect will be reading this book, I have lived all my life in the historical bubble of refrigeration. By its very nature, the refrigerator is a fermentation-slowing device. It enables food to maintain its freshness longer by limiting and slowing—via temperature regulation—not only the metabolic processes of microbes but also the enzymes present in the food that are poised to digest it. I call refrigeration a historical bubble because it has been available for only a few generations, predominantly in more affluent regions of the world where electrical power is readily available, and yet has powerfully distorted our perspectives on food perishability, instilling in us a fear of its absence; and given its high energy requirements, it seems uncertain whether refrigeration will always be so widely available and affordable. It behooves us to safeguard the living legacy of traditional food preservation techniques, including fermentation.

Fermentation can extend the life of food in several ways. First, the organisms that are being cultivated dominate in the food, thus crowding out and preventing the growth of many other bacteria. One of the mechanisms by which they protect themselves is the production of *bacteriocins*, proteins that are antibacterial against other closely related bacteria. Also, the fermentation organisms' metabolic by-products—primarily alcohol, lactic acid, and acetic acid, but also carbon dioxide and many others—have inhibiting effects on many microbial and enzymatic processes, thereby helping to maintain a selective environment that limits what can grow and supports food preservation.

However, not all ferments exist to primarily preserve food. For instance, wheat preserves better as dried grain than in the fermented form of bread. And even under refrigeration, tempeh is stable only a few days (longer tempeh storage requires freezing). Alcohol is an effective preservative, used to preserve grape juice (wine), and frequently used to preserve and deliver plant medicine (tinctures). But alcohol (unless concentrated by means other than fermentation) exposed to air ferments to acetic acid, transforming it into vinegar.

Acidification—by lactic acid even more frequently than acetic acid—is the primary means of food preservation by fermentation. "The advantages of acid food fermentations," according to food scientist and fermentation scholar Keith Steinkraus, are:

> (1) they render foods resistant to microbial spoilage and the development of food toxins, (2) they make the foods less likely to transfer pathogenic microorganisms, (3) they generally preserve the foods between the time of harvest and consumption, and (4) they modify the flavor of the original ingredients and often improve the nutritional value.[1]

Cabbage radishes

Preservation through acidification is the story of vinegar, pickles, sauerkraut, kimchi, yogurt, many cheeses, salami, and all sorts of other ferments eaten in different regions of the world. In each case, fermentation greatly extends the edible life of the raw food from which it is made.

To grasp the importance of fermentation in this regard, we must recognize that until quite recently, techniques for preservation were very limited. There were no refrigerators or freezers. In some locations, people worked with ice, but in most places this was not possible. Canning was not developed until the 19th century. Food could simply be kept in a dry and cool spot; or it could be actively dried (microbial activity is suspended without adequate water) using the sun, and/or gentle heat or smoke, and/or salt. Or food could be fermented. Working with mysterious, bubbling life forces, people could acidify foods and thereby create many exquisite—and lasting—delicacies.

Food preservation cannot be separated from food safety. For a preservation technique to be effective, it must preserve food reliably and safely. Indeed, acidification by fermentation is also a brilliant strategy for food safety. Rapid proliferation of acidifying bacteria makes it difficult, perhaps impossible, for pathogenic organisms to establish themselves, even if they are present. In addition to lactic and acetic acids, the acidifying bacteria produce other "inhibitory substances" including hydrogen peroxide, bacteriocins, and other antibacterial compounds.

Given recent large disease outbreaks traced to bacterial contamination of raw vegetables (typically from fecal runoff of factory farms), it might be fair to say that fermented foods are *safer* than raw foods. In a ferment, even in the case of contamination of the raw ingredients, the contaminating bacteria would have to struggle for survival in the presence of a stable community of acidifying bacteria specially adapted to the specific rich nutritive environment, and secreting acids and other protective compounds. In this environment, *Salmonella*, *Escherichia coli (E. coli)*, *Listeria*, *Clostridium*, and other foodborne pathogens cannot survive. This explains why hard cheeses made from raw milk are legal if they are aged at least 60 days, while fresher, softer raw-milk cheeses and raw fluid milk are not. The accumulation of acids created by the fermenting bacteria in the cheese renders it safe, so assuredly that even the food laws—which hold that raw milk is intrinsically dangerous—concede that the much-feared pathogens cannot survive the acidifying fermentation of hard cheeses.

In our cultural collective imagination, the food safety threat that looms largest is botulism, the rare but often deadly neurological disease caused by *botulinum*, "the most poisonous substance known to humans,"[2] a toxin produced by the bacterium *Clostridium botulinum*. Early symptoms of the neurological disease are usually blurred and double vision, followed by loss of motor skills: impaired vocalization; difficulty swallowing; and peripheral-muscle weakness. "If illness is severe," warns the US Centers for Disease Control, "respiratory muscles are involved, leading to ventilatory failure and death, unless supportive care is provided."[3]

The major reason we have even heard about this rare toxin is that it is associated with food preservation, specifically canning, a sterilization process that revolutionized food preservation in the 19th century, and is the diametrical opposite of fermentation. In fermentation, we rely upon native microbial communities, or cultures introduced in sufficient concentrations to assure success, to create an environment too acidic to allow the development of *C. botulinum* or other pathogenic bacteria. In canning, we apply heat in an attempt to kill off all microorganisms. Canning is vulnerable to botulism because it so happens that when stressed by heat, *C. botulinum* produces a spore that has an extraordinarily high tolerance to heat. Destroying this spore requires sustaining temperatures above the boiling point of water, between 240° and 250°F/116° and 121°C, which can be attained in a pressure cooker at 10 to 15 pounds per square inch. At normal boiling temperature of 212°F/100°C, destroying the *C. botulinum* spores can take as long as 11 hours![4] If the spores persist in a non-acidic medium after insufficient heating, they find themselves in an ideal environment: an oxygen-free vacuum, devoid of competition from other bacteria.

Although *C. botulinum* is a very common soil bacterium, botulism was an obscure disease until the advent of canning, when case reports skyrocketed. One dramatic headline-grabbing outbreak occurred in Oregon in 1924, when all 12 members of a family died from toxic home-canned string beans.[5] Stories like this take strong hold in the collective imagination and lead to generations of warnings, often very vague. Accidentally killing people with botulism is a fear I have heard repeatedly from people reluctant to try fermenting sauerkraut at home. But it is improperly canned foods, not ferments, that can harbor botulism (except in the case of meat and fish, which require specific precautions, covered in chapter 12). Plant-based ferments are generally safe, protected by their native or introduced organisms.

Most foods preserved by fermentation will not last forever. Our contemporary expectations of food preservation have been shaped by the technology of canning, along with subsequent developments in preservative chemicals, packaging, ultra-heat treatment, freezing, and irradiation. You can store canned foods in your storm shelter for decades while you await a big storm or the apocalypse. Not so for most ferments; there is a limit to how long different fermented foods will remain stable and retain their appeal. Exactly how long depends on the type of food; its pH, water activity, and salinity; the temperature and humidity of the environment; the way it is stored; and your tolerances. Fermented foods are alive and dynamic, and the microbial and enzymatic transformations that preserve them can eventually—depending upon storage conditions—yield to other organisms and enzymes. The sauerkraut eventually gets soft and mushy. If it is salt-free, or if it is made in summer heat, this will happen faster

carrots

than it would with salt, or in winter. But with an understanding of such dynamics, human cultures around the globe have used fermentation as an important strategy to preserve the surpluses of seasons with relative abundance to sustain them through times of relative scarcity.

Even as fermentation has receded in importance as a means of preserving food for later consumption, it has become more important with respect to another type of preservation: cultural preservation. "In the current food environment, traditional techniques take on a new meaning, so that their original function of nutritional preservation is being replaced by that of cultural preservation," observe Naomi Guttman and Max Wall.[6] For cultural revivalists, food preservation and cultural preservation are inextricably linked.

FERMENTATION AND HIV

I have frequently alluded in my writing and public speaking to the fact that I am living with HIV. As I wrote this book I marked the 20th anniversary of when I first tested positive, in 1991. I am so glad to be alive; and I remember many friends who were not as lucky. I wrote in *Wild Fermentation* (on the back cover) that "fermented foods have been an important part of my healing," and as a result many people have extrapolated that fermented foods are a "cure" for HIV/AIDS. I wish this were the case, but alas, it does not seem to be so.

Since a health crisis in 1999 I have been on anti-retroviral and protease inhibitor drugs. These drugs in no way negate or diminish the importance of nutrition, digestion, or overall immune function; in fact, in many people they impact specifically upon digestion. Live-culture foods have helped me maintain excellent digestive health. I also know from my research that live cultures in foods can stimulate various aspects of immunity. There has even been some research investigating whether probiotics can help elevate levels of CD4 cells, one of the markers of immune function that typically decreases over time in people with HIV.[10] I think live-culture foods can potentially improve almost anyone's health. But I emphasize that helping to maintain overall health is not the same as curing a specific disease.

The Health Benefits of Fermented Foods

Fermented foods, as a group, are highly nutritious and digestible. Fermentation pre-digests foods, making nutrients more bioavailable, and in many cases fermentation generates additional nutrients or removes anti-nutrients or toxins. Ferments with live lactic-acid-producing bacteria intact are especially supportive of digestive health, immune function, and general well-being. As I write, the *Proceedings of the National Academy of Sciences* has just published exciting new research establishing that gut bacteria influence immune responses far from the intestines, and specifically that they are associated with "productive immune responses in the lung" in response to influenza virus infection, and revealing "the importance of commensal microbiota in regulating immunity in the respiratory mucosa."[7] Bacteria in our gut, potentially enhanced by bacteria in foods (as well as probiotic supplements), can have far-reaching and profound impacts on our health. In my own healing journey, I have found that live-culture foods help me feel good all around and give me a proactive way to help myself, as well as others. However, this does not mean that live-culture fermented foods are panaceas.

Many miraculous claims have been made on behalf of particular fermented foods, but I think it is important to approach such claims with skepticism. For instance, I do not think that daily consumption of kombucha (sugar and tea, partially fermented) is likely to cure diabetes, as claimed by some web promoters. I think people with diabetes should use kombucha only in moderation, if at all, and perhaps get their live cultures from less sugary ferments such as sauerkraut and yogurt. The potential improvement of overall health does not necessarily ensure any particular outcome, and specific claims must bear scrutiny. In 2010, yogurt giant Dannon was found by the US Federal Trade Commission to have made "false and misleading claims" by suggesting in its marketing that its probiotic yogurt product line "reduces the likelihood of getting a cold or the flu" and "is scientifically proven to help with slow intestinal transit."[8] The FTC action forced Dannon to stop making these "unsubstantiated" claims and pay $21 million to the 39 states that had challenged them.[9]

In our culture of immediate gratification, we want magic-bullet cures, and enterprising marketers wish to oblige us. While I wish it were so, live-culture foods are not a cure for AIDS. And although consumption of yogurt, sauerkraut, miso, and other live-culture foods has been correlated with diminished cancer risks, I'm not convinced that any (or all) of them would be sufficient as primary treatment of an acute cancer.

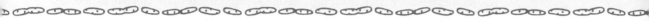

DIGESTIVE IMPROVEMENT

Leslie Kolkmeier

For years I have been diagnosed (wrongly) with IBS, celiac disease, and a variety of other attempts to explain my cranky gut. Recently I began making sauerkraut. My gut problems have nearly disappeared, and I am slowly adding back the occasional wheat product (a chocolate chip cookie and a brownie were my first tests, and a pizza is coming up next!). I think my natural probiotics had been wiped out by frequent rounds of antibiotics for Lyme disease, cardiac problems requiring antibiotics before dental work, and so on.

Well-being and healing are not simple phenomena attributable to any single determinative factor. Fermented foods are not *the* secret to health and longevity. Nor is exercise, nor a curious mind, nor an open heart, nor a wholesome diet, nor inner contentment, nor sexual bliss, nor regular bowel movements, nor restful sleep. But each of these, along with innumerable other factors, influences the overall state of our well-being. And fermented foods are part of the picture.

In this chapter, I will briefly describe the major nutritional and health benefits of fermented foods and beverages, summarize findings of the peer-reviewed scientific and medical literature, and try to answer some of the questions that have come up repeatedly, in my email and public presentations. It is the purported health benefits that are drawing many people to become aware of fermented foods as such. I do not have absolute answers. Scientific understandings of the role of bacteria in mediating and regulating physiological processes in our bodies are crude and rudimentary. Even less is understood about the dynamics of ingesting live cultures, how they interact with the indigenous populations, and how the mucosal intestinal linings function to mediate the bacterial balance, an important aspect of what we call our immune system. In the manner of contemporary scientific investigation, much of the research is corporate-sponsored and extremely narrow, measuring the impact of specific "probiotic" cultures, often proprietary strains, on various quantifiable biochemical markers, resulting in carefully guarded conclusions studded with caveats. How far can we extrapolate from that? Many basic facts and mechanisms remain unknown. But it seems that science is gradually confirming what traditional cultures always somehow just knew: that fermented foods are special foods, able to nourish us deeply and help keep us healthy.

Jiangs are fermented condiments—precursors to miso and soy sauce, though made from meat, fish, and vegetables, before beans—that were widely eaten in China more than 2,000 years ago. The 5th-century *Analects of Confucius* (*Lun Yu*) note that Confucius "would not eat a food without its proper *jiang*,"[11] and the Confucian classic *Chou Li* describes the duties of the "superintendent of fermented victuals."[12] William Shurtleff and Akiko Aoyagi, in their extensive historical bibliography on miso, *jiangs*, and other soy ferments, cite a 1596 source, *Bencao gangmu* (the great pharmacopoeia), which traces the word *jiang* to a document written in the year 150, which explains: "Jiang is like a military general who directs and can control the poison in food. It is just like a general controlling the evil elements in the population."[13] I'm not sure I approve of the metaphoric imagery, but it is a very early document clearly ascribing great power to this fermented food.

miso

The Chinese are not unique in associating fermented foods with good health. The Fur people of Darfur believe that *kawal*, a food made by fermenting a paste of the crushed green leaves of a plant also known as *kawal* (*Cassia obtusifolia*), prevents disease, and beyond that possesses mystical powers.[14] In many places, yogurt, kefir, and other fermented milks have traditionally been associated with good health and long life. Elie Metchnikoff, a Russian pioneer microbiologist, proposed in his 1907 book *The Prolongation of Life* that lactic acid bacteria in yogurt explained the unusual longevity of Bulgarian peasants. Ever since, people in many different parts of the world have deliberately sought out yogurt, kefir, and many other foods populated by lactic acid bacteria (LAB), as well as (in more recent times) probiotic supplements and "nutraceutical" formulations.

Broadly speaking, what I would consider to be the primary health benefits of fermentation, each of which will be explored below, are: (1) pre-digestion of nutrients into more accessible and bioavailable forms; (2) nutritional enhancement and creation of unique micronutrients; (3) detoxification and transformation of anti-nutrients into nutrients; and (4) live LAB cultures, present and alive in certain ferments, but not all.

Pre-Digestion

Fermentation is the digestive action of bacterial and fungal cells and their enzymes. Food may be preserved, but its composition is altered by the digestive processes of the organisms involved. Organic compounds are metabolized into more elemental forms. Minerals become more bioavailable, and certain difficult-to-digest compounds are broken down. In the varied soy ferments, fungi and bacteria digest the bean's prodigious protein into amino acids we can more readily assimilate. With milk, LAB convert lactose into lactic acid. Meat and fish are tenderized by the enzymatic digestion of fermentation.

Nutritional Enhancement

In the process of pre-digestion, many ferments accumulate increased levels of B vitamins, including thiamin (B_1), riboflavin (B_2), and niacin (B_3), as compared with the raw ingredients prior to fermentation. Vitamin B_{12} is controversial, as tempeh and some other plant source ferments once thought to contain high levels of B_{12} have been found instead to contain inactive analogues,[15] now known as *pseudo*vitamin B_{12}.[16] (Some contend that bacterial "contamination" of the pure *Rhizopus oligosporus* tempeh cultures in non-industrial settings accounts for B_{12} in traditional tempeh but not in the pure culture product.[17]) Fermentation increases availability of the essential amino acid lysine in cereal grains (more markedly in LAB-containing sourdoughs than in pure yeast fermentations).[18]

Various ferments create unique micronutrients, not present in the raw ingredients, produced by the fermenting organisms. For instance, the Japanese soy ferment *natto* contains an enzyme called *nattokinase*, which exhibits "very potent fibrinolytic activity . . . for managing a wide range of diseases, including hypertension, atherosclerosis, coronary artery disease (such as angina), stroke, and peripheral vascular disease."[19] New research has found that *nattokinase* also degrades amyloid fibrils and may be effective as a treatment for Alzheimer's disease.[20] In cabbage fermentation, phytochemicals known as glucosinolates are broken down into compounds including isothiocyanates and indole-3-carbinol, "anticarcinogens capable of preventing certain cancers," according to the *Journal of Agricultural and Food Chemistry*.[21] Who knows what other compounds as yet unrecognized by science may be present in all our varied ferments?

Detoxification

Fermentation can remove a variety of toxic compounds from foods, in some cases transforming them from anti-nutrients into nutrients. Certain food toxins, in sufficient doses, are dramatic poisons, like cyanide. The high-cyanide "bitter" cassava tubers (*Manihot esculenta*, also known as *yuca* and *manioc*) that grow in some regions of the world are detoxified if you peel and coarsely chop them, followed by several days of fermentation by simply soaking in water. (Note that the cassava/*yuca*/*manioc* that gets exported and is commercially available in most US cities is typically not bitter.) Similarly, many nuts, from acorns to Western Australia's macrozamia nuts,[22] must be soaked for days or even weeks to remove tannic or bitter compounds, inevitably fermenting in this process.

Some of the toxins in foods can be quite subtle. For example phytates— found in all grains, legumes, seeds, and nuts—function as anti-nutrients by binding minerals and thus rendering them unavailable for our absorption. During fermentation, the enzyme phytase releases minerals from their phytate bond, increasing their solubility and "ultimately improving and facilitating their intestinal absorption."[23] A 2007 study comparing availability of zinc and iron in *idli* batter (made from rice and lentils) before and after fermentation found that the process significantly increased bioaccessibility of both minerals.[24] Fermentation has been found to reduce naturally occurring nitrate[25] and oxalic acid in vegetables.[26] It has also been found to biodegrade certain pesticide residues on vegetables.[27]

"FERMENTATION MAY HAVE SAVED MY LIFE!"

Fermentation enthusiast David Westerlund, of Bellingham, Washington, accidentally harvested poison hemlock roots, thinking they were wild carrots, and fermented them. When he ate some, he got sick. "I noticed that my eyes were not tracking—basically as I shifted my eye muscles, they were delayed in responding. Scary. My head felt a bit tingly." But he did not experience any of the life-threatening symptoms, such as a racing heart, shortness of breath, or coma, warned of by a poison control phone line. "Fermentation may have saved my life," he reflects. "It definitely lessened the effects of the poison."

Fermentation has long been used as a strategy to make contaminated drinking water safe, by adding fermentable sugars and allowing a small accumulation of alcohol and/or acids to destroy the bacterial contaminants.

There have been some reports that miso may effectively remove heavy metals from our bodies, but unfortunately I have been unable to find any research documenting this claim. I hope it turns out to be true! Please, exercise caution. Do not assume that every toxic substance can be removed or transformed by fermentation, just because some can.

Live Bacterial Cultures

The pre-digestion, nutrient enhancement, and detoxifying actions of fermentation can be of nutritional benefit whether or not foods are cooked after fermentation, as with breads, fermented porridges, or tempeh (to name just a few examples). But in the case of foods and beverages fermented by lactic acid bacteria and then consumed without further cooking, the live bacterial communities themselves confer functional benefits. These live cultures, which I would say are the most profound healing aspect of lactic acid ferments, are only viable in foods that have not been subjected to heat exceeding around 115°F/47°C. Many packaged mass-produced ferments are pasteurized for shelf stability, thus destroying the live cultures. To receive the benefits of live cultures, you must obtain these foods unpasteurized, or make them yourself.

kimchi

Living lactic acid bacteria, which have always been present in foods, have increased in their dietary importance because of the multitude of chemicals present in our lives, some of which are valued specifically for their ability to kill a broad spectrum of bacteria, such as antibiotic drugs. After a round of antibiotics, researchers have found that "there are still persistent long term impacts on the human intestinal microbiota that remain for up to 2 years post-treatment."[28] Compound that with the growing levels of antibiotics present in our water supplies, along with chlorine, as well as the ubiquitous antibacterial cleansing products. Given the War on Bacteria so culturally prominent in our time, the well-being of our microbial ecology requires regular replenishment and diversification now more than ever.

One radical approach to this is direct implantation of bacteria into the colon, which in experimental application has been highly successful,[29] but the typical route of administration is oral ingestion. "Probiotic bacteria interact with and influence all cells within the gut," states researcher Karen Madsen in the *Journal of Clinical Gastroenterology*. "Mechanisms of probiotic actions include effects on luminal microbial ecology, modulation of immune function, and enhancement of epithelial barrier function."[30]

Most research published in recent decades documenting the benefits of ingesting live bacteria has focused on specific "probiotic" strains. Broadly defined, *probiotics* are microbes that confer some benefit to the organism that ingests them. Generally they are bacteria selected and cultured in laboratories, often from cells of human origin, on the theory that these strains are more likely to establish themselves in our intestines and confer benefit than the lactic acid bacteria native to traditional foods.

For decades, researchers have been establishing the broad benefits of probiotics. In 1952, the *Journal of Pediatrics* published a study establishing that "bottle-fed infants on formulas supplemented with L. acidophilus showed significantly larger gains in weight during the first month than did the controls."[31] Since then, hundreds more randomized double-blind, placebo-controlled scientific studies have verified benefits from ingestion of *specific* probiotics, for example: "Liver transplant recipients as well as patients with major abdominal surgery treated with *L. plantarum* 299 and oat fiber had significantly fewer bacterial infections and a trend toward shorter antibiotic therapy and shorter hospital stay";[32] or one presenting evidence "for the positive effects of consumption of *L. gasseri* PA 16/8, *B. longum* SP 07/3, *B. bifidum* MF 20/5 during at least 3 months in winter/spring on the severity of common cold episodes in otherwise healthy adults."[33]

In fact, the array of conditions for which probiotic therapy has been found to have some documented and quantifiable measure of success is quite staggering. Probiotics have been most definitively linked to treating and preventing diseases of the digestive tract, such as diarrhea (including that caused by antibiotics, rotavirus, and HIV[34]), inflammatory bowel disease[35], irritable bowel syndrome[36], constipation[37], and even colon cancer. [38] They have shown efficacy in treating vaginal infections.[39] Probiotics have been found to reduce incidence and duration of common colds[40] and upper respiratory symptoms[41] and to reduce absences from work.[42] They have been shown to improve outcomes and prevent infections in critically ill intensive care patients[43] and improve liver function in people with cirrhosis.[44] Researchers have documented efficacy of probiotic treatments to lower high blood pressure and reduce cholesterol,[45] reduce anxiety,[46] and increase CD4 cell counts in HIV+ children.[47] There is evidence that regular probiotic consumption can reduce dental caries in children.[48] In many other areas of human health, researchers are exploring theoretical applications of probiotics, including allergies,[49] urinary tract infections,[50] and the prevention of kidney stones,[51] periodontal disease,[52] and various cancers,[53] even where little hard data yet exists. Probiotics may "prove to be one of our most effective tools against new and emerging pathogens that continue to defy modern medicine in the 21st century," predicts a review in the journal *Clinical Infectious Diseases*.[54]

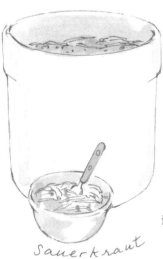

Sauerkraut

The precise means by which these bacterial cultures benefit us are not altogether clearly understood. Until immersing myself in the scientific literature in preparation for writing this book, my understanding of the benefit of the live cultures was that they essentially replenished and diversified intestinal bacteria. Ingested bacteria taking up residence in the intestines is the image suggested by Metchnikoff in 1907, and behind the subsequent healthful reputation of kefir, yogurt, and other traditional live-culture foods.

But it seems that actually the scenario is a bit more circuitous. A 2007 research review in *The Journal of Nutrition* summarized that current studies "demonstrate conclusively that ingested strains do not become established members of the normal microbiota but persist only during periods of dosing or for relatively short periods thereafter."[55] Microbiologist Gerald W. Tannock explains that Metchnikoff's theory "overlooked one of the most powerful forces in nature: homeostasis. . . . Because all of the ecological niches are filled in a regulated bacterial community, it is extremely difficult for [microbes formed in another place], accidentally or intentionally introduced into an ecosystem, to establish themselves."[56] Michael Wilson elaborates:

> The climax community that develops at each site will consist of microbes able to adhere to the existing substrata and utilize the available nutrients and is in a state of dynamic equilibrium as a result of the many interactions occurring between its constituent members. Any exogenous microbe attempting to colonise such a site will, therefore, be faced with a very difficult task, and the microbiota of that site is said to exhibit "colonisation resistance" as a consequence of its members having occupied all of the available physical, physiological, and metabolic niches.[57]

But that does not mean that ingested bacteria are not without great influence. It has been well established that bacteria can survive transit through the stomach's high acidity—particularly when buffered by food[58]—and in their passage through less densely populated regions of the digestive tract "they may constitute, albeit transiently, the dominant microbial population."[59] Like bacteria in general, the live cultures present in fermented foods are adaptable, are genetically fluid, and interact with their environment (our digestive tract, once we swallow them) in complex ways only beginning to be comprehended, and only through newly emerging methods of molecular analysis. The bacteria we ingest have elaborate interactions with our intestinal microbiota and the mucosal cells lining our digestive tracts, provoking multiple beneficial immune responses. "Both innate and adaptive immune responses can be modulated by probiotic bacteria," states the *Journal of Clinical Gastroenterology*.[60] Probiotics stimulate production of the antibody immunoglobulin A (IgA) and activate macrophages, lymphocytes, and dendritic cells.[61]

Can we extrapolate from the documented benefits of specific probiotic bacterial strains that naturally occurring bacterial populations used to ferment foods confer the same benefits? This is a hotly debated question. "The distinction between probiotics and live cultures is important relative to the presence or absence of data validating health effects in humans," notes Mary Ellen Sanders, a probiotics consultant and director of the International

pickles

Scientific Association for Probiotics and Prebiotics. "A recommendation that patients consuming antibiotics eat yogurt with live cultures is weak compared with a recommendation to consume a specific probiotic product that has been studied in human studies and shown to reduce antibiotic-associated side effects. Untested products still may have an effect, but cannot be recommended strongly."[62] Such is the voice of the probiotics industry.

Actually, traditional ferments have been studied, only not to the extent that probiotics have, at least somewhat because they do not offer the same degree of specificity (or proprietary sponsorship). Certainly, the most studied traditional live-culture food (and also the one most globally marketed) is yogurt. "Substantial evidence currently exists to support a beneficial effect of yogurt consumption on gastrointestinal health," asserts a 2004 review in the *American Journal of Clinical Nutrition*.[63] One refreshingly different study, published in the *Journal of Dairy Research*, looked at people who regularly ate live-culture foods—at least five portions per week of yogurt and cheese and at least three per week of other ferments. By analyzing blood and fecal samples collected at regular intervals through the study, researchers evaluated the influence of removing the fermented foods from the diet.[64] "The volunteers were asked to exclude from their diet any kind of fermented food or drink, such as fermented milk and dairy products including cheese, fermented meat, and fermented beverages like wine, beer or vinegar, and also any other kind of fermented food product such as cured olives." According to the researchers, "The dietary deprivation of fermented foods modified the gut microbiota and caused a decrease in immune response." After two weeks, the diets continued to be restricted, but participants were provided with yogurt each day for two more weeks, with half given standard live-culture yogurt, half yogurt fortified with probiotic strains. Interestingly, neither yogurt alone could fully restore participants to pre-restriction blood and fecal counts. This only occurred after they resumed their usual diets, with varied types of ferments. "It seems that other commercial starter strains and also wild-type lactic acid bacteria, which originate from the raw material or the environment, contained in other fermented products such as cheese or fermented meat contribute in an important way to the fermentive metabolism in the gut."

My thinking is that because of the genetic fluidity of bacteria (see chapter 1), the specific bacterial strains are not critical to maintaining healthy live-culture stimulation. What is more important is variety, diversity, and incorporating the bacteria native to different raw ingredients. Without denying that specific probiotic bacteria may turn out to be powerful therapeutic agents, it seems shortsighted to get too caught up in the search for perfect probiotic strains when we know how genetically fluid bacteria are. In bacterial populations, what we define as specific species and strains do not necessarily remain stable. "There are no species in prokaryotes," say microbiologists Sorin

unique ferments

Sonea and Léo G. Mathieu. "In complex consortia, incessant selective pressures select the best mixture . . . for the prevailing conditions."[65] Lactic acid bacteria in live-culture foods (or probiotics) increase the spectrum of genes available to our intestinal consortia, regardless of specific strains and whether they are able to permanently establish themselves.

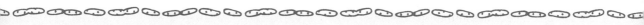

COMMON QUESTIONS REGARDING HEALTH BENEFITS OF FERMENTED FOODS

HOW DO LIVE-CULTURE FOODS AFFECT DIGESTION?

First of all, fermented foods are to varying degrees pre-digested, resulting in improved overall availability of nutrients. In live-culture foods, we ingest bacteria that help digest food and produce a multiplicity of protective compounds as they pass through our intestines. They and their various products enrich the microbial ecology of our intestines, enabling us to get more from our food and discouraging pathogenic bacteria by their presence. Many people find that their digestion improves as a result of incorporating live-culture foods into their diets. I have heard many anecdotal reports of improvements in digestion resulting from the regular ingestion of live cultures from people suffering from a broad range of digestive conditions, as varied as constipation, diarrhea, acid reflux, and many more serious chronic diseases. It appears that, as a group, foods with live lactic acid bacteria can help improve almost anyone's digestion, without any safety risk or huge expense. In some cases, these foods might, just might, be able to help improve or even resolve many varied health problems, acute or chronic. That said, individual responses will vary; and it's always good to introduce new foods, especially those containing live cultures, gradually and in small doses.

HOW DOES THE PH OF FERMENTED FOOD AFFECT THE BODY'S ALKALINE-ACID BALANCE?

Most ferments are acidic (with some exceptions, such as *natto* and *dawadawa*, chapter 11), yet sauerkraut, yogurt, and many other acidic live-culture ferments are actually considered to have an alkalinizing effect on us. The explanation for this apparent paradox is that the ferments make minerals (which are alkaline and alkalinizing) so much more accessible.

DO YOU HAVE TO AVOID ALL FERMENTED FOODS TO GET RID OF A *CANDIDA* OVERGROWTH?

Candida albicans is a fungus (yeast) that is a normal part of the human microbiota, found in most adult humans. A carbohydrate-rich diet can encourage its growth and increased prominence. The most important dietary modification you need to make to counter the *C. albicans* growth is restricting carbohydrate-rich foods, meaning not only sugar, grains, fruits, and potatoes, but also certain ferments made from them, such as bread, alcoholic beverages, vinegar, and possibly even kombucha. But to compensate for the deprivation, other live-culture ferments, based on less carbohydrate-rich foods such as vegetables or milk, even beans and meats, have lactic acid bacteria that can help to restore *C. albicans* to a more benign role.

CAN YOU EAT TOO MUCH FERMENTED FOOD?

Enjoy fermented foods and beverages in moderation. They have powerful effects and strong flavors and need to be respected. Eat them often rather than in large quantities. There is research indicating that high consumption of salty foods, including fermented ones, can cause many different problems. Ferments do not have to be salty or consumed in large quantities. Some research in Asia has suggested a correlation between high consumption of preserved vegetables and esophageal, nasopharyngeal, and some other cancers. Yet eating fresh fruits and vegetables has been found to reduce incidence of the same cancers.[67] Again, moderation and diversity must guide our diets. Finally, frequent consumption of highly acidic foods can erode tooth enamel. Rinse your mouth with water and brush your teeth after you eat!

CAN FERMENTED FOODS HELP CURE AUTISM?

I hear from lots of parents of kids with autism. For many of them, fermented foods are part of a dietary approach that they feel greatly helps their kids. The precise causes of autism remain elusive. Shifts in gut microbial ecology may be a factor in the dramatic rise of autism; nobody is exactly sure how or why. Live-culture foods can help restore health microbiota and thereby improve digestion, nutrient assimilation, and immune function. They may also aid the body in detoxifying mercury, another suggested factor in autism.[68]

Natasha Campbell-McBride, a British medical doctor whose son overcame autism, wrote the book *Gut and Psychology Syndrome*[69] in which she describes her son's recovery based upon a diet rich in live cultures and fatty acids, and without artificial ingredients, trans-fats and some other vegetable oils, sugar, gluten, or casein. Many other families have reported similarly positive results with the diet. According to McBride, restoring the health of the intestinal microbiota is key to recovery from not only autism but also a range of common psychological conditions including depression, attention deficit disorder, schizophrenia, and even dyslexia.

CAN FERMENTATION HELP WITH GOITROGENS?

I've been asked by people suffering with hypothyroid conditions if they should avoid ferments made from vegetables of the cabbage family, which are high in thyroid-suppressing goitrogens. The question many of them have is whether or not fermentation will break down the goitrogens in these foods. Unfortunately fermentation does not reduce goitrogens. If you need to avoid goitrogens for health reasons, I would recommend fermenting other types of vegetables, such as carrots and/or celery. Delicious ferments can be made from many types of vegetables beyond traditional cabbage and radishes.

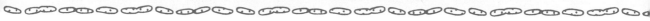

There are reasons to suspect that the genetic material even of lactic acid bacteria destroyed by heat may still be significant. The Hawaiian ferment *poi* (see *Poi* in chapter 8) is made from well-cooked taro corms, without the addition of a starter. The typical explanation is that enough lactic bacteria survive the heat to initiate the fermentation; but what if perhaps the bacteria themselves do not survive? Instead, perhaps their fragmented genetic remains provide the genetic starting point for airborne bacteria that find their way to the cooked taro. Similarly, as the days pass after baking sourdough rye bread, the bread continues to sour, suggesting that perhaps the genes of the sourdough bacteria are taken up by new viable bacteria that continue the sourdough's metabolism of carbohydrates into lactic acid. "For the most part, it is assumed that the active component of probiotic products is viable bacteria," noted a paper published in the *Journal of Nutrition* as part of a Symposium on Probiotic Bacteria. "However, the literature suggests several situations in which viability is not required."[66]

Eat a variety of fermented foods, some with live cultures. And while you're at it, eat a variety of plants. Make sure that at least some of the plants and the bacteria are wild. The range of plants and microbes under active cultivation is really quite limited. More different interactions—with varied phytochemicals, bacteria, and the compounds bacteria produce—stimulate us in functional ways. Diversity is its own reward.

Fermentation as a Strategy for Energy Efficiency

With fossil fuel supplies dwindling and requiring increasingly destructive extraction, rising global demand, and much uncertainty regarding availability, affordability, and safety of energy resources, we must consider the energy required by different foods. This means taking account of the energy embedded in the food's growth and transport, as well as the energy we use in our homes for refrigeration and cooking. Fermented foods can reduce the need for both refrigeration and cooking. As discussed at length previously in *The Preservation Benefits of Fermentation*, lactic acid ferments, on the whole, enable foods to enjoy some measure of stability outside of refrigeration. I regularly meet people who—for reasons of remote location, economic circumstances, or choice—live without refrigeration, and sauerkraut, miso, yogurt, hard cheese, and salami are among the kinds of foods these fridge-free folks eat. Envisioning a future where the refrigeration bubble could burst and average people could no longer afford to maintain refrigeration in the home, ferments such as these would become far more important.

Certain ferments also enable foods to be eaten with far less cooking. The most dramatic example of this is tempeh from soybeans. Cooking soybeans until they are soft takes about six hours of simmering, which takes a lot of fuel, whether you are heating with wood, gas, or electricity. To make tempeh, soybeans are cooked no more than one hour. After the fermentation, tempeh is usually fried; sometimes frying is preceded by steaming. In any case, post-fermentation cooking amounts to no more than 20 minutes. Altogether, cooking soybeans until they are soft enough to eat takes four times as much cooking time as making tempeh, and the unfermented beans are still far less digestible! Often, fermented meat and fish are not cooked at all. Because some of the transformations wrought by fermentation can substitute for or supersede some of the changes produced by cooking, fermentation can help extend fuel resources.

The Extraordinary Flavors of Fermentation

For as long as I can remember, I have been drawn to the lactic acid flavor of fermentation. Sour pickles (kosher dills) were what I most loved and sought out as a child, but I never turned down sauerkraut either. To this day, not just the smell but the mere thought of this lactic acid flavor triggers my salivary glands. As a rule, fermentation creates strong, compelling flavors.

Nor is lactic acid the only flavor of fermentation. Take a walk through any gourmet food palace and what you will see and smell are primarily fermented foods. I visualize myself walking into Zabar's, a New York City gourmet food wonderland I have visited since early childhood. The first food I see is olives, barrels of olives cured in different ways. (Raw olives are toxic and horribly bitter.) *Curing* is a broad term encompassing many different techniques of aging (even beyond food), but frequently involves fermentation. Olives are often cured by fermentation in a simple brine. Turning my back on the olives, I feast my eyes on a dazzling array of cheeses. Cheeses are not all fermented, but all the ones with strong flavors and aromas are, as well as hard cheeses and soft ones with runny textures. The enormous variety we find among cheeses is largely a result of the different bacteria and fungi developing in them, along with the conditions in which they age. To accompany the cheeses, there is a bakery, with breads in many different shapes, sizes, and flavors. Fermentation is what saves bread from being a dense brick, endowing it with texture, crumb, and lightness, as well as flavor. At the meat counter, fermented meats such as salamis, corned beef, pastrami, and prosciutto are prominent. Chocolate and vanilla are fermented, as are coffee and certain styles of tea. Wines and beers are fermented. So is vinegar. The flavors and textures of fermentation are beloved and celebrated and make up many culinary traditions' most prized delicacies.

Fermentation as a source of flavor enhancement is perhaps most pronounced in the realm of condiments. In many varied regions of the world, people use fermented condiments daily. What's special about condiments is that they make staple foods—potentially plain, monotonous, and dry—exciting. Sauerkraut and kimchi can be thought of as condiments, flavor enhancers and adorners of rice, potatoes, bread, and other plainer foods. Hamid Dirar estimates that "more than half of all the different fermented foods of the Sudan are used in the making of sauces and relishes to dress sorghum staple dishes. . . . These sauces and relishes play an important role in nutrition as they encourage the greater consumption of the staple, provide supplemental protein of high quality and probably supply an important portion of the vitamins of the diet."[70] Soy sauce and fish sauce are among the many fermented condiments of Asia. Inspiration for tomato ketchup, probably America's favorite condiment, came via Britain from Southeast Asia, imported as early as 1680, according to historian Andrew F. Smith.

> The ketchup that the British found was not a single, well-defined product. In today's Indonesia kecap (formerly spelled ketjap) simply means sauce and usually refers to fermented black soybeans with a roasted cassava flour. There are many other fermented kecap products: kecap asin (salty soy sauce); kecap manis (sweetened soy sauce); kecap ikan (a brown salty liquid produced by the degradation of fish material by enzymes); and kecap putih (a white soy sauce).[71]

While our contemporary American high-fructose-corn-syrup-based tomato ketchup is not exactly fermented, it, like most of our other contemporary American condiments—mustard, salad dressings, hot sauce, Worcestershire sauce, horseradish sauce, even mayonnaise—is made with vinegar, a product of fermentation.

Cheese can give us some insight into the extraordinary variety—in appearance, flavor, aroma, and texture—possible from the transformative action of fermentation. My favorites are runny cheeses, very ripe, very runny, very sharp, very fragrant. Sometimes other people are offended by the smell of the cheese that fills me with desire and would not for a moment consider putting it in their mouths. "The flavor of cheese can provoke ecstasy in some people and disgust in others," notes Harold McGee, author of the indispensable kitchen reference *On Food and Cooking: The Science and Lore of the Kitchen*.[72] There's no accounting for taste. Cheeses can be extremely dry and sharp, like Parmesan; or brined, like feta; or runny, like Brie. Cheesemaking (like all aspects of food production) evolved in so many quirky particular ways. Through the sheer variety of cheese we can view an aspect of culture in its infinite heterogeneous glory.

For people who are squeamish about stinky cheeses, it is usually because they associate the smell and appearance of the cheese with food that is rotting and no longer fit to be eaten. McGee describes fermentation as "controlled spoilage" and observes:

> In cheese, animal fats and proteins are broken down into highly odorous molecules. Many of the same molecules are also produced during uncontrolled spoilage, as well as by microbial activity in the digestive tract and on moist, warm, sheltered areas of human skin. An aversion to the odor of decay has the obvious biological value of steering us away from possible food poisoning, so it's no wonder that an animal food that gives off whiffs of shoes and soil and the stable takes some getting used to. Once acquired, however, the taste for partial spoilage can become a passion, an embrace of the earthy side of life that expresses itself best in paradoxes.[73]

Between fresh and rotten, there is a creative space in which some of the most compelling of flavors arise. Because the existence of such a creative space is so ubiquitous across cultures, there is no sharp, objective distinction between foods that are fermented and foods that are rotten. Referring to fermented tofu and Roquefort cheese, Sidney Mintz observes:

> Which is fermented and which is rotten may depend on whether a person has been raised to eat one or the other. Both are considered delicious by some people but spoiled, inedible, or worse by others. Hence, these two foods illuminate the power of culture and social learning to shape perception.[74]

Please do not take the idea that the boundary between fermented and rotten is blurry and slippery as a suggestion to start eating anything you would previously have rejected as rotten. Learning a sense of boundaries around what it is appropriate to eat is necessary for survival. But precisely where we lay those boundaries is highly subjective, and largely culturally determined.

If you grow up in the Arctic Circle, fish that has been mounded on or buried in the earth for months is a winter staple. But if you encounter this food for the first time as an adult it will probably look and smell to you like rotten fish. You may or may not be able to overcome your aversion, and in fact your body may or may not be able to tolerate the decomposed fish and the microbial community that is part of it. Like the stinky cheese, the fermented fish requires an acquired taste, and perhaps an acquired microbial ecology. One culture's greatest culinary achievement is sometimes another's nightmare. And usually, both involve fermentation.

As early humans expanded their range, they adapted to different climates, different foods, and different microorganisms, yielding wildly differing cultural particulars. Everywhere, the phenomenon of fermentation has been an important part of the story. It enables people to use and preserve food safely, effectively, and efficiently, as well as digest it better, get more nutrition out of it, enjoy it more, and stay healthy. For our continued well-being—as individuals, communities, and as a species—and our continued ability to adapt to change, we must revive and perpetuate the essential cultural practice of fermentation.

olives

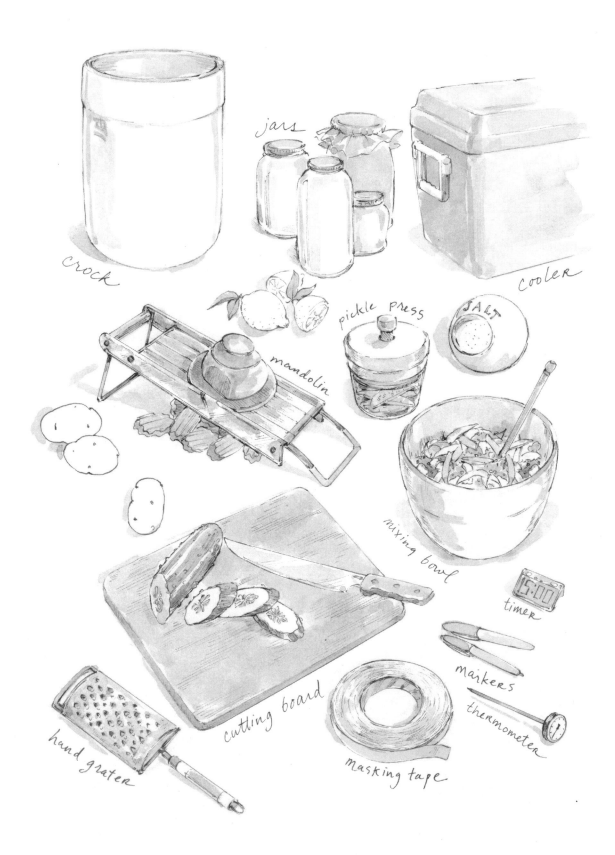

crock

jars

cooler

mandolin

pickle press

SALT

mixing bowl

timer

markers

thermometer

cutting board

hand grater

masking tape

CHAPTER 3

Basic Concepts and Equipment

*B*roadly speaking, *fermentation* is the transformative action of micro-organisms. Some definitions emphasize the role of enzymes, as it is through the action of enzymes they produce that cells digest and thereby transform nutrients. Indeed, certain ferments, such as *amazake* (see *Amazake* in chapter 10) or rice beers (see *Asian Rice Brews* in chapter 9), use molds as sources of enzymes, although the molds themselves do not grow. Biologists use a more specific meaning defining fermentation as anaerobic metabolism, the production of energy without oxygen. Most ferments—alcohol fermented by yeasts, and foods fermented by lactic acid bacteria—meet the biologists' more restrictive definition. But foods created by oxygen-dependent bacteria and fungi, such as vinegar, tempeh, and molded cheeses, are also widely understood to be products of fermentation.

 ## Substrates and Microbial Communities

The food we are fermenting is known in the literature as the *substrate*. It is both food for our microbial friends, and the medium upon which they grow. On any raw food that we wish to ferment, many different types of organisms are present. Microorganisms are never found in isolation; they exist in communities. "Mixed cultures are the rule in nature," writes mycologist Clifford W. Hesseltine.[1] Lynn Margulis and Dorion Sagan elaborate: "In any given ecological niche, teams of several kinds of bacteria live together, responding to and reforming the environment, aiding each other with complementary enzymes. . . . With other strains of bacteria always living nearby, ready to contribute useful genes or metabolic products, and to reproduce under favorable conditions, the team's overall efficiency is kept in top condition."[2]

It is the conditions of a particular ecological niche that determine which organisms will thrive there. The practice of fermentation largely consists of manipulating environmental conditions to encourage certain organisms and discourage others. For instance, a head of cabbage will never turn itself into sauerkraut. Left on a counter at ambient temperatures, a cabbage or any vegetable will eventually develop dark molds on its surfaces. Left long enough, these aerobic surface organisms can reduce a head of cabbage into a puddle of slime bearing no resemblance whatsoever to crunchy, tangy, delicious sauerkraut. Every vegetable is host to lactic acid bacteria, mold spores, and countless other microorganisms. The environmental manipulation that yields kraut rather than a puddle of slime is to submerge the cabbage under liquid and thereby deprive it of air and oxygen. In most cases, fermentation is as simple as this.

Wild Fermentation Versus Culturing

In the case of sauerkraut, people typically rely on bacteria that are present on cabbages and all raw vegetables. Fermentation based upon organisms spontaneously present on the food or in the environment is known as wild fermentation (also the title of my previous book about fermentation). The contrasting style of fermentation, in which specific isolated organisms, or established communities, are introduced to a substrate in order to initiate fermentation, is known as culturing (see *Fermentation and Culture* in chapter 1). Most fermentation cultures, also known as starters, involve simply transferring a small amount of an active or mature ferment into a fresh batch of its appropriate food nutrient (or *substrate*). This is how yogurt and sourdoughs are perpetuated. In the technical literature, this is referred to as *backslopping*. All introduced cultures had to have started as spontaneous wild fermentation events that people especially liked. Over time, people gained insight into the conditions that produced pleasing results, and techniques for perpetuating them were refined.

Certain fermentation starters have evolved into distinctive biological forms that reproduce themselves as cohesive communities. Kefir is a vivid example of this. Kefir "grains" or "curds" are rubbery blobs, polysaccharides inhabited by a community of some 30 distinct bacterial and fungal species.[3] The organisms coordinate their reproduction and spin their shared skin. And although these biological creations developed out of daily human interaction with milk, it is not possible to create a kefir grain from scratch. They reproduce in the nutritive medium of milk, and kefir begets kefir. This type of starter, evolved into a stable biological entity, is known as a symbiotic community of bacteria and yeast, or SCOBY. Kombucha mothers (sometimes erroneously described as mushrooms) are another example of the SCOBY phenomenon.

In order to maintain a culture over time, you must feed it regularly. Yogurt and kefir require milk; sourdoughs require flour or other forms of grains; kombucha requires sweet tea. Many cultures are descendants of ancient lineages, coevolved with their human keepers, fed regularly over more generations than anyone can count. They must be fed regularly, and while they can tolerate some neglect, they are vulnerable and can die of starvation. "At one point, I got to feeling that my fermentations were my pets, and then they were kind of taking over my life!" writes Elizabeth Hopkins, who tried maintaining eight different "kitchen pets" simultaneously before realizing that less can be more and scaling down. Fermentation is not about doing everything yourself. Find your niche, and seek out other fermentation revivalists. Share, trade, and co-create.

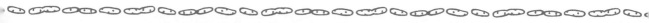

WILD FERMENTATION VERSUS LACTO-FERMENTATION VERSUS CULTURING

Some people have been confused by the different expressions used to describe fermentation processes, specifically *wild fermentation*, *lacto-fermentation*, and *culturing*. The truth is, these categories overlap. Wild fermentation specifically describes a spontaneous fermentation, initiated by organisms naturally present on the cabbage or grapes (or whatever food substrate), or coming via the air. Usually the nature of the substrate will determine what type of fermentation will occur spontaneously. If you are fermenting grapes, yeast will initiate an alcohol fermentation; if you are fermenting milk or vegetables, lactic acid bacteria will dominate and initiate a lactic acid fermentation, or lacto-fermentation in shorthand. So a wild fermentation is often a lacto-fermentation as well, but not always. Alternatively, a wild fermentation could also be an alcohol fermentation, an acetic acid fermentation, an alkaline fermentation, or (frequently) mixed.

Culturing usually means that a microbial starter of some sort (a packet of yeast, a SCOBY, a scoop of yogurt, whey, sauerkraut juice, et cetera) has been introduced, rather than relying upon organisms that are spontaneously present. The introduced cultures can be lactic acid bacteria, yeast, combinations, or others. Vegetables are typically done as wild fermentations. There are abundant lactic acid bacteria on all plant material, and if the vegetables are submerged, then molds cannot grow on them and lactic acid bacteria will. You can culture vegetables with whey or powdered starter cultures, but they are not at all necessary.

Selective Environments

Stuffing vegetables tightly into a jar so they are submerged under their own juices constitutes a selective environment. By excluding air, we make it impossible for molds to grow on the vegetables, which has the effect of encouraging lactic acid bacteria. Similarly, the air-locked carboy containing a fermenting alcoholic beverage serves to exclude air to prevent the growth of aerobic *Acetobacter* that transform alcohol and oxygen into acetic acid (vinegar). In contrast, to make vinegar or tempeh, oxygen is required, so air must freely circulate in the fermentation environment. Tempeh requires a warm environment, around 85–90°F/30–32°C. Yogurt does best in an even warmer environment, roughly 110°F/44°C, to get the heat-loving *Streptococcus thermophilus* and *Lactobacilli bulgaricus* to grow, but does not require oxygen. Much of the practice and technique of fermentation amounts to understanding the selective environment you want, and effectively creating and maintaining it.

LIFE, THE UNIVERSE, AND EVERYTHING: WHAT FERMENTATION TAUGHT ME

Lisa Heldke, professor of philosophy, Gustavus Adolphus College

◎ If the ancient Greek philosopher Heraclitus had been a yogurt maker instead of a river rat, his famous aphorism would have read, "You can't make the same yogurt twice." Flavor and texture vary batch by batch. It's a lesson in the importance of careful observation and meticulous technique—but also a lesson in the fact that observation and technique cannot change the weather in July or January, or the air of Minnesota or Maine. Now, I try to make something delicious each time, acknowledging that the qualities manifested by each batch of kombucha, or bread, or yogurt will be different, and that this is something to be celebrated. It's a tough lesson to learn for someone who is admittedly seduced by the siren song of uniformity.

◎ Rules alone cannot teach you how to do something. Written instructions are insufficient. Culturing food reminds me of this regularly. You can't learn it all from reading—whatever "it all" is. Set aside the book and "read" the ingredients; pay attention to them as if they matter. Put down the instructions and ask a human being for advice. Be prepared to be foolish, ignorant, naive, and wrong. Be grateful for the insights you are given—and don't complain because the teacher rambled. Life's truths cannot always be reduced to 12-point Times Roman.

◎ Even though they're insufficient, rules are good to follow. Culturing foods isn't a purely mechanical activity, but being a bit careful and meticulous (and systematic) about it will increase your chances of success tremendously. Not everything in life is a stir-fry—an endlessly flexible, infinitely adaptable dish. Some things are yogurt—fussy about the temperature difference between 108° and 115° [42–46°C]. (Consider your friends; some of them don't care if you show up an hour late for dinner, while others are going to be more than a bit peeved.) Pay attention. Learn the rules. Honor the one you're with.

◎ Mae West was wrong: Too much of a good thing is not wonderful. Kombucha fermentation can go too far (vinegar, anyone?). A tablespoon of yogurt culture is good, but a cup of it is disastrous. Two weeks at the ocean is not necessarily better than one.

◎ Fermented foods manifest one of my fundamental philosophical beliefs perhaps better than anything else in my life; in no other context am I so aware of the intricately participatory nature of reality; of the unpredictable interconnections between me and not-me. Other people experience this complex interconnectivity when they garden, or sail, or parent, or perform brain surgery. For me, it is encapsulated in a rubbery mat, stained brown and floating on top of a jar of tea. Yes, the mat is creepy and slightly malevolent. But treat it gently, for you and it are in a subtle, tenuous relationship, the parameters of which you are only beginning to discern.

Factors that people may seek to manipulate in creating selective environments for ferments include: oxygen access; carbon dioxide release; wateriness, dryness, or consistency; salinity; acidity; humidity; and temperature. Temperature can be very important. Some organisms can only function in a limited temperature range. Others, such as lactic acid bacteria, are more versatile, though it is important to understand that metabolism speeds up at higher temperatures and, consequently, fermentation proceeds faster and its products face faster perishability. Some organisms are *obligate* aerobes or anaerobes, meaning that they require oxygen all the time, or cannot ever tolerate it. Many organisms are *facultative*, meaning that they can exist and function in both aerobic and anaerobic environments.

Community Evolution and Succession

Every traditional fermentation practice involves communities of microorganisms. Over the past 150 years, microbiologists have isolated and bred many individual fermentation organisms, but it is only as communities of organisms that they have existed otherwise, and as evolved communities they exhibit the greatest stability and resilience over time. Microbial communities are dynamic and always shifting. When shredded cabbage is submerged under brine, one type of lactic acid bacteria, *Leuconostoc mesenteroides*, typically dominates at first; but as it produces lactic acid and alters the environment, *L. mesenteroides* is succeeded by *Lactobacillus plantarum*. Succession in a fermentation community can be likened to succession in a forest, where each dominant species alters light, pH, and other conditions that dictate what can grow and how well.

Yet for all the constancy of change in microbial communities, in some cases they exhibit extraordinary stability over time. "Compounds made by a mixture of microorganisms often complement each other and work to the exclusion of unwanted microorganisms," writes Clifford Hesseltine, who also notes that among the many advantages of mixed-culture fermentation starters, they "can be maintained indefinitely by unskilled people with a minimum of training."[4] In many cases, fermentation communities possess an internal balance among community members. Traditional yogurt cultures, for instance, can be perpetuated for generations, with proper care; in contrast, yogurt made from combinations of isolated pure cultures (as virtually all commercial yogurts are) generally loses its ability to produce yogurt after a few generations. Pure cultures in isolation are human inventions. "Pure culture fermentations are almost nonexistent," states microbiologist Carl Pederson.[5] In nature, and beyond the most controlled environments, microorganisms always exist in communities, and this is how people have always worked with them in the fermentation arts.

Cleanliness and Sterilization

Some of the contemporary literature of fermentation emphasizes chemical sterilization of equipment, and even of fermentation substrates, using sodium or potassium metabisulfite, popularly known as Campden tablets. In my own practice, I have never used these chemicals or aspired to sterile conditions. My motto is cleanliness, not sterility. It is certainly important to work with clean hands, utensils, and equipment, but in general sterile conditions are not necessary for fermentation.

William Shurtleff and Akiko Aoyagi offer helpful distinctions among clean, sanitary, and sterile conditions.

> A clean surface, one that is free of visible dirt, is obtained by washing. A sanitary surface, which is obtained by washing or spraying with a sanitizing or disinfectant solution, is free from most or all microorganisms, toxins, and other unhealthy substances. A sterile surface or substance, obtained by sterilization (as by pressure cooking, washing with alcohol, or heating in a flame), is completely free of living organisms.[6]

In my view, only certain specialized applications, such as producing sporulated pure culture starters, call for sterilization. I have had good success and no scary accidents in years of fermenting with mere cleanliness, using soap and hot water. I do periodically sanitize, wiping down surfaces with a vinegar solution, but only sporadically. Cleanliness and hygiene are important, fermentation or not.

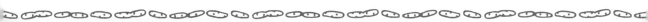

FERMENTATION INTUITION

Lagusta Yearwood

I cannot overstate how much fermentation has taught me on a practical level as a chef, but it's taught me something even more important as a person: trusting my instincts. Before I succumbed to the cult of fermentation, I wouldn't have considered myself an intuitive person. I was raised in a chaotic hippie household, and as a result I pretend I don't believe in "vibes" and "women's intuition." I like empirical evidence, I like a scrupulously clean and tidy kitchen, I like order and organization. I like recipes. I'm pretty uptight. Fermentation forces you to slow down and to "touch the process," as the animal rights activist and author Carol Adams has said. You must trust your instincts in order to successfully ferment anything. Fermentation is joyfully messy, wild, open-ended. You can follow the recipe precisely, but the larger truth is that there is no real recipe—only guidelines. No two people will make sauerkraut exactly the same, even if they follow the same recipe exactly. The air they are breathing (and thus changing) as they chop cabbage contributes to the flavor of the finished product. Fermentation is one of the most intensely personal things you can do in a kitchen—and because of this, you have no choice but to use your intuition (women's or otherwise), to go slow and feel the vibes in the air, to chop things by hand, to stir with your hands so you know exactly how much salt is enough by the way it makes the cabbage feel rough.

But generally sterilization is unnecessary. Incidental microorganisms that inevitably are found in non-sterile though clean environments cannot generally gain a foothold in a fermentation substrate. This is because the ferment either has its own indigenous microbiota (as in sauerkraut and traditional wines), or has had a critical mass of cultures introduced (as in yogurt, tempeh, and most contemporary beers). We are living in a microbial world, and these processes all developed under decidedly non-sterile conditions. Traditional mixed culture starters tend to be stable under favorable conditions. Only in the realm of propagating pure-culture mold spores, which tend to pick up more bacterial strains with each successive generation, have I found sanitization beyond mere cleanliness to be warranted.

Cross-Contamination

A question that comes up repeatedly among people who get inspired to experiment widely with fermentation concerns cross-contamination. Can your sauerkraut ruin your beer? Can your beer ruin your cheese? Or can your kombucha contaminate your kefir? My short answer to this question is that while different cultures may subtly influence one another through the air over time, typically this is not an issue. Alcohol makers wish to discourage *Acetobacter*, bacteria that ferment alcohol into vinegar. However, these bacteria are virtually everywhere, and the most effective way to discourage them is to protect your fermenting alcohol from air exposure. If you do this, then the vinegar fermenting in the same room should not be an issue.

I have experienced a vinegar mother developing on the surface of my "water kefir" (see *Water Kefir* in chapter 6), but then *Acetobacter* are fairly ubiquitous bacteria and the fermenting liquid was exposed to air. People have reported to me milk cultures that seemed to merge, but they usually have theories explaining it, such as shared utensils, that suggest possibilities other than contamination through the air.

Betty Stechmeyer, who co-founded a starter culture business, GEM Cultures, with her late husband Gordon and spent 30 years growing and selling fermentation starters, reports that for all those years she propagated several different sourdoughs, several different milk cultures, tempeh starter, and more in one 12-by-12-foot/3.7-by-3.7-meter kitchen. "Pretty primitive and simple, eh?" Betty claims that even propagating and selling these cultures over several decades, she never experienced cross-contamination. I cannot guarantee that cross-contamination among cultures is impossible, but it is not a likely occurrence, and I encourage enthusiastic experimentalists to ferment to your heart's content without worry of cross-contamination.

cutting board

Water

Many of the ferments discussed in the chapters ahead call for water to be added. But not all water is the same. The biggest problem with water, from a fermentation perspective, is the presence of chlorine. Chlorine is added to municipal water supplies specifically to kill microorganisms. If you add heavily chlorinated water into mixtures you wish to ferment, you may find that the chlorine prevents fermentation altogether, or slows, changes, or inhibits it. If you are working with chlorinated tap water, it is best to remove the chlorine. You can use filters to remove chlorine from water. Or you can boil the water in an open pot; the chlorine will evaporate. The only drawback of this method is that you need to cool the water down to body temperature before you can add it into a mixture that contains the live cultures we are trying to encourage. If you can plan ahead a day or two, leave chlorinated water in an open vessel with large surface area and allow chlorine to evaporate. If you are inclined to test water, you can buy simple chlorine measuring kits at pool supply shops.

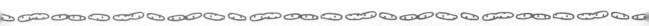

TAP WATER

Chris Chandler, Oakland, California

One thing I learned the hard way is never to add yeast to tap water that hasn't been allowed to sit long enough to allow the chlorine to evaporate. I've always used filtered water, but one time the filter failed as I was mixing it up, and in haste, I finished off with tap water and added yeast almost immediately. Which killed them promptly.

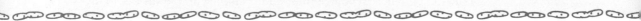

Unfortunately, new, more stable forms of chlorine—called chloramines—are increasingly being used in water systems. Chloramines—produced by mixing chlorine with ammonia—are valued because they are less prone to dissipation than simple chlorine. Chloramines cannot be boiled out, or evaporated at ambient temperatures. Evidently charcoal filtration systems can remove them, given sufficient contact. Some homebrewers use Campden tablets to neutralize chloramines. These tablets, consisting of sodium and/or potassium metabisulfite, are widely available from beer and winemaking suppliers but, as described previously, are primarily used to sterilize equipment, as well as the sweet liquid prior to adding yeast. I have no experience with this. If your ferments seem sluggish, one important factor could be your water. Inquire with your water supplier as to whether your water contains chloramines.

Salt

Many fermentation processes call for using salt. Limited saltiness, or salinity, is one way of creating a selective environment to encourage the growth of certain microorganisms, most often lactic acid bacteria, which are fairly salt-tolerant. At higher levels of salt, only specialized halophilic bacteria can survive.

Not all salts are the same. "Most discussions of salt ignore the issue of salt processing," points out Sally Fallon Morell. "Few people realize that our salt—like our sugar, flour, and vegetable oils—is highly refined; it is the product of a chemical and high-temperature industrial process that removes all the valuable magnesium salts as well as trace minerals naturally occurring in the sea."[7] Standard table salt in the United States has iodine added, to replace the iodine and other minerals stripped out of it, as well as various chemical anti-caking agents. Since iodine has antimicrobial properties, and the anti-caking agents can cause darkening and cloudiness, some of the literature suggests avoiding standard table salt for fermentation. The usual alternative suggestion is to use pickling, canning, or kosher salts, which do not contain iodine.

I typically work with unrefined sea salts. Because one of the important nutritional benefits of fermentation is making minerals bioavailable, I have come to the conclusion that it makes sense to ferment with salts containing a broad spectrum of minerals, rather than sodium chloride alone. Interestingly, among the trace minerals found in unrefined salt is iodine, but in organic forms via tiny marine life, and without any inhibiting effect on the fermentation. In fact, having had the opportunity to ferment vegetables with every possible kind of salt handed to me by workshop organizers, I have observed that lactic acid bacteria seem tolerant to a wide variety of salts, including iodized table salt, and are not particularly picky.

In most ferments, including vegetables, salting can be done to taste, without any need for measuring. In other cases, more specific salt proportions may be required for safety and effective preservation. For instance, with curing meats, adequate salt and curing salts are necessary for safety. And in ferments such as miso and soy sauce, which age for many months or even years, insufficient salt can lead to putrefaction rather than controlled fermentation.

Through the book I have tried to indicate where salting to taste is appropriate and where more precise measurements of salt are recommended. An average level tablespoon of salt weighs about ½ ounce/14 g. But if the salt is fine, it will weigh a little less; and if the salt is coarse, it will weigh a little more. For measuring salt, weight is much more accurate than volume, which can vary considerably with different grinds and densities. Taking two grinds I keep in my kitchen, a cup of coarse salt weighs over 7 ounces/200 g, while a cup of fine salt weighs less than 6 ounces/170 g. A difference of this magnitude is generally not critical in terms of safety, but it can be significant in terms of flavor, microbial environment, and perishability. A small kitchen scale can be very helpful.

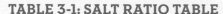

TABLE 3-1: SALT RATIO TABLE

This is a *very* general guide, intended for quick reference. Read the appropriate sections for more thorough and nuanced information.

VEGETABLES

Dry-salt method	1.5–2 percent weight of veggies, or roughly 1½–2 teaspoons/pound
Brine method	5 percent weight of water,* or roughly 3 tablespoons/quart
Grains	1½–2 percent weight of dry grains, or roughly 1½–2 teaspoons/pound

MISO

Long-aged misos	13 percent dry weight of beans and grains, or roughly ¼ cup/pound
Short-term misos	6 percent dry weight of beans and grains, or roughly 2 tablespoons/pound

MEATS

Dry-cured meats	6 percent weight of meat, or roughly 2 tablespoons/pound
Brined meats	10 percent weight of water,* plus 5 percent sugar, or roughly 6 tablespoons salt and 3 tablespoons sugar per quart
Salamis	2–3 percent weight of meat, or roughly 1 tablespoon/pound

* For quick reference, water weighs approximately 2 pounds per quart/1 kg per liter.

Salinity level is most often expressed as a percentage w/v, meaning weight of salt (in grams) per volume (in ml) of what it is being dissolved into, such as water. So, for instance, to achieve 5 percent salinity in a liter (1,000 ml) of water would take 50 grams of salt. Since a liter of water weighs 1 kilogram, really w/v is no different from w/w, which may be easier to conceptualize. So any quantity of water we want, measured in any units, may be weighed and multiplied by the desired salinity level to calculate salt to add. Occasionally brine salinity is expressed in salometer degrees (°SAL): 0° SAL means no salt; 100° SAL means full saturation of salt, as much as water can hold, 26.4 percent salt at 60°F/16°C; and the values in between indicate densities of salt saturation. Thus 10° SAL is 10 percent salt saturation or 2.6 percent salt; 20° SAL is 20 percent saturation or 5.2 percent salt, and so on.

Darkness and Sunlight

In most traditions, although not all, fermentation is generally practiced protected from direct sunlight. The high levels of ultraviolet radiation in direct sunlight can destroy or inhibit many organisms. In the rare instances in which fermentation specifically does take place in the sun, such as some traditions of cucumber pickling (see *Sour Pickles* in chapter 5), often the rationale is that the sunlight, hitting the surface of the ferment directly, prevents surface molds and thus creates an advantageous selective environment. In addition to impacting upon microbial ecology, sustained direct sunlight can diminish nutrients in the food that is being fermented. My general rule of thumb is to keep ferments away from direct sunlight. However, this does not mean that they must be in total darkness. I keep almost all of my ferments in the kitchen, protected from direct sunlight, but still illuminated by indirect light. The only process in which I make an effort to protect the food from even indirect light is malting grains, not a fermentation process in itself, but essential to the fermentation of beers (see chapter 9). Sustained access to even indirect sunlight initiates photosynthesis in the young sprouts, which turn green as their sweet flavor gives way to more bitter compounds. These I still do in the kitchen, but with towels draped over the jars to protect them from light.

Fermentation Vessels

The need for fermentation vessels has driven much human inventiveness. Lucky for us in the 21st century, we do not need to reinvent pottery, glass-making, corks, air locks, or threaded lids. You really do not need any special equipment to get started fermenting. Look around your home, and scavenge recycling centers, and you will find vessels, such as glass jars in which foods were packaged, that you can use for fermentation. A glass jar will suffice as a vessel for most ferments. But as your fermentation practice expands, you might want to acquire some more specialized equipment. In this section, we will review different types of equipment required for various ferments and examine the pros and cons of different options, materials, shapes, and sizes.

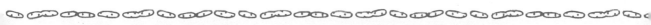

FERMENTATION PHILOSOPHY
Jonathan Samuel Bett

Fermentation is just wild enough to give you a safe sense of creative chaos without the anxiety of larger, more involved creative projects that require a more bracing investment of time and money. Anyone, anywhere can ferment. It takes perhaps three dollars of ingredients and equipment to make a good amount of sauerkraut, and even less money if you get creative about your sources. I can imagine someone asking a deli for a used glass jar, Dumpster diving for a head of cabbage, and taking salt packets from a fast-food restaurant and making a zero-overhead head of sauerkraut! The low investment necessary for fermented foods makes it all the more fun to indulge in them, paying the extra dollar for a locally grown heirloom vegetable or buying an antique crock or new glass jar to house your projects.

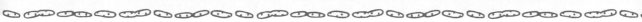

Differently shaped vessels offer different functional benefits and challenges. For a solid food, like sauerkraut, a wide mouth is important, wide enough to get your hand or a tool inside. For aerobic processes such as making kombucha or vinegar, in which the fermentation is most active at the surface where access to oxygen is greatest, you also want a wide vessel. Once wines or meads are vigorously bubbling, if you wish to ferment to dryness, move them to narrow-necked vessels, fairly full, with an air lock, so as to minimize surface area where aerobic vinegar production could occur. The requirements of the ferment, as best you understand them, balanced with what you can find determine the best vessel to use.

Jar Method

A jar filled with any raw food submerged under liquid will ferment. I like to save jars of all sizes, with their lids; the wider the mouth, the better. The smallest ones I do not use as fermentation vessels, but rather to hold finished ferments in order to share them.

There are many ways you can use a jar in fermentation. Mix flour and water in a jar (or in a bowl) to start a sourdough. In this case, when you are trying to catch some organisms from the air to supplement what is already on the flour, and aeration stimulates yeast growth, you don't need the lid on the jar. Instead use a cloth, towel, coffee filter, or other barrier that will keep flies out but allow airflow and with it both oxygen and microbial life. In the case of sourdough, though, neither the oxygen nor the airborne organisms are essential, and it can grow in a sealed jar as well. Some ferments require a steady flow of fresh oxygen. If you ferment kombucha or vinegar in a jar, you'd better leave the top off, since the kombucha and vinegar need air, and only fill the jar partway, so the surface area will be higher in proportion to the volume. As with the sourdough, use a light breathable cover to keep flies and mold spores away.

Many ferments, such as sauerkraut or cultured milks, do not require either oxygen or microbes from the air. These may be fermented in sealed jars. However, in many cases, if you seal a jar containing an active ferment, be aware that pressure may build from the production of CO_2. With yogurt you need not be concerned, but if you ferment vegetables or beverages in a sealed jar, you usually need to release pressure, or it can build to the point where jars explode. Leave the jar on the kitchen counter, where you will see it daily, gauge pressure by the bulging top, and release pressure by loosening the lid, as needed. Alternatively, you can place the lid loosely on the jar so that pressure will be released. Or you can drill a small hole in a lid to release pressure, or fit it with a plastic air lock from a beer- and wine-making supply store (see *Alcohol-Making Vessels and Air Locks* later in this chapter) and a rubber gasket so that it will seal tightly. You can even purchase an apparatus as just described.[8]

If an acidic ferment sits for a long period in a jar with a metallic lid, the lid may corrode. In this situation, I use a plastic top, or a small piece of parchment paper or waxed paper, as a barrier between the ferment in the jar and the lid. Others have described lightly coating the interiors of lids with coconut oil to prevent corrosion. You can also use jars for what I call the "open crock method," described ahead in *Crock Method*, using two jars, selected so that the small one fits inside the mouth of the larger one. I've also heard of people creating ceramic, glass, or even plastic disks to fit inside jars to weigh down the vegetables.

Ana Antaki, a fermentation enthusiast from Maine, wrote to tell me about the virtues of using bail-top clamped jars for fermenting vegetables. These are jars with glass tops held down by levered wire clasps, with rubber gaskets to assure a tight seal. Ana writes:

> I have been using them for 3–4 years now, for a wide range of lacto fermented items, and cannot say enough good things about them. I have not lost one single batch, and they keep for a long time. These bottles are reasonably priced and eliminate the "maintenance" that accompanies the lacto-fermentation process. As the food ferments, pressure builds up inside the closed bottle. When the pressure inside is greater than it is outside, the gasket will release either the gas, or brine from inside the jar. But, it does not allow anything from outside the container to come back inside. In effect, a gas seal will be created so that even if the brine level falls below the level of the vegetables, there is no mold or spoilage inside the bottle. Once you seal the bottle to begin the fermentation, DO NOT open it again, until you are ready to eat.

You may find old jars in this style, in which case you may need to replace rubber gaskets (easy to find with an Internet search), or contemporary ones such as Kilner, Fido, or Le Parfait brands.

Crock Method

Jars are ideal vessels for small batches, but for fermenting at a larger scale, I generally use ceramic crocks, usually with a simple cylindrical shape, which I have collected in sizes ranging from about ½ gallon to 12 gallons (2–45 liters). The straight-sided cylindrical shape of these crocks gives large surface area and easy access and makes it very easy to bear weight down on the ferment and thereby keep it submerged. When I make a fruity mead, I mix my honey water in a crock, then add berries and stir, stir, stir until the mix gets vigorously bubbly. Frequent stirring distributes the yeast-covered fruit and brings it into contact with more of the honey water; stimulates yeast growth by oxygenation; and incorporates airborne organisms that land on the surface. I cover the crock with a cloth to keep flies away but leave the crock open to air circulation.

When I make sauerkraut, I cover the chopped salted vegetables with a plate that fits inside the crock and sits on the surface of the vegetables, then weigh the plate down, usually with a gallon-size jug full of water, to keep the vegetables submerged under their juices and thereby protect them from oxygen. Finally, I cover the whole setup with a cloth to keep flies out. Often, I tie a string around the cloth to secure it.

In the case of sauerkraut and other vegetables, the ferment is anaerobic and does not require oxygen. The benefit of the open crock is that pressure does not accumulate, and the kraut is easily accessible so I can smell, see, and taste it as it develops. The drawback of this method is that access to oxygen can enable aerobic molds and yeasts to form on the surface of the ferment. When this happens to me, I just scrape or skim the growth off the surface, along with any discolored layer, and discard. Beneath the surface, the kraut is still fine. But some people do not like to have to scrape mold from the surface and prefer using lidded vessels. "I have found that putting cloth over ferments is a surefire way of attracting microorganisms and molds for which you did not send an invitation!" writes enthusiast Patricia Grunau. Every vessel and method involves trade-offs. Some air-locked crock designs are discussed in *Crock Lids*.

Lots of old crocks are hidden in barns and cellars; my first crock was one I found in an old barn. Many family heirloom crocks have been appropriated for non-food uses, such as umbrella stands or vases. Old crocks can command high prices in antiques shops, and some people worry about lead leaching into food from old glazes. There have been documented cases of lead poisoning in which ferments in lead-glazed vessels were implicated.[9] I have never personally observed erosion of glazes in my crocks, but others have reported such erosion. If you have an old crock you are concerned about, you can test it using easy lead-testing kits widely available on the Internet.

New crocks, on the other hand, generally use lead-free glazes. Many potters I have met over the years are experimenting with making crocks, and I urge readers to support local artisans when you can. The crock-producing capital of the United States seems to be Roseville, Ohio, where the Robinson Ransbottom company produced glazed ceramic crocks from 1900 until 2007, succeeded by the Burley Clay Company and Ohio Stoneware Company. Some old-time hardware and houseware shops sell their crocks. It's usually cheaper to buy crocks from a local source than to buy them on the Internet and have them shipped, as shipping charges will often approach the cost of the crock. When I searched on the web, I found that you can buy Ohio Stoneware crocks at Ace Hardware's site[10] and they will ship them to a local Ace outlet for free. If you know other fermentation enthusiasts, organizing a bulk purchase of a pallet of crocks directly from the manufacturer can greatly reduce costs.

The biggest problem with ceramic crocks is that they are so fragile. They are heavy when empty, much heavier when full, and can easily crack. A small hairline crack does not necessarily destroy a crock, however. The most important functional characteristic of a crock is that it hold water. You can test whether a hairline crack leaks by filling a crock with water, marking the fill line, and observing it over a 24-hour period. Some people have

crock

expressed concern over organisms that could be harbored in such cracks. In an empty crock, hairline cracks often become visible by the molds that grow out of them. Scour such crocks with vinegar and/or hydrogen peroxide, then wash with hot soapy water. The microbial reality, either in a spontaneous ferment (such as sauerkraut) or a culturing situation, is that the critical mass of fermentation organisms will easily dominate the incidental environmental molds. Don't worry too much about them.

It is possible to repair crocks with leaking cracks. Gary Schudel of Toledo, Ohio, wrote that he stopped his old crocks from leaking by melting beeswax and propolis, which the bees use to seal their hives, into the cracks from inside the crocks using a soldering iron. Propolis "may actually work better than wax," he wrote later. Ethnobotanist William Litzinger reports that the Tarahumara people of northern Mexico repair their ceramic fermentation *ollas* using pine resin or resinous substances produced by insects. "Resins are melted into place and make very good seals." He also reports that leather strips are used to reinforce the vessels, preventing further cracking. "Wet leather strips are applied to the ollas that when dry will tighten around the olla."[11] This seems key to protect against the outward pressure that is exerted upon the crock when it is filled.

Crock Lids

A crock may or may not have a lid; or may, in fact, have two. Lids may be interior lids, which fit inside the crock and rest upon the food being fermented, to keep it submerged. Or they may be exterior lids, which cover and enclose the crock. Sometimes crocks are made and sold with fitted lids; other times people use flat wooden disks, or improvise with such common household items as plates or (only as an exterior lid) pot tops. If you fill a crock with vegetables relatively full, and then weigh them down, unless you have a very flat dense weight, the weight will protrude above the top of the crock. In my typical home setup, I place a plate inside the crock atop the vegetables, and weigh it down with a 1-gallon jug filled with water. I have also used hardwood disks and rocks as weights. If you use rocks, be sure to use hard smooth ones that are not limestone, which can dissolve in an acidic environment. It's tempting to make the interior lid as tight a fit as possible, but leave at least a small margin, so that if the crock tapers inward (as many do), you won't get your lid wedged inside your crock, or risk breaking your crock with it. (I've done it.) If you make an interior lid out of wood, be sure to leave extra space for the wood to expand in the brine. "I wish I had known that the homemade oak lids I made to put inside my crocks would expand so much in the brine that they would sometimes break the crock in two," reflects fermenter Alyson Ewald. To cover a crock with a jug sticking out of it, I use a cloth. In summer, when flies are most abundant, I tie a string around the cloth to secure it tightly. Flies landing on your ferments can result in maggots crawling out a few days later.

Another approach that I have seen people use successfully, at every scale from small jars to huge barrels, is to fill a plastic bag with water and let that serve as both weight and lid. Gravity forces the water enclosed in the flexible plastic to spread and cover the full surface of the fermenting food, effectively cutting off air access. "The bags are much easier to manage and set up and adjust as necessary than trying to use plates and jars filled with water," writes fermentation enthusiast Rick Otten. To avoid water leaking into the ferment and diluting it, use a thick plastic or multiple layers. Some people fill the bag with brine, in case it leaks into the vegetables. Functionally, this is an excellent solution; the only drawback is that it brings the food into prolonged contact with plastic, discussed ahead in *Plastic Vessels*.

Different Crock Designs

The cylindrical shape seems to be the most popular crock design in the United States, but in other parts of the world people work with varied shapes. In Asia, people generally work with crocks in a sort of potbelly shape. The Korean tradition of ceramic fermentation crocks is called *onggi*. My friend and neighbor Amy Potter in Dowelltown, Tennessee, has been making gorgeous crocks of her own design. Amy's crocks are ever so slightly potbellied, with two lids: a thick and heavy interior lid that functions as a weight on the ferment and an outer lid to keep flies out. I've collected and seen many other gorgeous creative crock designs handcrafted by ceramic artisans. A few different styles are pictured in the color insert. See *Resources* for potters' websites.

To reiterate a point I will make repeatedly throughout this book, there is no single method or vessel or style for fermenting. This is a natural phenomenon that people have harnessed in myriad different ways. Don't be afraid to try a different shape vessel. And don't feel like you need some standard-issue shape. Just as the fermentation revival is about reclaiming food in our communities, we have the technology and the talent to produce fermentation vessels in our communities. Collaborate with a potter and improvise. And scavenge. When I find myself in thrift stores, I always peruse the housewares section for potential fermentation vessels, such as food storage canisters, cookie jars, bowls, vases, or crock pots. Do not let lack of a specialized vessel inhibit your fermentation practice.

One crock design that has received much attention is the water-locked moat style, usually imported from Germany, sometimes from Poland or China. These crocks are designed with a moat around the mouth, which you fill with water, and a fitted top that goes into the filled moat. This effectively prevents fresh air from getting into the ferment, while allowing pressure to release. The German Harsch brand crocks also come with two semicircular weights for keeping vegetables submerged. This design is very effective for preventing aerobic surface growth. The only disadvantage of this design is that it is only effective at preventing mold if you leave the crock sealed, and you defeat its purpose if you open the crock repeatedly to look, smell, or taste—which I really like to do. No engineered solution is perfect; each design has its benefits and drawbacks.

Metal Vessels

In general, it is best to avoid fermenting in metallic containers, at least for the acidic ferments. The reason is that the acids, as well as the salt typically used in many of the acidic ferments, corrode metals, and the corrosion goes into the food. Theoretically, stainless steel resists corrosion. Stainless-steel vessels manufactured for the wine industry are being used by some commercial enterprises for fermenting vegetables, without corrosion (see *Scaling Up* in chapter 13). However, it is important to understand that unlike the industrial-grade solid stainless steel used in specialized products such as this, most household stainless steel has just a thin stainless coating, and corrosion can occur anywhere it gets scratched. You *can* serve ferments in metal, or store them for short periods, but it is best to avoid metal for the prolonged contact typically required of a fermentation vessel. Enameled pots are another story, as the enamel protects the metal from corrosion. Check carefully for nicks in the enamel. If unblemished, these may safely be used as fermentation vessels.

Plastic Vessels

Plastic, a material embodiment of our time, can be functionally effective for fermentation, but it also has its drawbacks. Prime among the disadvantages of plastic vessels are the chemicals that may leach from the plastic into your fermenting food or beverage. The known chemicals of greatest concern that leach from plastics into food are endocrine-disrupting phthalates, which have been linked to "incomplete virilization" in male rodents exposed to them as fetuses, and to problems in male reproductive development in many species.

The journal *Environmental Health Perspectives*, which reported that polyethylene terephthalate plastic bottles (PET or PETE, Number 1) used for water and soft drinks can leach phthalates, summarizes that "a growing literature links many of the phthalates with a variety of adverse outcomes, including increased adiposity [fat] and insulin resistance, decreased anogenital distance in male infants, decreased levels of sex hormones, and other consequences for the human reproductive system, both for females and males."[12] A report by the National Toxicity Program of the US National Institutes of Health cautiously concurs, expressing "concern" that exposure to the phthalate known as DEHP "may adversely affect male reproductive tract development." Fetuses and infants are most vulnerable; ironically, infants exploring the world with their mouths tend to have the greatest exposure, thanks to the fact that "DEHP is ubiquitous in the environment" via flooring, building materials, cosmetics, perfumes, hairsprays, and other everyday products. But most human exposure is via foods and beverages that have been in plastic containers.[13]

Fortunately, the food-grade 5-gallon buckets I've most often seen used as fermentation vessels—previously having contained cooking oil, mayonnaise, pickles, and other bulk supplies for food service establishments—are high-density polyethylene (HDPE, Number 2), which does not contain phthalates or bisphenol A (BPA), another plastic chemical of concern. Nonetheless, other chemicals may be migrating into food from the HDPE. Who knows? Generally, I don't use plastic as a primary fermentation vessel, although I do sometimes pack my finished ferments in plastic. I collect the barrel-shaped gallon-size plastic barrels in which olives are often imported to reuse as leak-resistant vessels for traveling with sauerkraut or other ferments.

The plastic that I use that is of the greatest concern is the reuse of number 1 water and soft drink bottles. The *Environmental Health Perspectives* study found that "the concentration of phthalates in the contents of PET bottles varies as a function of the contents of the bottle, with phthalates leaching into lower pH products such as soda and vinegar more readily than into bottled water." Furthermore, *National Geographic's Green Guide* reports that although PET is "a safe plastic if used only once . . . as number 1 bottles are reused, as they commonly are, they can leach chemicals," although they do not specifically identify phthalates.[14]

I frequently reuse 1- to 3-liter plastic soda bottles, and fill them with partially fermented beverages I wish to carbonate. Sometimes I'll bottle most of a batch in glass, but use one plastic bottle, just to gauge how pressurized the bottle becomes, by feeling how the plastic yields (or doesn't) when I press it. This enables me to know when the ferment is adequately carbonated, at which point I can refrigerate it to slow continued fermentation. Unchecked carbonation can result in dangerous explosions (see *Carbonation* in chapter 6). How do you weigh potential developmental problems in fetuses and infants against the danger of glass bottles exploding in your face? It depends upon your situation. As someone who is not pregnant or living with an infant, I sometimes opt for the practical benefits of storing ferments in recycled plastic containers. If I were pregnant, trying to get pregnant, or living with an infant, I would probably risk the exploding bottles and stay away from the plastics (or just enjoy easy, safe, non-carbonated beverages).

 ## Wooden Vessels

For large-scale fermentation, wooden barrels make excellent vessels. The barrel I use, which I acquired from the Jack Daniel's distillery for $75, was originally used to age whiskey and has a capacity of approximately 55 gallons/200 liters. I use it for radish kraut, and it takes about 440 pounds/200 kg of vegetables to fill it. When I bought the barrel, it had only a single small hole (called a bung) in its side. For it to be useful for fermenting kraut, I had to cut out one of the ends and plug the bung. I found a tapered wooden bung plug, which works perfectly, via the Internet.[15] A skilled or determined woodworker could easily fashion an appropriately shaped plug.

I use the barrel exactly as I use a crock. After it is filled, I place two semicircular hardwood boards on the surface of the vegetables, then I weigh them down using either two jugs of water (one on each board) or a crock filled with water. Finally, I cover the whole setup with a cloth. Wood grains definitely harbor microbes, but lactic acid bacteria on all vegetables easily dominate the protected environment under the brine. During the long slow winter fermentation, surface molds develop; I skim off and discard, along with any discolored or mushy vegetables at the exposed edges, and the vegetables protected under the brine remain fine. As I harvest the kraut through the winter and spring, the exposed moist wooden sides of the barrel mold completely, and I always have to compost the exposed edges of the radish kraut. Even so, the kraut protected under brine is appealing and delicious, month after month.

Canoa

Another type of wooden vessel used for fermenting alcoholic beverages is a *canoa*. This is a hollowed-out log, laid on its side like a canoe (the word *canoe* being derived from *canoa*). "The hollow-log fermentation container, known as a '*canoa*,' is always situated to the east of the God house," reports ethnobotanist William Litzinger.[16]

> Before the first measure of water is poured into the canoa, it is carefully inspected for obvious cracks and holes. Sometimes small woodboring insect larvae will make holes in the canoa. These holes are plugged using spines from a low palm that grows in the forest understory. If the holes are too large to be plugged with palm spines, or if there are splits in the canoa from drying, the cavities are filled with resin collected either from the copal tree (*Prorium* spp.) or from Pine (*Pinus* spp.) which grow at higher elevations directly to the south of Naha. The resin is applied by placing small pieces of it over the area to be patched and igniting it with a match so it will burn and melt into the cavity.

The desire for alcoholic beverages has inspired incredible creativity and inventiveness.

Gourds and Other Fruits as Fermentation Vessels

Before there were glass jars or any pottery vessels, there were gourds. Gourds have been used as fermentation vessels for thousands of years by many cultures around the world.[17] To hold water or ferments, gourds must be dried, opened, cleaned, and waxed. They may be left outside in the elements to dry, or dried faster in an indoor heated space. Sometimes gourds dried outdoors exhibit exquisitely beautiful mold patterns. "Mother Nature is the best artist," says my gourdist friend Jai Sheronda, quoting our mutual friend Dan Harlow, who grows gourds for his Vermont farm stand. As it dries, the gourd's outer skin may or may not peel off. The gourd is dry when it feels hollow, and the seeds inside rattle when you shake it. Then you can open and condition your gourd.

You need to create an opening in your gourd large enough to fit your hand inside. Some gourds have thin enough skins that you can cut through them with a knife or box cutter. With others you may need to use tools such as a tiny Dremel saw blade, or drill small holes to perforate the opening, then smooth the edges with a knife and sandpaper. Remove the seeds (which you can replant) and any loose flesh. Then smooth the inside as best you can, by scraping and sanding. Finally, melt beeswax and rub it into the interior surface. Test the gourd with water to make sure it doesn't leak. If it does, dry and apply more wax.

I have also made short-term sauerkrauts and kimchis in a variety of large fruits and vegetables, including watermelon, pumpkin, and eggplant. These are fun and dramatic presentations for the ferments, but as vessels they are far from ideal because they deteriorate rapidly, fermenting themselves and thereby losing the ability to hold liquids.

Baskets

Although I have never seen it done, there are references in the literature to fermentation in tightly woven baskets. Anthropologist Henry Bruman, who studied indigenous ferments of Mexico, cites a 16th-century Spaniard's report from central Mexico: "They have no vessels of pottery or wood, but only a sort which they make of fiber so closely woven that it will hold water. In these they make the wine."[18] Perhaps beeswax or some plant resin is applied to seal the tightly woven basket? Check out the basket-molded tempeh featured in *Making Tempeh*, chapter 10.

Pit Fermentation

I have no personal experience with fermenting in pits, but in the interest in creating a compendium of cultural information relevant to the fermentation arts, I think it is important to mention that simple holes dug into the earth have also been used as fermentation vessels. I have already referred to fish fermented in pits in Arctic regions (see *The Extraordinary Flavors of Fermentation* in chapter 2). In the Himalayas, *gundruk* and *sinki*, fermented greens and radishes (see *Himalayan Gundruk and Sinki* in chapter 5), are traditionally prepared in pits 2 to 3 feet (up to 1 meter) in both diameter and depth. "The pit is cleaned, plastered with mud, and warmed by burning. After removal of the ashes, the pit is lined with bamboo sheaths and paddy straw." The pit is filled with radishes, then "covered with dry leaves that are weighted down by heavy planks or stones. The top of the pit is plastered with mud and left to ferment."[19]

In the mountainous Austrian region of Styria, whole cabbages have historically been buried in pits without salt in a process known as *grubenkraut*. A Slow Food Presidium seeking to revive the practice describes the process:

> The pits varied in shape (round, oval, square) and could be lined with stone or larch wood. The pits were required to be of a significant depth—around four meters—and the cabbages had to be arranged in a certain fashion in the bottom of the pit to ensure they would not freeze. The bottom of the pit was first covered with straw (traditionally it was cumin scented straw), then a layer of cabbage leaves and then the whole heads of cabbage, turned down and stacked in layers. The cabbages were covered with a wool cloth and topped with more straw, and the pit was closed with a wooden lid, weighed down by large stones (at least 100kg). Before being placed in the pit, the cabbages were blanched in boiling water for several minutes in a large iron pot. This process would change the leaf color from green to white and had several functions: to sterilize the cabbages; to help the cabbage expand a little; and to facilitate the start of fermentation. When removed from the pit, each cabbage (whose volume reduces by half during fermentation) is stripped of its outer leaves, washed, and sliced finely.[20]

hand grater

Similarly, in Poland, reportedly into the 20th century, "it was customary to pickle cabbages in special ditches, which had their sides covered by wooden planks," reports ethnologist Anna Kowalska-Lewicka.[21]

The United Nations Food and Agriculture Organization reports that in the South Pacific and other tropical regions, "pit fermentations are an ancient method of preserving starchy vegetables," and continues:

> Root crops and bananas are peeled before being placed in the pit, while breadfruit are scraped and pierced. Food is left to ferment for three to six weeks, after which time it becomes soft, has a strong odour and a paste-like consistency. During fermentation, carbon dioxide builds up in the pit, creating an anaerobic atmosphere. As a result of bacterial activity, the temperature rises much higher than the ambient temperature. The pH of the fruit within the pit decreases from 6.7 to 3.7 within about four weeks. . . . The fermented paste can be left in the pit and removed as required.[22]

Keith Steinkraus et al. report that "foods preserved in pits can last for months or years without deterioration," serving "as a reserve to prevent famine in time of drought, warfare, and hurricanes, and as food for seafaring expeditions." They further describe South Pacific pit preparation:

> The type of soil and its drainage are important considerations in the selection of a pit site. The sides of the pit have to be firm so that soil does not fall into the pit. To that objective the sides of the pit may be pounded or the pit

may be lined with stones. A family pit may be 0.6 to 1.5 m deep and 1.2 to 2 m wide and hold 5 or more breadfruit. Community pits may hold 1000 breadfruit . . . the pit is lined with dried banana leaves and then the green banana leaves are folded and arranged in a circular manner with their sides overlapping and extending above the pit. At least two or three layers of banana leaves are necessary to prevent contamination with soil. The washed food is then placed in the pit, the green banana leaves are folded over the food, additional dried banana leaves are added to the top, and then stones are placed on the top of the pit.[23]

Do not allow lack of an ideal vessel limit your fermentation practice! Take inspiration from these ancient pit fermentation traditions from geographically disparate location, and don't be afraid to improvise.

Pickle Presses

Pickle presses are mechanical devices designed to press vegetables in order to force the juices out of them, and then keep them submerged. I have seen Japanese-manufactured plastic ones and have heard of presses fitted to barrels for making sauerkraut. When I searched the words "kraut press" online, all I could find was a patent granted in 1921 to Ignatz Glanschnig for "new and useful improvements in kraut presses." Personally, I am quite content with the lower-tech methods of weighing down vegetables described earlier, but I do find human ingenuity to be infinitely fascinating, and these are clever inventions created for fermentation.

Vegetable Shredding Devices

You do not need to buy any special device to chop vegetables for fermentation. A knife is perfectly adequate and may be supplemented by a hand grater. Of course, you may use any shredding device you like, including food processors and mandolins. I have a kraut board, which I like to use for large batches. This is a large wooden board with three diagonal blades parallel to one another. With each slide of the cabbage or other vegetables over the blades, they shred three thin slices. Once you get a good rhythm going, it shreds vegetables very quickly. But watch your fingers! After watching a series of helpers injure themselves, I got a stainless-steel mesh glove to use it more safely. For large-scale production, continuous-feed food processors can be invaluable, and there are also specialized industrial machines for shredding cabbage.

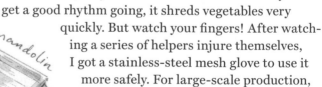

mandolin

Pounding Tools

When fermenting vegetables, it's helpful to bruise vegetables and break down cell walls, to release the vegetable juices. At a small scale, I recommend squeezing vegetables with your hands in a bowl to accomplish this. If you produce large or frequent batches, you will want some sort of tool. Any sturdy, blunt wooden object will do, such as a baseball bat or 2x4 board. An Oregon chapter of the fermentation-positive Weston A. Price Foundation is handcrafting and selling a wooden tool they call "the kraut pounder."[24]

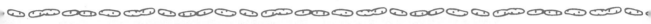

STRATEGIC STORAGE OF FERMENTS

Keep protecting ferments from air after fermentation. Even if I ferment vegetables or miso in crocks, I transfer it to jars to share and keep in the kitchen to eat from. Once the jar is half empty, it's half full of air. In warm weather especially (but even in the fridge), the ferment becomes increasingly vulnerable to molds when there is more air in the jar. So when your jar gets to the half-empty point, move its contents into a smaller jar that will now be full and devoid of significant air to feed mold growth.

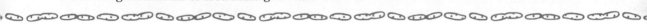

Alcohol-Making Vessels and Air Locks

There is much information, and much equipment, available for home alcohol makers. Some of it can be used to create downright sublime beverages. However, I like to continually remind myself of how well people have provided themselves with meads and wines and beers without a lot of the technology now available. You can ferment alcohol with nothing beyond what has already been discussed. A jar or crock (or gourd), along with honey and water, will suffice.

Alcohol fermentation typically gets vigorous at first, actively bubbling and foaming. But as fermentation slows—while the sugars are only partially converted into alcohol—bubbling subsides and the surface of the ferment becomes vulnerable to the growth of *Acetobacter*, bacteria that convert alcohol to acetic acid (vinegar). Historically, and still in many places to this day, alcoholic beverages have often been drunk only partially fermented, lightly alcoholic, still sweet, and sometimes sour. *Acetobacter* needs oxygen and begins growing on the surface of the beverage, where liquid meets air. To ferment to dryness (converting all the sugars to alcohol), especially with slow honey- and fruit-based ferments (as opposed to faster grain-based ones), minimizing surface area and blocking access to air helps avoid souring.

A *carboy* is a jug-shaped fermentation vessel, with a narrow neck. By filling it to the narrow neck, you minimize the surface area of your ferment exposed to air. The reason you can't just plug the mouth of the carboy is that the fermentation, even in its slower phase, still produces CO_2 that will build pressure until the plug shoots out (or the vessel explodes). An air lock is a plastic contraption that enables pressure to release from the carboy while protecting it from the flow of oxygen-rich air outside. These are made in a few different designs, each requiring the addition of water, which blocks the airflow, but CO_2 pressure from fermentation can push through the water to be released. You can find air locks at beer- and wine-making supply shops. If you can't find one locally, the Internet is full of them. Air locks cost just a couple of dollars and are used in tandem with special corks. The cork (typically rubber) should fit snugly in the mouth of the jug or carboy; it has a smaller hole for the air lock itself, which needs to be filled (usually to a marked level) with water. Because water can evaporate over time, if you leave a ferment in a carboy for more than a month or so, periodically check the water level in the air lock and add water as necessary.

In the absence of a manufactured air lock, there are a few ways you can create your own. The easiest method is to fit a balloon or condom on the fermentation vessel. Pressure will blow it up, and once it expands beyond a certain point, it will typically leak slowly rather than explode. But keep an eye on it, because it could explode or be forced off. If you have some thin plastic tubing, you can also make an easy air lock. Find or create a cork that fits your vessel, and drill a hole in it to accommodate the tube. Insert the tube into the cork, and run it into a container holding water. Pressurized CO_2 will force itself out as bubbles through the water, but the ferment will be protected from atmospheric air. Alternatively, you can use clay to fashion a stopper around the tube.

Beer makers use an additional vessel called a *lauter-tun*, which filters the liquid wort extraction from the grains after mashing. Manufactured *lauter-tuns* are available from beer-making supply shops, and many homebrew books contain plans for improvisational homemade units.

 ## Siphons and Racking

Rather than pouring alcoholic ferments from one vessel into another, or into bottles, typically people transfer them by siphoning. The advantage of siphoning is that you can leave behind the sludge of dead yeast (called *lees* in wines and *saké*; *trub* in beers) that accumulates at the bottom of the fermentation vessel. A siphon can be simple flexible tubing, or that same tubing enhanced by various accessories, such as a firm "racking tube," giving you greater control over the position of the siphon in your vessel, and a hose clamp to close and open the siphon. To siphon, I place the vessel from which I wish to siphon on a relatively high surface, then leave it so the sludge, disturbed by moving the vessel, has a chance to settle. Place the receiving vessel on a lower surface (often the floor), and place the siphon so that it is situated in the clearer liquid above the sludge. I always have a glass nearby for a taste while I'm transferring. To start the siphon, I stand up, suck on the hose until I taste the ferment, and then crouch down and let it go into the new vessel.

Not everyone approves of this method. One visitor to my website was offended: "Just the thought of siphoning wine/beer by mouth is disgusting and unsanitary. When I rack or bottle I wear a mask and gloves, and use a .02 micron sterile filter on ALL openings that can allow air to come into contact with the liquid." You can use a simple inexpensive pump if sucking on the siphon disgusts you, or if you are bottling in any kind of commercial operation.

Racking is simply siphoning the ferment from one vessel into another. Typically during a long wine or mead fermentation, people like to rack the ferment primarily in order to leave behind the lees. The lees are edible and nutritious, but we have developed a cultural preference for clarified beverages, and many people prefer to minimize the yeasty flavor the lees impart. The aeration of the siphoning can also restart a fermentation that appears to be "stuck." After you a rack a ferment and leave behind the lees (along with some of the ferment), you will have less of the ferment and thus an emptier vessel with more airspace. I typically add extra honey water or sugar water (mixed in the same proportion I started with) to make up the difference, so the surface area of the ferment in the vessel continues to be minimized.

Bottles and Bottling

If you do not wish to age or carbonate your fermented beverage, you can serve it right out of the fermentation vessel. This is the low-tech way, how most indigenous cultures do it. But often, people prefer to transfer their ferments to bottles, for storage, serving, and aging. The first consideration in bottling is which type of bottle. Wine bottles are corked but cannot hold much pressure. Beer bottles are capped and can hold some pressure but usually are not used for years-long aging. Champagne bottles are thicker than wine bottles, in order to hold more pressure, and typically corks are wired in place for the same reason.

You can easily scavenge wine and beer bottles at recycling centers everywhere. You cannot get an airtight seal crimping a cap on a screw-top beer bottle, so forget the screw tops and collect the round smooth-top beer bottles. For champagne bottles, go scavenging after New Year's. Wine bottles require a corking tool, while beer bottles require a crimping bottle-capper apparatus. These can be purchased at wine- and beer-making supply shops, with the most basic designs costing around $15, and many more elaborate and more expensive choices. There are plans for building your own capper in the excellent *Alaskan Bootlegger's Bible* by Leon Kania.

Bail-top bottles are another excellent option. These elegant heavy-duty bottles each have a clamp and reusable cap, fitted with a rubber gasket, attached. Grolsch beer comes in them, and they are available at beer- and winemaking supply shops. What is especially great about these bottles is that they are designed for reuse, and you can seal them without any special tool. If the gaskets wear out or get lost, they are easily replaced.

These are the classic bottle types used for fermented beverages. As with crocks, ceramic jugs for holding beverages may be handcrafted. If you are bottling for immediate use or short-term storage, you can also use other random beverage bottles for your fermented beverages, such as liquor bottles (some of which are extremely distinctive) or even plastic soda bottles. No need to be bound by tradition.

When bottling, always have enough bottles for your whole batch clean and ready to fill before you start siphoning. Once the siphon is flowing, the whole process can go very quickly. Do it in a place that will be easy to clean up, as spills are common, and spilled alcohol is sticky. Be ready to stop the flow with a clamp, or by holding your finger over the end of the tube, or by crimping the tube. Fill each bottle up to where the neck narrows, leaving just a little airspace.

The conventional wisdom in the fermentation literature is to sterilize everything with chemicals: bottles, corks, caps, and siphons. As described earlier, my motto is cleanliness, not sterility. Sterility is a myth, not achievable in our homes, nor desirable. The alcohol (or acidification) is its own protection. So long as it is kept from prolonged access to oxygen, which would spur vinegar production, it will be okay. Wash bottles with dish soap and hot water. Be sure to rinse well. Boil caps or plastic corks. Traditional corks should not be boiled, as it can hasten their disintegration. Instead, boil water, remove from heat, then submerge corks in the near-boiling water. For aging, I would recommend buying new corks. You can reuse intact corks for short-term bottling.

The big question in corks is whether to use the traditional cork material from a Mediterranean oak tree (*Quercus suber*) or ones made of plastic. Many wineries are switching to plastic or screw tops to avoid what is known as cork taint, which can occur when cork molds react with wine, imparting a musty odor. I've worked with both plastic and cork, and I don't have a strong preference. I'm more drawn to natural materials and have not experienced anything I could identify as cork taint. But I'm also not a purist and am not averse to working with plastic when I feel it's appropriate.

Rumors that corks come from an endangered tree are untrue. In fact, cork harvesting is not only sustainable—the trees are not killed when cork is harvested, and the cork rapidly regenerates—but the cork industry is credited (by the World Wildlife Federation) with protecting millions of acres of forests in Southern Europe and northern Africa that are critical habitats for a number of endangered species.[25] Bottles corked with natural corks should be stored on their sides to keep the corks moist; if they dry out, they may disintegrate.

Some avid beer makers avoid bottling altogether by conditioning and serving their beer in kegs rather than bottles. This can save much time and work but requires its own set of specialized equipment, beyond the scope of my expertise.

thermometer

Hydrometers

Hydrometers are tools for measuring the specific gravity of a solution. *Specific gravity* is the ratio of the density of the solution to the density of water. The specific gravity of the solution you are about to ferment can tell you its alcohol potential, and the specific gravity of a fermenting solution can tell you whether unfermented sugar (further alcohol potential) remains. That said, I have hardly used hydrometers in my years of mead fermentation. But they are inexpensive and easy to use, and many home fermenters swear by them.

Thermometers

Many fermentation processes require maintaining a particular temperature range, or cooling cooked ingredients to some moderate temperature before culturing. While you can train yourself to recognize certain temperatures using your senses, as fermenters have done throughout history, a thermometer is a very helpful tool. I use two different types. One is a simple dial thermometer, available almost anywhere; the other is a digital thermometer with a sensor attached by a cord (designed as a meat thermometer with a readout outside the oven). The corded thermometer is great for monitoring incubation spaces (see *Incubation Chambers*, below) because it enables you to see the temperature inside without opening (and thus cooling) it.

Cider and Grape Presses

If you have access to large quantities of fruit—particularly apples, pears, and grapes—a well-designed press enables you to get the most out of it. A press generally encompasses a mill (or grinder) as well as a press. The mill grinds the fruit against a jagged surface, tearing it apart into a pulp. Then you press the pulp, called *pomace*, using a screw-type or hydraulic press. If you buy or create a press, go with heavy-duty materials—pressing juice from fruit requires force and repetition. Good presses cost hundreds of dollars and therefore would be a great resource for a community to share. One household can own and maintain it, and make it available, for a fee if necessary, or for a share of the juice. This year we had a bumper pear crop, and I helped my friend Spiky press more than 25 gallons/100 liters of juice using our friends Merril and Gabby's press. They got fresh pear juice and perry (fermented pear juice) for their neighborliness.

You can always improvise. With grapes, you can crush them with your (scrubbed) feet in a tub, and they are soft enough that you can get a good bit of the juice out of the pulp by an ad-hoc press. For apples or pears, you can use an electric juicer, but most household models are not designed for high volumes or continuous use. If you don't have the technology for juicing, there are other ways to work with fruit, such as infusing the fruit flavor in honey water to make a fruity mead, or in sugar water to make country wine (see *Fruit and Flower Meads* and *Sugar-based Country Wines* in chapter 4).

Grain mills

I use my grain mill to crack beans in two for tempeh, and to crack grains coarsely for porridges and beers, more often than to grind grain into fine flour for baking bread. My grinder is as basic as they come, a roughly $35 model known as a Corona Mill. It grinds between two grooved steel plates and was originally designed for grinding cooked corn into *masa* flour. I have ground grains in it for bread, but it is very hard work. A mill with a larger flywheel, such as the Country Living grain mill, is much more efficient for hand grinding. The people I know who regularly bake multiple loaves of bread from fresh-ground flour generally use electric mills. If you have a stone grain mill, do not use it for soybeans, as the oil from the beans will gum up the grinding stones.

Steamers

Many of the Asian traditions of growing molds (see chapter 10) and fermenting grain-based alcoholic beverages (see chapter 9) require grains or soybeans to be steamed *above* water rather than boiled *in* water. The difference can be significant, especially in terms of growing molds. I have used a number of different steaming systems. Most often, I use stacking bamboo steamers, available at many Asian grocery stores. They work best if you have a pot that they fit upon tightly. Alternatively, they can sit in a wok. The reason I prefer them on a pot is that a pot can hold plenty of water for them to steam for hours, if need be, while a wok must constantly have water added to it, since there is much less volume capacity for water beneath the steamers. With stacking steamers, the bottom steamers get filled with steam before the top steamers, so it is a good idea to shuffle them around a few times through the process to get even steaming.

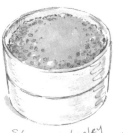

Steamed barley

Another steaming option, particularly helpful in the case of soybeans, which otherwise take five to six hours to cook, is to steam in a pressure cooker. Some pressure cookers come equipped with a hanging steamer basket; I've improvised in a big canning steamer by placing an upside-down colander in the water in the bottom of the pressure cooker and placing another colander containing the soybeans on top of that.

Incubation Chambers

Incubation involves keeping an environment warm so as to encourage development that requires a particular temperature range. This is what a hen does by sitting on her eggs, or what a hospital does for premature babies. Certain ferments require maintaining an environment warmer than normal ambient temperatures. Historically, people have incubated these near heat sources, wrapped in blankets, or even by taking them to bed and using the body to keep them warm. The history of fermentation consists of clever improvisation to simulate some observed condition. With simple household technologies available to us in the 21st century, we can easily create effective incubation chambers.

In creating incubation chambers, it is important to understand that some of the ferments requiring incubation also require airflow, whereas others do not. (Aerobic molds are covered in *Incubation Chambers for Growing Molds* in chapter 10.) Incubation for ferments not requiring air—such as yogurt and *amazak*é—is simpler, because minimizing airflow is in itself a means of maintaining temperature. The way I usually incubate these ferments is in an insulated cooler (which in this case is used as an insulated warmer). Insulated coolers come in many different shapes and sizes. The smallest one you can find that will fit your ferment will be most effective at maintaining the desired temperature. Often I will ferment yogurt or *amazak*é in a gallon-size jar and incubate it inside a round insulated unit designed for serving lemonade or coffee. Other times I ferment these in several quart-size jars incubated together in a rectangular unit. A related method is to incubate directly in a thermos.

The key to incubating in insulated coolers is preheating them. If you put your 110°F/43°C milk with yogurt starter into a cold cooler, the temperature will quickly drop. If, on the other hand, you add it to a cooler already warmed to the target temperature, it will hold the temperature for hours. I preheat insulated coolers simply by filling them with hot water before I begin final preparations on the ferment, so they heat for at least 15 minutes. Then I pour out the still-warm and -clean water (reusing it for dishwashing), add the ferments, and close the cooler. If there is extra space inside the insulated chamber, you can fill it with jars of warm water. You can also add insulation by wrapping the whole thing in blankets.

Other suitable incubation improvisations include: your oven (or microwave), turned off, heated simply by an incandescent lightbulb or a bottle of hot water (it may need to be propped open); a dehydrator; fermenting on a heating pad (usually with a towel or other buffer from the heat); or fermenting on or near a heat source or vent. Use a thermometer to make sure you are in the target range. Don't feel like you need to go out and buy an incubator. Use tools and objects in your midst, and be creative, like our ancestors were, about how to use them.

Curing Chambers

Just as certain ferments require warmer-than-ambient temperatures, others require cooler temperatures for a long, slow curing period. Ferments requiring cave-like curing conditions include cheeses and dry-cured meats. An actual cave, or an effective root cellar that maintains a roughly even earth temperature, is an ideal curing environment. Unfortunately, most people do not have ready access to such spaces. A wine refrigerator, typically calibrated to about 55°F/13°C, is the easiest option for creating a curing chamber. But a more versatile option is to plug any refrigerator into an external temperature controller (see below).

Temperature Controllers

Temperature controllers, also known as thermostats, are devices that turn electricity on or off at a set target temperature. If you plug a heat source into it, such as an incandescent lightbulb or a space heater, it can maintain a warm temperature by turning the flow of electricity on if the temperature falls below the set value. If you plug a refrigerator into it, it can maintain a cool temperature by turning the flow of electricity on if the temperature rises above the set value. For long periods of curing or incubation, these can be invaluable.

The most versatile model I've used, with a long sensor extension and a 0° to 255°F/-18° to 124°C temperature range, was the "Yet Another Temperature Controller" gifted to me by its designer, fermentation enthusiast Mikey Sklar. He and his partner have "become infatuated with fermentation," he writes, "so much so that we developed a gizmo to assist with it," which they sell online.[26]

I've worked with two other manufactured models. The Lux Programmable Outlet Thermostat is a good value at approximately $40. Its major limitation is a very short temperature sensor, so it must be placed inside the chamber. The other model I've used and like is a brand called SureSTAT, which I found at a greenhouse supply website for about $50. Many other thermostats and temperature controllers can easily be adapted with an outlet and sensor by anyone with electrical wiring savvy.

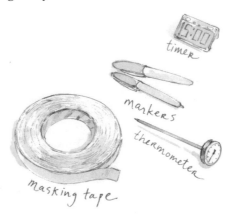

timer

markers

thermometer

masking tape

Masking Tape and Markers

Label your ferments! Masking tape and indelible markers are indispensible kitchen tools for the fermentation revivalist. Write what you are fermenting, the date, and the projected date of its completion. A journal for details and observations about your experiments is a wonderful resource too, but marking the jars and crocks themselves is essential.

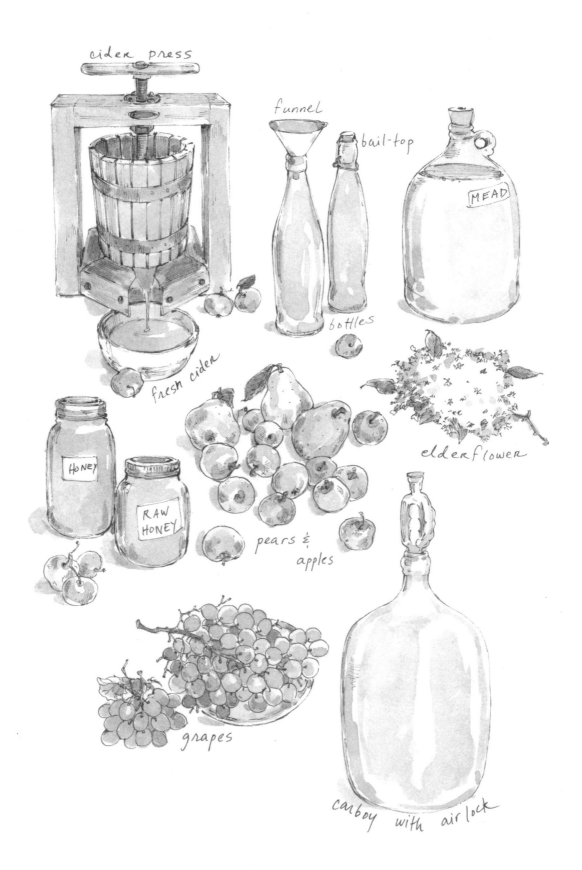

cider press

funnel

bail-top

MEAD

bottles

fresh cider

elderflower

HONEY

RAW
HONEY

pears &
apples

grapes

carboy with airlock

CHAPTER 4

Fermenting Sugars into Alcohol: Meads, Wines, and Ciders

*A*lcohol is a magical substance with the power to temporarily transport us outside of ourselves. When I drink, I feel a welcome lightness, at least fleetingly. Alcohol can make worries and inhibitions disappear, and embolden us to speak freely; it is a social lubricant and sexual catalyst. Alcohol is also a holy sacrament, both in indigenous traditions around the world and in some of the major world religions. As Patrick McGovern observes, "Wherever we look in the ancient or modern world, we see that the principal way to communicate with the gods or the ancestors involves an alcoholic beverage, whether it is the wine of the Eucharist, the beer presented to the Sumerian goddess Ninkasi, the mead of the Vikings, or the elixir of an Amazonian or African tribe."[1]

In moderation, drinking has been shown to promote health and lengthen life span.[2] In many human cultures, the B-vitamin synthesis that occurs in alcoholic beverages during fermentation has been nutritionally significant; when puritanical colonial governments outlawed certain indigenous fermented beverages, some native cultures experienced nutritional deficiency diseases for the first time as a direct result.[3] In excess, however, alcohol can lead to nausea, vomiting, passing out, debilitating illnesses, and even death, and sometimes the feelings caused by alcohol lead to impulsive behavior people later regret. For many people, alcohol use can become a problem, causing unacceptable behavior or addictive dependence. All of this is testament to its powerful nature.

The process of yeasts fermenting sugars into alcohol is a natural phenomenon that does not require human intervention. It happens in damaged or overripe fruits; it happens in honey that gets diluted by water; it happens when plant saps drain out of the plant. Many animals have enjoyed inebriation from spontaneous natural fermentations. What is a uniquely human cultural achievement is that we learned how to manipulate conditions to make this fermentation happen on our own terms.

In fact, there is broad consensus that alcohol was the earliest form of fermentation consciously practiced by human beings. And while it can be produced by precise methods requiring considerable skill, fermenting alcohol is not rocket science.

As I prepared to write this chapter, my neighbor Jake showed up one evening with some of his week-old wine. He had dissolved sugar into water, to taste (without measuring), and added an array of chopped-up ripe fruits fresh from a supermarket Dumpster, with no yeast except what was on the fruit. He stirred the mix frequently as it fermented in a bucket. The wine was fresh, light, sweet, bubbly, and already quite perceptibly alcoholic. A few days later, I pulled out a bottle of six-year-old plum mead. The initial fermentation of the mead—six years back—was not so different from Jake's wine. In a ceramic crock, I had mixed raw honey with unheated water at a ratio of 4 parts water to 1 part honey. Then I added fresh whole small plums and stirred frequently over the course of about a week, during which time the mixture became vigorously bubbly. I tasted some then, but most of it I strained and transferred to a 5-gallon carboy (I could have used any narrow-mouthed vessel), air-locked, and left to ferment for about six months until the visible action stopped. I then racked it (see *Siphons and Racking* in chapter 3) into another air-locked carboy, left it to ferment another six months, bottled it, and aged it in the cellar. The six-year-old mead was drier (less sweet) and considerably stronger than Jake's week-old wine but also required all those additional steps, and all those years of passing time.

There are many different ways to approach making alcoholic beverages. The elaborate steps involved in fermenting to dryness and aging can be well worth it. But they are not necessary in order to ferment alcohol. Fermentation processes are ancient rituals that humans have been practicing since long before the dawn of history, although we do not and probably cannot know the exact origins of alcohol. "Whoever seeks the origins of wine must be crazy," wrote a Persian poet a thousand years ago.[4] However, we can be pretty sure that the Neolithic practitioners of fermentation were not typically aging their ferments for years. Fermenting fruits, honey, sugar, or plant saps into alcoholic beverages can be extremely simple. They were utilizing technology such as pottery vessels— cutting-edge at the time, but common household items today. And while the contemporary literature of home alcohol making tends to emphasize chemical sterilization, specialized yeasts, and elaborate gadgetry—and these methods can yield fine beverages— they are not necessary. What you will find in this chapter are extremely simple, low-tech methods for creating alcohol, not much different from how people have been doing it for thousands of years. I will cover alcoholic beverages from simple carbohydrates: fruit, honey, sugar, and plant saps. The beer chapter (chapter 9) explores the somewhat more involved processes required to ferment alcohol from the complex carbohydrates of cereal grains and starchy tubers.

Yeast

Yeasts are the organisms that ferment sugars into alcohol and carbon dioxide. They give us alcoholic beverages and bread. Although yeasts are single-cell fungi not visible to the human eye without a microscope, their actions—the bubbling action in fermenting liquids and the rising action of fermenting dough—have been visibly observed throughout the evolution of language. The English word *yeast* (like the Dutch equivalent *gist*) derives from the Greek word *zestos*, meaning "boiling hot." Fermentation definitely is zesty! Interestingly, the word *fermentation* comes from the Latin *fervere*, also meaning "to boil." While yeasts do not technically boil liquids in the sense that we use the word today, the effect of both heat and fermentation on liquids is to produce bubbles. It's easy to understand these two bubbly phenomena's common linguistic heritage. The French word for yeast, *levure*, derives from the Latin *levere*, to raise, while the German *hefe* comes from the verb *heben*, to lift. Bubble, raise, and lift; that's what our eyes can see yeasts doing.

Fermentation yeasts were among the first microorganisms to be identified, isolated, and named. As a result of this, along with their economic importance, they are among the most studied of microbes. The most famous yeast (and the one most studied), known as *Saccharomyces cerevisiae*, is the one predominantly used in alcohol fermentation and baking. *S. cerevisiae* and many other yeasts, much like the cells of our bodies, are capable of both anaerobic fermentation and oxidative respiration. In the oxidative mode, yeasts grow and reproduce much more efficiently but do not produce alcohol.[5] Vigorous stirring stimulates yeast proliferation by providing aeration. However, alcohol accumulates only in the fermentative mode, without oxygen. But some aeration is critical; yeast growth "stops after a number of generations in the complete absence of oxygen," note Phaff, Miller, and Mrak in their book *Life of Yeasts*. Biosynthesis of two compounds essential for yeast growth (*ergosterol* and *oleic acid*) requires oxygen, though low concentrations are sufficient.[6] So the yeast can ferment without oxygen for a while, but eventually it requires another dose of oxygen in order to go on fermenting. This explains why racking—siphoning the ferment from one vessel into another, which aerates it—restarts "stuck" fermentation. In addition to multiple modes of metabolism, yeasts exhibit multiple modes of reproduction. They may be self-fertile (homothallic) or reproduce sexually (heterothallic), and many are both at different times.[7]

S. cerevisiae was the first eukaryotic genome to be completely sequenced, so thoroughly studied that it is frequently cited as the eukaryotic "model system." Yet despite all the research into the genetics of *S. cerevisiae*, its natural history and habitats are little understood.[8] In nature, yeasts are frequently found in association with plants, on fruits, leaves, flowers, and exuded sap. There is considerable seasonal variation, with the highest populations in the summer.[9] According to Phaff, Miller, and Mrak, "Insects are probably the most important vectors in the distribution of yeasts in nature."[10] The origins of the specific species *S. cerevisiae* have been hotly debated. Some researchers have arrived at the conclusion that *S. cerevisiae* evolved exclusively in association with human activities and is *not* otherwise found in nature. "On the basis of incontrovertible experimental support from the numerous surveys carried out on the yeast ecology of various natural and man-made environments associated with grape must fermentation, we must exclude a natural origin for *S. cerevisiae*," assert microbiologists Ann Vaughan-Martini and Alessandro Martini.[11]

Other researchers have come to quite different conclusions, noting that *S. cerevisiae* has been isolated in such diverse environments as mushrooms, oak-tree-associated soils, and beetle guts.[12] Recent study of beetle digestive tracts has found more than 650 distinct yeasts, at least 200 of which were previously unidentified, along with *S. cerevisiae*.[13] An analysis of *S. cerevisiae* gene sequences from dozens of different human and natural habitats determined that the domesticates "have been derived from natural populations unassociated with alcoholic beverage production, rather than the opposite."[14]

In any case, alcohol-producing yeasts (whether or not they are *S. cerevisiae*) are plentiful in nature. Some can keep producing alcohol to concentrations as high as about 20 percent; others can tolerate no more than about 3.5 percent alcohol; most function between those two extremes.[15] In this book, I emphasize wild fermentations, using only naturally occurring yeasts. The quickest, easiest, and most straightforward way to ferment a sugary liquid into alcohol may be to culture it by adding yeast. Hundreds of yeast lineages are commercially cultivated, now genetically modified as well, and available for sale through specialty suppliers. We who are blessed and cursed with so many consumer options have many exceptional yeasts from which to choose. However, it is helpful to understand that most (if not all) fermentable sugars, in raw form, are already populated by yeasts. Getting them to grow and produce alcohol is pretty easy. A yeast far less famous than *S. cerevisiae*, *Kloeckera apiculata*, frequently dominates the early stages of spontaneous fermentation of fruit juices, even grapes. Yeasts capable of fermentation are everywhere, even if they are not the number one global superstar monoculture species. "Yeasts are a bottomless reservoir of biodiversity, with more to offer than the classical handful of species traditionally used or studied," conclude Vaughan-Martini and Martini.

Simple Mead

Mead is honey wine. It can be flavored in infinite variation, and many of the fruits and other botanical flavorings you can add to it also serve as sources of yeasts and yeast nutrients. The rest of this chapter discusses different plants that people have fermented into alcohol, with and without honey, but first we'll start with the most utterly simple ferment there is, mead, which simply requires that you dilute raw honey with water. Raw honey contains abundant yeasts. (Pasteurization or cooking kills them.) The yeasts are inactive so long as the honey's water content remains at or below 17 percent (as it is in fully mature honey). But increase the water content just a little bit beyond that and the yeasts wake right up. According to the US Department of Agriculture, "above 19 percent water, honey can be expected to ferment even with only one spore per gram of honey, a level so low as to be very rare."[16]

You can dilute the honey however much you like. My typical proportion, measuring by volume, is 1 part honey to 4 parts water. For a lighter mead (or if I'm adding a large amount of sweet fruit), I'll dilute each part honey with 5 to 6 parts water. The Polish mead makers I met at Terra Madre, the international Slow Food gathering, make a mead they call *pultorak*, in which they mix each part honey with just half its volume of water (and age it for a minimum of four years). Lacandon *baälche* makers in Mexico dilute each part honey with as many as 17 parts water. Within these broad parameters (and even beyond them), you can experiment with proportions and find what you like.

I always add cold or room-temperature water to raw honey. If working with municipal water systems, dechlorinate water (see *Water* in chapter 3). Many recipes call for boiling everything. This is fine if you will be adding yeasts, but if you are expecting the honey to be the source of yeasts, keep it raw. To get the yeasts going, mix the honey with water. You can do this in a jar with a tight lid, or in a wide-mouth vessel. Thoroughly dissolve honey in water by vigorous stirring or shaking. Be persistent if necessary. Leave the vessel capped, or cover it to keep flies away; any covering, from a cloth to a tight-fitting lid, is okay. If your honey is *not* raw, good air circulation is necessary, because the air is the source of the yeasts landing on the surface of the ferment. Otherwise, constant air circulation is not necessary, but at this stage poses no problem. Stir or shake, vigorously and frequently, several times a day for a sustained couple of moments. In an open vessel, I like to stir rapidly in one direction to create a downward-pulling vortex; then I reverse it and create a vortex in the opposite direction. This rapidly aerates the solution (in the biodynamic style) and helps stimulate yeast growth. After a few days of frequent stirring, you will start finding the honey water with bubbles on the surface and an effervescent release when you stir. You can also do this in a sealed jar, with vigorous shaking; be sure to open the lid and release pressure, which can build dramatically. Keep shaking and stirring a few more days and the bubbles will build into a formidable force. I find the slow, steady buildup tremendously exciting.

Once you have vigorous bubbling, keep stirring or shaking daily. After a week or 10 days, you will notice that bubbling begins to subside. The fermentation of honey starts and peaks quickly but will continue slowly for many months. Honey contains both fructose and glucose, but the glucose ferments much more quickly (which you're seeing in the first few days of bubbling). The fructose fermentation is much slower, however, and takes place over months. You can drink your mead once rapid glucose fermentation peaks and slows, if you like, partially fermented, with most of the glucose converted to alcohol, but the fructose will still be mostly intact. Or you can ferment the mead fully, and age. See *Simple and Short Versus Dry and Aged* ahead in this chapter for a fuller discussion of your options for how to proceed from here. The easiest option is to avoid all the further complexity and additional steps by just enjoying your mead young and fresh. This is how most people throughout time have enjoyed their meads and other alcoholic beverages.

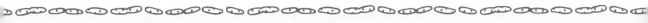

MEAD WITH BEESWAX CAPPINGS

Michael Thompson, Chicago Honey Co-op

We often use beeswax cappings for mead since these are what we have after extracting honey. (The cappings hold the honey in cells in the hive and must be cut away to release the honey; they are always dripping with honey.) We estimate the volume needed per water volume and taste for preferred sweetness. When transferring the mead to a fresh vessel after the first week of fermenting, we strain the cappings from the ferment, lay the wax out to dry on newspapers overnight, and use it for candles or body products. The mead holds a special flavor from this process.

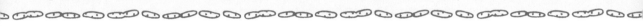

Botanical Enhancements to Mead: *T'ej* and *Baälche*

Mead has had many different names in different places over time. In Ethiopia, mead is known as *t'ej*, a name I used in *Wild Fermentation*. *T'ej* is traditionally made with twigs and leaves of *Rhamnus prinoides*, also known as *gesho* or woody hops. Like *t'ej,* many traditional meads are distinguished by the addition of plant ingredients. Sometimes these are simply for flavor; sometimes, to incorporate tonic, medicinal, or psychotropic qualities. Plants can also be sources of yeast to speed fermentation, or to initiate it in a sterile medium, such as pasteurized honey, pasteurized fruit juices, or refined sugar. In addition to flavors and yeasts, botanical ingredients can contribute acids, tannins, nitrogen, and phytochemical "growth factors" that stimulate yeast growth. "Honey, particularly light yellow honey, is deficient in nitrogen and growth factors needed by yeasts," explains food scientist and fermentation scholar Keith Steinkraus. "The rates of fermentation of all honeys can be increased by addition of nitrogen and growth factors."[17] Steinkraus reports that in village *t'ej* production, honey "is either collected from wild nests or produced in traditional barrel-type hives, and thus contains broken combs, wax, pollen, and bees. The belief persists that crude honey makes a better mead than refined honey."[18] I concur in this belief, as pollen, propolis, royal jelly, and even dead bees and wax provide more diverse nutrients to sustain the fermentation. Another characteristic noted by Steinkraus distinguishing *t'ej* production is that "the fermentation pot is smoked so that the t'ej will have a desired smoky flavor."

The mead the Mayan-descended Lacandon people of Chiapas ferment is called *baälche*, which is also the name of the tree *Lonchocarpus violaceus*, the bark of which is always used as an ingredient in this mead. *Baälche* is fermented in a hollow log vessel described in chapter 3 called a *canoa*. Ethnobotanist William Litzinger's PhD dissertation documented the techniques and rituals of *baälche* fermentation; he reports that the Lacandon mix honey and water together in the *canoa* at a proportion of approximately 17 parts water to each part honey, judging by color, and add a considerable quantity of bark.

Measuring (and serving) is done in a special ceramic "pot of the wine god." In Litzinger's documentation, the *baälche* maker reported that his pot "was given to the great grandfather of his great grandfather." Litzinger tested samples scraped from the pot interior and found high counts of *S. cerevisiae*. "The vessel is an important manifestation of an ancient cultural heritage," he observes. "Also, it has made possible a very long continuity in the presence of a single strain of *S. cerevisiae* in the Lacandon fermentation system."[19]

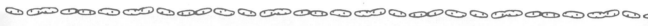

MEAD-MAKER ALCHEMIST

Turtle T. Turtlington

We humans have made quite a lot of hype around yeasts, these invisible little elves. Stories abound of how it was up to the shaman or medicine woman of a village or tribe to produce the sacred brews, and there was much chanting and dancing around needed, in order to invite into the jars the proper spirit. Many people, upon finding a "spirit" they liked working with, would place branches or logs, of either spruce or birch, at the bottom of their fermenting vats; the yeasts would dig into the wood to find the sweet saps, thus making it easy for a brewer to transfer the friendlies to another fermentation vat. It was even common for parents to give a log loaded with the family strain of wine yeast as a wedding gift. Talk about heirloom!

And so here we stand, just barely into the 21st century, rediscovering our roots as herbalists and brewers, witch doctors and alchemists, asking ourselves, "What is tradition?" And when it comes to yeast and brewing, there is no definable answer. It's all traditional, from packages of Montrachet and Premier Cuvée to the all-around classic "Champagne Yeast." Each brings its own flavor, its own style, each selected and bred for different characteristics. Each passed from brewer to brewer, through the millennia to this day. And we have the strains floating about us, same as they ever were, wild and mysterious! Descending from the heavens, alighting upon our meads, working their magic and then vanishing till needed again.

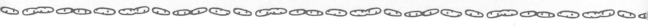

Like all traditional fermentation processes, *baälche* production and consumption are practiced with elaborate ritual. The *baälche* makers mark the removal of foam from the active ferment by holding kernels of special sacred symbolic corn in their palms over the *baälche* while moving their hands over it in a clockwise circular motion, and then they similarly bless the utensils and the cups used in drinking. Finally, they place the corn kernels with the skimmed-off foam in a plantain leaf with other sacraments, and the *baälche* maker folds the leaf into a package, goes into the forest, and buries it as an offering to the deity of death. Indigenous fermentation practices are thoroughly enmeshed in broader understandings about death, life, and transition. Those of us who have no such received tradition have to discover and reinvent these practices and give them meaning as best we can. In reclaiming fermentation, we can take back more than the mere substance of our food and drink. Through fermentation, we can reconnect ourselves to the broader web of life, in spirit and in essence , as well as the physical plane.

Fruit and Flower Meads

My own mead making is very often inspired by the abundance of some fresh seasonal fruit. Fresh fruits are covered with fermenting yeasts, especially those with edible skins. Most fruits are also acidic, and some contain tannins, both helpful to yeasts (in moderation). The greater the concentration of fruits, the faster yeast activity will be evident, and the stronger the fruit's influence will be on flavor. If possible, I would recommend using organic or unsprayed fruits rather than those grown using chemical pesticides, but I can testify that many intrepid Dumpster divers ferment their abundant conventional agriculture bounty into perfectly wonderful ferments.

With berries and small fruits, I just add them whole into the honey-water mixture. With larger fruits, if the skins are inedible, I peel them, then chop the fruit coarsely to increase surface area and facilitate infusion of sugars and phytochemicals into the fermenting solution, and I sometimes remove seeds or cores. Some people I've met routinely crush fruits in their ferments. This works too. I stopped doing this many years ago after my biodynamic farmer friend Jeff Poppen explained his philosophy of fermenting fruit: "It's the *essence* of the fruit you want, not the substance." Indeed, after a week bubbling in an alcohol-producing solution, berries and other small fruits, or chunks of larger fruits, typically have little sweetness or flavor left in them if you taste them. I don't worry about the proportion of fruit. The more fruit the better, except perhaps in the case of highly acidic fruits, such as lemons, where less may ferment better than more. My proportion of water to honey varies with the concentration of fruit: with just a little fruit I'll typically use 4 volumes water to each volume honey; with lots of fruit I'll further dilute, adding about 6 units water to each unit of honey. I fill my wide-mouth vessel with fruit, and then add honey water to cover it. And remember, always leave a little space at the top for expansion.

For flowers, it is important to only use flowers that are edible and taste good. Don't assume a flower tastes good just because it smells good! Some classic flowers to ferment are dandelion, rose petal, and elderflower. Try passionflower, marigold, nasturtium, or yarrow. The more flowers you use, the stronger the flavor will be. (Note: You can pick a small amount at a time and freeze them until you have enough.) For best flavor, remove petals from the

grapes

stems and green sepals, which can taste bitter. With flowers, yeast can be helped by the addition of some acidity, such as a little bit of citrus juice, and some tannins from raisins. I typically use flowers raw to incorporate their yeasts, exactly as I use fruit; but some people boil them to extract flavors, or steep them in hot water. There are many methods.

With a high concentration of fruit and/or flowers, aided by frequent stirring, fermentation starts quickly. Then proceed as for simple mead, above, stirring frequently. Once bubbling builds up, it will lift the fruit or flowers above the fermenting liquid. Frequent stirring is necessary to mix it back in, keep extracting flavor, and prevent it from molding. I cannot overemphasize: Stir, stir, stir.

After about a week of vigorous bubbling, and certainly by the time bubbling begins to noticeably subside, it's time to strain out the fruit. (Flowers can be strained sooner, since they are so comparatively small.) Place a mesh strainer, or a cheesecloth-lined colander, over your target vessel. Then pour or scoop the fruity fermenting liquid through it. Definitely taste the fruit. If it still has flavor, enjoy it. Eat it and share it. Use it to start a fermented fruit salad (see *Fermented Fruit Salads*). Pour some sugar water over it and make a fruit scrap vinegar. If the flavor seems spent, feed it to your chickens or your compost pile.

Now you have big decisions to make about your fruity or flowery mead. Taste a little to help you decide. Enjoy it now, sweet and young, if you like. Or ferment it further, as detailed in the following section.

Simple and Short Versus Dry and Aged

Meads and other fermented beverages can be enjoyed "green," meaning young, and by extension only moderately alcoholic; or they can be fermented longer to convert more of their sugars into alcohol, and once they have higher alcohol levels and are no longer actively fermenting, they can be bottled and aged for years or even decades. I have come to enjoy the smoothness that develops over years of aging. But for people first experimenting with fermentation, I strongly recommend enjoying some green. You do not need to delay gratification for years. Once you do it a few times and get comfortable with the process, you can start making bigger batches and aging them.

Some fruits lend themselves better to shorter-term ferments than aging. They tend to be sweet, soft fruits prone to rotting quickly, such as cantaloupes, watermelons, papayas, and bananas. "One time I was making cantaloupe wine with very ripe cantaloupes," writes fermentation enthusiast Olivia Zeigler. "On the second morning, it was really smelling wonderful, and I thought, 'I'll just come back tonight and strain it out.' Ten hours later it was rotten. Just disgusting." The lesson: "The smell will tell you when you've got it just right; don't leave it any longer!"

If you decide to continue fermenting a batch, transfer it to a narrow-necked jug-shaped vessel. The point of the narrow neck is to minimize surface area, so if necessary top off the liquid with more honey water, so that the surface of the solution reaches the narrow neck. If you are happy with the level of sweetness of the batch, mix new honey water in the same proportions you used earlier. If you wish to make it sweeter, use more honey; less sweet, use less or just add plain water.

Once the jug or carboy is filled to the narrow neck, air-lock. This is simple technology to protect the surface of the ferment from oxygen in the air. The reason for this is the widespread presence—especially in ferments based on spontaneous yeasts and the motley company they are likely to keep—of bacteria called *Acetobacter* that metabolize alcohol and oxygen into acetic acid. While the fermentation is vigorous, there is a constant release of carbon dioxide to prevent *Acetobacter* from growing on the surface. But as fermentation slows and the surface stills, there is greater opportunity for *Acetobacter* to grow. By protecting the ferment from air circulation, air locks diminish the risk of vinegar development and enable us to ferment much longer. There are several ways to improvise air locks, described in *Alcohol-Making Vessels and Air Locks* in chapter 3.

After a couple of months, your vessel full of mead will seem to have stopped fermenting. This does not necessarily mean that fermentation is complete. Honey especially can be very slow to ferment. When you can no longer perceive bubbling, it is time to rack your mead. This means siphoning it into another vessel, as described in *Siphons and Racking*, chapter 3. Typically, when fermented beverages are racked, the dead yeast accumulation on the bottom of the vessel, called lees, is left behind. The lees is vitamin-rich and can be cooked into soups, breads, or casseroles.

bail-top

If you leave behind the lees, and taste a bit of the mead (how can you not?), you will not have as much volume after racking. But you still want the mead to fill the vessel up to the narrow neck. As you did when you first transferred the mead to the narrow-necked vessel, top it off with new honey water as needed. Then air-lock. The ferment should start gently bubbling again. The brief aeration of the ferment stimulates further fermentation by giving yeasts enough oxygen for respiration to synthesize essential compounds (ergosterol and oleic acid) that allow them to go on fermenting. After another few months, once the second round of fermentation appears to have stopped, you can bottle your mead. (See *Bottles and Bottling*, chapter 3.)

Once it is bottled, you can age your mead for weeks, months, or years. The higher the ferment's alcohol concentration, the greater the potential for storing it long-term. It's fun to sample ferments over time and see if you can perceive how they change. Sometimes they become *much* better after years have passed. I had a batch of strawberry mead that tasted nasty when I bottled it. I couldn't bring myself to throw it away, but I didn't touch it for about three years. It's really delicious now. Stored fermented beverages continue to develop through various slow chemical reactions after fermentation has ceased.

Continuous Starter Method

If you can get into a rhythm of mead making, you can keep adding a cup or two of actively fermenting, vigorously bubbly mead to the next new batch. In this way, you could do small batches in a continual progression. This is how many traditional ferments have historically been perpetuated, through a long unbroken lineage. You can take short breaks from your routine. If you have a fermentation-slowing device in your home (also called a refrigerator), use it to slow down your starter's metabolism; if not, find a cool dark spot. But don't leave it too long. To keep it vigorous, it needs regular use, just like a sourdough (see *Sourdough: Starting One and Maintaining It* in chapter 8). This is how a spontaneous ferment evolves into a starter culture: through persistent engagement. Share starters with a network of others. You can back one another up if and when someone else's starter dies, or loses its vigor. Continuous rhythms can be extremely challenging in our fast-paced culture of mobility.

Herbal Elixir Meads

Meads can possess many powerful and magical botanical qualities. Any plants you can use for well-being or healing, you can ferment into mead or other types of alcoholic beverages. Ayurvedic medicine uses fermented beverages known as *arishtas* and *asuvas* as means of delivering botanical medicine. "These products in general possess preservative properties, potentization of the drug due to biotransformation mediated by native microbes, improvement in drug extraction and drug delivery."[20] Much herbal medicine in our time is dispensed as *tinctures*, which are plant extracts in distilled alcohol. As a vehicle for plant medicine, alcohol is both a solvent and a preservative, extracting phytochemicals into a stable medium. But the alcohol need not be distilled; as an alternative, we can preserve and share plant medicine by incorporating medicinal plants into herbal elixir meads and wines.

I first heard the phrase *herbal elixir mead* from my friend and teaching partner Frank Cook, who died in 2009. Frank was a devoted plant explorer, who traveled the world on a quest to meet plants and healers of broadly diverse locales. He walked across both California and North Carolina foraging. He had a mission to get to know each of the 500 plant families, which he quite nearly accomplished despite his early death at age 47 and not finding his green path until age 30. Frank was a gifted teacher, who loved to share what he knew, and constantly took people out on educational plant walks, telling stories of the plants and challenging people to look beyond "the green wall" by becoming conscious of plants and engaging with them. "Eat something wild every day" was one of his mantras that I have adopted. "Don't be an end user" was another. Take what you learn and become a teacher. Spread valuable knowledge.

Frank and I came together over our shared passion for mead making. He frequently made mixed herbal infusions of plants he found on his walks, to enjoy as teas, and to mix with honey to ferment. He called these ferments herbal elixir meads. Frank would typically make an herbal infusion as follows: He would bring water to a boil, then remove it from the heat, add a mix of the day's wildcrafted herbs, stir, cover, and leave for a while. For roots, barks, or mushrooms, he would boil the woody plant material in a decoction. He would drink and share some as a tea while warm, then cool the rest to ferment. Frank was emphatic about only working in 1-gallon/4-liter batches, because he found that modest scale so much easier to work with than the typical homebrew 5-gallon size. He would add about 3 cups of honey for a gallon batch then add water as necessary to fill the gallon jug. Usually he would leave in plant material as it fermented.

When I first met Frank, he would add a packet of yeast to the mixture, but as a result of our collaborative teaching experiences, he increasingly came to use wild yeasts. Remember, to get wild yeasts, be sure to use *raw* honey, cool your infusion to body temperature before adding the honey, and start it in a wide-mouth vessel, so you can stir, stir, stir to get wild fermentation going. You can also save some of the plant material to add raw as another yeast source. The source of yeast in the Ayurvedic fermented herbal preparations, for example, is the "fire flame" flower, *dhataki* (*Woodfordia fruticosa* Kurz).[21]

Just as so many different plants can be fermented in this way, plants can also be introduced in many different ways. You could skip the infusion altogether and simply add harvested plant material raw to honey water and stir, as for fruit, above. As another possibility, plants can be preserved using honey as a solvent and preservative. Then you can enjoy flavored medicinal honeys and dilute (as for simple mead) to ferment.

Need some inspiration for plants to use? Go for a walk outside and get to know your herbal neighbors. Some of them will be perfect. The sidebar lists some of the herbal elixir meads sampled at two mead circles in Black Mountain, North Carolina, in 2006 and 2007. Frank was a regular participant in these circles and took great pleasure in the growing circle of mead makers with elixirs to share. Though he's gone, the circles continue, invoking his spirit in their ritual of creation, sharing, and inebriation.

elderflower

HERBAL ELIXIR MEADS PRESENTED AT MEAD CIRCLES, IN ASHEVILLE, NORTH CAROLINA

(Abridged from lists compiled by Marc Williams)

- Apple
- *Ashwaganda*, Red Clover, Bilberry, *Hipala*, Sweet Birch
- Astragalus, Lychee, *Rymania*, Jujube, *Schisandra*, Ginger, Licorice, Tangerine, Ginseng
- Astragalus, Red Peony, Jasmine, Green Tea
- Birch, Pineapple Sage
- Birch, Sassafras, Maple
- Birch, Yarrow, Red Clover
- Black Balsam, Goldenrod
- Black Birch, Red Spruce
- Blackberry, Chai, Juniper
- Blueberry
- Chaga
- Chaga, Ginseng
- Chamomile, Dandelion, Hibiscus, Elderberry
- Chrysanthemum, Gogi Berry
- Clary Sage
- Coffee, Yarrow, Thyme, Cardamom, Cinnamon, Clove
- *Cornus kousa*
- Dandelion
- Dandelion, Burdock, Fig, Cinnamon, Chicory
- Darjeeling Tea, Sage, Licorice, *Gotu Kola*, Chai, Lap Sang
- Fig, Chocolate Chip, Dandelion, Chicory, Burdock, Cinnamon
- Ginger
- Ginger Curry
- Ginger, Turmeric, Sassafras
- Goldenrod, Ginkgo, Red Clover
- Green Tea Chai plus Black Tea, Raisin, *Pedicularis*, Cumin, Vanilla
- Ground Ivy
- *Gruit* (contains 30 different plants and mushrooms)
- Hawthorn Mead
- *Hexastylis* spp., *Osmorhiza* spp.
- Hibiscus, Lemongrass, Ginger
- Kaviana Mead: Kava Kava, Damiana
- Lemon, Blueberry, *Pedicularis*, Lemon Balm
- Maitake
- Mango, Rose Conjou Tea
- Mint
- Mint, Mugwort, Wineberry
- Mugwort
- Nettles, Dandelion, Hyssop
- Nettles, Lemon Balm, Rosemary, Lavender, Yarrow

- Nettles, Rosemary, Yarrow, Nutmeg, Pea Shoots
- Nettles, Sassafras
- Nettles, Yarrow, Lemon Balm, Red Clover
- Passionflower, Damiana, Hawthorn, Rose Petal
- Paw Paw, Goldenrod, Sunshine Wine
- Peaches, Plums, Apple, Elderberry, Grape
- Pine, Juniper, Mushroom
- Red Pear, Pennyroyal
- Roasted Chicory, Chaga, *Aplenatum*, Heather, Sassafras
- Roasted Dandelion
- Rosemary
- Sassafras, Birch
- Sassafras, Dandelion
- Sassafras, Holly, Yellow Root
- *Smilax*, *Hexastylis*, Cayenne, Sparkleberry
- Stevia, Nettles, Mint
- White Oak Bark
- Wild Ginger, *Pipsissiwa* Leaves, Spice Bush Leaves and Roots
- Wild Grape, Wild Ginger, Toothwort, Yarrow
- Wineberry, Sassafras
- Wineberry, Shiso
- Wormwood
- Yarrow
- Yarrow, Coffee, Thyme, Clove, Cinnamon, Cardamom
- Yarrow, Fennel, Lemon Balm
- Yarrow, Lemon Balm, Lemongrass
- Yarrow, Mint, Stevia, Motherwort
- Yellow Root, Sassafras, Elderflower

Wine from Grapes

Wine is simply grapes, juiced and fermented. Grapes possess an ideal balance of sugars, acids, and tannins to support yeast growth, so it is easy to fully ferment grape juice into a strong alcoholic beverage to store, age, and ship around the world. In addition, the skins of grapes are covered with a whitish bloom, visible to the eye, that includes yeasts. I had the good fortune a few years ago of being present for the grape harvest at Pratale, a small farm in Umbria, in central Italy. About 10 of us spent the morning picking grapes, nice full clusters of several different varieties, some green-skinned, some dark purple, almost black. We mixed the grapes together, and as we continued to pick, a mule named Otello hauled the boxes of grapes to the farmhouse where the wine was to be made.

The first step of the process, after gathering, is crushing the grapes. At Pratale, they had a clever old mechanical device for this. The device had two wooden rollers, with interlocking grooves. A hand crank turned the rollers.

Above the rollers was a wooden hopper, which we kept filling with grapes. As we cranked the rollers, the grapes passed between them, emptying, crushed, into a vessel below. In a classic scene from the 1950s television hit *I Love Lucy*, Lucille Ball accomplishes the same thing by stomping on grapes in a tub with her feet. This is a viable low-tech approach.

What the crushing yields is a mass of grape skins, stems, and pulp in grape juice. At Pratale, once the grapes were crushed we were ready for lunch (accompanied by the previous year's wine, of course). When we returned to the grape juice two hours later, it was a bubbling froth. Ripe grapes are so yeast-rich that vigorous fermentation starts almost immediately. For white wines, you must quickly strain out the skins and other solids and ferment the juice alone. For red wines, you leave the fermenting juice with the skins, which darken the wine and contribute tannins. At Pratale, my hosts Etain and Martin were making red wine. They left the fermenting grapes in open vessels to ferment for the first few frothy days, then strained the liquid, pressed the remaining juice from the grapes, and transferred the fermenting wine to air-locked vessels. They could have drunk it then if they wished, lightly fermented. In Turkey, people enjoy a lightly fermented grape juice they call *sira*, still very sweet and bubbly, with about 2 percent alcohol. In Germany, this young partially fermented grape juice is known as *federweisser*. But Etain and Martin prefer to ferment theirs a few months, to dryness, before bottling. Their process was extremely simple, and the wine it produced was wonderful, and a daily staple in their lives.

Grapes make wonderful wine, but any fruit can be fermented into alcohol. Wine from grapes emerged as the global favorite from the Zagros Mountains, in a region encompassed today by Armenia and Iran. According to Patrick McGovern:

> The world's first wine culture—one in which viniculture, comprising both viticulture and winemaking, came to dominate the economy, religion, and society as a whole—emerged in this upland area by at least 7000 BC. Once established, the wine culture gradually radiated across time and space to become a dominant economic and social force throughout the region and later across Europe in the millennia to follow. The end result over the past ten thousand years or so, since the end of the Ice Age, is that the Eurasian grape now accounts for some ten thousand varieties and 99 percent of the world's wine.[22]

McGovern describes the dynamics of how the Canaanite culture, beginning as early as the 2nd millennium BC, spread wine around the Mediterranean: "They applied a similar strategy wherever they went: import wine and other luxury goods, befriend the rulers by presenting them with specialty wine sets, and then wait until they were asked to help in establishing native industries."[23]

Wine has been a symbol of status, frequently associated with elites, while other indigenous ferments or beers were what common people drank.

According to Tom Standage, in *A History of the World in Six Glasses*, "Romans took Greek connoisseurship to new heights. . . . Wine became a symbol of social differentiation, a mark of the wealth and status of the drinker . . . the ability to recognize and name the finest wines was an important form of conspicuous consumption; it showed that they were rich enough to afford the finest wines and had spent time learning which was which."[24]

Today grape cultivation has spread to every continent. A few years ago I flew from Northern California to Croatia. In both places I was struck by the endless monoculture of manicured rows of trellised grapevines. And the grapes themselves are almost always propagated by cloning existing vines, giving rise to genetic uniformity. "Because there has been very little sexual reproduction [of grapes] over the last eight millenniums, this [genetic] diversity has not been shuffled nearly enough," reports *The New York Times*.[25] In sexual reproduction, genes are continually recombined, yielding occasional improvements, such as pest resistance. Grapes and wine are well and good, but monocultures and genetic uniformity both are inherently unhealthy, because they diminish biodiversity and increase vulnerability to disease and pests.

One of the great challenges of reviving local food is to avoid simply replicating the most popular globalized products and instead to develop strategies to turn what grows most easily and abundantly in each region into products that satisfy our cravings. People almost everywhere have traditions of turning fruits and other available carbohydrates into alcohol. Lovely as wine may be, we do not need grape vineyard monocultures everywhere in order to satisfy our desires.

Cider and Perry

Cider is fermented apple juice. Perry is fermented pear juice. The varieties of both fruits that we eat are typically grown from trees cloned from particular cultivars that people found especially pleasing. The vast majority of what grows from seed produces fruits generally considered either too small, too mealy, or too astringent to be enjoyed as food; these fruits have traditionally been fermented into cider and perry.

The only thing challenging about fermenting apples or pears is pressing the juice out of them. The best way is a cider press (see *Cider and Grape Presses* in chapter 3). Cider presses use a two-part process: first milling fruit into what is called *pomace*, then pressing pomace into juice. Sometimes milled pomace is left to sit for a few hours, or a few days, before pressing, which can develop color and flavor, and reduce tannins in astringent varieties. You can also use any electric juicing contraption, though if it heats the juice above about 113°F/45°C, yeast will be killed. You can certainly ferment this anyway, like commercial apple or pear juice. The difference is that fresh unheated juice is raw and very rich in yeasts, while excessive heat kills yeasts.

If you have raw fresh-pressed juice, just let it do its thing. It will soon start to bubble. You can leave it in a wide-mouth vessel and stir to stimulate yeast growth. Transfer to a narrow-necked jug or carboy once fermentation becomes vigorous. Or you can put it right into a jug or carboy and watch the inevitable fermentation build without your active participation.

If you use pasteurized juice, which has had its natural yeasts killed by heat, you need to introduce yeasts into it. Only use juice that is free of preservatives, which can prevent or inhibit yeast growth. The easiest way to introduce yeasts in our time is by adding a packet of yeast. Or you can actively draw yeast from the air, by placing juice in a wide vessel where it will have a large surface area exposed and stirring frequently. But my favorite way to get the pasteurized juice fermenting is to add some fresh raw apples or pears to it, with skins. Quarter, remove cores, and coarsely chop. And then stir, stir, stir until bubbling starts and gets vigorous. Then strain, transfer to jug or carboy, and continue to ferment.

In the early days of fermentation, cider and perry often "boil over," with foam spilling out. For this reason, it's important that you do not insert your air lock immediately into the jug or carboy, as this initial foaming will likely spew through or dislodge it. Instead, place jug/carboy in a sink, tub, pot, or tray to catch any overflow, and place any flat disk (such as a jar top) on top, or cover loosely with plastic wrap. After a few days, when foaming subsides—or at any point from then on—you can enjoy very lightly fermented, bubbly cider or perry. If you wish to bottle cider or perry for storage, clean up the foam residue from the interior edges of the vessel (or transfer to a clean vessel), then air-lock. Ferment air-locked for a month or two, until bubbling slows and cider clears. Rack and ferment another month or two. Then bottle. If you wish your cider/perry to be carbonated, add about 1 teaspoon/5 ml of sugar, or ¼ cup/60 ml fresh sweet cider per quart/liter at the bottling stage so fermentation will continue, at a very limited scale, in the bottle. Beware of adding too much sugar or unfermented juice at the bottling stage; bottles can overcarbonate and even explode.

This year we made perry with tiny pears so astringent they could not be eaten. We had always regarded those trees and fruits as ornamentals, but when I met English perry makers at Terra Madre, I learned from them that they use old astringent varieties, and the fermentation greatly reduces their astringency. This perry was not suitable to drink lightly fermented, but given a full fermentation of several months and some aging, it is terrific. The remaining astringency gives it a feeling of extra dryness, as in red wine. This year we fermented the astringent pears alone, to prove that fermentation would diminish the astringency. Next year we'll try mixing the different pear varieties together, which is how most people approach cider and perry.

pears &
apples

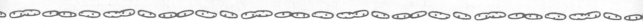

LIFELONG CIDER MAKER

Ann Peluso, Limerick, Maine

My specialty has been hard cider. I will admit that I learned the crude technique at Quaker boarding school. Everyone there stuffed gallons of cider in the clothes closets: open jug, pour some out, leave the lid raised on one side, then let it sit in the closet until it stopped bubbling. Now I brew about 100 gallons a year just like I did in high school. After three weeks under the dining room table, they go to shelves in the garage. That's it. My husband says he is the great awe at work because his wife brews. I seem to be some sort of folk hero there. I have shared the rudimentary technique with all the farm markets in the area, the orchards where I get cider, my adult piano students, and my credit union. So far very few believe it is possible except my main apple grower, who may know more about it than I do, but isn't saying. I took him a sample, he drank down the whole thing in one gulp, and proclaimed it very good. I feed the dregs to our ducks. They have a high niacin need, and poultry feed may not cover it in the winter. I drink down to the almost-dregs, because I need the vitamins too.

Sugar-Based Country Wines

As with cider and perry, the biggest obstacle to fermenting other fruits into alcoholic beverages is juicing them. Even with a juicing machine, it is both labor- and energy-intensive to juice fruit. Many traditional fruit-based ferments have relied upon cooking fruit down into a thick syrup, then diluting with water. For instance, this is how the Papago and several other peoples of northwestern Mexico and the southwestern United States ferment the fruits of the *sahuaro* (saguaro) cactus. After the fruits are knocked down from where they grow atop tall cacti, the pulp is "scooped out with the thumbs," according to Henry Bruman. "After a process of boiling, straining, and boiling down, there remained a brownish syrup and a mass of fiber and seeds. The syrup, when mixed with from one to four times its volume of water and allowed to stand in earthen jar, readily fermented into an intoxicating beverage."[26] The resulting saguaro beverage is known among the Papago as *navai't* (pronounced *na-wait*).

Usually when I make fruit-flavored ferments, I don't bother either juicing or cooking pulp down into a syrup. The far easier method is to simply infuse the fruit in honey water (as described in *Fruit and Flower Meads*) or sugar water. Sugar has two great advantages: It is cheap and easy to find, and its flavor is neutral enough that it will not rival the flavoring you add. As with honey-based meads, proportions of sugar can vary. For a strongly alcoholic beverage that will ferment a long time, you might want to use as much as 3 pounds/6 cups (1.5 kg/1.5 liters) sugar per gallon/4 liters; for a shorter-term, lighter ferment, or one with a heavy concentration of fruit, you might want to use as little as half as much sugar.

A general term for an infusion of fruit, flowers, vegetables, herbs, spices, or any other flavoring in a sugar solution is *country wine*. In the United States, early settlers "brought with them an English tradition of using substitute ingredients whenever necessary," writes historian Stanley Baron, who found documentation of alcoholic beverages made in the colonial United States with persimmons, pumpkins, and Jerusalem artichokes.[27] As with any ferment, there are many ways to approach country wines. I simply dissolve sugar in cold water. Many books say to add sugar to boiling water and cook it into a syrup, but I have not found this to be necessary. Then I typically add raw fresh or dried fruit (or flowers, vegetables, herbs, spices, or other flavoring), stir, stir, stir, and proceed exactly as I do with mead. Sometimes people cook flavorings with sugar water or steep them in boiled sugar water. Depending upon whether the flavoring agent contains acids or tannins, many people add citrus for acidity and/or raisins or black tea for tannins. Recipes are everywhere once you start seeking them out. There is no single best way to make country wines; this is an improvisational art that people successfully practice in many different ways.

If you approach a country wine as a wild fermentation, bear in mind that unlike raw honey, crystalline sugar has been cooked in its processing and so will not contain live yeasts. Raw flavorings can serve as sources of yeasts. If everything is cooked, an open vessel with a broad surface area is essential to incorporate airborne yeasts that land on the surface. Or add a packet of yeast or starter from an earlier batch that is still active. In any case, stir, stir, stir. Country wines can be enjoyed young, as soon as vigorous fermentation subsides, or transferred to an air-locked vessel and fermented to dryness.

Alcoholic Beverages from Other Concentrated Sweeteners

The techniques described above for fermenting with sugar and honey can be used with other sweeteners, such as maple syrup, sorghum, agave, jaggery (palm sugar), rice syrup, or barley malt. (Just to give you an idea of how incredibly varied are the sources of sugar that people have successfully fermented into alcohol, James Gilpin in the United Kingdom has been fermenting alcohol from the urine of diabetics, which, due to their disease, contains high levels of unmetabolized sugar.[28]) Stevia and artificial sugar substitutes will not ferment; yeasts can only ferment alcohol from carbohydrates. The above-mentioned sweeteners are all cooked in the processes that concentrate them into shelf-stable, commercial forms. Therefore they do not contain viable yeasts. Yeast must be introduced in the form of raw fruits, or a packet of yeast, or with a broad surface area exposed to fresh air and frequent stirring. I definitely advocate small experimental batches before attempts to ferment gallons and gallons.

Fermented Fruit Salads

Fruits can be fermented into alcohol in solid form as well. Fermentation enthusiast Mark Ericson recalls that his pastor grandfather always had a jar of "friendship fruit" fermenting on the kitchen counter: "Typically canned fruit, fruit cocktail, canned peaches, etc. fed with white sugar. People share a cup of starter and recipes so others can start their own batch." As with most ferments, the starter helps get fermentation going. Fresh fruit will also introduce yeasts, as will a pinch of packaged yeast and/or frequent stirring. Sugar pulls juices out of the fruits, making a mash of fermenting juice and flesh. In a large jar with a lid, mix together fruit and sugar. Many recipes call for sugar equal in weight with fresh fruit, but I encourage you to experiment with less. In the early stage, until yeast activity is evident, do not seal the jar, but rather cover it with a cloth to keep flies away while still maintaining air circulation. Stir frequently. Once it is bubbling, seal the lid on the jar and continue to stir frequently, which also opens the jar and prevents pressure from building. Store the jar out of direct light, but where you will not forget about it.

Taste at each stirring to evaluate progress. You can enjoy either fermented lightly or more fully. Enjoy as a fruit salad, dessert topping, or chutney, salsa, or stuffing ingredient. You can also find recipes for fruitcakes with fermented friendship fruit starters. Once you have a ferment like this going, you can easily perpetuate it by continuing to feed it fresh fruit and sugar.

A variation on this idea is a German tradition known as *rumtopf*. In this fermented fruit salad, the fruit-sugar mixture is topped off with a little rum or brandy. Let the fruit and sugar sit a few hours (so the sugar can pull juices out of the fruit) before adding just a tiny bit of liquor. Traditionally people add layers of fruit, sugar, and liquor as different fruits ripen, and let the *rumtopf* mature for a few months to enjoy as a winter holiday treat.

Plant Sap Ferments

Beyond fruits and grains (for beers, which I discuss in chapter 9), the form of plant sugar most fermented into alcohol around the world is sap. To be honest, I do not have much personal experience fermenting fresh saps. But decades ago, as a 23-year-old traveling in West Africa, I sampled many fine palm wines, which are popular in tropical regions with abundant palm trees. And my exploration of the literature suggests that in many regions of the world, the primary source of sugars that people ferment into alcohol comes from the saps of various trees and other plants.

"Apparently, most palm saps can yield wine," reports Keith Steinkraus. "Fresh palm sap is generally a dirty brown, but as yeasts multiply in it, it becomes pale and eventually milk white and opalescent."[29] Patrick McGovern describes palm tapping he observed in Africa:

> At the top of the tree, the tappers skewer male and female flowers, bind them up so that there is a steady flow of sap, and attach a gourd or other

container to collect the sap. A healthy tree can produce nine or ten liters a day and about 750 liters over half a year. . . . Because the sap has already been inoculated with yeasts by insects eager to consume the milky, sweet exudates, the fermentation process is self-starting. Within two hours, palm wine ferments to about a 4 percent alcohol content; give it a day, and the alcohol level goes up to 7 or 8 percent.[30]

Palm wine ferments fast and is drunk soon thereafter. According to the United Nations Food and Agriculture Organization (FAO), "Palm wine has a very short shelf-life. The product is not preserved for more than one day. After this time accumulation of an excessive amount of acetic acid makes it unacceptable to consumers."[31]

Ethnographer Henry Bruman, who documented indigenous fermentation traditions of Mexico and Central America, reported another method used by people in Chiapas, who would fell a palm tree and carve out a hole of 1- to 2-quart/liter capacity in the remaining trunk of the tree. "The flow of sap would continue for a week or two. The sap, which was withdrawn once or twice a day, was consumed when it was judged sufficiently fermented."[32]

When coconut palm sap is fermented, as is commonly practiced in India and Sri Lanka, it is known as toddy. "The sap is collected by slicing off the tip of an unopened flower. The sap oozes out and can be collected in a small pot tied underneath the flower," according to the FAO report. "The toddy is fully fermented in six to eight hours. The product is usually sold immediately due to its short shelf-life."[33]

Bamboo also has sap that can be fermented. According to the FAO, areas of eastern and southern Africa enjoy a fermented bamboo sap beverage called *ulanzi*. The report describes *ulanzi* as a "clear, whitish drink with a sweet and alcoholic flavour," prepared as follows:

The bamboo shoots should be young in order to obtain a high yield of sap. The growing tip is removed and a container fixed in place to collect the sap. . . . The raw material is an excellent substrate for microbial growth and fermentation begins immediately after collection. Fermentation takes between five and twelve hours depending on the strength of the final product desired.[34]

Green cornstalks (maize) can be similarly pressed into a juice, which can be fermented as is, or boiled down into a syrup. An ethnographic team writing in the 1930s, W. C. Bennett and R. M. Zing, reported that: "After the leaves are removed, the stalks are taken to a large hollow boulder and pounded with oak sledges. Then the juice is squeezed out of the stalks by means of a clever device, *mabihímala*, invented for this purpose." The *mabihímala* consists of a net woven from yucca fiber, with a stick through each end, one stick to hold between the feet, the other twisting in both hands, to wring the juice out of the beaten stalks.[35]

Sugarcane juice also readily ferments. I've had excellent spontaneous fermentations of raw cane juice, light and bubbly; I've also read about traditions that concentrate the sap by cooking it down, for instance in *basi* from the Philippines, where sugarcane is believed to have evolved. Sorghum stalks, grown in the southeastern United States, are pressed into juice, which is typically cooked down into a syrup known as sorghum molasses; fresh sorghum juice or diluted sorghum molasses can be similarly fermented.

A further source of sweet fermentable plant saps is desert succulent plants. In Mexico, people continue an ancient tradition of fermenting the sap of the agave (also known as century plant or maguey) into a beverage called *pulque*. Each plant can yield hundreds of quarts/liters of fermentable sap, known as *aguamiel* (honey water). The pulque process begins after nearly a decade of plant development, when plants develop flowering stalks called *quiotes*. The first step in extraction is called *capazón*, or castration, which involves removing the tight central cluster of leaves, thus exposing the developing flower bud, which is removed. The castrated plant is then left for months or even years, during which the bud continues to swell with sap but not grow. Then the exposed surface of the castrated bud is punctured, mashed, and left to rot for a week or so, after which it is easily removed. According to Henry Bruman, "This process creates both an irritation to the plant that stimulates the flow of sap and a cavity in which the sap may collect. . . . The constant flow necessitates the removal of the aguamiel usually twice and occasionally three times daily."[36] Aguamiel may be drunk sweet, fermented into *pulque* (traditionally using hides as vessels), or boiled into syrup for use as a sweetener. "Pulque differs in flavor and texture from most other kinds of beers and wines," notes William Litzinger. "It often has a slimy appearance due to the presence of a *Bacillus* species which forms slime sheaths of cellular strands."[37] "It is sweetish and acidy at the same time and curiously refreshing," writes Diana Kennedy.[38]

Another way that agave and other plants have been turned into both food and alcohol is by harvesting and roasting their stems. To make the beverage *mescal*, roasted agave stems or "hearts" are pounded to a pulp and mixed with water; later this slurry is strained and pressed, then boiled. After cooling, it ferments in four to five days.[39]

A final fermentable plant sap to consider is that of deciduous hardwood trees. In Poland, people have traditionally tapped and fermented the early-spring-rising sap of birch and sometimes other trees into a lightly alcoholic beverage called *oskola*.[40] Maple sap too can be fermented. Although I have diluted maple syrup and successfully fermented it into alcoholic beverages, I have been unable to find any reference to a traditional practice of fermenting the sap directly. Henry Bruman notes that the Iroquois tapped maple and birch trees, drank the fresh sweet saps, and cooked them into syrups. "That they should not at some time have allowed some unboiled sap to stand around for a few days

carboy with airlock

until it fermented and then not have tasted it, noticed the new flavor, and experienced the result of imbibing it in quantity is almost inconceivable," he comments. "Yet, if that event took place it made no impression on the culture of the tribe."[41]

Carbonating Alcoholic Beverages

Any mead, wine, cider, or perry can be bottled to make a sparkling beverage. Carbonation is a matter of trapping in the bottle carbon dioxide produced as a by-product of fermentation. The critical factor in carbonating beverages is making sure there is just a small amount of fermentable sugar in the beverage at the point of bottling, for if there is too much sugar to ferment in the bottle it can easily overcarbonate, resulting not only in the loss of a significant proportion of the liquid to volcanic spewing, but potentially dangerous explosions. As I report in graphic detail in relation to bottling still-sweet carbonated soft drinks (see *Carbonation* in chapter 6), active ferments sealed in bottles when they still have significant sugar to fuel continued fermentation can explode like bombs, with disfiguring and life-threatening results.

For this reason, before bottling, the beverage should be fully fermented; this means fermenting until fermentation stops, racking into another vessel, and fermenting further until it stops again. Then, when you are ready to bottle, add a small amount of sweetener—about 1 teaspoon/5 ml of sweetener per quart/liter of beverage—and stir to dissolve, before bottling. This modest addition of fermentable sugars will restart fermentation, at a controlled scale, in the bottle.

Beverages intended for carbonation need to be bottled in bottles capable of holding pressure. In standard wine bottles, the building pressure of carbonation will simply force the cork out. Crimp-topped beer bottles, bail-top bottles, and champagne bottles are designed to hold pressure. Many soda, juice, and other beverage bottles with tight caps may also be used. (For more bottle and bottling information, see *Bottles and Bottling* in chapter 3.) Allow at least two weeks for fermentation in the bottle for carbonation to develop in mature, dry alcoholic beverages. Chill sparkling beverages before opening to minimize loss of beverage to foam.

You can bottle partially fermented beverages and carbonate them, but, as I will keep reiterating, be aware of the potential danger of excessive carbonation and exploding bottles (see *Carbonation* in chapter 6). Ferment in the bottle for much shorter time periods, often just a day or two. I would recommend always bottling at least one bottle of such batches in a plastic soda bottle. Monitor the plastic bottle daily (or more frequently if it is particularly vigorous or warm) by squeezing to feel how pressurized it has become. Once it feels pressurized, after just a few days at typical indoor temperatures, refrigerate to slow fermentation and enjoy your beverage. Young ferments still carbonating in the bottle should be enjoyed quickly rather than stored for the future.

Mixed Source Legacy

The world of fermented alcoholic beverages clearly extends far beyond the typical choices of wine or beer. Our challenge is not simply to learn the techniques for replicating the most popular globalized forms of fermentation; instead, we must channel the ingenuity of our ancestors in identifying carbohydrate sources abundantly available to us and working with them. Fermented beverages need not be made from a single carbohydrate source. The 9,000-year-old alcohol remains identified on pottery from the Chinese archaeological site at Jiahu reveal a beverage fermented from the sugars of grapes and hawthorn fruits, honey, and rice.[42] Much of the evidence of early fermentation around the world suggests mixed carbohydrate and yeast sources, as do many surviving indigenous fermentation practices. Our agricultural and fermentation monocultures have yielded wonderful products, but alcohol can be fermented from any carbohydrate source. Resilience and versatility demand that we embrace our legacy of fermenting mixed carbohydrate sources as we reclaim fermentation as part of the broader revival of our formidable powers of creation through renewed regional food self-sufficiency.

Troubleshooting

Ferment never started bubbling

Stir, stir, stir. Stirring distributes and spreads yeast activity, and oxygenation stimulates yeast growth. If the only source of yeasts is the air (no raw ingredients), stirring incorporates yeasts landing on the surface. If your space is cool, fermentation will start and proceed more slowly. Seek a warmer microclimate in the house, if possible, or be patient and wait for warmer weather. Finally, check your water source. Water should be dechlorinated before use in fermentation; as described earlier, chlorine at sufficient concentrations will kill yeast. Filter water, boil it in an open vessel, or leave the water a couple of days for chlorine to evaporate before using. Check with your water system to see whether your tap water contains chloramines, new forms of chlorine that are not volatile and cannot be boiled or evaporated off.

Mold developed on the surface of your ferment

Gently skim the mold off surface. If this is not feasible, siphon from below the mold into another vessel, leaving the mold behind. In the early stages of a wild fermentation, it is imperative to stir frequently. Stirring disturbs the surface, and if it's done with enough frequency it makes it impossible for molds to develop. Usually mold is a sign of insufficient stirring.

Your ferment tastes like vinegar

Fermented alcoholic beverages exposed to air will inevitably turn into vinegar over time; acetic-acid-producing bacteria known as *Acetobacter* are present everywhere. These bacteria need oxygen in order to grow. In the earliest stages of fermentation, yeasts will always dominate in a sugary liquid. And during the most vigorous period of fermentation, even in an open vessel with a broad surface exposed to air, the constant release of carbon dioxide at the surface protects it from vinegar development. The potential for vinegar development comes later, as fermentation subsides. Drink beverages fermented in open vessels quickly, as fermentation subsides, or they turn into vinegar before long. If you intend to ferment all the sugars into alcohol, transfer to a narrow-necked jug or carboy, air-locked, to complete fermentation. If your ferment tastes like vinegar, somewhere along the line it was not effectively protected from prolonged air exposure.

Vinegar is not such a bad consolation prize. A delicacy in its own right, vinegar is great for condiments, pickling, salad dressings, marinades, and more. If your alcohol has gone partway to vinegar and you wish to coax it the rest of the way, transfer it to a vessel where it can spread out and expose a large surface area to air (with a cloth draped over to keep flies away). See *Vinegar* in chapter 6 for more information.

Fermentation stopped but the ferment is still sweet and not very alcoholic

This is known as "stuck" fermentation. Often racking—siphoning the ferment into another vessel, which aerates it—is adequate to restart fermentation (see *Siphons and Racking*, chapter 3). If the ferment has been in a cool spot, moving it to a warmer spot can often restart fermentation. Sometimes the addition of small amounts of acids (citrus or other fruit juice) or tannins (raisins, tea) can give yeast essential nutrients and stimulate yeast activity. All yeasts have maximum alcohol tolerances, limiting the potential of how much alcohol they can produce, and for some wild yeasts this tolerance may not be very high.

When should you transfer the ferment to an air-locked vessel?

It can be confusing deciding how long to ferment in an open vessel before transferring to an air-locked vessel, and how long to ferment in the air-locked vessel before bottling. An open vessel facilitates frequent stirring to get yeast active. Once yeast activity is vigorous, the ferment may be transferred to a narrow-necked, air-locked vessel. Generally, if there are botanical ingredients infusing into the ferment, they are strained out before transfer to an air-locked vessel. In this case, I'll usually let the ferment bubble with the botanicals for a few days before transferring.

Once air-locked, I'll leave the vessel ferment to ferment for at least a few months. When it appears that fermentation has stopped, it's time to siphon it into another vessel to try to restart stuck fermentation. If it never restarts, or if it bubbles for a while and then stops again, it is ready for bottling.

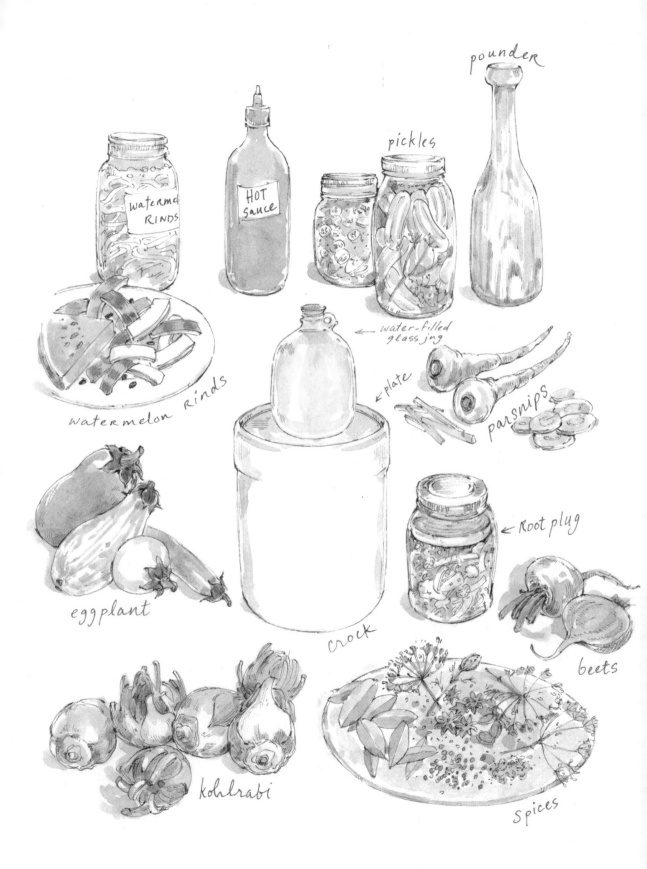

pounder

pickles

watermel RINDS

HOT sauce

← water-filled glass jug

← plate

parsnips

watermelon rinds

eggplant

crock

← Root plug

beets

kohlrabi

spices

CHAPTER 5

Fermenting Vegetables (and Some Fruits Too)

*T*here is an underlying unity to all vegetable fermentation: By keeping vegetables submerged under liquid, you create a selective environment where molds and other oxygen-dependent organisms cannot grow, thereby encouraging acidifying bacteria. Beyond this simple technique, in all the particulars of what, where, when, and how, approaches to vegetable fermentation can be quite varied and quirky. Some traditions wilt vegetables, either in saltwater brine or in the sun; others pound or bruise fresh vegetables. Some people ferment a single vegetable, while others mix a dozen different vegetables together, perhaps along with spices, fruit, fish, rice, mashed potatoes, or other additions. Some people ferment theirs for just a few days; others for weeks, months, or even years. Some ferment in sealed jars; others in open crocks; others in specially designed vessels. Some ferment in cellars or buried crocks; others on balconies or in garages; still others right on their kitchen counters. Some ferment in the protection of darkness; others directly in the sun. Most traditions work with the bacteria native to the vegetables; some add various starters. There is no single way of accomplishing this task that has been so widely interpreted in varied regions by different cultural traditions, and incorporated into infinite unique secret family recipes, passed down through the generations, with periodic adjustments and adaptations.

Fermenting vegetables is the ideal way to begin a fermentation practice in your life. It is very easy; it can be enjoyed fairly quickly; it is extremely nutritious and beneficial to health; it is delicious and a satisfying accompaniment to any meal; and it is intrinsically safe. Sometimes people are afraid to try fermentation for fear of accidentally getting the wrong bacteria growing and potentially sickening or even killing themselves and others. At least in the realm of raw plant materials, this fear is unfounded. "As far as I know, there has never been a documented case of food-borne illness from fermented vegetables," states Fred Breidt, a microbiologist for the

US Department of Agriculture who specializes in vegetable fermentation. "Risky is not a word I would use to describe vegetable fermentation. It is one of the oldest and safest technologies we have."[1]

In light of recent outbreaks of foodborne illnesses traced to spinach, lettuce, tomatoes, and other raw vegetables, I think it would be fair to say that fermented vegetables are *safer* than raw vegetables. For even given some freak incident of contamination, the incidental pathogenic bacteria could never compete with the native lactic acid bacteria populations, and the acidification that rapidly develops in fermenting vegetables would destroy any surviving pathogens. Lactic acid bacteria offer a strategy for safety and preservation that is present in all vegetation.

Some people are concerned about the safety of fermenting garlic because there have been reports of botulism from garlic preserved in olive oil. But preserving a vegetable in olive oil is very different from preserving the same vegetable under water or its own juices; specifically the environment becomes far more anaerobic. When garlic is preserved in brine or mixed with other vegetables, botulism is not a concern. If you wish to preserve garlic in olive oil, a simple step to ensure safety is to marinate the garlic in vinegar to acidify it first, thereby making it an inhospitable environment for *C. botulinum*, the bacteria that produces the botulism toxin.

Lactic Acid Bacteria

Lactic acid bacteria (LAB), most commonly *Leuconostoc mesenteroides*, are found on all plants, though in relatively low numbers, averaging below 1 percent of plants' microbial populations. "As soon as the plant is harvested, the number of microorganisms increases," according to a team of biologists. "This is a result of more nutrients becoming available from the cellular contents of ruptured tissue. Besides the increase in total number, the distribution among different types of microorganisms changes."[2] Aerobic bacteria dominant on the living plant are replaced by "facultative anaerobes," including various lactic acid bacteria, among them *L. mesenteroides*. If vegetables are submerged, *L. mesenteroides* initiates fermentation.

L. mesenteroides is described as *heterofermentative*, meaning that in addition to its primary product, lactic acid, it creates significant quantities of secondary products, including carbon dioxide, alcohol, and acetic acid. Homofermentative LAB are those producing nearly exclusively (at least 85 percent) lactic acid.[3] The homofermentative bacteria are more specialized and are better able to tolerate low pH (high acidity). The noticeably heavy CO_2 production in the earliest stages of vegetable fermentation is due to heterofermentative activity. As that activity acidifies the environment, the population shifts toward acid-tolerant homofermentative LAB, such as *Lactobacillus plantarum*, which characterize later stages of vegetable ferments.[4] "The success of the sauerkraut fermentation depends primarily upon the symbiotic relationships of the heterofermentative and homofermentative lactobacilli."[5]

A critical aspect of the action of lactic acid bacteria is its self-protection: "The lactic acid they produce is effective in inhibiting the growth of other bacteria that may decompose or spoil the food," according to the United Nations Food and Agriculture Organization report, *Fermented Fruits and Vegetables: A Global Perspective*.[6] This is why lactic acid fermentation is such an effective strategy for food preservation and safety. LAB are not found exclusively on plants. "The lactic acid bacteria are a diverse group of organisms with a diverse metabolic capacity," states the UN report. They are among the first bacteria newborn babies are exposed to in childbirth. Infants continue to have lactic acid bacteria exposure through breast-feeding. "Every person in the world has contact with lactic acid bacteria," state a team of microbiologists. "From birth, we are exposed to these species through our food and environment."[7] Given the constant assault on our intestinal bacteria by antibacterial chemicals (see *The War on Bacteria* in chapter 1), we need the *replenishment* of lactic acid bacteria populations and genetics that are present in fermented vegetables and other products of fermentation by lactic acid bacteria.

Vitamin C and Fermented Vegetables

The tradition of preserving vegetables by fermentation became so widespread because in temperate regions of the world, historically, there were no fresh vegetables available in winter. Fermentation of vegetables is primarily a strategy for extending the season by preserving vegetables for winter consumption. Vegetables contain critical nutrients, prime among them vitamin C; therefore a balanced winter diet is facilitated by fermentation. Chinese philosopher Confucius wrote, in the 6th century BC: "Having *yan-tsai* [salted vegetables], I can survive the winter."[8] Two millennia later, the British sailor Captain James Cook was famously credited with conquering scurvy (vitamin C deficiency) by bringing barrels of sauerkraut with him to sea and feeding it to his crews daily.

While the fermentation process does not contribute *additional* vitamin C (as it does with B vitamins, see *The Health Benefits of Fermented Foods* in chapter 2), it does *preserve* vitamin C by slowing down its loss. A 1938 study undertaken by the New York State Agricultural Experiment Station demonstrated that "the loss of vitamin C begins only after the fermentation process . . . has been completed and the production of carbon dioxide has practically ceased." The study concludes that the post-fermentation loss of vitamin C "is due more to a loss of the protective atmosphere of carbon dioxide than to any other factor."[9] Even if nutrients are not fully preserved forever, keeping more of them longer is valuable.

Kraut-Chi Basics

Kraut-chi is a word I made up, a hybrid of *sauerkraut* and *kimchi*, the German and Korean words for fermented vegetables that we have adopted into the English language. The English language does not have its own word for fermented vegetables. It would not be inaccurate to describe fermented vegetables as "pickled," but pickling covers much ground beyond fermentation. Pickles are anything preserved by acidity. Most contemporary pickles are not fermented at all; instead they rely upon highly acidic vinegar (a product of fermentation), usually heated in order to sterilize vegetables, preserving them by destroying rather than cultivating microorganisms. "For pickles, fermentation was the primary means of preservation until the 1940s, when direct acidification and pasteurization of cucumber pickles was introduced," writes Fred Breidt of the USDA.[10]

My vegetable ferments are usually concoctions that do not fit any homogeneous traditional ideal of either German sauerkraut or Korean kimchi. But of course, everything I've learned about sauerkraut and kimchi reveal that neither of them constitutes a homogeneous tradition. They are highly varied, from regional specialties to family secrets. Nonetheless, certain techniques underlie both (and many other related) traditions, and my practice is a rather free-form application of these basic techniques rather than an attempt to reproduce any particular notion of authenticity.

In a nutshell, the steps I typically follow when I ferment vegetables are:

1. Chop or grate vegetables.

2. Lightly salt the chopped veggies (add more as necessary to taste), and pound or squeeze until moist; alternatively, soak the veggies in a brine solution for a few hours.

3. Pack the vegetables into a jar or other vessel, tightly, so that they are forced below the liquid. Add water, if necessary.

4. Wait, taste frequently, and enjoy!

Of course there is more information and nuance, which the rest of this chapter explores, but really, "Chop, Salt, Pack, Wait" is what most of it amounts to.

Chop

Every rule has exceptions. Even though the basic kraut-chi process above starts with "Chop," it is not necessary to chop or grate vegetables in order to ferment them. If vegetables are to be fermented whole, or in big chunks, they are typically fermented in saltwater brine, buried in other chopped or grated salted vegetables, or in some other pickling medium. What chopping and grating do is create more surface area, which facilitates pulling juice out of the vegetables so they can be submerged under their own juices. That is our objective. Without exposing surface area, it is impossible to pull juices out of vegetables. The more finely chopped or grated they are—the more surface area is exposed—the faster and easier it is to pull water out of them, and the juicier the vegetables will be; but coarse chopping, or mixed textures, is good too. I usually tell people who help me chop veggies: "Chopper's choice." Be flexible when you can.

Salt: Dry-Salting Versus Brining

Like chopping, salt is not absolutely necessary for fermentation. Some traditions of fermenting vegetables, such as those of the Himalayas, mostly ferment vegetables without salt (see *Himalayan* Gundruk *and* Sinki, ahead). Some people believe (I do not) that vegetables fermented without salt contain more beneficial bacteria than those fermented with salt. And some people have been given a medical directive to avoid salt. Vegetables can be fermented without any salt. But with even a modest amount of salt, ferments generally taste better, maintain a more pleasing texture, and have the potential to ferment longer and more slowly.

Salt facilitates vegetable fermentation in a number of different ways:

- ◎ Salt pulls water out of the vegetables, through osmosis. This is part of getting the vegetables submerged under their own juices.

- ◎ It makes vegetables crispier by hardening plant cell compounds called pectins and keeps them crispy by slowing the action of pectin-digesting enzymes in vegetables that eventually make vegetables mushy.

- ◎ By creating a selective environment, salt narrows the range of which bacteria can grow, giving the salt-tolerant lactic acid bacteria a competitive advantage.

- ◎ Salt extends the potential for preservation by slowing the fermentation, slowing the pectin-digesting enzymes, and slowing development of surface molds.

Since fermented vegetables have been such a critically important food for survival in many cold temperate places, the fact that salt enhances preservation means that historically ferments have often been heavily salted. In some traditions, ferments have been salty enough to warrant soaking and rinsing before eating. The problem with this approach is that the soaking leaches not just salt but other nutrients as well.

I do not generally measure the salt when I ferment vegetables, although many people do. I salt lightly as I chop vegetables, then mix together, taste, and add more salt if necessary. It is always easier to add salt than to remove it. Salt can be diluted by adding more vegetables without salt, or by adding water. Excess water can be poured off, and with it salt will be removed.

There are two broad methods people use to salt vegetables for fermentation: dry-salting and brining. Dry-salting is simply sprinkling salt on vegetables. This is the method I use most often. Brining involves mixing salt with water—the mixture is the brine—and submerging vegetables in it. The dry-salting method requires that vegetables be chopped or shredded, for only with lots of surface area exposed can the salt pull water out of the vegetables. If vegetables are to be left whole, or in large pieces, the brine method is more appropriate. Some traditions use hybrid methods, such as submerging vegetables for a short wilting soak in a strong brine, or heavily dry-salting vegetables, leaving them to sweat, then rinsing them to remove excess salt. (More on brining to come.)

For the dry-salt method, commercial manufacturers typically work with salt proportions ranging from 1.5 percent to 2 percent by weight, or roughly 1.5 to 2 teaspoons of salt per pound/500 g of vegetables. In *Wild Fermentation*, I recommended 3 tablespoons of salt per 5 pounds/2.3 kg of vegetables. Many people have told me they found that to be too salty. Try less. Measuring salt by volume rather than weight is inexact, as different grinds of salt will yield very different weights for a given volume.

In considering how much salt to use in your fermented vegetables, it is helpful to understand the dynamics of salt in the fermentation environment. Salt essentially slows fermentation and enzyme activity and thereby prolongs preservation potential. Temperature also impacts upon the speed of fermentation, which is slower in cool temperatures and faster in warm temperatures. Therefore, in summer heat, I typically use more salt in order to slow down fermentation; in winter I use less. If I'm fermenting vegetables intending to preserve them for months, I use more salt; if I'm making a batch for an event next week, I use less.

Another aspect of salting vegetables for fermentation is what type of salt to use. Not all salts are the same (see *Salt* in chapter 3). I typically work with unrefined sea salts containing many trace minerals, made bioavailable by the fermentation. Some sources suggest avoiding iodized salts, which can darken vegetables and make brine cloudy. But really, you can ferment vegetables with whatever salt you have on hand. Having had the opportunity to ferment vegetables with every possible kind of salt handed to me by workshop organizers, I have observed that lactic acid bacteria seem tolerant to a wide variety of salts and are not particularly picky.

Pounding or Squeezing Vegetables (or Soaking in a Brine)

Once vegetables are chopped and salted (or not salted, if you prefer it that way), bruising them helps to further remove water, so that we can submerge them under their own juices. Cells function to hold water. Bruising the vegetables breaks down cell walls and facilitates the release of juices. At a small scale, up to say 5 gallons (20 liters), I find it easiest and most pleasant to do this by simply squeezing vegetables with my clean hands. I like working with my hands. (At my workshops, it's always easy to find enthusiastic volunteers for this job.) You can also pound vegetables with a clean heavy blunt tool: a baseball bat, a 2-by-4 board (make sure the wood is not pressure-treated!), or a specialized tool elegantly crafted for just this purpose (see *Pounding Tools* in chapter 3). At a large scale, people have often stomped on the vegetables with their feet. Squeeze, pound, or stomp until vegetables are dripping wet. Pick up a handful and squeeze, and vegetable juice should be expressed.

In the Asian tradition, rather than pounding as described above, people typically wilt vegetables by soaking them in brine for a time. This accomplishes the same objective in a different way, with less work but more time and more salt. Vegetables are soaked in salty brine for several hours or longer— just a few hours in a very salty brine, longer in a moderately salty mix—then drained before mixing with spices. See the *Kimchi* section for details on this method.

Pack

Once vegetables are nice and moist, through bruising or soaking, they can be further salted or spiced, if desired, and packed into vessels. (See chapter 3 for more discussion on different types of vessels.) Whether you seal them in a jar or ferment them in a crock, stuff vegetables into the vessel tightly so that air pockets are forced out and liquid rises, submerging the vegetables. If the vegetables are not fully submerged, press hard on them a few times to see if you can force a little more juice out. If you keep pressing, or leave the bruised vegetables under a weight for a few hours, more juice will come out. If the vegetables are not fully submerged by the next morning, or if at any point it seems that water has been lost (in an open crock due to evaporation), simply add a little dechlorinated water. Getting the vegetables submerged is the most critical factor for success in vegetable fermentation.

In the salty brine environment, the vegetables have a tendency to float, much like our bodies in the ocean. In a crock, people generally place a weight upon the vegetables to force them down and keep them submerged (see *Crock Method* in chapter 3). One method of accomplishing this in a jar is to cut a chunk of a root vegetable, or the heart of a cabbage, into the shape of a plug or a disk to place on the surface of the vegetables protruding just a bit from the mouth of the jar. Forcing the lid down and securing it will have the effect of pushing down the plug and the vegetables, keeping all but the plug itself submerged. Some people have fashioned small ceramic or glass weights for this; and a South African company is producing a plastic insert it calls the ViscoDisc to keep vegetables submerged in jars. If your weight or plug does not cover the entire surface, resulting in vegetables floating on the surface, don't worry. This is not a problem. If some vegetables on the surface begin to discolor from oxidation, or develop surface molds, simply remove and discard them.

If you are sealing your ferment in a jar, remember that the fermentation process will produce considerable CO_2, which will build pressure inside the jar. Brine may be forced out of the jar through the threads; jar tops may be contorted by the pressure seeking release; jars have even been known to explode. Release pressure daily in the first few days of fermentation, when CO_2

production will be greatest, by simply loosening the jar lid for a moment. After a few days, CO_2 will continue to be produced, but at a much slower rate.

How Long to Ferment?

Waiting is the hard part. Much of the contemporary literature assumes that we require immediate gratification and recommends fermenting vegetables only two or three days. Certainly, after two or three days the vegetables have begun to be transformed. Taste some at this point. But understand that this is not the full potential of fermented vegetables. Traditionally, fermentation has been a strategy for preserving vegetables for a season or longer. As the days and weeks pass, flavors meld, acidification increases, and textures change. Taste your developing ferment at frequent intervals. Try it at two weeks, and if you have any left, at two months.

I cannot tell you when your kraut-chi will be best. You will have to be the judge of that. Some people love the mild flavors and crunchy textures of an immature "green" ferment after just a few days. Others prefer the flavors of more mature, longer-aged versions. In warm weather or a heated environment, fermentation will proceed faster than in cooler temperatures. "Lower temperatures—at least under 70°F/21°C, preferably under 65°F/18°C, ideally 50–60°F/10–15°C, make for superior products," writes April McGreger, who ferments vegetables commercially in Carrboro, North Carolina, under the label Farmer's Daughter Brand. I've found that by compensating for warmer temperatures with shorter fermentation times, wonderful ferments are possible even at warmer ambient temperatures.

Steinkraus et al. report at length on the influence of temperature:

> At the low temperature of 7.5°C [45°F], fermentation is very slow. *L. mesenteroides* grows slowly attaining acidity of about 0.4% in about 10 days, and an acidity of 0.8 to 0.9% in a month. . . . The kraut may not be completely fermented for 6 months or more or until the temperature rises. . . . At a temperature of 18°C [65°F] with a salt concentration of 2.25%, a total acidity of 1.7 to 2.3% will be attained . . . in about 20 days. At higher temperatures, i.e., 23°C [73°F], the rate of fermentation will be greater so that a brine acidity of 1.0 to 1.5% may be attained in 8 to 10 days. . . . At a still higher temperature of 32°C [90°F] the rate of fermentation may be very rapid and an acidity of 1.8 to 2.0% may be attained in 8 to 10 days. . . . The flavor of the kraut will be inferior. . . . It will have a poorer shelf life.[11]

Salt also influences fermentation speed. I generally make ferments saltier in summer heat to slow down fermentation; less salty in winter.

Some people approach the question of readiness in a strictly utilitarian manner, asking: When is the ferment healthiest? Or: When does it contain the highest number of bacteria? My general impression from reading is that the numbers and concentration of lactic acid bacteria in a vegetable ferment typically follow a bell curve: Populations grow after vegetables are submerged, build to a peak, then decline at high levels of acidity. In addition to the numbers fluctuating, the types of lactic acid bacteria shift as the fermentation proceeds. Rather than thinking about an optimal time to maximize benefit, I believe it makes sense to eat fermenting vegetables at intervals throughout their process, as a way of diversifying our bacterial exposure.

Whenever you judge your batch of kraut-chi to be ready, moving it to the refrigerator will slow its continued fermentation to an imperceptible pace. Similarly, in a cool spot, such as a 55°F/13°C cellar, vegetables that have been salted and acidified by fermentation can be stable for years. Visiting the Flack Family Farm in northern Vermont, I was treated to delicious still-crunchy three-year-old kimchi from a barrel in the cellar. Ferments can also last for years hidden in the back of the refrigerator.

In warmer temperatures, fermented vegetables are not quite as stable, because eventually pectin-digesting enzymes will activate, making the ferment lose its texture and get mushy. Fermentation enthusiast Hyla Bolsta reflects, "Sometimes a good thing needs to be eaten and finished because it doesn't stay crisp forever, just as in our lives, sometimes we have to do it now, because if we wait, things can get mushy, murky, slimy, etc." Personally, I'm not crazy about fermented vegetables after they get mushy, but some people prefer them that way. I've met several Austrian people who have expressed a preference for soft kraut, and Vickie Phelps wrote to tell me that her partner's dental work makes it impossible for him to eat crunchy vegetables and so he likes when the ferments get soft. If you desire the ferment to go soft quickly, use little salt and ferment in a warm spot.

I ferment vegetables in a barrel in the cellar for six months every year, put up in November and eaten through the winter and spring. But by July, with hot summer temperatures, the vegetables lose their crunchiness and get mushy. Vegetables can be fermented deliciously in the tropics or in a heat wave, but they develop fast and don't last for long. The elegance of this is that fermentation preserves vegetables longest in precisely the places where the growing season is shortest and preserved vegetables are most important.

Many people like to can their sauerkraut to preserve it after fermentation. This can be done, but at the sacrifice of live-culture benefits.

 ## Surface Molds and Yeasts

The technique of submerging vegetables is a strategy for encouraging the growth of lactic acid bacteria by protecting the vegetables from oxygen, the presence of which promotes the growth of fungi, including both molds and yeasts. An inevitable aspect of this technique is the edge, where (in an open vessel) the surface of the liquid under which the vegetables are submerged typically comes into contact with oxygen-rich air. The meeting at this boundary of the nutritious vegetable juices and the air encourages a rich biodiversity, where molds and yeasts frequently develop. Surface growth is common and normal; it should be removed, but it is not cause for alarm and it does not ruin your fermenting vegetables.

The aerobic yeasts that develop are distinct from the molds, though a surface layer of yeast can become a layer of mold. The yeast layer that frequently develops on the surface of fermenting vegetables is known as Kahm yeast. *The Life of Yeasts* describes:

> During the lactic acid fermentation . . . a characteristic fermentative yeast flora develops in the liquid. . . . When the sugar is used up and the pH has dropped because of lactic acid production by the lactic acid bacteria, a secondary, oxidative yeast flora develops on the surface of the liquid in the form of a thick, folded layer of yeast.[12]

The Kahm yeast layer is beige in color, with a dramatic texture, something like waves or a plate of spaghetti. Mold typically develops as a white film at first. It is not important to be able to distinguish between Kahm yeasts and molds. Surface discoloration can be caused by simple oxidation as well. Any growth or discoloration that develops on the surface of your fermenting vegetables should be removed.

To get rid of surface growth, gently remove weight from the ferment. Use a wide stainless-steel spoon to get under the mold, and skim it off as best you can. Depending on how wet or dry the ferment is, you may need to remove the plate or interior lid in order to skim growth off. Sometimes it is not possible to remove all the mold, because as you attempt to remove it, the mold dissipates and little bits are left remaining. If this happens, remove most of it, as much as you can, and don't worry. As long as the mold is white it is not harmful. If other color molds start to grow, do not eat them. Bright colors often indicate sporulation, the molds' reproductive stage. To prevent spreading the spores, gently lift the entire mold mass from your ferment. Fortunately, the occasional colorful molds I have encountered (always preceded by white molds) were cohesive and easily removed in their entirety.

The longer you allow a mold to grow on the surface of your ferment, the deeper its mycelia penetrate. Molds can digest pectins, leading to mushy vegetables. Eventually, the vegetables can come to taste like mold. Molds can also digest lactic acid, lowering the acidity of the ferment that enables it to be effectively preserved.

Remove mold or other surface growth, as best you can, as soon as you notice it. After removing mold, evaluate the texture of the underlying vegetables. If the vegetables near the surface have been softened by mold growth, remove and discard.

Some people like to use outer cabbage leaves as a barrier between the shredded vegetables and the surface. In a jar, simply fold a leaf to fit. In a larger vessel, most people who do

watermelon rinds

this arrange leaves in an overlapping circle or spiral. Fermentation enthusiast Lisa Milton wrote describing another technique:

> I use the outside cabbage leaves that I would normally compost; wash them thoroughly and roll them up very tightly to a cigar shape. Then I place them side by side on top of the veggie mixture. When the veggies are nice and fermented, I remove the rolled up cabbage leaves and toss them. Often times I will find mold growing on top of the cabbage but the veggies are not affected at all.

Another strategy some people use to protect the surface of the ferment from air exposure is covering it with a layer of olive oil.

The most effective way to avoid surface growths is to protect the surface of the ferment from exposure to air. People do this with heavy plastic bags filled with water or brine that can spread to cover the full surface of a vessel; or with specially designed crocks or jar lids. See *Crock Lids* and *Different Crock Designs* in chapter 3 for a full discussion. If you are fermenting in an open vessel, be aware that water can evaporate, especially in a dry climate or a heated space. Check fluid levels periodically and add water as necessary. If you peel mold off a dry top layer of vegetables, you may need to also compost the top layer of vegetables. Remove any vegetables that seem dry or discolored. Keep veggies submerged!

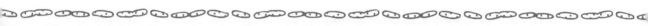

IT GETS BETTER

Luke Regulbuto and Maggie Levinger make and sell fermented vegetables in Northern California under the label "Wild West Ferments."

We often hear stories of people throwing away whole batches, because it smells or looks bad at first sight. We have found beautiful kraut under a moldy maggot-infested top layer—it was delicious. People should know that an offensive odor often decreases and sometimes even disappears once a crock is packed into jars and refrigerated.

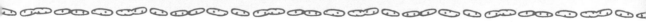

 ## Which Vegetables Can Be Fermented?

Shredded cabbage is certainly not the whole story. The simple process of vegetable fermentation is extremely versatile; there is no vegetable that cannot be fermented. That is not to say that all vegetables will ferment equally well, or that all vegetables will taste good fermented. Some vegetables get mushy faster than others during fermentation (cucumbers, summer squash); these vegetables I only use in small batches that I eat quickly rather than aging them. Dark green leafy vegetables rich in chlorophyll (kale, collards, and other greens) will develop a very strong characteristic flavor during fermentation, which you may or may not like. Anneke Dunnington, of southern coastal Oregon, writes, "I personally am terrified of what happens when I try to ferment kale . . . every time it ends up smelling like the worst dead thing I have ever smelled." I limit dark greens to minor ingredients in mixed vegetable ferments. In that context I find them to be delicious; when they stand alone their flavor is too strong for me. Rick Chumley, of Tennessee, writes that his favorite batch mixed half kale and half cabbage into "Supergreen Sauerkraut."

The most popular vegetables to ferment for long storage are cold-weather vegetables that are harvested late in the season as temperatures are cooling, such as cabbages or radishes. The significance of cool temperatures is that they facilitate a slow fermentation and long storage. Vegetables harvested and fermented in summer heat tend to ferment fast and do not lend themselves as well to long-term storage.

Personally, I especially love to ferment root vegetables, including radishes, carrots, turnips, beets, parsnips, rutabaga, celery root, parsley root, and earthy burdock. A large proportion of beets, being so sugary, can encourage a yeasty fermentation, and produce thick, syrupy brine. But Marcee King writes, "I love fermented beets with horseradish, onion, garlic, and dill." Typically I scrub but do not peel root vegetables. The stems of leafy vegetables, such as chard and bok choi, often discarded during preparation, also ferment well. Celery does too. If you enjoy okra, try fermenting some. I usually use okra whole, mixing them with shredded vegetables. That way their sliminess remains mostly enclosed within them, so the people (like me) who enjoy that can, while others can simply avoid the okra. If you chop the okra with other vegetables, the whole batch can take on okra's slime (yum).

All kinds of peppers ferment well: sweet or hot, fresh or dried, smoked or roasted (more on peppers in hot sauce later). So do eggplants. Some people salt and drain the eggplants first; personally, I have found that the bitterness of the eggplants is removed by fermentation. People ferment tomatoes, green and red; brined green tomatoes, which can get very sour, are a Jewish delicatessen staple. In addition to all varieties of cabbages, brussels sprouts, cauliflower, kohlrabi, broccoli, and other *Brassica* vegetables ferment beautifully. So do other greens, such as chard (especially their stalks), as do fresh green, yellow, or purple beans. I've enjoyed fermented fiddlehead ferns, bamboo shoots, pumpkins and winter squash, *nopales* (cactus pads), and shiitake and other mushrooms. My friend Nuri E. Amazon writes that spaghetti squash in a brine with lots of garlic is "one of the best ferments ever." Brined watermelon rinds rival cucumbers as sour pickles in both flavor and texture. Corn too can be fermented as a vegetable.

parsnips

Dawn Beeley wrote from Italy about her experiences fermenting artichokes. "I only used the hearts and sliced them very thinly . . . they turned out great . . . even my 13 month old and four year old ate them." Jerusalem artichokes, no relation but rather delicious, earthy, starchy tubers (*Helianthus tuberosus*), sometimes known as sunchokes, also ferment beautifully, and the fermentation digests the inulin (a long-chain carbohydrate) in them that can give people gas (though inulin is considered "prebiotic" because it feeds our intestinal bacteria so well, hence the gas). The biggest challenge with using Jerusalem artichokes is cleaning their knobby nooks and crannies. "I find it helps to break them apart as much as possible and then blast them with a hose for a couple rinses," advises Anneke Dunnington.

You need not limit yourself to cultivated vegetables. Lagusta Yearwood (and others) rave about fermenting wild spring ramps (otherwise known as wild leeks, or, in the UK, as ramson). "Ramps, with their funky potency, are ideally matched with the fermentation process—those magical bacteria simultaneously tame and heighten the bright *umami* richness of those beautiful wild greens." "Eat something wild every day" was the advice of my friend Frank Cook as he encouraged people to get to know and interact with common plants around them. I try to visit the garden every day to "graze" on weeds as well as vegetables. While I'm not always sure where the weeds end and the wild edibles start, sometimes I incorporate them into my ferments, though typically as minor elements.

In Eastern Europe, an umbelliferous weed known as *barszcz* in Slavic languages (*Heracleum* spp.) has historically been fermented and used in soups, giving us the soup called borscht in English, now typically made with beets. Leda Meredith, author of *The Locavore's Handbook*, writes in an email: "I like mixing in foraged ingredients such as garlic mustard seed, spicebush berries, and wild ginger." Finnish fermentation enthusiast Ossi Kakko describes ferments featuring stinging nettles, whole dandelion flowers, dandelion leaves, plantain leaves, and lamb's-quarters. "Some more bitter leaves can turn mild through fermentation," he observes. Maria Tarantino, an Italian fermentation experimentalist who lives in Belgium, elaborates that "very bitter leaves generally release a bouquet of flavors in the fermenting crock, as if the bitterness opens up to more subtle components." Of the wild herbs she has tried, "so far the most amazing was wild sea fennel (in Italian *critmo*), a cactus-like plant that grows on the rocks at the seaside and which is already slightly salted. The flowers are very bitter but if you wait long enough the hard edge softens. Another favorite is *egopode* [*Aegopodium podagraria*, known in English as ground-elder, goutweed, or snow-in-the-mountain], a plant that has celery-like stems that are perfumed and exotic."

Seaweed is a delicious mineral-rich ingredient to add to ferments. I prepare seaweed by covering it with just a little water and squeezing it with my hands. After a few minutes the seaweed hydrates and becomes soft and pliable. I chop the hydrated seaweed and add it, along with any extra juice, to other vegetables. Kraut maker Elizabeth Hopkins suggests using kelp or other green seaweeds rather than reddish dulse. "Dulse completely disintegrated and turned my otherwise palatable ferment into a brown sewage-looking mess," she writes. "Should have definitely used kelp."

Fruits can be another exciting addition. Eastern European traditions often add apples, raisins, or cranberries to sauerkraut. You could also add hints of citrus fruits or juice. Or other fruits: berries, pineapples, plums. Luke Regalbuto, a California kraut maker, reports: "Dried fruit in kraut, for example dried blueberries, hold up much better in the crock than fresh ones." Greg Olma adds quinces to his sauerkraut: "Every 5 lbs., I add the pickling salt, about a cup of sliced and cleaned quinces with a pinch of coriander seed, a few whole cloves, some black peppercorns, a few allspice berries, and a pinch of fennel and anise seeds." I love to add seasonal berries, and shredded green papaya when it comes my way, to vegetable ferments. Nuts too can embellish fermented vegetables; I especially like the textural variation they contribute.

In the Korean tradition, fish are often added to vegetables in the preparation of kimchi. Raw small fresh or dried fish, shrimp, oysters, and other fish are added, as well as fermented fish sauce. The raw fish transforms during acidification; in the fermented kimchi, as in citrus-cured *ceviche*, the fish develops the appearance and texture of cooked fish. In some inland regions of Korea, meat and meat stock are also used in kimchi.

Fresh vegetables can be supplemented with mung or other bean sprouts, rice or other cooked grains, potatoes steamed, mashed, or fried, and other cooked ingredients. I tried a delicious edamame kimchi with steamed green edamame (a type of soybean, served in the pod) among the more commonly found vegetables. I've thrown the crusty remains of fried potatoes into kraut with very pleasing results. A friend of mine even added peeled hard-boiled eggs to a mixed vegetable ferment, and after absorbing red from beets, they were not only tasty but beautiful. When incorporating cooked foods, cool to body temperature before adding. And because cooked foods generally do not contain significant lactic acid bacteria, they are rarely fermented alone, without some sort of raw ingredient for culturing. Still, as a minor element in a mostly raw mix, they work fine.

kohlrabi

You can ferment vegetables past their prime and beginning to soften or wilt. If there is any mold on the surface, cut it away and discard. Fermenting is not the same as rotting. Be judicious. The worst kraut I ever made was from a box of pre-shredded cabbage, carrots, and onions from Kentucky Fried Chicken, intended for coleslaw. My friend MaxZine, a dedicated food rescuer, obtained several such boxes from a local food bank's distribution and gave me one. The veggies were not rotted at all, but I suspect that they must have been sprayed with some kind of preservative chemical, because the fermentation appeared not to proceed at all, and it tasted awful. Nonetheless, fermentation is a great strategy for Dumpster divers, gleaners, and others who find themselves with abundant supplies of vegetables others have rejected.

In general, I would advise against adding additional ingredients to a batch of kraut-chi that has been fermenting for a while. The older vegetables can begin to soften just as the newly added vegetables are developing their flavor. If you have a fresh supply of vegetables, start a fresh batch. It's fine to have several batches at different stages of development fermenting simultaneously.

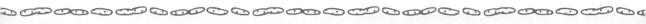

NORTHEAST KINGDOM KRAUT-CHI

Justin Lander, East Hardwick, Vermont, in the Northeast Kingdom

After a few years of experimenting with kitchen sink mixed vegetable ferments (known as MVF in our house), I decided to try to make a regionally appropriate Northeast Kingdom Kimchi. The main inspiration for the recipe came while working in a friend's sugar bush [another name for maple forest], where at the end of sugaring season ramps grow abundantly. Mixed in the ramps there are large patches of wild ginger. These two ingredients are the base. Then I add dandelion greens and roots, burdock root, salt, and sometimes dried hot pepper from the previous year. I let it ferment for several weeks. The exciting thing about this stuff is that it comes out sweet and perfumey. It's almost a dessert kraut.

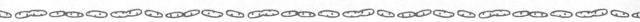

Spicing

The spicing of fermented vegetables is similarly versatile. Vegetables can be fermented unadulterated, mildly spiced, or as strong as you can take it. Kimchi is typically spiced with hot peppers, ginger, garlic, and onions, scallions, shallots, or leeks. Often the hot pepper is added in the form of powder or flakes, though it can also be used fresh, dried, or as hot sauce. German tradition often spices sauerkraut with juniper berries. Caraway, dill, and celery seeds are other popular sauerkraut herbs. In El Salvador, *curtido* is spiced with oregano and hot pepper.

Functionally, most of the traditional spices used in fermentation, mentioned above, act as mold inhibitors. This does not mean that molds cannot ever grow in their presence, just that they slow mold growth. If two open crocks are placed side by side in the same environment, with the same vegetables and the same salinity, differing only in the addition of spices to one, the spiced batch will always be slower to develop surface molds than the plain unspiced batch. Another mold inhibitor and spicy ferment ingredient is nasturtium leaves.

Feel free to depart from tradition. Turmeric adds a great flavor and color, as well as antioxidant, antiviral, and other medicinal qualities, to fermenting vegetables. Cumin is lovely in a ferment, as is lightly toasted oregano. People have written to me citing black pepper, coriander, fennel, fenugreek, and mustard seeds as favorites. Some of the flavors of fresh herbs tend to be somewhat volatile, so they may not persist over the period of a long fermentation, but in shorter ferments they can be delicious, and it can't hurt to try.

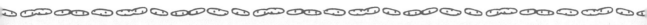

FERMENTED HERB MIX

Monique Trahan lives in western Massachusetts on a "farmlet" with gardens, dairy goats, chickens, and pastured pigs, "within sight of the biggest shopping center in town."

I make fresh herb salad dressing mix in late summer and fall and use it all winter. I use whatever is growing in abundance, but my favorite is mostly basil, lots of oregano, parsley, scallions/chives, garlic, and a bit of hot pepper. Chop/mince (I use the chopping blade on my food processer), add brine (salty is good with this as it is used as a flavoring ingredient), and ferment at room temperature for three days or so. Then move it to the fridge for storage (although we are building a root cellar this year). It is so easy to plop a spoonful into a cruet with vinegar and olive oil for a quick dressing, or into some drained kefir for a creamy dressing or dip. It can also go into soups and such for a very quick jolt of summer. I call it "Seasons of Refreshing," and it is a hit with guests.

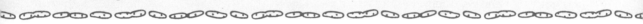

Sauerkraut

The best-known style of fermented vegetables in the United States and much of Europe is sauerkraut. Sauerkraut consists primarily of shredded cabbage and salt. Often the shredded cabbage is spiced with juniper berries or caraway seeds. In some traditions, fruits such as apples or cranberries are added. I met a woman whose grandmother was from a town in Poland where everyone added mashed potatoes to their sauerkraut. The potatoes take on the flavor of the sauerkraut and lend it a distinctive varied texture. (Be sure to cool the mashed potatoes before adding.) I often mix red cabbage with the white cabbage to yield bright pink kraut. It is actually quite possible to add many varied minor ingredients while still maintaining the essential qualities of sauerkraut by making sure it is made mostly from shredded cabbage. The process is the generic kraut-chi method, with dry-salting.

One iconic sauerkraut is the Bavarian style, in which the sauerkraut is made with caraway seeds and served sweet, typically mixed with sugar and warmed before serving. Another traditional German sauerkraut variation is *weinkraut*, made with the addition of sweet white wine. "What a miracle that turned out to be," recounts Judith Orth, of New Hampshire. "The fermentation process transformed a lousy wine into a lovely subtle elusive flavor . . . everyone's favorite batch by far."

Many traditions of kraut making (and fermentation more broadly) use the phases of the moon to determine the best time to prepare it. A woman who lives near me in Readyville, Tennessee, shared with me her grandmother Ruby Ready's sauerkraut recipe. "The secret, of course, is to make it in the light of the moon—while the moon is growing—and that way it will never shrink or get dark." Folklore traditions being widely varied, I have also encountered conflicting advice, suggesting that the best time to make sauerkraut is when the moon is waning.[13] To be honest, I have made sauerkraut throughout the moon's phases and have never observed any differences based on that.

The techniques of sauerkraut have already been covered. I have been struck through the years by the number of stories people have shared about the significance of sauerkraut in their lives. For instance, Lorissa Byely of Indianapolis, Indiana, writes:

> My parents were born and grew up in Russia. I learned from my dad that after WWII, he (age 8) and his family literally survived on sauerkraut and potatoes for a year. There really was no other food and he is still healthy today at 70 (and still loves sauerkraut).

Christina Haverl Tamburro, of Andover, Connecticut, reports that "One of my great-grandmothers, who came to Bridgeport in 1908, was so kraut obsessed that a cabbage cutter was the only thing she brought with her to this country, besides a few clothes in a sack. My great aunt is still using the cutter." Many barns, basements, and attics hold similar old kraut shredding boards, and crocks, which were so vitally important to people's lives in the past but have fallen into disuse. Find them, clean them up, and put them back to work!

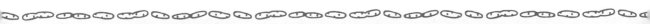

THE CASE OF THE KRAUT CALLED HOOCH

My friend D spent some time in a federal prison. D likes to eat well and decided to try to make sauerkraut. She did it by rinsing off the prison coleslaw, salting it, and weighing it down with an orange. Unfortunately, when it was discovered by guards, they accused her of trying to make "hooch." Her mother wrote to me: "They immediately confiscated it, tested and analyzed it for content and scent (the preliminary 'breath test' registered nothing), but, still determined she was absolutely making hooch with illegal contraband, they wrote her up, required her to submit a written statement explaining herself, and charged with her with making liquor." At the hearing, "D clearly presented her facts and intention and they understood her to be truthful, especially after reviewing all her previous dietary requests. Her charges were changed from a major to a minor offense (nothing to darken her prison record) and D was sentenced to 1 day of segregation." D has long since been released and can ferment to her heart's content (and her belly's) at home.

Kimchi

Kimchi is the iconic food of Korean culture. "I cannot think of a single food from any other country that is half as important to a nation's culinary traditions as kimchi is to Korea's," writes Mei Chin in *Saveur*.[14] A major South Korean newspaper called the 2010 failure of the cabbage crop there, and the resulting kimchi shortage, "a national tragedy."[15] When the country sent its first astronaut to the International Space Station in 2008, he traveled there with a specially developed kimchi. "Three top government research institutes spent millions of dollars and several years perfecting a version of kimchi that would not turn dangerous when exposed to cosmic rays or other forms of radiation and would not put off non-Korean astronauts with its pungency," reports *The New York Times*.[16] Scientists feared that in space, radiation could cause dangerous mutations to the bacteria that inhabit kimchi, which are so beneficial on Earth. "The key was how to make a bacteria-free kimchi while retaining its unique taste, color and texture," according to Lee Ju-woon of the Korean Atomic Energy Research Institute. Meanwhile here on Earth, those bacteria and their metabolic products have been credited with curing the avian flu.[17]

I have received a steady trickle of email since the publication of *Wild Fermentation* from people frustrated that my recipes did not produce a kimchi they regarded as authentic. "Kimchi is so hard!" writes Elizabeth Hopkins. "I've tried at least four times and have never got a romping, spicy, fizzy, truly-kimchi-tasting ferment. I've followed your recipe in *WF*, and while it was a tasty jarful, it was certainly not kimchi." Never having visited Korea, my personal knowledge of kimchi is fairly limited, but one of the lessons I have learned is that kimchi is made in a mind-boggling variety of styles. In her excellent cookbook *Growing Up in a Korean Kitchen*, Hi Soo Shin Hepinstall describes some of that variety:

> Korean kitchens create more than one hundred kinds of kimchi, using everything from cabbage to watermelon skin and even pumpkin blossoms in summer. Each family's kimchi has its own unique flavor, but the basic process is to salt the vegetable, firming it up by extracting its liquid, locking in the original flavor. A mixture of spices is then introduced and the vegetable is fermented, creating its distinctive character. The most important spices are fresh and powdered hot red peppers, which give the kimchi its biting zest and help seal in its freshness, and crushed garlic and green onions, which enhance its flavor and help to sterilize it. Additional flavor-builders may include ginger, fruits, nuts, and seafood such as salted shrimp and anchovies, fresh oysters, pollack, yellow corvina, skate, and live baby shrimp, or even octopus and squid. Green seaweed, chŏnggak, may be added to help retain freshness; in the mountainous region of the northern provinces, where seafood is not available, beef broth is used instead.[18]

In *Saveur*, Mei Chin waxes:

I have tasted subtly flavored kimchis made from mushrooms or burdock root, light and crunchy ones made with soybean sprouts, meaty ones made with tender chunks of pumpkin, and luxurious ones made with young octopus. Kimchi can be mild, like tongchimi, or water kimchi, a combination of ingredients like cabbage, Asian pear, pine nuts, whole chiles, and pomegranate seeds floating in a tangy brine. It can also be eaten before it is allowed to ferment, as with geotjeoli, or "salad," kimchi, which consists of raw leaves of cabbage dressed with kimchi fixings, a kind of coleslaw that heats the belly as it cools the throat. In all of these forms, kimchi is curiously refreshing, not just because of its heat, which shoots straight to the brain, but also because it effervesces on the tongue. Kimchi serves the same purpose in a Korean meal that palate cleansers serve in a Western one: when you are tired of eating, you take a bite of it, your eyes and mouth water, and you have the energy to begin eating again.[19]

"Wow, there are just *so* many," effuses Chris Calentine, an email pen pal of mine from Indiana who married into a Korean family, when I ask about varieties of kimchi he has encountered.

Although kimchi is made in diverse styles and with varied ingredients, there are some common patterns. Kimchi recipes typically call for pre-soaking vegetables in salty brine (3 to 6 hours in a brine of 15 percent salt by weight, or 12 hours in a 5 to 7 percent salt brine[20]). Often, vegetables are turned or stirred a few times during their soak. Alternatively, chopped vegetables may be dry-salted, fairly heavily, and left to sweat a few hours, turned, mixed, and agitated; followed by a thorough rinse to remove excess salt. *The Kimchee Cookbook*, the most comprehensive book on the topic that I have found, explains:

Salting is a process that allows the seasoning to penetrate the food gradually. Today, salting is done in one day; in the past, it took place over a period of three, five, seven, or even nine days. The vegetables were moved from container to container of salted water, each with a brine solution of a different strength. It was considered that the longer the process took and the slower the salt was absorbed, the deeper the taste of the kimchee.[21]

Another feature that distinguishes kimchi recipes is the use of hot pepper in dried flake or powder form. Furthermore, pepper and pureed ginger, garlic, onion, and any other spices are typically mixed with a starchy base into a paste. The starchy base—like thin porridge or gruel—is a mixture of flour (usually rice flour, but wheat or other flours work fine) and water, mixed together cold at a proportion of around 1:8, or 1 cup water to 2 tablespoons flour, then gently heated and simmered for a few minutes, with constant stirring, until the liquid begins to thicken. You could also soak rice (or oats or other grains) and cook with extra water into a thin *congee*. After cooling rice paste to body temperature, add pepper flakes and pureed garlic-ginger-onions. Mix thoroughly. Taste and adjust the seasoning as desired. Then mix the sauce with rinsed vegetables. After the ingredients are well mixed, taste and add salt or other seasonings as desired. Taste and adjust again after a day or two.

While kimchi may be extremely spicy, it is also made in varieties with little or no spice. "Not all kimchi is hot," writes Chris Calentine. "Many varieties, called *mul* or water kimchi, have no hot peppers, or very little." Echo Kim emailed to tell me about her "white" kimchi, with lots of radishes and no hot pepper at all in the starchy base. "It's considered a cooling summer kimchi, it's sweet." Of course, every rule may be broken. "My mom puts in a little red pepper flakes so that it has a zesty tang and it turns a light milky pink. That's her special touch/flair."

A further quality characterizing many popular styles of kimchi is limited acidity. This requires a shorter fermentation time and/or fermentation in a cooler spot. "Tests show that the best taste is attained after 3 days of fermentation at 20°C [68°F] with 3 percent salt," report a team of Korean academics. In the succession of organisms that characterize vegetable ferments from the early-stage *Leuconostoc mesenteroides* to the later, more acid-tolerant *Lactobacillus plantarum* (see *Lactic Acid Bacteria* earlier in this chapter), kimchi is typically associated with the early-stage activity. "The data indicate that *L. mesenteroides* is the important microorganism responsible for kimchi fermentation, whereas *Lactobacillus plantarum*, which is considered to be responsible for making sauerkraut, deteriorates the quality of kimchi."[22]

The fizziness associated with some kimchis is a result of heavy carbon dioxide production in the early stages of fermentation. As the environment becomes more acidic, continued fermentation produces less CO_2. A good way to get a fizzy kimchi is to ferment it in jars for one to three days at room temperature; then seal the jars and store in the refrigerator for a couple of weeks, where fermentation continues slowly and the kimchi accumulates trapped CO_2, resulting in effervescent release when the jars are opened.

Chinese Pickling

Kimchi, sauerkraut, and most other styles of fermented vegetables are widely recognized as having been inspired by practices that originated in China, where diverse traditions of vegetable fermentation continue. In that vast nation, each province is associated with specific vegetable ferments. Some of the styles call for starters, including *chiang*, similar to Japanese miso, and *qu*, the Chinese mixed fungal and bacterial culture essential to rice beverages and many other ferments (see chapter 10, *Growing Mold Cultures*). Some styles are dry-salted, while others are fermented in brine. Some vegetable ferments use thin rice gruel (*congee*) as a medium, or add starchy water that has been used to wash rice.[23]

China has an incredible array of specific regional styles, of which I know very little. The most descriptive information I've found in English comes from the writings of an English woman, Fuchsia Dunlop, who studies Chinese cuisine. In her book on Sichuan cuisine, *Land of Plenty*, Dunlop writes:

Pickled vegetables are fundamental to the spirit of Sichuan cooking. Every household has its *pao cai tan zi*—a rough earthenware pot with a rounded belly and narrow neck, and a lip that functions as a water seal. In the darkness within, crunchy vegetables soak in a pool of brine, with a splash of rice wine and a selection of flavorings that probably include brown sugar, Sichuan pepper, and ginger, with a few pieces of cinnamon stick, cassia bark, and star anise. The vegetables come and go, replenished every day or two with fresh supplies, but the pickling brine, or mother liquor, goes on, they say, forever. With each new batch of vegetables, a little salt and wine is added, and the spices and sugar are renewed from time to time But the rich, aromatic liquid base goes from strength to strength as the years, or even generations, pass. . . . Sichuan pickles are often used in cooking, but they are also eaten with rice porridge for breakfast and as a refreshing palate cleanser at the end of almost every other meal.[24]

From a paper Dunlop presented at a conference we both attended, I learned about an amaranth stalk ferment from the city of Shaoxing, which I was inspired to try with the gorgeous red amaranth that has naturalized in my garden.

The stalks are gathered when they are more than a metre tall, and their twigs, leaves and woody bases are discarded, leaving an even, green central section that is then cut into pieces a couple of inches long. After washing, these pieces are soaked for a day or so in cold water, until the water becomes frothy, and then washed again and shaken dry. They are then sealed into a clay jar (known locally as a *beng* 鬏) and left in a warm place to ferment. There's an art to timing the fermentation: if it is insufficient, the stalks will be too hard to eat; if it is too advanced, the pulp and skin of the stalks simply dissolves away, leaving nothing but fibrous tubes in a filthy liquid. After a few days (the precise time depending on the ambient temperature), the stalks will have softened and a 'special fragrance' will be detectable at the mouth of the jar. At this point, saltwater is added, and the stalks sealed into their jar for another couple of days, by which time they are ready to eat.

I used a glass jar. And the amaranth stalks were delicious, not much different in flavor from my beloved sour pickles, only more miraculous in being made from a part of a plant typically discarded as inedible. In addition to turning an otherwise inedible stalk into a tasty fermented delicacy, the brine produced by fermenting amaranth stalks (*lu*) can be used as a medium for fermenting other things, including pumpkin, other vegetables, and tofu (see *Fermenting Tofu* in chapter 11). Dunlop explains the importance of fermented vegetables in the region: "Many of the origin myths of Shaoxing's fermented delicacies tell tales of extreme poverty, and of the accidental discovery of ways of using fermentation to make spoiled, inedible or overlooked odds and ends of produce taste striking and delicious."[25]

I wish I knew more and could provide more than a cursory glimpse of the broad, dynamic, and living tradition of Chinese vegetable fermentation, which spawned all the other styles I know better. What an extraordinary gift to human culture! The diversity of the Chinese traditions has been a source of inspiration to many distinct cultural traditions and serves to reaffirm the extraordinary adaptability and applicability of the simple idea of storing vegetables under liquid to promote the growth of lactic acid bacteria.

Indian Pickling

Indian pickling, which of course is not a singular unified tradition at all, has a couple of unusual distinguishing features. One is the use of oils, including mustard oil, sesame oil, and others, depending upon the region; another is the tradition of fermenting the pickles outside under direct sunlight. At least in the case of mustard oil, the oil is thought to inhibit the growth of certain yeasts, molds, and bacteria, thereby helping to establish a selective environment for fermentation and effective preservation and safety. To use mustard oil, heat it until it starts to smoke, then allow it to cool before adding to vegetables, in order to burn off some of the component erucic acid and reduce the oil's pungency.[26] Many contemporary Indian pickle recipes use vinegar rather than fermentation, but a search through recipe books or online will yield many varied styles, both fermented and not.

A blogger named Siegfried[27] caught my attention with a write-up of a hot pepper pickle inspired by Madhur Jaffrey's *World-of-the-East Vegetarian Cooking*.

> Cram hot peppers, sliced into rounds, into a mason jar. My favorite was a combination of serranos, jalapeños, banana peppers, and poblanos. Salt them as you go and add some seasonings (we like black mustard seeds ground coarsely and fresh ginger, chopped finely.) Heat oil (we like mustard oil)—not much, only about two tablespoons. Pour over peppers and place lid on. Don't boil the jar. Leave on a sunny ledge for a day or two. Shake jar several times per day, more if liquid doesn't cover them entirely. The peppers should shrink some. Add lime juice—a few tablespoons—and leave in the sunny place. (Bring them in at night if your sunny place is outside.) Continue to shake to ensure even pickling! Once they have soured to your liking (a week? two? longer?) refrigerate to slow the fermentation. They are wildly sour and addictive.

I tried a batch as Siegfried described and it exploded with flavors: sour from the fermentation, hot from the peppers and mustard, and salty. I use it—sparingly—as a condiment, and it enhances whatever I put it on.

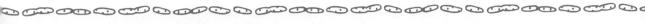

CONSERVA CRUDA DI POMODORO (RAW TOMATO PRESERVES)

Sergio Carlini, Italy

This recipe, which uses a wild fermentation, has been used for hundreds of years in Italy, and I prepare it every year. However, because of the new European regulations it is not (of course . . .) still seen on market shelves.

Tomatoes (ripe, washed, and with any rotting parts removed) are squeezed in a large plastic bin. Fermentation occurs spontaneously, quite similar to the alcoholic one, in an acidic environment and supported by lactic acid bacteria and molds. The bin must be *not* completely full and must be covered by a canvas or a net (to keep insects away). The mass bubbles, and the solid parts come to the surface, and become covered by a white mold. Stir twice daily, mixing in the mold. After four to five days (depending on temperature), the fermentation stops completely. Remove solids floating on the surface and pass them through a low-tech machine that separates the peel and seeds. [In the United States, this device is sometimes marketed as a Squeezo.] The pulpy flesh is the part to keep; the peel and seeds go to the compost. Strain pulp in a fine mesh or cotton bag, tied closed with string, and hang to drip liquid for a day. The bag may become covered externally by mold; if so remove by "shaving" with a spoon, and discard. Also "shave" the inside of the bag, to separate the pulp, now reduced by hanging. Retie the bag and place it between two wooden boards or panels, clean and dry, and weigh down, evenly, to press it and remove further water. Press for a few days, until the pulp has the consistency of firm dough. Mix in 25–30 percent salt. A few hours later, knead the dough. It is very salty and concentrated and has to be used in very (very) small quantities. The yield in weight is about 8 percent of the tomatoes you start with. The preserve is usually stored in a jar, where it can be kept unrefrigerated. In the past, when really firm, it was preserved for months enveloped in paper. This concentrate is then used as needed through the winter, added to vegetables and meats for tomato-based sauces.

Fermenting Hot Sauce, Relishes, Salsas, Chutneys, and Other Condiments

All varieties of hot peppers may be preserved by fermentation. The method is extremely simple, exactly the same as the sauerkraut method. Remove the stems from peppers. Chop them. Add salt to taste, or approximately 2 percent by weight. Add garlic, other spices, or other vegetables if desired. Ferment a month or longer, keeping the peppers submerged and skimming off mold if necessary. Liquefy in a food processor. Use as a seasoning in cooking or as a raw condiment. "Commercial hot sauce with factory-farmed peppers soaked in cheap vinegar will never taste the same again," warns Rick Otten. "I make an heirloom hot sauce, a fermented chili-garlic sauce (think *sriracha*), and a fermented version of the Southern pepper vinegar sauce for greens," writes April McGreger, who sells her ferments as Farmer's Daughter Brand in Carrboro, North Carolina. "I am forever in awe of the complexity in the flavor of a fermented pepper."

Like hot sauce, relishes are typically preserved in vinegar but may be fermented instead. Salsas and chutneys are typically eaten fresh or stored in the refrigerator but may also be fermented. If you're following recipes, omit (or greatly reduce) the vinegar. Salt the vegetables and spices, and ferment under their own juices. Add whey, kraut juice or pickle brine, or other starters if desired. Similarly, tomato ketchup, *ajvar* (a delicious roasted pepper and eggplant condiment from the Balkans), mustard, and other condiments may be made by fermentation. Reduce or omit the vinegar, and replace it (after cooling cooked sauce) with live-culture starters.

Himalayan *Gundruk* and *Sinki*

In the Himalayan Mountains, in Nepal, India, and Bhutan, people ferment vegetables in a distinctive manner, wilting the vegetables in the sun before fermentation; fermenting without salt; and finally, drying fermented vegetables for storage. Mustard greens, radish greens, and other greens of the *Brassica* family fermented in this manner are called *gundruk*; radish roots are called *sinki*. Vegetables are fermented in jars or crocks, or in pits plastered with mud hardened by fire (see *Pit Fermentation* in chapter 3).

To prepare vegetables for *gundruk* or *sinki*, wilt them in the sun for two or three days. Bring them inside at night to protect from dew, and turn them periodically to expose different surfaces. For *gundruk*, shred or chop leafy greens; pound, squeeze, or crush them; and stuff forcefully into the fermentation vessel. As with other vegetable ferments, the objective is to get them submerged; add water if necessary to cover the vegetables. Ferment the vegetables for a week or longer, then remove the leaves from the jar, sun-dry for several days, and store dry. To use *gundruk*, soak the dried leaves in water for about 10 minutes, squeezing out excess moisture. Then fry them in oil with onions and spices, and boil them into soup. For *sinki*, dip wilted radishes in water, then stuff them whole into the fermentation vessel, with added water if necessary. *Sinki* is typically fermented longer than *gundruk*, about three weeks. After fermentation, chop the radishes into small pieces, dry for several days in the sun, and store dry. Use *sinki* in soups just like *gundruk*.[28]

Considerations for Salt-Free Vegetable Ferments

The general kraut-chi method can be adapted for fermenting without salt. Personally, as I've said before, I think ferments made with just a tiny bit of salt taste much, much better than those with none; but if you wish to avoid all salt, you can still enjoy fermented vegetables. As described earlier, salt slows the fermentation process, inhibits other bacteria and molds, and slows the enzymes that digest pectins and make vegetables go soft. Without these functions provided by salt, salt-free ferments are typically fermented for much shorter periods of time; two or three days is plenty. Taste daily, and refrigerate when your ferment tastes ripe to you.

Other mineral-rich ingredients can provide at least a portion of the beneficial functions of salt. Seaweed is an excellent source of minerals. Kelps, kombu, arame, and hijiki all work great; some have complained that dulse disintegrated. Soak seaweed in a little water to rehydrate. Press it under water and squeeze. Chop rehydrated seaweed and add to the ferment along with soaking water. Seeds such as caraway, celery, and dill seeds are also mineral-rich. Celery juice is as well; the best salt-free kraut I have made incorporated celery juice. I juiced a few stalks of celery, diluted the thick juice with an equal quantity of water, and mixed this liquid with vegetables to ferment. Another approach is to use whey or another starter for salt-free ferments, to introduce acidity, as well as a concentration of lactic acid bacteria that speed acidification. See the discussion of starters later in this chapter.

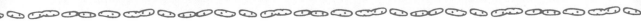

VINEGAR PICKLING VERSUS FERMENTATION

Although vinegar is a product of fermentation, most vinegar pickles use hot vinegar as a means of sterilizing vegetables. In these pickles, fermentation is prevented by this heat treatment, combined with high levels of acidity in the vinegar. Some brining recipes call for a relatively small proportion of vinegar, what I would call hybrid pickles. Vinegar in a small proportion, and added at ambient temperatures, will not prevent fermentation. In this context, vinegar is a flavoring and a means of creating a slightly acidic selective environment in which fermenting lactic acid bacteria can flourish.

Pulling water out of the vegetables—typically facilitated by salt—can be a challenge when fermenting without salt. Vegetables to be fermented without salt need more bruising, by pounding or squeezing, than salted vegetables. It can also help to expose more surface area, chopping vegetables more finely. With or without salt, the primary objective remains the same: to get vegetables submerged under liquid. Add whey or water as necessary.

Salt also functions as one of the ways of making the fermentation environment more selective, giving the salt-tolerant lactic acid bacteria a competitive advantage over other bacteria that are also present. In salt-free ferments, some people squeeze lemon or lime juice into the vegetables so that acidity will create a selective environment.

Brining

In contrast with the dry-salt method, in which salt is typically used to pull water out of vegetables in order to ferment them under their own juices, brining involves preparing a saltwater solution to cover the vegetables. In the Asian tradition, vegetables are often soaked in strong brine for a limited time, to wilt them and leach bitterness from greens, then packed into a vessel to ferment. In the European tradition, cucumbers, olives, and other whole vegetables or large chunks of vegetables are fermented directly in brine. "Nothing could be simpler than the age-old method of salt-pickling," writes Anne Volokh in *The Art of Russian Cuisine*.[29]

Brines can be flavored with many spices beyond salt. Recall that many spices function as mold inhibitors. They also contribute bacterial cultures. Garlic is a popular pickling spice. If it turns blue during fermentation, do not be alarmed; that is a harmless reaction due to compounds called anthocyanins in some varieties of garlic, which can turn garlic blue as an acid reaction to traces of copper in your water.[30] Dill is another classic pickling spice, in any form: fresh flowers, seed heads, dried seeds, or leaf. Try smoked or other hot peppers, shallots, tarragon, coriander seed, cloves, fenugreek, horseradish. "I love how using 'pickling spice' makes it taste Southern, and adding some sliced lemon or lime or oranges or even raw apple cider vinegar to pickle brines can shift the flavor profile in a different direction," says April McGreger. "I made some garlicky, fermented Vietnamese-style pickled carrots with sliced limes, lime leaf, bird chilis, and lemongrass. I try lots of different flavor variations." Aylin Öney Tan writes that in Turkey, where she lives, dried chickpeas are often added to brines (as well as breads) as a sort of starter. "A handful is added to pickles to activate fermentation," she explains.

Brined sour pickles (also known as kosher dills) and brined olives are addressed in the following section. Whole or halved brussels sprouts also ferment beautifully under brine. Try brining radishes, turnips, cauliflower, carrots, onions, string beans, peppers, burdock, eggplant, watermelon rinds— any vegetables you like. Tender early-summer grape leaves can be brined, then later stuffed with spiced rice or other fillings for *dolma*, *sarma*, and other tasty hors d'oeuvres.

Volokh's cookbook contains a recipe for cucumbers brined in a pumpkin (exactly as described below, only inside a pumpkin). What she recommends as a usual vessel is a 1-gallon oak barrel. Wouldn't it be nice to get those back into production! Her recipe for brined tomatoes got me to try brining ripening but not fully ripe tomatoes. In the past I had brined only green tomatoes, which are crispy but very sour. Fully ripe tomatoes get mushy very quickly. The ripening tomatoes were a happy in-between, sweeter than brined green tomatoes, but maintaining a pleasing crispiness, especially when lightly fermented just a few days. Volokh has recipes for brined apples, lemons, and watermelon, described in *Lactic Acid Fermentations of Fruit*.

Whole cabbages are brined, typically in big barrels, in Croatia, Bosnia, throughout the Balkans, and Romania. After fermentation, leaves can be removed from the cabbages whole for stuffing, or cabbages may be shredded into kraut. "This is a fun and simple preparation that is great for storing bulk amounts of cabbage, and there are many wonderful traditional variations on the recipe," write Luke Regalbuto and Maggie Levinger, who traveled extensively in Eastern Europe investigating fermentation techniques before starting their business, Wild West Ferments in California. "Unfortunately, we have found that this ferment creates a particularly nasty smell that we can only liken to dirty diapers. We love stuffed cabbage leaves, and so we have found that we prefer to ferment whole cabbage leaves removed from the core." I've also buried whole cabbages, usually with the cores removed to facilitate brine penetration, in shredded cabbage or other vegetables. Luke and Maggie write that they encountered something similar in the Carpathian Alps of Romania, called *muraturi asortate*, meaning "assorted pickles," which involved fermenting whole heads of cabbage in a brine with other vegetables.

Torshi (from the Persian *torsh*, meaning "sour") are vegetable pickles enjoyed in Iran and throughout much of the Middle East, Turkey, and the Balkans. Astrid Richard Cook, who lived in Kuwait, reports that vegetable pickles called *torosh* accompanied every meal there.

> It is a very basic recipe and always includes cucumbers, carrots and turnips, although I have also seen it with cauliflower. Basically they chop the vegetable in large chunks (it's eaten with the fingers or occasionally a fork or spoon). You add in salt, lemon juice and water and allow it to ferment. Our Iranian friends make a couple gallons of it at a time and they say it will last several years.

Many contemporary torshis are vinegar-based. Bulgarian ethnologist Lilija Radeva notes that "pickling in vinegar was very rare among the Bulgarians until the 20th century," and describes the simple brining method for making *tursii*: "Green tomatoes, green or red paprika pods, carrots, and—in the southern regions—small unripe pumpkins, honey-dew melons, watermelons and cucumbers, are soaked together or separately in salt water.

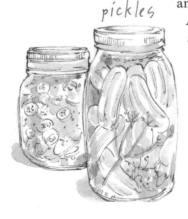

pickles

After fermentation they are are eaten with mush, meat dishes, and other meals, and often simply with bread."[31] Karmela Kis, who, with her husband Miroslav, graciously hosted me when I visited Croatia, sent me a recipe for an old Serbian style of fermenting vegetables called *tursija*, in which whole paprikas (sweet peppers), green tomatoes, and cucumbers are brined, spiced with hot peppers and horseradish.

As with dry-salting, I typically do not measure the salt in my brines. I salt to taste. You want to mix brine fairly strong, since it will be diluted by the vegetables that go into it. Estimate required brine quantity as about half the volume or weight of your vegetables. Add as little brine as possible to the vegetables, packing them tightly and pressing down under brine. Salt in brine will pull water from the vegetables and the amount of brine will increase. Salt will diffuse into vegetables gradually. Taste the brine after a day or two and adjust the salt by adding more, if necessary, or water if the brine is excessively salty.

Discussions of brine strength in the literature typically express salinity as a percentage indicating weight of salt in proportion to water. A brine of 5 percent means you use 5 percent salt relative to the weight of the water for the brine. (You need a scale to measure this.) A liter of water weighs exactly 1 kilogram. A quart weighs roughly 2 pounds; a gallon roughly 8 pounds. Calculate salt by multiplying the weight of the water quantity by brine strength; in the case of 5 percent brine, 0.05. For a quart of 5 percent brine, this comes to 1.6 ounces of salt to add to a quart of water (50 grams of salt to a liter). If you don't have a scale, 1.6 ounces of salt comes to approximately 3 tablespoons (a bit more with fine salt, a bit less with a coarse). Although brining recipes vary widely, 5 percent is a good brine strength to use as a starting point. While 5 percent salt would be extremely high in sauerkraut or kimchi, it is important to understand that 5 percent brine yields a much lower-salt product, because once the vegetables go into the brine, they absorb salt and release juices, thereby diluting the salt concentration by more than half.

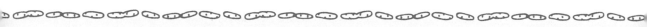

BRINED OKRA

Lorna Moravec, West, Texas

By far my most spectacular success was with okra. And in the hot Texas summer, I mean, it made quick. Even woody, tough okra that would not have been too good fried or in gumbo was just heavenly when fermented in brine for a couple of days. It was super easy. I just jammed the okra pods into mason jars. The shoulders held them down. I crammed a few garlic cloves and jalapeños down in amongst them and poured in the brine. Man! We ate them up so fast!

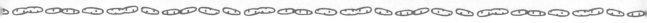

Compared with the much saltier "salt-stock" style of brining, which saturates vegetables with salt to prevent microbial and enzymatic transformations, followed by a desalinating soak before consumption, 5 percent is considered a low-salt brine. "Brines of low salt concentration favor the rapid formation of a relatively high amount of total titratable acid and the development of a relatively low brine pH," concludes a 1940 study by the North Carolina Agricultural Experiment Station. "Brines of increasingly higher initial salt content favor correspondingly retarded rates of acid formation, lower total quantities of acids produced, and higher . . . pH values."[32]

The best thing about fermenting vegetables in brine is having lots of extra brine. Pour some into a pitcher and enjoy shots as a digestive tonic. Use it as a starter for seed cheeses (see *Cultured Seed and/or Nut Cheeses, Pâtés, and*

Milks in chapter 11), a live-culture acidifier for soaking grains and legumes (see *Soaking Grains* in chapter 8), a flavoring in salad dressings or marinades, or a base for soups. Brine is a precious, tasty, and nutritious resource.

Sour Pickles

It is brined sour cucumber pickles that got me interested in fermentation in the first place. As a kid in New York City I'd frequently enjoy a pickle as a satisfying (and cheap) after-school snack. The garlic-dill-lactic-acid flavor of pickles is something I have always loved and craved. As soon as I started making sauerkraut and thinking about fermentation, it was only natural that I try fermenting cucumbers into sour pickles.

The sour pickles I grew up with in New York, known in many places as kosher dills, are iconic symbols of Eastern European Jewish cuisine. In fact, they and all things pickled are prominent in cuisines across Eastern Europe. Polish ethnographer Anna Kowalska-Lewicka explains that "the peasant diet contained only minimal quantities of meat and consisted almost exclusively of vegetables, flour, and buckwheat—all with a bland taste." In her analysis, by adding a different flavor and greatly broadening the palate, the sour flavors of fermentation did more than simply preserve food.[33]

I learned from Jane Ziegelman's book *97 Orchard: An Edible History of Five Immigrant Families in One New York Tenement* that the taste for pickles among Jewish immigrants was cause for alarm and moral judgment. "The excessive use of pickled foods destroys the taste for milder flavors, causes irritation, and renders assimilation more difficult," writes Boston dietitian Bertha M. Wood in her 1922 book *Foods of the Foreign-Born in Relation to Health*.[34] John Spargo, author of *The Bitter Cry of the Children*, sought to understand why Jewish children so frequently spent their lunch pennies on pickles. "It would seem that the chronic underfeeding creates a nervous craving for some kind of stimulant which the child finds in pickles. The adult resorts to whiskey very often for much the same reason."[35]

In our time, pickles are more frequently celebrated than condemned. I have attended many pickle festivals, at which Americans of varied ethnicities celebrated the pickling traditions of their people. Sour pickles are more appropriately viewed as healthy, live-culture digestive stimulants than as dangerous moral hazards.

Fermenting cucumbers is more challenging than most other vegetable ferments. Cucumbers are extremely watery, and subject to fast decomposition by pectin-digesting enzymes. And while cabbages and radishes typically mature in cool weather, cucumbers grow in heat, which speeds both fermentation and enzymatic digestion. Because of these factors, it is easy to have fermented cucumbers get mushy, which is not a pleasing texture for most people.

To keep cucumbers crunchy, I suggest adding grape leaves, oak leaves, cherry leaves, horseradish leaves, or other tannin-rich plant materials (even a tea bag or green banana peel). Harold McGee writes that using unrefined sea salt "improves crispness thanks to its calcium and magnesium impurities, which help cross-link and reinforce cell-wall pectins," which he points out is also how pickling additives such as alum or calcium hydroxide work.[36] There are many other ideas on how to keep cucumber pickles crispy; for instance, fermentation enthusiast Shivani Arjuna writes: "Adding some slices of carrot along with cucumber will keep the cucumber crisper." A Russian woman in one of my classes recalled seeing cucumbers blanched briefly in boiling water prior to brining to maintain crispiness. Fred Breidt et al. report that in commercial production, calcium chloride is added to brine (0.1 to 0.4 percent) to maintain crispness during storage.[37] People have used many varied strategies to accomplish this sometimes elusive goal.

Add lots of garlic and dill. There's no need to even peel the garlic; I just add whole heads cut in half cross-sectionally, and the garlic infuses into the brine. For dill, flowers or seed heads are ideal, but seeds and/or greens are fine. Horseradish (roots and/or leaves) and hot peppers are great, also. For best results, ferment small pickling cucumbers of fairly uniform size. Prepare cucumbers just before brining by soaking in cold water (even ice water), scraping away any residue of the flower blossoms on the ends of the cucumbers, and gently rubbing off the spines. For sour pickles, mix 5 percent brine, roughly 3 tablespoons of salt per quart/liter of water, as described previously. For shorter-fermenting "half-sours" or *malossol* ("little salt" in Russian), use weaker brine, around 3.5 percent, or 2 tablespoons of salt per quart/liter of water. For French-style *cornichons*, use tiny cucumbers of the *cornichon* variety, and spice 5 percent brine with tarragon, garlic, and peppercorns. Submerge cucumbers and other ingredients under brine. Use a plate or other modest weight to keep vegetables submerged, as they will tend to float.

Many Eastern European pickle recipes call for floating a slice of rye bread in the brine. Fellow pickle lover Ira Weiss, who grew up on the Lower East Side of Manhattan in the 1950s—when "there was a pickle stand on every third corner"—reports that his Hungarian-Romanian-born mother made her pickles with a slice of rye bread on top of the brine. But after much experimentation, Ira concluded that the rye bread made no difference and discontinued the tradition.

Spices

Ira does recommend another practice he learned from his mother: fermenting cucumbers in a glass jar near a window, so it gets some direct sunlight, which he reports "helps eliminate the formation of scum (mold)," because "ultraviolet light is a good disinfectant." Ira's mother's advice is echoed in a textbook account of commercial cucumber fermentation, "commonly done in 8,000- to 10,000-gallon, open-top, plastic or fiberglass tanks that are located out-of-doors so the brine surface is exposed to sunlight. The UV radiation in sunlight is relied upon to kill aerobic surface yeasts."[38] Many fermentation traditions insist on fermenting in the dark, but it can work well both ways.

If you are fermenting cucumbers when temperatures are hot, averaging above roughly 77°F/25°C, ferment just a few days before eating or moving to refrigeration. In cooler temperatures, you can ferment cucumbers longer, but taste frequently and refrigerate at the first sign of softening. As cucumbers ferment, their skin color changes from bright green to a darker olive green and their interiors change from white to translucent. Half-sours are eaten still somewhat bright, in transition. As the pickles absorb salt from the brine, the cucumbers' specific gravity increases while the brine's decreases, resulting in the pickles sinking rather than floating. Store live fermented cucumber pickles in the refrigerator unless you have a root cellar or other spot that stays below 60°F/16°C.

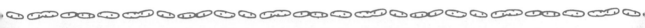

EXPERIMENTALIST SPIRIT

Barb Schuetz, Viroqua, Wisconsin

I love, love, love carrots fermented with radishes in the sour pickle brine and spices. The radishes lend a beautiful color to the brine but also add a unique flavor and a bit of a bite to the carrots. I've also made a kraut with green cabbage, onion, garlic, radish, and a large amount of carrot, and it's perfect. I enjoy experimenting; I throw just about anything within grasp into kraut and I haven't had an unpleasant batch yet. I also like to play with textures and shapes, even mixing it up within the same batch.

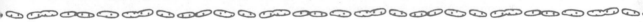

Brining Mushrooms

Frequently people have asked me whether mushrooms can be fermented. I have occasionally fermented mushrooms, especially shiitakes, mixed with other vegetables. Fermentation experimentalist Molly Agy-Joyce of River Falls, Minnesota, wrote to tell me about her kimchi with crimini mushrooms: "The ginger and hot pepper flavors mingled really well with the mushrooms." But I have never fermented mushrooms as a primary ingredient.

Polish ethnographer Anna Kowalska-Lewicka writes that in Poland, historically: "Almost all varieties of edible mushrooms were pickled in the villages, *Lactarius deliciosus* [saffron milk cap] being considered the best. . . . Mushrooms were pickled similarly to cabbage, and were highly regarded as an addition to warm dishes or bread."[39] Anne Volokh has an extremely simple recipe for brined mushrooms in *The Art of Russian Cuisine* (1983). She calls for 1 pound/500 g of mushrooms, 2 tablespoons of non-iodized salt, peppercorns, caraway seeds, garlic, dill, and optional horseradish, black currant, or sour cherry leaves. Mushroom stems are trimmed to ½ inch/1 cm, and spices (except salt) are mixed together. Then mushrooms are packed into the fermentation vessel, caps down. "Sprinkle each layer with salt and every other layer with the spice and herb mixture." Leave with a weight bearing down, to force water out of the mushrooms. Volokh recommends fermenting at room temperatures for a day or two, then refrigerating for 10 to 14 days. These fermented mushrooms, she writes, "are the perfect accompaniment for vodka."[40]

Finnish fermentation enthusiast and teacher Ossi Kakko, who describes himself as a "researcher on the horticulturalist gatherer way of life," advises using a starter to ferment mushrooms. For starters, he recommends fermenting birch sap ("it has phosphorous and calcium which are not present in mushrooms"), *rejuvelac* fermented from soaking sprouted grains in water (see *Rejuvelac* in chapter 8), or extra brine from a previous batch of fermenting vegetables. "Drop whole mushrooms into fermented liquid and keep 'em in warm room temperature for three days. Their texture softens and they just melt in your mouth! Superb vibrations throughout the body-mind-soul!"[41]

Ossi says to use mushrooms "that can be eaten without special preparation"—he specifically mentions chantarelles, boletus, horns of plenty, sheep polypores, funnel chantarelles, morels, and hydnum species—while Volokh's recipe calls for "small mushrooms" without any specificity. At least with wild mushrooms, the type of mushroom could have some bearing on the appropriateness of fermenting them. A group of mycologists included me in a round-robin email conversation they were having on the question of fermenting mushrooms. Leon Shernoff, editor of *Mushroom the Journal*, expressed concern that bacteria associated with some mushrooms could create toxic compounds in a fermentation context. "Hen of the Woods, for instance, is fine raw . . . but after a few days in the refrigerator, the surface bacteria multiply to the point where doing this gets you a burning mouth and throat." Because so little research has been done on mushroom fermentation, I would recommend cautious experimentation.

I have heard other concerns about fermenting mushrooms. Some people worry about hydrazine and other volatile toxins that are present in many mushrooms, typically removed by cooking. "I doubt that fermentation per se breaks down hydrazine," writes Shernoff. But because of hydrazine's volatility, "to the extent that the fermentation liquid dissolves hydrazine it will evaporate preferentially and thus be reduced in the finished product."[42] There is also the question of whether the compound chitin, of which mushroom cell walls are composed, is made digestible by fermentation. Chitin is regarded as indigestible raw but digestible after cooking. There is some research suggesting that chitin in another chitin-containing substance—shrimp shells—becomes more digestible as a result of fermentation,[43] but none that I have found specifically in regard to mushrooms.

 ## Brining Olives

In their raw state, olives are horribly bitter and toxic, due to the presence of the compound oleuropein. Before olives can be eaten, they are always cured to reduce oleuropein. Curing is a broad category encompassing many different methods of aging, leaching, and ripening. There are many different styles of curing olives, many (but not all) of which involve fermentation.

I have no access to raw olives and no personal experience curing them. In fact, until quite recently I did not like to eat olives. If they were cut into small pieces in food I would tolerate them, but I would always avoid whole olives or big pieces. Then I started challenging myself to try them. And I have found that I love some olives.

Olives grow in mild Mediterranean-type climates; California, Italy, and Croatia are where I have encountered them. The fruits are harvested from trees in late autumn or early winter. "For those of you living in olive country, there's no reason not to forage for your own olives," writes blogger Hank Shaw. "In most places, they are free for the taking."[44]

There is much information in books and on the Internet detailing various olive-curing methods. The sources from which I have gleaned information lead me to conclude that the simplest method is to ferment them. For a quicker cure (one month or several), you need to somehow break the skin of the olive: gently cracking them with a mallet, slicing into them, halving, or piercing. Curing whole intact olives takes much longer, eight months to a year, as the bitter oleuropein leaches out much more slowly.

If you choose to crack or pierce the olives, get them under water right away to prevent discoloration due to oxidation. Soak in lots of water. Change the water every day, or even more often if water darkens quickly, for about two weeks, or until the bitterness is gone. Then place the olives, with spices, in 5 percent brine, just as with cucumbers. People use many different spices. "Always bay leaves and coriander," writes Hank Shaw. "Beyond that I improvise: citrus rind, black pepper, chiles, oregano, rosemary, sage, garlic, Sichuan peppercorns, etc. Go easy, though: Olives should taste like olives—slightly bitter, firm and rich." Use a plate or other modest weight to keep olives submerged. Taste periodically and evaluate. After a few weeks, or longer, when they're sufficiently ripe, enjoy or store in the refrigerator.

Whole intact olives take longer to cure, eight months to a year. In such a long ferment, the surface typically becomes moldy. Remove surface growth as it forms; the submerged olives are fine. When the brine becomes dark with leached oleuropein, drain the olives, discard the brine, and mix fresh brine. Don't add spices until a few months have passed and most of the bitterness has already been leached. Whole fermented olives generally retain their crunchiness better than olives with broken skins.

Dilly Beans

Fresh green (or yellow or purple) beans preserved with dill are known as dilly beans. I grew up eating my father's excellent dilly beans, and to this day, every time I visit him, he pulls out a jar of them to share, and we enjoy them as a crunchy, sour, and light snack while dinner cooks. My dad pickles his dilly beans by stuffing beans in a wide-mouth canning jar with dill, garlic, chili peppers, salt, and celery seed; pouring a boiling mix of half vinegar, half water over them; sealing and heat processing by boiling in a hot-water bath for 10 minutes. Dilly beans may also be fermented under brine. Mix 5 percent brine (roughly 3 tablespoons of salt per quart/liter of water) and submerge beans in it, along with lots of dill and garlic. Fermentation time will vary with temperature.

Some of the literature recommends cooking beans before fermenting. "They contain a toxic substance called phasin, a protein that interferes with digestion and decomposes when heated," according to Klaus Kaufmann and Annelies Schöneck. "Never eat raw beans on a salad plate!" they admonish, recommending boiling beans for 5 to 10 minutes in salted water before eating or fermenting.[45] Having enjoyed raw string beans all my life, without noticeable toxicity, it's hard for me to worry about phasin. I've only found a few references to phasin as a toxin that cite any specific sources. One is a 1962 citation of a 1926 German study in which "mice were unable to grow on the isolated protein (*phasin*) of the white bean (*Phaseolus vulgaris*) unless it was cooked."[46] This hardly seems relevant; a string bean isn't a white bean, and we are not mice being fed a diet of exclusively an isolated protein derived from it. It probably is not healthy to eat just an isolate of any single food, including beans. The other reference I found was from botanist James Duke, who summarizes a report from a German medical journal in 1979:

> After eating only a few raw beans (*Phaseolus vulgaris*) or dried beans (*P. coccineus*), three boys, 4 to 8 years old rapidly developed symptoms of poisoning, notably sickness and diarrhea. Phasin, a toxalbumin destroyed by cooking, was considered responsible. All boys had normal aminotransferase values and parenteral treatment with fluid and electrolytes led to complete recovery in 12 to 24 hours.[47]

Note that the boys ate raw beans *or* dried beans. That really is a significant distinction. Dried beans definitely contain toxic anti-nutrients (see chapter 11), and in some varieties fresh "green" beans do too. Only certain varieties of beans are eaten green, even cooked. And fermentation is generally an effective means of removing such compounds and transforming them into other benign or even nutritious forms. It's hard for me to worry about fermenting raw string beans. Nonetheless, I have tried Kaufmann and Schöneck's method of precooking the beans, and despite my initial skepticism (since the lactic acid bacteria present on raw vegetables are destroyed by cooking), the blanched beans fermented beautifully, thanks to the presence of raw garlic and dill with lactic acid bacteria still intact.

 ## Lactic Acid Fermentations of Fruit

Various fruits have already been mentioned in this chapter as minor ingredients of vegetable ferments, but it seems appropriate to devote a section to lactic acid fermentations of fruit. Typically sugary fruit and fruit juice will spontaneously ferment into primarily alcohol (and then acetic acid if exposed to air) rather than lactic acid. (Chapter 4 details different methods for fermenting fruit into alcohol.) Ferments mixing fruits with vegetables generally contain both yeasts and lactic acid bacteria. In fruit kimchi, fruit is mixed with salted and spiced vegetables; fruits ferment primarily into alcohol and acetic acid while vegetables ferment primarily into lactic acid. To enjoy fruit kimchi with fruit still somewhat sweet, eat or refrigerate after just a few days' fermentation.[48]

Yeast activity can be inhibited by heavy salting, or overpowered by the addition of lactic acid starter cultures such as whey. One popular lactic acid fermentation of fruit is salted lemons and limes. Madhur Jaffrey's book *World Vegetarian* contains a simple recipe for Moroccan-style salted lemons, calling for 2 pounds/1 kg of lemons and 9 tablespoons of salt. Cut the lemons into quarters lengthwise, leaving them attached at the bottoms. Remove the seeds and "rub the lemons with most of the salt, inside and out, closing them up again so they look whole." Use a quart jar as a vessel. Sprinkle salt into the bottom of the jar, then add the salted lemons one by one, pressing down to force the juice out of the lemons, until they are all in the jar, submerged under brine. Ferment three to four weeks, until the lemon skins have softened completely, then refrigerate. "Both the skin and pulp add sourness," notes Jaffrey, "but it is a special, mellow sourness with echoes of an ancient world."[49] Salting of lemons varies quite a bit among recipes. Another recipe I found used much less salt: 4 tablespoons for 10 pounds/4.5 kg of lemons. Once again, there is not a single way of doing this. You can similarly ferment limes, oranges, or other citrus fruits. In fact, Sally Fallon Morell writes that "originally marmalade was a lacto-fermented food," in which oranges were pressed into large casks with seawater.[50]

Another example of a heavily salted fruit ferment is the Japanese pickled plum known as *umeboshi*. The salty and sour fermented plums are used as both seasoning and medicine in Japan. Aveline Kushi, the Japanese author of several macrobiotic cookbooks, recounts a Japanese adage: "Eat one *umeboshi* plum before taking a journey and you will have a safe trip."[51] The ume plums (*Prunus mume*) are harvested green, not fully ripe. The red color of *umeboshi* plums comes from the leaves of perilla, also known as beefsteak plant, or *shiso* in Japanese (*Perilla frutescens*). My friend Alwyn de Wally, who spent time 40 years ago living with the Katsuragi family in a farming village in southwestern Japan, recorded in his journal his host-mother's method of pickling *umeboshi* plums.

> For every 1½ quarts/liters of plums you'll need 1 pint/½ liter of sea salt and 3.5 oz/100 grams perilla leaves (about 50 leaves) plus another 2 tablespoons of sea salt. In Japan, the plums to be used are gathered in mid-June when they are beginning to turn yellow but are still green. Fully ripe plums will disintegrate in pickling.

Wash the plums well and leave to stand overnight in clear water. Then drain off the water and put the plums and salt in alternating layers into a crock. Put a heavy rock on top of the last layer of plums. A day or two later, when enough liquid has been drawn off the plums (by the salt) to cover the plums completely, remove the rock and put a cover on the crock. Wait about 20 days. When you expect to have three good, hot days without rain, drain the liquid (umeboshi vinegar) off the plums and put the plums outside to dry in the sun. They should be spread out in a single layer, ideally on propped-up baskets or screens so that air can circulate above and below them. Leave them spread out like this for three days and nights. During that time, mix two heaping tablespoons of salt into the perilla leaves and squeeze by hand until you've expressed all the (purple) liquid you can. (The liquid is thrown away.) Then add the leaves to the sun-dried plums as you put the plums back in the crock. Pour back in enough of the plum-vinegar to cover the plums completely (the remaining vinegar can be used in cooking), and put the lid on the crock again.

The following summer, remove the plums again, dry in the sun for one day, and put in jars for storage without the vinegar. These are real umeboshi. They will be very salty at first but will gradually become less salty and more delicious.

Fermentation enthusiast Andrew Donaldson wrote to me raving about cranberries fermented in brine, which he mixed at a proportion of 2 tablespoons salt per quart/liter of water. In the mountainous regions of Bulgaria, cranberries are preserved with "only water poured over them"—no salt—and "they are remarkable for their good flavour," according to ethnologist Lilija Radeva.[52] Anne Volokh, in her book *The Art of Russian Cuisine*, has recipes for brining apples and watermelons. For the apples, she mixes a sweet brine, dissolving 3.5 tablespoons/50 ml of sugar and 1.75 tablespoons/25 ml of salt in 3 quarts/3 liters of water, and mixing in 6 tablespoons/90 ml of rye flour. Then, in a gallon vessel, Volokh layers whole tart cooking apples, on their sides, with tarragon and sour cherry leaves, pours the brine over them, weighs them down, and covers. She ferments the apples at room temperature for a few days, then moves them to a cellar or refrigerator for a month or longer. For watermelon, she uses only small melons (3.5 pounds/1.5 kg or smaller) and ferments them whole in 5 percent brine (see *Brining*, earlier in this chapter), spiced with whole cloves and cinnamon sticks, for 40 to 50 days at cellar or refrigerator temperatures. She describes the brined watermelons as having an "incomparable, cool, prickling, sweet-and-sour taste."[53]

Fruits can also be fermented with vegetables. Earlier we touched upon small proportions of fruit mixed into mostly vegetable ferments,

← water-filled glass jug

← plate

crock

and just the reverse can be done as well. Rick Chumley wrote me about his pineapple mango chutney, combining and fermenting for a few days chopped pineapple and mango, along with radishes, onions, cilantro, lime juice, tarragon, ginger, and black pepper, salt, and whey as a starter.

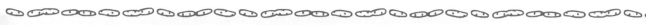

LOCAL ROOTS CAFÉ BLACK MISSION FIG BUTTER

Rives Elliot

(makes 1 quart/liter)

4 cups/1 liter dried black mission figs
1 tablespoon/15 ml sea salt
¼ cup/60 ml whey
¼–½ cup/60–125 ml raw honey, to taste
Water, as necessary

1. Destem the figs and soak for 1 hour in warm water.

2. Process all the ingredients together until smooth in a food processor. Add water as necessary at this point to allow the processor blades to blend smoothly, and not overheat.

3. Pour the mixture into your 1-quart/liter mason jar. If necessary, add water and stir until the fig butter reaches within 1–1½ inches/2.5–4 cm of the brim.

4. Seal the jar tightly with the lid, and leave at room temperature for 2 days (or until bubbly), then transfer to the top shelf of your refrigerator. In 3 weeks to a month, it will be sufficiently delicious; eat within 2 months.

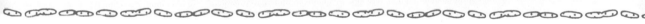

Fruit ferments can be cultured with whey, sauerkraut, or kimchi juice, or any other lactic acid bacteria starter. Sally Fallon Morell has a number of recipes in this vein in her book *Nourishing Traditions*. Rives Elliot, who founded Local Roots Café, a locavore restaurant in Roanoke, Virginia, made a delicious lacto-fermented raw fig butter that stands out in my memory (see the sidebar). Really, you could take any raw or cooked fruit concoction (cool it down to body temperature if it's cooked), add a live lactic acid bacteria starter, and ferment. Just be sure, if you ferment fruit with lots of sugar in jars, to release pressure from the jars, because with so much sugar there is the potential of building considerable pressure and exploding jars.

Kawal

Kawal is made by fermenting the leaves of a wild leguminous plant also known as *kawal* (*Cassia obtusifolia*), used as a flavoring and meat substitute in Darfur, Sudan. "*Kawal* is a food of some of the very poorest Africans," writes Hamid Dirar, who adds that it is "shunned by the elite who consider it unfit for modern social life because of its repugnant, fetid odour that lingers on the fingers for hours."[54] Nonetheless, *kawal* is spreading across Sudan. "The displaced carried with them the know-how of *kawal* preparation and use to areas where the raw material, the wild legume, is found in abundance but the inhabitants were not aware of the fermentation process."

The process for making *kawal* is pretty straightforward. Leaves are harvested when plants are fully grown, but still green and tender, as flowers and seedpods first begin to develop. Harvested leaves are cleaned of debris and beaten into a green paste with a mortar and pestle. *Kawal* is typically fermented in a clay pot (*burma*) buried in the ground. A cool kitchen or cellar would be fine. The green paste is packed into the vessel, and the surface covered with green sorghum leaves, which are weighed down by stones.

> Every 3–4 days the jar is opened, the now yellow and dry sorghum leaves removed and the contents of the burma thoroughly hand-mixed and repacked . . . [with] fresh sorghum leaves. . . . Within a week or so the fermenting *kawal* develops a characteristic strong odour which stays with it until it is consumed. . . . Two signals herald the maturity of the fermenting *kawal*. The first is the appearance of a yellowish pickle on the surface of the paste, and the second is a drop in temperature of the paste from the warmer temperature of active fermentation to that of ambience. At the end of the fermentation the separated juice is reincorporated into its mother paste, which is in turn kneaded well and crushed between the fingers. The paste is next fed into small, irregular balls or flattish cakes which are then sun dried for 3–4 days . . . [55]

The dried *kawal* cakes can be stored for a year or more. They are traditionally mixed with water for sauces, though "urban people use ground *kawal* by sprinkling it on the food much like pepper."[56]

Adding Starters to Vegetable Ferments

All vegetables are pre-inoculated, with native lactic acid bacteria adequate to initiate fermentation. In my own practice, I have found the bacteria on vegetables to consistently produce successful and delicious ferments, and almost all the varied traditions of fermenting vegetables that I have learned about rely upon bacteria present on the vegetables. You do not need any special cultures in order to ferment vegetables. Nonetheless, many people prefer to add cultures—selected strains and/or concentrated populations of lactic acid bacteria—to speed or better control fermentation. In addition to commercially available laboratory-bred bacterial strains, people use mature sauerkraut juice or brine, kombucha, kefir, or whey as starters.

The idea of adding starter cultures to vegetables has been investigated by researchers for nearly a century, since early in the emergence of the field of microbiology. Most research has concluded that in this context starters are "impractical and unnecessary, since the organisms responsible for fermentation occur naturally in adequate numbers, and . . . proper fermentation will occur if temperature and salt concentration are suitable."[57] Typically in such research, what constitutes suitable conditions are a salt concentration of approximately 2 percent and a temperature around 65°F/18°C.

Where starter cultures have been found to be effective is in ferments with lower salt concentrations. "We have shown that fermenting with 50 percent less salt results in increased variability among many quality factors, including unpredictable softening and generation of off-flavors," reports a 2007 study in the *Journal of Food Science*. "Addition of *L. mesenteroides* starter culture provided the appropriate fermentation regardless of salt level, ensuring the production of high quality sauerkraut."[58] Note that the problems attributed to low-salt ferments are aesthetic considerations of texture and flavor, rather than safety. Compensating for low salt levels with shorter fermentation times can prevent these flavor and texture degradations. With or without starters, regardless of salt level, fermentation of raw vegetables is intrinsically safe.

I have periodically added mature brine to a new batch of vegetables, without observing any dramatic difference in fermentation speed or product quality. But pickle-making enthusiast Ira Weiss strongly recommends it: "Adding a cup of the finished brine to a fresh batch of brine and cukes acts as a very effective starter and will reduce fermentation time. At about 72°F/22°C, the pickles become full sour in 4–5 days instead of 7–10." In my research, I came across several references in the literature discouraging this practice in sauerkraut. The United Nations Food and Agriculture Organization report summarizes:

> The efficacy of using old juice depends largely on the types of organisms present in the juice and its acidity. If the starter juice has an acidity of 0.3% or more, it results in a poor quality kraut. This is because the cocci [*Leuconostoc mesenteroides*] which would normally initiate fermentation are suppressed by the high acidity, leaving the bacilli with sole responsibility for fermentation. If the starter juice has an acidity of 0.25% or less, the kraut produced is normal, but there do not appear to be any beneficial effects of adding this juice. Often, the use of old juice produces a sauerkraut which has a softer texture than normal.[59]

I have heard about people similarly using mature kombucha liquid as a starter, and even people using kombucha mothers to cover the surface of the vegetables.

A popular website devoted to kefir, created by an Australian kefir aficionado named Dominic Anfiteatro, promotes the idea of using excess kefir grains—either traditional kefir grains for culturing milk, or what are known as water or sugary kefir grains, or both—to culture vegetables. He blends the granules with a little carrot and apple juice and mixes the resulting "kefir grain emulsion" in with the vegetables, with or without salt, to ferment. "The process is very flexible," writes Dom on his website,

> for you can either use whole kefir grains, putting these first at the bottom of the container and then again half way up the container when half of all ingredients are put in the brewing container. Or, kefir grains may be blended with water or fresh fruit/veggie juice and mixing the mash or emulsion with the pounded ingredients, then filling the brewing container with the fresh ingredients. Or, a few kefir grains may be pounded together with amounts of fresh veggies, and filling the brewing vessel as you go. Any of these methods produce a superior kefirkraut in little time, all of the time![60]

The homemade starter culture in most widespread use for fermenting vegetables is live-culture whey. This is the starter advocated by Sally Fallon Morell. Whey is the liquid that separates from the fatty curds when milk curdles. Depending upon how the milk curdled, whey may or may not contain live cultures. For instance, if milk is heated and then acidified by the addition of vinegar, whey will result—but because the milk was heated, the whey will not contain live bacteria. Similarly, whey protein powders marketed to bodybuilders contain no live cultures. Only if milk is cultured, and then curdled by acidification or rennet enzyme action without heat, or raw milk is allowed to spontaneously acidify, will the resulting whey contain live bacteria.

The easiest sources of whey are kefir and yogurt. Kefir will spontaneously separate after two or three days of fermentation, and whey can be simply poured off; be gentle, or the curds and whey may reintegrate. With yogurt, place a colander over a bowl, line it with several layers of tightly woven cheesecloth, and scoop yogurt into it. Then gather the corners of the cheesecloth, and gently and evenly lift them; whey will begin to drip out into the bowl. Find a hook, nail, or other spot where you can hang the yogurt-filled cheesecloth as whey continues to drip out of it. The longer you leave it hanging, the firmer the yogurt becomes and the more whey accumulates.

In addition to these homemade starters—which amount to harnessing already vigorous microbial activity and moving it into a new substrate—there are a number of laboratory-bred starter cultures commercially available. As an experiment while working on this book, I tried a starter produced by Caldwell Bio-Fermentation Canada. I shredded 2 pounds/1 kg of cabbage and added 1.8 percent salt. Then I cultured half with the Caldwell starter, and let the other half spontaneously ferment, as I usually do. The batch with starter definitely exhibited a more dramatic initial decrease in pH, but while the control did not acidify quite so quickly, it too came into the safety zone (pH below 4.6) in less than 24 hours. Both batches tasted good and had similar texture.

beets

I continue to regard the use of commercial starter cultures as unnecessary, even though they can speed fermentation and acidification. The central criticism I have of them is how they are generally marketed, which is by exploiting fear and exaggerating the risk associated with spontaneous fermentation. Caldwell Bio-Fermentation states on its website that spontaneous fermentations of vegetables "can even be risky."[61] When I questioned this, they sent me a study they conducted with the Canadian government comparing ferments using starters with spontaneous ferments. The study confirmed the idea that pH drops faster with a starter, which I do not contest; but it also made blanket statements not supported by the findings of the study, such as: "The indigenous flora of the vegetables . . . can contain molds, yeasts or even pathogens, which may cause health risk."[62] Indeed, vegetable flora may contain all these elements, and yet because of the predictability of acidification, and the resulting suppression of pathogens, they pose no risk, except in a purely theoretical way. Recall the statement from the USDA's vegetable fermentation specialist, Fred Breidt: "There has never been a documented case of foodborne illness from fermented vegetables. Risky is not a word I would use to describe vegetable fermentation." Use starter cultures if you wish, but do not do so from a place of fear. The spontaneous fermentation of vegetables, for all its variability, is a safe process, proven by the tests of time.

Liquid Forms of Vegetable Ferments: Beet and Lettuce Kvass, Cultured Cabbage Juice, *Kaanji*, and *Şalgam Suyu*

Mostly vegetables are fermented in a solid state, generating liquid, but in modest proportions. This liquid has strong flavor and can be drunk as a powerful digestive tonic. *Joy of Cooking* (1975 edition) calls sauerkraut juice "a decoction for heroes."[63] By fermenting vegetables in a high proportion of water, vegetable nutrients infuse into the liquid, resulting in delicious sour live-culture tonic beverages.

Beet kvass (also known as beet *rassol*, meaning brine) is a fermented infusion of beets in water, lightly salted. I usually make beet kvass in a quart jar. Chop a large beet or two small ones into ½-inch/1 cm cubes. Cover with water to mostly fill the jar. Add a pinch of salt, and whey or other starters if you like. Ferment a few days; exactly how many days depends upon temperature, specific ingredients and ratios, microbial ecology, and flavor preferences. Taste daily. When it starts to develop a deep, dark color and a pleasing strength, strain out the beets. You can enjoy beet kvass just like that, as a beverage; use it as a base for borscht; or lightly carbonate by transferring the liquid to a sealable vessel that can hold a little pressure, sealing, and leaving a day more at room temperature. Sally Fallon Morell suggests adding a little whey to the beet water and writes that beet kvass is "an excellent blood tonic, promotes regularity, aids digestion, alkalinizes the blood, cleanses the liver, and is a good treatment for kidney stones and other ailments."[64]

Lettuce kvass is made just like beet kvass, only replacing the chopped beets with chopped lettuce. I heard about lettuce kvass from two Canadian women who have been piecing together the story of it. Gail Singer grew up in Winnipeg, the granddaughter of Romanian Jewish immigrants, and the daughter of a father who made many kinds of pickles, including lettuce pickles, which he called *salata*. Years after his death, she became interested in lettuce pickles and could find no information. Through the Internet she found some other people with memories of lettuce kvass or pickles, and she found food historian Alexandra Grigorieva, a Russian immigrant to Canada. "Right now the proof that such lettuce dishes ever existed consists of about 30 testimonials, including Gail's, all of them belonging to Jewish culture," writes Grigorieva, who mapped and charted the details of the testimonials she and Singer collected. "The only persons who are aware of this dish hail from Jewish families mostly from just a few certain regions of Ukraine within the Pale of Settlement." Grigorieva views these ferments as practical strategies to remove the bitterness of lettuce, sometimes known in Yiddish as *shmates* (rags). She describes lettuce pickles and lettuce kvass as "variations on the same theme (with vinegar and light brine versions often criss-crossing and merging)." Lettuce kvass, a "slightly greenish refreshing lettuce drink," is made by fermenting "roughly torn lettuce leaves in slightly salted and sometimes subtly sugared water with dill and garlic," according to Grigorieva.[65]

The reason so little is remembered of the tradition is that the *shtetl* culture that spawned it was displaced and annihilated. "No wonder we have so few memories of what must have been once a summer staple all over Ukraine either in pickled or in *kvass* form. . . . The few people that still persevere with these culinary traditions mostly live well away from the original *shtetl*-land of their families in Israel, Canada, the United States, Russia, and even Germany."[66]

Cultured cabbage juice is another fermented vegetable in liquid form, though really it is an infusion rather than a juice. To make it, fill a blender with chopped cabbage, then cover the cabbage with water, until the blender is about two-thirds full with water. Blend into a slurry and pour into a crock, jar, or bowl. Repeat a few times for a larger batch. Cover and ferment, with or without salt. Ferment a few days, tasting daily. When it tastes ripe, strain out the cabbage (which you can incorporate into food, feed to animals, or compost). The liquid is cultured cabbage "juice."

I heard about cultured cabbage juice before I specifically developed my interest in fermentation. It was among the many home remedies legendary in the early AIDS treatment underground movement. For people with a disease characterized by wasting away because they are unable to keep food down, liquid infusions were important sources of live cultures and vegetable nutrients, sometimes resulting in dramatic improvements. A 1995 compilation of dietary and other tools for living with AIDS called *How to Reverse Immune Dysfunction* praises "the amazing benefits of cultured cabbage juice," and advises drinking ½ cup two or three times a day.[67]

Kaanji is a delicious spicy Punjabi beverage made by fermenting carrots and mustard seeds in water with salt. It calls for burgundy-colored carrots; if you don't have those, try adding a beet to your carrots. Slice vegetables into matchsticks. Use about ½ pound/250 g vegetables and ½ cup/120 ml ground mustard seeds, along with 2 ounces/57 grams/¼ cup salt, with ½ gallon/2 liters of water. Ferment in a covered vessel in a warm spot for about a week. Strain the veggies out of the liquid and serve chilled.

Şalgam suyu is a Turkish beverage and another vegetable ferment in liquid form—a brine from fermented purple carrots and turnip. My friend Luca took me to a Turkish restaurant in London to try this. I loved it. We drank it with *raki*, an anise-flavored liquor (each in separate glasses), and they complemented each other perfectly.

Tsukemono: Japanese Pickling Styles

Japanese pickles—called *tsukemono*—are produced in an extraordinary variety, especially notable for the diversity of media—beyond the typical water and salt—in which they are pickled. Vegetables are pickled in miso; *shoyu*; *saké* lees, the residual rice and yeast from *saké* making; *koji*, the cultured rice used in both miso and *saké* (see *Making* Koji in chapter 10); and rice bran. "Japanese naturally fermented vegetables tend to have flavors distinctive to one family or shop, or at least to one district, sometimes different from one hamlet to another within the same village," writes Richard Hayhoe, a US-raised American fermentation enthusiast who married a Japanese woman and has lived for many years in Japan. "The flavors tend to have adherents, and are often the result of cultures, recipes, and practices handed down from generation to generation within an extended family, and sometimes subject to quite a bit of debate."

Like fermentation practices everywhere, the traditional methods of Japanese pickling have been in decline; but there is also a revival under way. Eric Haas, a fermentation enthusiast who spent time traveling in Japan, reports:

I was somewhat surprised and saddened by how few people make their own veggies, and how chemical-infused the grocery-store varieties have become. Example: I met one old woman in the middle of nowhere who made pickles according to the traditional style, organic and chemical-free. We got to talking, and it turns out she doesn't like the traditional pickles. She's only been making them for a few years, ever since some man from the big city drove into town and started asking people to make things the traditional way, contracting them out to live the traditional-rural fantasy (that many Japanese seem to be increasingly interested in). She only eats pickles from the grocery store, full of chemicals that "make it taste better." The people I met who were doing the really cool traditional stuff—like fermented veggies—were mainly mid-twenties to mid-forties, disenchanted with the pace of conventional Japanese city-culture, striving hard to make a life for themselves outside of the noise. Sound familiar?

The same countervailing processes are of course happening in the United States, with food traditions being supplanted by homogenized industrial products, then the resulting void catalyzing cultural revival to reclaim those traditions. Don't let food traditions disappear; be part of the culture of revival!

Miso pickles (*miso-zuke*), *shoyu* pickles (*shoyu-zuke*), *koji* pickles (*koji-zuke*), and pickles in *saké* lees (*kasu-zuke* or *nara-zuke*) are all pretty straight-forward, once you create or obtain the medium itself. *Shoyu* pickles are easiest, since it is a liquid. *Shoyu* may be mixed with rice vinegar and/or *saké*, then simply poured over vegetables in a jar. In all the others, with solid pickling media, sliced or whole small vegetables are layered with the medium so that each piece of vegetable is completely surrounded by the pickling medium and not in contact with other vegetable pieces. Like sauerkraut, it helps to keep the vegetables weighed down, although at a small scale they can be made in a jar or other small vessel without weight. The different pickling mediums can also be combined—into, for instance, miso and *saké* lees pickles—and other flavorings, such as *saké*, may be incorporated.

Usually vegetables for any of these pickling techniques are first dried somewhat, through salt pressing (dry-salting vegetables and weighing down for 24 to 48 hours) or air-drying. In this way, there is less dilution of the pickling medium by vegetable juices. Miso pickles are generally fermented the longest, sometimes for years, although they are transformed and delicious after just a few days. As vegetables are harvested from the pickling pot, miso (flavored by the vegetables) may be used in soups, sauces, and other cooking. *Saké* lees pickles are also generally fermented for months or years. *Koji* pickles, which are very sweet, are usually fermented for the shortest time, just a few days to a week. Prior to burying in *koji* (or *amazaké*), vegetables are usually salt-pressed.

The Japanese pickles that I have made the most are rice bran pickles, *nuka-zuke*, because I really love their rich multilayered flavor. For these pickles, vegetables are buried in rice bran, the most nutrient-dense part of the rice, which gets removed in milling white rice. Wheat bran or other grain brans may be used instead or in addition. In the Japanese tradition, house-holds generally purchase whole-grain rice and bring it themselves to a mill, where they specify how much bran to remove. Ten percent would be lightly polished, 30 percent would be typical white rice; the highest-grade *sakés* use rice more than 50 percent milled. Customers go to the mill with a bag of brown rice and return home with two bags: one of rice and one of bran. Find fresh bran if possible, and refrigerate until you make your *nuka* pot, as bran is oily and can go rancid.

I like to gently dry-roast the bran in a cast-iron pan until it becomes aromatic, and then transfer the roasted bran to a crock, which I aim to fill roughly halfway with bran. Then add salt. Recipes I've seen are all over the place on salt, ranging from roughly 5 percent to 25 percent of the weight of bran. I prefer the lower end of spectrum, but as with other vegetable ferments, salt to taste, and remember that it is much easier to add more salt if desired than to dilute it. The uniqueness of each *nuka* pot is the combination of flavorings in the bran. I like to use powdered mustard, strips of kombu seaweed, shiitake mushroom, hot peppers (with stems and seeds removed), garlic, gingerroot, miso, and a little *saké* or beer.

Next, add water. In my recipe in *Wild Fermentation*, I called for quite a bit of water (6 cups/1.5 liters of water plus 1 cup/250 ml of beer) for 2 pounds/1 kg of bran, so that the bran is saturated with water, and water rises when the bran is weighed down, resulting in a wet, sludge-like texture that produces delicious pickles. I've received some feedback through the years that *nuka* is generally much drier than that. "The nuka pickles I saw in people's homes used a much drier medium," writes Eric Haas. I first learned the *nuka* process from Aveline Kushi's *Complete Guide to Macrobiotic Cooking*, and her recipe calls for 2 cups of water per pound of *nuka*, along with weighting the *nuka* so that water rises to the top. Most of the other recipes I have found call for much less water and no weight.

The most detailed information I've found on *nuka* is in Elizabeth Andoh's beautiful book *Kansha: Celebrating Japan's Vegan and Vegetarian Traditions*. Andoh, who moved from the United States to Japan more than 40 years ago, writes that "My neighbors were surprised at first (shocked, really) to discover that I kept pickle pots at all, but have since become willing and enthusiastic 'babysitters'. . . . Cultivating a *nuka* pot has provided me with special access to the lives of many Japanese women—pickle bonding across an otherwise difficult cultural divide."[68] Andoh describes the nuka mix as "a stiff paste," and her recipe calls for using roughly a quarter as much liquid (water along with beer or *saké*) as rice bran, by volume (1¼ cups/300 ml liquid for 1 pound/500 g bran, which measures to 4 cups/1 liter).[69]

Before vegetables are buried in the *nuka* pot, they are generally salt-rubbed in a technique called *ita-zuri*. With coarse salt in the palm of one hand, roll the vegetable around in the salt for a moment, rubbing its skin with the abrasive salt. This begins the breaking down of the skin of the vegetable and the release of fluids. If this causes any foamy white release of bitter compounds from the vegetables (*aku*), rinse them before burying in the pickling medium.

Start out your *nuka* pot by adding just a single vegetable at a time. Make sure the vegetable is completely covered by bran. Smooth out the surface of the *nuka*, and wipe any residual bran from the sides of the vessel. Cover the *nuka* pot with a cloth to allow it to breathe while also keeping flies and dust out. The next day, remove the first piece of vegetable, stir the *nuka* pot with your clean hand, and add another salt-rubbed vegetable. Repeat several times with one vegetable at a time, until the harvested vegetables start to have a distinctive pickled flavor. Andoh calls this "conditioning" the *nuka* paste. "Lapsed time is necessary for the paste to be ready, and rather than leave the pot empty, which would increase the time it takes to get the good bacteria going, you need to add something to it."[70]

Once the *nuka* crock is cultured, you can bury more vegetables in it. They can be whole or chopped into bite-size pieces, and fermented for different lengths of time. Andoh describes her *nuka* rhythm:

> In the spring and fall, an active pot ripens vegetables into flavorful pickles in 8 to 12 hours. I typically put vegetables in my pot after breakfast to enjoy for dinner the same night. When daytime temperatures rise above 80°F/27°C, the vegetables will take only 6 hours (often less) to reach maturity, which means I can put vegetables in the pot in early afternoon and still enjoy them for dinner. If I must be out of the house all day during warm weather, I put the vegetables in the pot the night before, remove them in the morning, and then refrigerate them with the paste still clinging to them. That night, I rinse off the paste and serve them. When temperatures drop below 45°F/7°C, it will take at least 15 hours, or possibly 20 or 24 hours, to achieve a ripe flavor. In the cold months, I add the vegetables to the pot at night after dinner to enjoy the following evening. If the vegetables remain in the nuka paste after they have reached maturity, they turn very sour. *Furu-zuké*, as these "old pickles" are known, have their fans (much like the folks who like very sour dill pickles).[71]

I'm one of those people who love *furu-zuké*. Experiment with length of fermentation and figure out what you like best.

As you harvest vegetables from the *nuka* pot, take care to brush as much of the *nuka* bran as you can from the vegetables back into the crock. With proper maintenance, a *nuka* crock can be used in perpetuity. The key to maintaining a *nuka* pot is to mix it every day. You will need to add salt periodically, since salt absorbs into the vegetables and migrates out with them over time. Other flavorings and the bran itself also need occasional refreshing. If you go away, store the *nuka* paste in the refrigerator.

One final, very special Japanese pickle is *takuan*, whole daikon radishes pickled in rice bran for six months, a year, or longer, yielding delicious pickles with a delicate, earthy quality. To start, hang daikon radishes in the sun to dry for one to two weeks with their tops intact. Hanging them in front of a sunny window is easiest, if possible. If you hang them outdoors, bring them in each evening so they are not wet by dew. As the daikons dry out, they become much lighter and also flexible. Once you can easily bend them, they are ready for pickling. Trim away leaves (save them for the top of the crock) and then roll each daikon root back and forth on a flat surface with your hands and press to soften any hard spots.

Following a recipe posted online by a blogger,[72] I pickled the radishes in 15 percent bran and 6 percent salt, based on the weight of the radishes (much diminished by the drying period). This involved weighing the radishes and calculating and then weighing out appropriate amounts of bran and salt. If you do not have a scale, that comes to roughly 2 tablespoons of salt and ½ cup of bran per pound/500 g of dried radishes. Mix the bran and salt, along with dried persimmon skins (for color), if available, a few pieces of kombu, and some chili pepper or *saké* if desired. Spread a thin layer of the pickling mixture at the bottom of your crock, then a layer of daikons, which can curl and contort with their new flexibility. Stuff any small pockets between daikons with their leaves, aiming to leave as little airspace as possible. Cover the daikon layer with another thin layer of pickling mixture. Then another layer of radishes, another layer of bran pickling mix, and so on, making sure to finish with a layer of the pickling mixture. Cover the top layer with the remaining daikon leaves, then a plate and a heavy weight. Secure a cloth over the top, and leave to ferment in a cool spot for at least a season, or as long as several years.

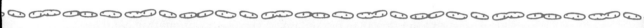

IDEAS FOR COOKING WITH FERMENTED VEGETABLES

◎ Marinate and/or stew meat in them and their brines; the acidity and bacteria help tenderize meat. *Bigos* is a Polish style of stewing meat in sauerkraut; *choucroute garni* is an Alsatian style.

◎ Pancakes: Kimchi pancakes are frequently found in Korean cuisine; incorporate any finely shredded vegetable ferment into savory sourdough pancakes (see *Flatbreads/Pancakes* in chapter 8).

◎ Soup: *Kimchi jigae* (kimchi soup) is a Korean staple. Sauté onions, vegetables, and bite-size pieces of pork belly or other meat, if desired; once the onions and meat are browned, add kimchi and continue to sauté a few minutes. Then add stock, tofu, and soy sauce, and bring to a boil; adjust the seasonings and enjoy. *Shchi* is a comparable Russian soup, made with sauerkraut (or sometimes just unfermented cabbage). Russian cuisine also uses pickle brine (*rassol*) as a soup base, especially for cold summer soups. Beet kvass can be used as base for borscht. Fermented vegetables can be either a central element or a minor flavoring agent in soups, or used as a garnish.

◎ Pierogi, strudels, pies, and dumplings: Sauerkraut is a classic stuffing for pierogi and savory phyllo dough pies and strudels. Similarly, Korean cuisine features kimchi-filled dumplings. In the Balkans, whole fermented cabbage leaves serve as wrappings for *sarma* (stuffed cabbage).

◎ Cakes: Like buttermilk or sourdough, sauerkraut can be used as the acidic element to react with alkaline baking soda in baking. Community cookbooks from areas with histories of German settlement frequently include recipes for sauerkraut cakes.

Cooking with Fermented Vegetables

I have emphasized eating fermented vegetables raw, because I believe that their most profound nutritional benefit is the live bacterial cultures in them, which are destroyed by cooking. Yet in the cultures in which they evolved, fermented vegetables are frequently used in cooking as well. As long as you make sure to eat some of the ferments raw, there is no reason not to enjoy them cooked too.

Laphet (Fermented Tea Leaves)

Laphet (also transliterated as *lephet* and *lahpet*) is an unusual vegetable ferment—leaves of the tea plant (*Camellia sinensis*), pickled to be eaten—from the Southeast Asian nation of Burma. Adele Carpenter, of San Francisco, California, who first brought them to my attention, writes: "They are an extremely delicious salty pickled pulp, served with fried nuts and seeds and lemon as a salad at Burmese restaurants." To make *laphet*, fresh tea leaves are steamed for about an hour, then spread on bamboo mats and hand-mashed. The mashed leaves are then packed into a vessel—traditionally a bamboo-lined pit—heavily weighted to expel air and compress the leaf mass, and fermented from several months to as long as a year.[73] The travel diary of a tea importer explains how to eat *laphet*: "The pickled (sour-tasting) tea leaves are mixed with ginger, garlic, chilis, oil, and salt and all eaten together."[74] My friend Suze sent me a package of *laphet* imported from Burma that she found at a market in Philadelphia. "This stuff is quite honestly one of my favorite dishes of all time," she wrote. I made a salad of lettuce and *laphet*, seasoned as described above. It was an explosion of flavor. The friends I served it to oohed and aahed and returned for another taste. Suze is growing tea on her Alabama farm but has to wait for the shrubs to mature a few years before she can attempt *laphet*.

Troubleshooting

Ferment is or isn't foaming

Don't worry. Foaming is common, especially in the first few days of fermentation. Skim persistent foam off the surface and discard. Foaming slows down very quickly and can be imperceptible. It is entirely possible that you will never notice any bubbles. It's okay.

Ferment develops yeast or mold surface molds

Surface growth is very common. Do not be alarmed. Do not compost your kraut. Skim off the mold as best you can, and don't be concerned if a little of it dissipates. See *Surface Molds and Yeasts* for a lengthier discussion.

Ferment is too salty

Add a little water, mix it around for a moment, and taste. Repeat if necessary. If you need to add a lot of water, pour off the excess. If you add just a bit, treat it as extra sauerkraut juice. In some traditions, vegetables are fermented with lots of salt and then rinsed before eating. Extra salt can preserve veggies longer, but the problem with rinsing is that you also rinse away nutrients and bacteria.

Ferment has a strong odor

Fermenting vegetables emit strong odors. This is normal and generally not a problem. If you or those you live with are bothered by the smell, you can try fermenting in a semi-outdoor ventilated space, provided that it not get wet or excessively hot or cold. Fermenting in jars is another approach. When you release the pressure as described earlier, just do it out the window. Greg Large ferments vegetables in an air-locked vessel, with a plastic tube venting the bubbles that come through the air lock right out the window. "The result was no smell at all in the house and no mold."

A truly putrid smell can indicate a number of problems and is typically accompanied by long-growing, deep-penetrating surface growth of some sort that needs to be removed. Many times, I have removed top layers that were obnoxious and offensive in their smell and appearance from long-fermenting barrels and crocks full of vegetables, only to discover gorgeous, mouthwateringly aromatic, delicious kraut-chi a few inches below.

Ferment is mushy, not crunchy

Unless inhibited by low temperatures, high salinity, tannins, and/or other factors, enzymes in vegetables will eventually, given enough time, break down the pectins that give vegetables their crunchiness. This will happen fastest in watery vegetables like cucumbers and summer squash. But given enough time, especially in conjunction with warm temperatures or low salinity, even cabbage can go soft. It's perfectly safe to eat soft; some people even prefer it that way.

Ferment is slimy, with thick, viscous brine

Sometimes fermenting vegetables develop thick, gooey, viscous, almost ropy brine. In some cases, this is a fleeting stage of development; as successive metabolic processes proceed, the sliminess disappears. In other cases, the batch remains slimy. "The production of slime in sauerkraut has never been thoroughly investigated," according to the *Microbiology of Fermented Foods.*[75] Another technical reference, *Modern Food Microbiology*, states that "slimy kraut is caused by the rapid growth of *L. cucumeris* and *L. plantarum*, especially at elevated temperatures."[76] My experience corroborates the idea that slimy krauts most often develop in warmer-than-ideal fermentation temperatures. Wait for cooler weather and try again.

Ferment turns pink

Pink kraut is great if the color comes from red cabbages, radishes, beets, or fruit. But sometimes kraut from white cabbages turns pink due to a pigment produced by yeasts, typically present in kraut, in an environment in which salinity is greater than about 3 percent. The pink kraut is perfectly safe to eat.[77] In large commercial vats of sauerkraut, improper distribution of salt can result in areas of pink kraut (indicating excessive salt) and areas of soft kraut (indicating insufficient salt).[78]

Maggots are crawling in your ferment

It is imperative to protect food you are aging from flies. Otherwise they will find it and lay eggs on it, and when the eggs hatch, you will find maggots crawling out of your food. I protect fermenting crocks from flies with old sheets or other finely woven cotton fabrics; in the summer months, when flies are most plentiful, I tie a string around the cloth to secure its edges. If you do find maggots in your kraut-chi, there is no need to panic or discard the whole batch. As they hatch on the surface of a ferment, maggots migrate up and out of the food; they do not burrow farther down. Remove the top inch or so of the fermenting vegetables, and go as deep as necessary until you reach kraut-chi with no sign of maggots, no discoloration, and a pleasant aroma. Be sure to wipe the interior sides of the vessel to remove any lingering maggots or eggs. And don't forget to secure a cover to protect the kraut-chi from more flies landing on it.

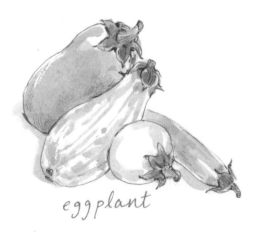

eggplant

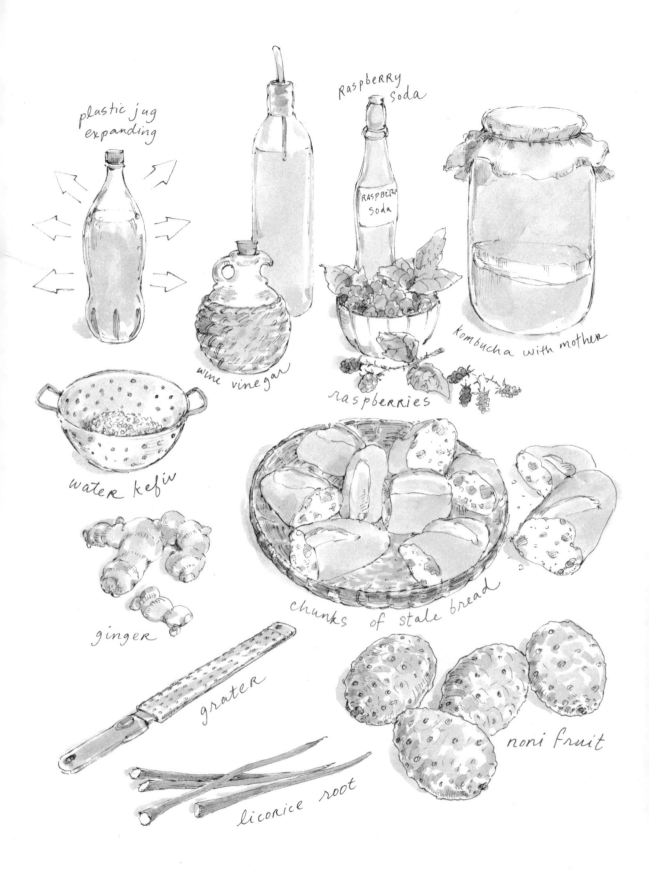

plastic jug
expanding

Raspberry soda

RASPBERRY soda

Kombucha with mother

wine vinegar

raspberries

water kefir

ginger

chunks of stale bread

grater

licorice root

noni fruit

CHAPTER 6

Fermenting Sour Tonic Beverages

S̸our tonic beverages comprise a broad group of ferments that I have only recently begun to conceptualize in a unified way. In *Wild Fermentation*, I included a recipe for sweet potato fly, a lightly fermented beverage from Guyana made with sweet potatoes, in the dairy chapter (because whey was the starter); Russian kvass in the grain chapter; ginger beer in the wine chapter; and shrub in the vinegar chapter. Kombucha, which I had no idea what to do with, ended up in the grain chapter, oddly enough, since it is made with tea and sugar but no grains whatsoever.

Now I can see that all these beverages, and many others—including specific beverages produced in long continuous traditions by peoples around the world, as well as newfangled variations being created by revivalists—are varied manifestations of a common theme: They are tasty beverages, somewhat acidic, somewhat sweet, and in some cases lightly alcoholic, teeming with live lactic acid bacteria (among others), and generally regarded as healthful and tonic. *Tonic*, according to my old *Webster's Collegiate Dictionary*, means "invigorating; refreshing; bracing." This group of beverages—soft drinks, if we may reclaim a corrupted phrase—certainly exhibits those qualities.

Most, but not all, of these beverages require starter cultures of some sort. Once you get them going, they are all self-perpetuating. They make the most sense as a continuous rhythm, in which you keep starting new batches with the previous batch; or, to think of it another way, you keep feeding the culture. I think that for people wanting to incorporate simple natural rhythms into their lives, as well as the health benefits of live bacterial cultures, the sour tonic beverages offer many mouthwatering, thirst-quenching possibilities, and boundless opportunities for experimentation and innovation.

Some starters, such as ginger bug (see *Ginger Beer with Ginger Bug*) or sourdough starter (see *Sourdough: Starting One and Maintaining It* in chapter 8), can be easily started in your kitchen with common ingredients. In other cases, such as kombucha and water kefir, the starters are communities of bacteria and fungi that have evolved into distinctive physical forms, which are large enough for us to see, handle, and transfer from batch to batch. These entities are known as SCOBYs, symbiotic communities of bacteria and yeast, which coordinate their reproduction and produce a shared skin. To enjoy these ferments, you must first obtain the cultures. Fortunately, they grow with use, so enthusiasts are always eager to share them. *Resources* lists a number of international culture exchanges—people with SCOBYs to share, listed geographically—as well as relevant information on commercial sources. An online search will turn up many other sources, both commercial and more informal. After you obtain these cultures and grow them for a while, you are likely to find yourself with an abundance of SCOBYs to share. Spread the cultures, and the cultural revival!

It's hard to say with any exactitude what the alcohol content of any of these beverages may be when you make them. They all have the potential to be at least lightly alcoholic, especially if sealed in a jar, thus favoring anaerobic activity. If you wish to minimize this, in order to make beverages appropriate for children or someone who is avoiding alcohol, ferment for as short a time as possible. This enables fermentation to create carbonation along with probiotic bacteria and limited acidity but forestalls the accumulation of significant alcohol. A small amount of alcohol production, below the legal limit for non-alcoholic beverages of 0.5 percent, is negligible and generally cannot be perceived; common foods and beverages, ranging from bread to orange juice, often contain such traces of alcohol.[1]

Carbonation

All these beverages may be carbonated, if desired. Personally, I love carbonated beverages. Growing up in our time, how could any of us resist the allure of their omnipresence, their insidious marketing, their addictive sweetness and stimulation, and the satisfying sensations of the explosive bubbles going down our throats? Before there were tanks of compressed CO_2 to carbonate sweet syrups into sodas, there was the natural carbonation produced by fermentation.

Carbonation is the release of trapped carbon dioxide. Ferments from open vessels may be lightly effervescing if they are highly active, but if you wish to carbonate a beverage, wait until fermentation is actively progressing (as evidenced by vigorous bubbling), then transfer and seal it in bottles that can hold some pressure, such as bail-top bottles, beer bottles with crimp caps, or soda bottles. Then let the bottles ferment, but only for a short time—in some cases measured in hours, depending upon temperature and level of fermentation activity. Refrigerate and enjoy.

Carbonating sweet beverages can be dangerous! It is imperative that you understand this. A vigorously active ferment trapped in a bottle has the potential to explode. When alcoholic beverages are naturally carbonated, such as champagne or beer, typically the fermentation is completed to the point at which all the sugar has been converted to alcohol. A tiny amount of sugar is then added to "prime" the bottles, enough to create carbonation, but not enough to explode bottles. It's different when beverages are bottled only lightly fermented, with a good proportion of sugars still intact, as these tonic beverages are typically enjoyed. The remaining sugar has considerable potential to ferment and produce CO_2 once bottled, leading to the possibility of excessive carbonation, which can be dangerous. Bottling must be done with care and attention.

This is not meant to scare anyone, just to create awareness. Moderate carbonation enhances and enlivens these tonic beverages. High-pressure carbonation results in wasted beverages and explosive bottles. Wasted beverages are sad, but no big deal. Recently, my friend Spiky opened a bottle of our friend Gonoway's ginger beer at a swimming hole on a hot day.

> On the hot country roads, then hiking down into the river gorge, I looked forward to the moment I'd pull it out of the bag and surprise our friends with it. The moment came, and I popped the top. It thudded like a big marching-band drum, and a geyser of ginger beer shot up over our heads. What a thrilling sight! Collectively, like kindergartners, everyone groaned. I suppose we might feel grateful that the glass hadn't exploded in my bag, but we could only stare at the puddle of ginger beer on the rocks—almost the entire contents of the bottle—with dismay.

Watching your fermented beverage spew all over may feel tragic, but exploding bottles can hurt, disfigure, or even potentially kill people. Missouri fermentation enthusiast Alyson Ewald made water kefir "fruit beer" from grape juice, bottled it in glass bail-top bottles, and set them on top of her refrigerator (a warm microclimate) to ferment overnight. Alyson awoke around 7 AM to the sounds of bottles exploding. Her partner Mark was standing near the fridge, and their daughter Cole was 10 feet away. Alyson reports:

> Everybody was unscathed, though Mark had tiny glass crystals scattered across his bare back. There were glass splinters on every surface in the house, not to mention grape soda. We found chunks of glass the size of marbles on the other side of the bed and across the sheets, a good 30 feet from the explosion. It is utterly miraculous that we didn't even bleed, even as we mopped and wiped and swept it all up for the next two hours. . . . Maybe someone will avoid a hospital trip because of our experience.

I have also heard the stories of people who were not so lucky. Rhode Island fermentation enthusiast Raphael Lyon writes: "A few weeks ago, a friend of ours was seriously injured by an exploded glass bottle of what was some kind of ginger beer or root beer . . . pretty much all bombs unless really carefully watched or refrigerated."

Part of the problem is that it is difficult to gauge the pressure building in glass bottles. One traditional way of gauging carbonation is to add a few raisins to each bottle of a ferment you are seeking to carbonate; as the contents of the bottle carbonate, the raisins float to the top. In my practice, I have come to bottle these still-sweet fermenting beverages mostly in plastic soda bottles. Even if I bottle most of them in glass, I bottle some in plastic. The benefit of plastic bottles, in this context, is that you can feel how pressurized they have become by squeezing the bottle and gauging resistance. If the plastic bottle easily yields, it has not pressurized; if it is firm and resists pressing in, it has pressurized and should be refrigerated before more pressure builds, or enjoyed quickly.

Another safety measure I recommend is to wrap your bottles of fermenting sweet beverages in towels to buffer any potential explosion. To minimize mess and reduce losses of beverages to spewing when bottles are opened, chill bottles before opening, and open them over a clean bowl in a sink so the bowl can catch at least some of the beverage if they spew. Begin by opening bottle gradually, and if you see a large quantity of foam start to rise, screw the cap back down and wait a moment. Then begin to open again, and as foam rises tightly close. Repeat this process a few times, until the beverage is no longer so pressurized, and you can open without spewing foam. Carbonation enhances these beverages in moderation, but in excess it results in waste and dangerous explosions. Be careful!

Ginger Beer with Ginger Bug

Ginger beer is a classic flavor of homemade soda. It can be made lightly gingered, like most commercial ginger ale, or as spicy as you can take it, using lots of ginger. A ginger bug is a simple ginger beer starter (it can also be used as a starter for other beverages) made from ginger, sugar, and water. Ginger beer can also be made with many different types of starters; see *Water Kefir* and *Whey as a Starter*.

A ginger bug could not be easier to start: Grate a bit of ginger (with skin) into a small jar, add some water and sugar, and stir. Stir frequently, and add a little more grated ginger and sugar each day for a few days, until the mixture is vigorously bubbly. Gingerroots are rich in yeasts and lactic acid bacteria, so ginger bugs usually get bubbly quickly. However, many people have reported that their ginger bugs never get bubbly. My theory is that most of the ginger imported into the United States has undergone irradiation, thus destroying its bacteria and yeast. Foods marketed as organic cannot be irradiated (according to the US Department of Agriculture's organic standards), so for best results make ginger bug with organic ginger, or ginger from a known, non-irradiated source.

Once your bug is vigorously bubbly (or you have one of the other starters), prepare a ginger decoction that will become your ginger beer. I like to make a concentrated decoction that cools to body temperature as it is later diluted with cold water. To make such a concentrate, fill a cooking pot with water measuring about half the volume of ginger beer you wish to make. Add finely sliced or grated ginger, using 2–6 inches (5–15 cm) of gingerroot (or more) for each gallon/4 liters of ginger beer you are making (though only half this volume is in the pot). Bring to a boil, then gently simmer the ginger, covered, for about 15 minutes. If in doubt about how much ginger to add, experiment. Start with a smaller amount, taste after boiling (and diluting), and if a stronger flavor is desired, add more and boil another 15 minutes.

After boiling the ginger, strain the liquid into an open fermentation vessel (crock, wide-mouth jar, or bucket), discarding the spent ginger pieces (or leave the ginger in and strain later). Add sugar. I usually use 2 cups of sugar per gallon (of target volume, still requiring more water), but you might like it a little sweeter than I do. Once sugar is dissolved in hot ginger water, add additional water to reach the target volume. This will cool your sweet ginger decoction. If it feels hot to the touch, leave it a few hours to cool before adding ginger bug or other starter. If it feels no warmer than body temperature, go ahead and add ginger bug or other starter. Add a little lemon juice too, if you like. Stir well. Cover with a cloth to protect from flies and leave to ferment in the open vessel, stirring periodically, until the ginger beer is visibly bubbly, anywhere from a few hours to a few days depending upon temperature and the potency of the starter.

Once your ginger beer is bubbly, you can bottle it. If you wish to minimize alcohol content, bottle it quickly, and give it a short time to ferment in the bottle. If you prefer a more alcoholic brew, leave it to ferment for several days before bottling. Observe daily and bottle after bubbling has peaked and begun to slow down. Either way, in bottling, *always* be aware of the possible dangers of overcarbonation. Leave bottles to ferment at ambient temperatures until they become carbonated. Gauge carbonation with a plastic soda bottle. When it resists squeezing between your fingers and no longer yields easily, it is carbonated. Refrigerate bottles to cool and prevent further carbonation. Ginger beer will continue to slowly ferment (and pressurize) in the refrigerator, so enjoy it within a few weeks.

I've also made starters from other similar rhizomes, specifically turmeric and galangal, with wonderful results. I made raw soft drinks with each of them by placing grated roots into a bottle with light sugar water, and leaving to ferment about a week. Sparkly and delicious!

Kvass

Kvass is a lovely, refreshing, effervescent sour beverage usually made from old bread. It is traditional in Russia, Ukraine, Lithuania, and other countries of Eastern Europe, where mobile kvass wagons can still be found, especially in summertime. Kvass is so iconic in this region that other types of sour beverages are also called kvass—beet kvass, for instance, or tea kvass, a name for kombucha. According to Elena Molokhovets, author of the 1861 Russian cookbook *A Gift to Young Housewives*, at that time drinking kvass was "a culture-laden act that helped to define one's Russianness."[2] Similarly, today in Russia, kvass is being marketed with an appeal to nationalistic pride. An Internet blogger translated a Russian news report: "Local drink producers advertise their products as patriotic alternatives to Western drinks. One of them even chose a patriotic name: Nikola, alluding to *ne kola* [not Cola]. In the last year they even launched an 'anticolanization' campaign against colanizing Western soft drinks."[3]

The only starter needed to make kvass is a sourdough starter, easy to start from flour and water (see *Sourdough: Starting One and Maintaining It* in chapter 8). If your starter is not vigorously bubbly, feed and stir it for a few days before you start your kvass. Or you can use a packet of yeast to start kvass instead.

The primary ingredient in kvass is bread, usually old, dry, and hard bread (though fresh bread works fine too). Traditionally, kvass is made primarily from rye bread, but bread from wheat or other grains can be used. Periodically the scavengers in my life show up with big bags of discarded loaves. Bakeries often give away their bread at the end of each day; and supermarket Dumpster divers often find bagged loaves past their "best by" date. Chop bread into large chunks, and dry in a warm oven for about 15 minutes. Meanwhile, boil water, enough to cover the bread.

I usually start kvass in an open ceramic crock, but a large cooking pot works fine for the pre-fermentation stage. Once the bread is dry, transfer to a vessel. Add a little dried mint or other herbs. Pour boiled water over the bread and mint, enough to cover all the bread. The bread will float and rise with the water level, so press down to gauge when you have added enough water. Leave a plate on top of the bread to weigh it down and keep it submerged. Cover the crock with a cloth to keep flies off, and leave overnight.

In the morning, strain and press the liquid from the bread solids. The way I accomplish this is by lining a colander with a few layers of cheesecloth. I scoop the soggy bread from the crock into the colander, then as it fills I gather the corners of the cheesecloth together, twist and wring out the liquid, and then knead the ball of cloth-encased soggy bread from different angles, trying to force out liquid. I squeeze as much as I can (not necessarily every last bit), then dump the spent bread, place the cheesecloth back in the colander, and continue until all is strained.

Then I measure the liquid (less than the water you added, as it is impossible to press it all out), transfer it to an appropriate-size jar or crock, and for each gallon/4 liters add a pinch of salt, about ½ cup/125 ml of honey or sugar, the juice of a lemon, and ½ cup/125 ml sourdough (or water kefir or a packet of yeast), and stir thoroughly. Cover the kvass mixture with a cloth and leave to ferment a day or two, stirring when you can.

Once the kvass is bubbling vigorously, it is ready to bottle. Bottles will pressurize rapidly; review the earlier recommendations and cautions for

stale bread

carbonating sweet beverages. Often in less than 24 hours my bottles of kvass have become highly carbonated. A traditional way of gauging the carbonation of kvass (like the other carbonated beverages described previously) is to place a couple of raisins in each bottle, which rise to the top as the kvass carbonates. Once bottles of kvass are carbonated, transfer to the refrigerator to slow continued carbonation. Enjoy kvass as a refreshing beverage, or use as a base for cold summer soups like *okroshka*.[4] If you get into a rhythm of regular production, you can leave out the sourdough starter and use some bubbly kvass as the starter for the next batch. Any of the beverages in this chapter can be self-perpetuated in this way.

There are many other sour tonic beverages enjoyed around the world based on grains. Many indigenous beers, covered in chapter 9, are sour as well as mildly alcoholic. Others are included in chapter 8 on fermenting grains and starchy tubers. I have included kvass here because it is so unique, so different in technique from most other grain ferments, and so iconic as a sour beverage.

Tepache and Aluá

Tepache is a Mexican soft drink, historically made from corn, but in its contemporary manifestation usually made from fruit. *Aluá* is the name for a very similar group of lightly fermented beverages enjoyed in northeastern Brazil. Making these is essentially the same as starting a fruit-infused wine—sugar water plus fruit, as detailed in chapter 4—only it is fermented more briefly. "Various fruits such as pineapple, apple and orange are used," reports the UN Food and Agriculture Organization on *tepache*. "The pulp and juice of the fruit are allowed to ferment for one or two days in water with some added brown sugar. . . . After a day or two, the *tepache* is a sweet and refreshing beverage. If fermentation is allowed to proceed longer, it turns into an alcoholic beverage and later into vinegar."[5] One popular flavor of both *tepache* and *aluá* is pineapple, made by simply mixing pineapple peels in sugar water. Mix sugar water to taste, using sugar as little refined as you can find, or honey or other sweeteners. In tropical heat, 24 hours of fermentation typically suffices; in cooler temperatures, fermentation will take several days. Evaluate by tasting. After a brief fermentation it is bubbly and light; a few more days and it gets more alcoholic; a few more and it starts to be very vinegary.

Karen Hurtubise of North Carolina has a raspberry farm and makes a raspberry soft drink exactly this way, which her kids call "raspbubble." Karen dissolves 1 cup/250 ml of honey in 3 quart/liters of water and adds a quart/liter of fresh raspberries. She ferments the mix for about three days before transferring to the refrigerator. She says her kids prefer it to commercial soda.

Typically, *tepache* is prepared as a wild fermentation without any starter beyond the raw fruit. Sometimes granules called *tibicos* or *tibis* are used, the same or functionally similar to water kefir grains (see *Water Kefir*).

FRUIT KVASS

Hannah Springer, from her blog at www.healthyfamilychronicles.blogspot.com, and inspired by Dr. Natasha Campbell-McBride, author of Gut and Psychology Syndrome

Pick out a combination of fruit, berries, and fresh herbs or spices that you think would go well together, and get started. In a 1-quart/liter wide-mouth mason jar combine the following (be sure to use organic ingredients for the best fermentation results):

⊙ A big handful of berries

⊙ One sliced "core" fruit (such as apple or pear)

⊙ A tablespoon of grated ginger

⊙ ½ cup/125 ml raw-milk whey

⊙ Enough filtered water to fill the jar

Combine all ingredients, top off with water, place a weight of some sort on top of the fruit to keep it submerged, and close tightly. Keep on the counter in a warm-ish place for three days, before transferring to the fridge. You can top off the bottle with filtered water and a splash of whey when it gets low, until the fruit is all used up.

This recipe can be varied by using different fruits, citrus juices, fresh herbs, or even vegetables.

Mabí/Mauby

Mabí, also known as mauby, is a tonic beverage popular on some of the islands of the Caribbean, made from a sweetened decoction of the bark of a tree also known as *mabí*, or in English soldierwood (*Colubrina elliptica*). One account of the etymology of the name *mabí* is that it comes from Creole for the French *ma biere* (my beer).[6] I first heard about *mabí* from Norysell Massanet, who lives in Puerto Rico and mailed me some *mabí* bark to experiment with and provided some guidance:

> Although I found several recipes for mabí on the web (they all call for cinnamon and ginger, and I just couldn't find those flavors in my taste buds' memory), today I spoke with the Mabí Lady, at our organic market in San Juan, who only uses the bark and sugar, and she said something that made sense to me: "You have to try it and it is in the process of making it that you will develop your own recipe." Beautiful!

> Norysell worried that I would not be able to make *mabí* without mature *mabí* as a starter, but starters are largely interchangeable, so I tried using

water kefir as a starter and produced a delicious, bubbly beverage. Compounds in the *mabí* (saponins) hold the bubbles and produce a foamy head. The bittersweet flavor of *mabí* really spoke to me, but never having tasted anyone else's *mabí*, I had no reference point.

Then in 2010 I was invited to teach at the Virgin Island Sustainable Farming Institute on the island of St. Croix, and at the Saturday-morning market there I was thrilled to finally encounter *mabí*, though on St. Croix and other Anglophone islands it is mostly known as mauby. The mauby was dark and bubbly, produced in small batches as an informal cottage industry, and sold in recycled juice and liquor bottles, bulging with pressure. I bought a couple of bottles from a St. Croix mauby maker, who allowed me to photograph her but refused to divulge the specific spice mix in her recipe: "A woman's got to have her secrets," she told me.

I was able to bury a small bottle of *mabí* in my luggage, and I have been making *mabí* the traditional way ever since, using mature *mabí* as the starter. A friend brought me some more *mabí* bark, purchased at a convenience store in Alabama, and I found a source on the Internet where I was able to purchase a 5-pound/2.3 kg bag. I boil a handful of the bark in water for about half an hour, usually alone, sometimes with star anise, ginger, cinnamon, nutmeg, or mace. Then I add sugar and more water, to taste. Because of the bitterness of the *mabí* bark, I make it pretty sweet; I'd recommend 3 cups of sugar per gallon/4 liters as a starting point, and adjust to taste. Norysell recommends using muscovado sugar, although I have mostly used evaporated cane juice. My friend Brett Guadagnino talked to a mauby maker in the British Virgin Islands who added a pinch of salt. One Internet recipe I found, posted by Cynthia, a Guyana-born woman transplanted to Barbados, called for making a *mabí* concentrate by boiling *mabí* bark and other spices in a small quantity of water, then adding that to a gallon of sugar water.[7]

Like all fermentation traditions, *mabí* varies in its particular details. Once the mix cools to body temperature, add the starter and stir. At least that's what I do. Cynthia's recipe uses no starter whatsoever, but describes how to "brew" the *mabí*: "Using a large cup, dip into the mixture, fill the cup and then pour it back into the container. Do this for at least 3 minutes." Ferment the *mabí* a few days, stirring or "brewing" periodically. Once the *mabí* gets bubbly, bottle it, and allow it to ferment another day or two, until the bottles become pressurized. Refrigerate and serve chilled for a refreshing, bubbly, bittersweet treat.

Water Kefir (aka *Tibicos*)

Water kefir is one of many names used to describe a versatile culture that can be used to ferment any carbohydrate-rich liquid. I usually use it to ferment sugar water with some fruit in it for flavor, but I've also used it to ferment honey, fruit juices, coconut water, and soy, almond, and rice milks. The culture—also known as *tibicos* or *tibis*, sugary water grains, Tibetan crystals, Japanese water crystals, and bees wine—is a SCOBY, a symbiotic community of bacteria and yeast, which appear as small whitish translucent granules and grow quickly when fed regularly. Water kefir is not directly related to kefir, the ancient culture from the Caucasus Mountains used to ferment milk. It would seem that because they are similar in form, people perceived them as related, even though they are distinctly different. A study of the microbial flora of sugary kefir grains found that they "consisted chiefly of lactic acid bacteria and a small proportion of yeasts."[8] One particular bacterium, *Lactobacillus hilgardii*, was found to produce the polysaccharide gel that forms the home of the fermenting community.

Fermenting with water kefir is extremely simple. Typically, I mix sugar water, to taste, in a wide-mouth glass jar. Try 2 cups of sugar per gallon/4 liters of water as a starting point, but many people prefer to ferment a sweeter solution. To that I add the water kefir grains (about 1 tablespoon/15 ml per quart/ liter) and usually a small amount of fresh or dried fruit, and ferment usually for two to three days. The vessel can either be sealed airtight, or loosely covered to allow air circulation. Water kefir does not need oxygen, but it's not inhibited by it. After about two days, I remove the fruit (typically floating at the top), strain the fermenting solution through cheesecloth to remove water kefir grains, and transfer the fermented solution into sealable bottles. Then I prepare a new sugar solution for the grains and seal the bottles of fermented water kefir, leaving the sealed bottles to carbonate as they continue to ferment at ambient temperatures for another day or two, monitoring the pressure and moving pressurized bottles to the refrigerator to prevent overcarbonation. Water kefir color will shift with different sweeteners and added ingredients, as will growth rates and grain sizes.

water kefir

Like any SCOBY, water kefir requires regular attention, feeding, and care. Typically it should be fed fresh sugar every two days— in cold spaces, every three days. Left too long unfed in acidic solution, the organisms that compose the grain will die, and the grains themselves will literally pickle. Water kefir works best if you can get into the rhythm of a regular routine. If you go away, leave water kefir grains in a fresh sugar-water solution in the refrigerator. If you go away for longer than a couple of weeks, they may not survive, so you might want to have someone feed them periodically. You may also dry water kefir grains for long-term storage (or as a backup), either in the sun or in a dehydrator. Store dried grains in the refrigerator for longest survival. People have also reported freezing water kefir grains for storage of up to several months; to do this simply rinse the grains, pat them dry, and freeze in a sealed bag.

Water kefir will ferment any type of sugar, or other sweeteners, such as honey, maple syrup, agave syrup, rice syrup, or barley malt. Stevia and other non-carbohydrate sweeteners will not ferment. Many people ferment coconut water using water kefir. Coconut milk and nut, seed, and grain milks can also be fermented in this way. Herbal infusions or decoctions can be sweetened and fermented with water kefir. Fruit juices, provided they are not too acidic, can also be fermented by water kefir. Missouri fermentation enthusiast Alyson Ewald describes her water kefir practice of fermenting pure grape juice: "The grape juice ends up completely explosive, like champagne." Her family calls the fermented fruit juice fruit beer. "Like root beer, only made from fruits instead of roots; and because, like root beer, it's basically a soda or soft drink, albeit an oh-so-slightly and deliciously alcoholic one. Fruit beer. Rolls right off the tongue." For highly acidic juices, such as pineapple or citrus juices, dilute a small proportion of juice (around 25 percent) with sugared water.

Water kefir can be used to ferment many different types of sweet liquids. One I tasted was coffee-flavored! Try herbal elixir ferments with sweetened sun teas, infusions, and decoctions. Be aware that it can be difficult to separate water kefir grains from teas and small bits of plant material, and that some herbs with antimicrobial compounds may inhibit the kefir grains. Fermentation enthusiast Favero Greenforest of Washington developed an innovative two-stage system in which he maintains the grains themselves in sugar water with just a slice or two of fruit, which he calls the "starter" and feeds every couple of days. He then adds the starter to various other sugary solutions. "In a gallon-size jar, I make a sugar solution and add whatever fruit I want to use, then add the starter solution, leaving the kefir grains in the starter jar. That way I keep track of them and they don't get lost. The resulting ferment works great, and I don't have to worry about losing the SCOBYs."

Various factors can influence the growth rate of the water kefir SCOBY. Dominic Anfiteatro, an Australian fermentation enthusiast whose website[9] is the Internet's most comprehensive source of information about all forms of kefir, has documented 48-hour water kefir SCOBY weight increases ranging from 7 percent to 220 percent. Dom recommends adding ginger to increase growth, and using less refined forms of sugar, or adding molasses. He also observes that mineral-rich "hard" water promotes water kefir SCOBY growth, while distilled water, or water purified using an activated carbon filter, can retard growth. If hard water is not available, Dom recommends adding ⅛ teaspoon of baking soda per ½ gallon/2 liters. Another mineralizing idea of Dom's is to add a small amount of crushed eggshells, limestone, or ocean coral to the fermenting solution. Too much, however, can cause the development of a slimy texture in the water kefir.

The more traditional name of water kefir appears to be *tibicos*, a Mexican culture. According to some reports, *tibicos* are derived from the fruits of cacti in the genus *Opuntia*. Ethnobotanist William Litzinger reports that "*Tibicos* commonly are found to develop naturally beneath the epidermis of ripe cactus fruits, and in the residue left in the fermentation vessel shortly after the main portion of a batch of wine [*colonche*] is removed."[10] I've tried this without success; but then, I

Raspberry soda

RASPBERRY soda

raspberries

was not working with freshly picked fruit, so I am not ready to disregard this information, from a source I have generally found to be thorough and reliable. It could be that only the fruit of a particular *Opuntia* variety produces these masses, or some other specific condition.

In 1899, the *Journal of the Royal Microscopical Society* published a report on the culture (recorded as *tibi* grains) in which M. L. Lutz describes them as:

> spherical transparent masses resembling boiled rice-grains. These vary in size from a pea to a pin's head. They ferment sugar-water and produce a light agreeable beverage. Microscopical examination shows that the tibi grains are composed of bacilli . . . and yeasts. . . . The fermentation occurs only by the co-operation of the two organisms, either alone being insufficient.[11]

Evidently, Lutz and probably others before him brought the *tibi* grains back home, and they have continued to spread and be propagated. Exchange, migration, and adaptation can render origins extremely murky. The 1978 book *Life of Yeasts* describes the "*tibi* konsortium" as being Swiss:

> This popular Swiss drink is a sour, weakly alcoholic, carbonated liquid, made by fermentation of a 15% cane sugar solution to which dried figs, raisins, and a little lemon juice have been added. The inoculation is done by adding a number of tibi grains. These consist of a capsulated bacterium and a yeast that live symbiotically. The combined action produces lactic acid, alcohol, and CO_2. The tibi grains multiply during fermentation and can be transferred to a subsequent batch.[12]

It took me a long time to figure out that water kefir is *tibicos*. There are other similar cultures, such as "ginger beer plant," so named and used in England. Ginger beer plant (GBP) was a subject of scientific investigation and an 1892 report in the *Philosophical Transactions of the Royal Society of London*. The author, H. Marshall Ward, describes the microbiology of the ginger beer plant but confesses to be utterly clueless as to its origins:

> Professor Bayley Balfour states: "it is said the Ginger-beer Plant was introduced into Britain by soldiers from the Crimea, in 1855;" but so far as I can discover this was mere conjecture, and it is not to be taken as an accepted piece of history. Dr. Ransome informs me, in a letter dated April, 1891, "some say it was brought from Italy," but this, again, I have failed to substantiate more definitely. The whole question as to whence it was first derived, in fact, is enshrouded in mystery.[13]

For a while, I had come to the conclusion that GBP was also *tibicos*, and that both were the same thing as water kefir. Then my friend Jay Bost, an ethnobotanist very interested in fermentation who had recently been given *tibi-cos* by a friend in Mexico, sent me a link to the website yemoos.com, which was selling cultures of both *tibicos* and ginger beer plant. I wrote to them to inquire about how distinct the two cultures really are. "We've noticed many differences," explained Nathan and Emily Pujol, the couple who propagate the cultures and run the site:

> Both respond very differently to the same recipe (using control tests etc.). . . . Also both have a much different appearance to the discern-ing eye—GBP being more round, murky and much tinier, tibicos being more jagged, clear and quite a bit larger. We've also noticed that with the occasional "odd-ball" grains, tibicos will always be exceptionally large and triangular, whereas GBP will form an almost spiral torpedo shape. I have never seen either form the shape of the other—it seems very specific to the culture.

Indeed, when Nathan and Emily sent me samples of the two cultures, I could plainly see that visually they are quite distinct. I now believe that the first "water kefir" grains I was given were actually ginger beer plant, and only later, after those had died of neglect, did I get *tibicos*, though without seeing them side by side I did not notice a difference. Functionally, the major differ-ence between the two cultures seems to be that the *tibicos* ferment faster than the ginger beer plant, and need to be fed more often.

Another place where similar SCOBY granules are reported is Sudan. Hamid Dirar, author of *The Indigenous Fermented Foods of the Sudan*, describes a fermented honey beverage in Sudan called *duma*, fermented using grains known as *iyal-duma*. "The grains are visible to the naked eye and have flattened and irregular shapes, varying in diameter from 2 to 6 mm [up to ¼ inch]," reports Dirar.[14] They consist of both yeast and bacteria, in an elabo-rate configuration. Under microscopic examination: "The yeast were noticed to be invariably surrounded by tangles of a chain-forming, heavy slime-producing, fat bacterial rod. The long chains of the bacterium, encapsulated in thick slime, actu-ally engulfed each of the yeast cells and seemed to keep the yeast aggregate together."[15]

ginger

Duma is produced by different families as a cottage industry. Dirar writes: "The grain line owned by each family has descended from past generations of the family to the present generation as a business secret not to be relin-quished to strangers. Each family claims that its grains are better fermenters of duma than those of other families." Many brewers claim that duma grains only derive from previous duma grains, while "others describe ways and means by which the grains can be raised from natural sources," usually roots of the *dalieb* palm (*Borassus aethiopum*) in honey water.[16]

Perhaps you have access to *dalieb* palms or *Opuntia* cacti and figure out how to obtain grains from them. Perhaps in some wild fermentation you will find a precipitate and then discover that it grows and ferments, as the pioneer developers of all these cultures presumably did in the speculative prehistoric past. Otherwise, you will have to obtain water kefir (or ginger beer plant, or *tibicos*; not *duma* so far as I have found) grains from commercial sources or from people who are already using them (see *Resources*). Regular use of these grains results in rapid proliferation. Everyone working with them ends up with more grains than they know what to do with. There are people out there with water kefir grains, and many other cultures, willing to freely and enthusiastically share them. When you find fellow fermenters who can provide you with desired cultures, make an effort to build relationships of sharing information and mutual aid. The Internet can be a powerful resource for networking, with online trading posts and many opportunities to post messages to targeted groups of people with similar interests. Use your quest for water kefir grains and other cultures as an opportunity to make connections and build community. The bacteria and yeasts are the primary actors in fermentation, but their growth and spread are the result of human actions and interactions. Be creative and persistent in your cultural revival efforts.

Whey as a Starter

Whey is the thin liquid that separates from curds when milk curdles or sours. The curds are coagulated fats and other solids. Whey is a nutritive by-product of cheesemaking, as well as yogurt and kefir making. (Dairy fermentation is addressed in chapter 7.) For our present purposes, whey can be used as a starter for naturally carbonated sodas and other sour tonic beverages. It can be produced in many different ways, but if produced by means of heat, it will not contain live cultures. Whey derived from cultured- or raw-milk products without high heat is, of course, populated by abundant microbial communities.

The most vigorously active whey starter is from kefir (dairy kefir, not water kefir), because the kefir community includes yeasts as well as lactic acid bacteria. In the first day of fermentation, kefir typically does not curdle, but after two or three days it does, with milk fats floating to the top, then eventually sinking. Before consuming kefir, typically I shake the jar to reintegrate the curds and whey; but if you want to use the whey, gently pour some off. It makes the most vigorous starter when it is freshly fermented, though it can be stored in the refrigerator for weeks or months.

To ferment a beverage using whey, simply add whey to the beverage base in a proportion of roughly 5 to 10 percent by

draining whey from curds

whey

volume. So for a quart/liter, use about 2 to 3 ounces (¼ cup) or 50 to 100 ml of whey. The beverage base can be sweetened water with fruit; a sweetened herbal infusion or decoction; or fruit juice. Mix whey into the sweet liquid you wish to ferment, and leave to ferment about 24 hours, until the beverage is bubbly, then transfer to sealable bottles and seal. Leave sealed bottles at room temperature another 24 hours or so, until pressurized, then refrigerate. As always, beware excess pressure and avoid explosions! Serve chilled.

Roots Beer

A traditional root beer is a sweetened and fermented decoction of flavorful plant roots. Contrary to the commonly known singular "root" beer, various roots have been and can be used. As a matter of fact, mixing together more than one type of root yields a better flavor than a single root alone. My friend Frank Cook reported that when he visited Jamaica he encountered (plural) roots beers, containing the roots of many different plants, rather than singular root beer.

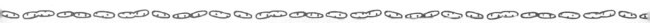

ELROY'S JAMAICAN ROOTS BEER

Frank Cook

Jamaica is famous for its roots beers made by Rastafarian bushmen. During my journey there I had several opportunities to slow down with bushmen and learn a bit about the process they use in making their brews and the plants they incorporate. When making the brews, the bushmen used a range of different plants, and the number of ingredients was significant to them energetically. I did not learn the deeper meanings behind this, but I understood that certain numbers were important to the bushmen.

One bushman, Elroy, I feel indebted to for slowing down and letting me take in how he brewed. He went out and harvested a bunch of plants including Jamaica's second most famous plant, Jamaican sarsaparilla root. I recognized about half the plants he used. They included (Latin names when known are in parentheses): Jamaican sarsaparilla (*Smilax*) root; strongback (*Cuphea*) root; shuteye marker (*Mimosa*) plant; dandelion (*Senna*) plant; coconut (*Cocos*) root; guava (*Psidium*) root; vervain (*verbena*) plant; chainy root; bloodwrist plant; hug-me-close root; tan pan root; jack saga root; long liver; cold tongue; dark tongue; dog's tongue; search-me-heart; soon-on-the-earth; God's bush; devil has whip; water grass; raw moon.

Elroy fills a pot with all this, adds water, and then he splits open five green bananas and lays them across the top for iron. He cooked all this on an open fire for two hours. Then he added honey and poured it into bottles. In about three days one could start drinking them and they would be good for a week or so (if they lasted that long!) before they turned to vinegar. I tried a number of different ones when I was there and enjoyed their vitality and flavors.

In my own roots beer practice, I have brewed root mixes that revolve around sassafras, because it has a pleasant flavor and is abundant in the woods where I live. But I always add other roots, most often ginger, licorice, and burdock. Sarsaparilla (*Smilax regelii*) is another traditional ingredient. I encourage you to experiment with proportions and other combinations. Decide how much roots beer you want to make (your target volume), and measure half that amount. Boil roots in measured water to create a concentrate. The advantage of boiling the roots in only half the water is that it's easy to cool, by adding the remaining water cold. After boiling roots for at least an hour, add sugar. I usually use 2 cups of sugar per gallon (based on the target volume), but you might like it a little sweeter than I do. Once sugar is dissolved in the hot root decoction, add the remaining half of the water cold, to reach target volume. Taste and add sugar if necessary. Adding water will cool your sweet decoction. If it still feels hot to the touch, leave it a few hours to cool before adding starter. If it feels no warmer than body temperature, go ahead and add starter. Starter can be water kefir, ginger bug, whey, yeast, or a previous batch of roots beer.

Ferment a day or two, until the mixture is vigorously bubbly, then transfer to bottles, seal, and ferment another day or two until bottles are pressurized. Then chill to slow continued fermentation (always heeding the caution against overcarbonation and explosions) and enjoy.

 ## *Pru*

Pru is a tonic beverage from Cuba. It is made from a variety of botanical sources, most commonly a mixture of several, including *Gouania polygama* bark and stem, *Pimenta dioica* (allspice) fruits and leaves, and *Smilax domingensis* or *Smilax havanensis* rhizomes. A team of ethnobotanical investigators describe its preparation as follows:

> Stems of *G. polygama* are cut lengthwise in two or four parts, thus exposing the inner wood; sometimes the bark is peeled away. The stems should be fresh and used for one decoction only. The rhizome of *S. domingensis* is cut into little pieces (*ruedas*) that can be boiled two or three times, while the leaves of *P. dioica* should be dried and can only be used once. During the day, the roots, stems and leaves are steeped in a large pot for about two hours until the water comes to a boil (some *pruzeros* turn off the fire when the water starts boiling while others leave the pot for another 10 or 15 minutes and then turn it off). Then, vegetal parts are removed and the decoction is strained two or three times through a cloth (some use a woolen cloth) and left all night to cool. In the morning, sugar and a fermentation starter (called *madre*) are added to the decoction, which then must be stirred with a wooden spoon to obtain rapid and homogeneous fermentation. *Madre* is previously fermented *pru* that is two to three days old that has an unpleasant vinegar-like taste. It probably contains bacteria, fungi

and/or yeasts responsible for the fermentation process. All *pruzeros* use it as a starter to enhance fermentation and to speed-up the production process since, without madre, *pru* making would take 72 hours instead of 48. Each time that pru is produced, producers store the *madre* necessary for the next fermentation process. According to the data collected, traditionally *pru* was not prepared with *madre*: it is now widely used. . . . After the addition of sugar and *madre*, *pru* is stored in bottles which are tightly capped and put into the sun (in a patio or on the roof of a house) all day long to ferment. . . . The complete consensus of our informants about the importance and necessity of fermenting *pru* in capped bottles may represent an adaptation to "modern" food habits of the Cuban population: the resulting effervescence makes *pru* seem more like an industrial soft drink.[17]

Traditionally, *pru* has been produced and consumed only in eastern Cuba. After the 1991 collapse of the Soviet Union and the ensuing economic crisis in Cuba, "industrial soft drinks disappeared from shops and homes, to be replaced by locally available traditional beverages. Thus, *pru* spread westward" and is now available throughout Cuba.[18]

Sweet Potato Fly

Sweet potato fly is a really wonderful traditional tonic beverage from Guyana, on the northern coast of South America. It's a big hit whenever I make it. I've made sweet potato fly using various starters, including water kefir, whey, and ginger bug. The major ingredients are sweet potatoes and sugar. For a gallon/4 liters, I use two large sweet potatoes and 2 cups/500 ml of sugar. You may like it a little sweeter. Grate sweet potatoes into a bowl; then remove starch by covering the grated sweet potato with water, stirring, and pouring off now cloudy water. Repeat until the water pours off clear.

You could just cover the grated sweet potato with a gallon of water, mix in sugar to taste, and add starter to make a simple fly. Or you can dress it up a bit. I learned to make sweet potato fly incorporating lemon, eggshell, and what I call the Christmas spices: cloves, cinnamon, nutmeg, and mace. For a gallon, use one or two lemons, juice and grated rind. The mace is cooked into water; bring about a teaspoon of mace (fresh or powdered) to a boil in a couple of cups of water. Then remove from the heat, cool by adding cold water, and add to the sweet potato mix. Add a few whole cloves and a pinch each of ground cinnamon and nutmeg. The eggshell seems to neutralize sourness, and, as noted in the water kefir section, encourages starter growth if you are working with water kefir grains. Clean an eggshell, crush into small pieces, and add to mix.

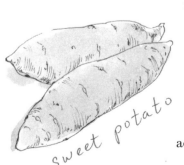

sweet potato

Culture sweet potato fly with whey, ginger bug, or water kefir. If you use water kefir, note that if you add the grains it will be very difficult and tedious to separate them from the grated sweet potatoes. Either use sugar water cultured with water kefir grains rather than the grains themselves, or use cheesecloth to create a tea-bag-like enclosure for the water kefir grains, for easy removal.

Ferment the sweet potato fly for a day or two; then, after the mix is good and bubbly, you can strain into sealable bottles. Leave sealed bottles at ambient temperatures another day or two, until the bottles become pressurized; then refrigerate before they get overcarbonated and potentially explosive.

Inventive Soda Flavors

Sweet potato fly, ginger beer, roots beer, fruit beer—indeed, any of these tonic beverages can, when carbonated, be thought of as natural sodas. There is no flavor that cannot be made into a carbonated beverage. The basic formula is sweetened water (with sugar, honey, agave, maple, sorghum, fruit juice, or any carbohydrate sweetener) plus flavoring (fruit, herbs, essential oil), plus culture, fermented for a short time, then sealed in a bottle and fermented for a little more time until pressure builds, indicating carbonation.

Here are a few flavors people who have written to me raved about:

- ◎ Carrot juice fermented with ginger. "It was just about the most delicious drink I've ever had," writes Mike Ciul of Philadelphia.

- ◎ Ginger, cinnamon, clove, nutmeg, and molasses fermented with water kefir "make a lovely gingerbread-flavored soda-like thing," writes Bev Hall of Hillsboro, Tennessee.

- ◎ Pine needle: When Erin Newell WWOOF-ed in Japan, she stayed on a farm where a pine cider called *mitsuya* was served every day. "It's made by stuffing a jar full of pine needles and then topping it up with sugar water." Add a starter to this infusion and bottle it, and you get a pine-flavored soda.

- ◎ Coconut water goat kefir: "I mixed some of my fermented coconut water with goat kefir [see chapter 7] and added a few berries and let sit overnight," writes my friend Destin Joy Layne of Brooklyn, New York. "It's fizzy and creamy and absolutely delicious!"

- ◎ Three Stone Hearth, a "community-supported kitchen" in Berkeley, California, makes natural sodas in many unusual flavors, including "antique rose" and several different hibiscus combinations.

- ◎ "Honeysuckle, blueberry-lemon verbena, lemon-rosemary, and strawberry-rose geranium are favorite fermented herbal soda flavors," of April McGreger, who ferments vegetables commercially in Carrboro, North Carolina, and still experiments for fun.

Experiment, invent, go wild! Just beware the dangers of overcarbonation.

NISHANGA'S SODA FLAVORS

Nishanga Bliss is an acupuncturist and nutritionist in the San Francisco Bay Area, who authored the book *Real Food All Year* (New Harbinger 2012). Nishanga has also been teaching classes in fermenting natural sodas, and she sent me this list of some of her favorite flavors:

- Hibiscus and Schizandra, with and without Rose Hip
- Goji Berry and Rose Hip
- Elderberry, Goji Berry, and Hibiscus
- Strawberry and Scarlet Queen Turnip
- Lemon and Rosemary
- Blackberry and Hibiscus
- And a client has made her own, by prescription from me for heartburn symptoms, fresh Calendula Flower and Bee Pollen

Nishanga says: "I usually use evaporated cane juice or honey for the sweetener. For starters, I've been using yogurt whey, water kefir grains, encapsulated probiotics (!), and most recently, ginger-turmeric bug. Adding fresh grated turmeric root to ginger bug gives it a lot more bubble power (sometimes too much), but if you use half the amount of ginger in the bug it doesn't alter the flavor much."

Smreka

Smreka is a wonderful light juniper berry soft drink from Bosnia that I learned about from Luke Regalbuto and Maggie Levinger, who traveled around Eastern Europe seeking hands-on education with traditional fermentation methods (and now sell fermented foods and beverages in the San Francisco Bay Area as Wild West Ferments). Luke and Maggie encountered *smreka* at a particular establishment they happened into in Sarajevo. "*Smreka* did not seem to be widely consumed around Bosnia," they wrote to me. They believe the place where they had it was Muslim-owned because the "*smreka* was served in lieu of any sort of alcohol." The *smreka* they were served was cold out of the fridge, with a heaping spoonful of sugar. (I enjoy mine unsweetened at room temperature, and with some carbonation from being sealed in a bottle.) "When we inquired about the beverage and its contents they just kept saying '*smreka*' (which means juniper berry) as if that was the only ingredient, which seemed preposterous to us, as it tasted so dynamic and delicious, and there appeared to be something else in there (white stuff at top of bottle) but indeed it is just the juniper and some sort of yeast (wild of course)."

Smreka could not be easier to make. All you do is add juniper berries to water in a jug or jar, no sugar at all. I have picked juniper berries in the western United States and used them in sauerkraut. I've made *smreka* with dried juniper berries I bought from a bulk herb supplier, and it worked fine. Most junipers, including the common *Juniperus communis*, produce berries that are tasty and safe to use; a few species, notably the Eurasian *J. sabina*, produce berries that are regarded as toxic. If you harvest juniper berries from a new place, taste one before you harvest a bunch, and spit it out if the taste is harshly bitter. Only use berries with a mild, pleasant flavor.

I use 2 cups/0.5 liter of berries for 1 gallon/4 liters of water. Cover with a cloth, or cap loosely to allow pressure to release; alternatively, cap tightly and relieve the pressure every few days, yielding a carbonated beverage. Leave this to ferment about a month, less in hot weather. The berries float to the top, slowly infusing color and flavor into the water, and beginning to bubble. Shake or stir a couple of times a week. Within about a week, the *smreka* develops a lovely light flavor; as a few weeks pass, the fermenting action builds in vigor. "When all the berries have sunk to the bottom the *smreka* is ready," according to Luke and Maggie,[19] though I typically start enjoying mine sooner, and then give them a second go-round of water, less this time, to just cover the berries.

Noni

Noni is the fruit of the tropical tree of the same name, Latin name *Morinda citrifolia*, native to Southeast Asia. It is believed to have traveled to Hawai'i with the earliest Polynesian settlers. Ripe *noni* has an intensely cheesy flavor. Throughout its range, *noni* is used medicinally and as a dye. As a food, in Hawai'i and elsewhere, *noni* fruits were primarily famine food, otherwise fed to pigs; in other places, they were more commonly eaten. The Latin name *Morinda* is derived from *morus*, Latin for "mulberry," and indeed the fruit roughly resembles a mulberry in shape. In Hawai'i, where I have encountered *noni*, it is frequently used medicinally. "Traditionally, Hawaiians used medicinal *noni* primarily topically, not internally, and considered the plant to have cleansing properties—of the blood, intestines, and other body systems," according to an anthropological account.[20] I developed a staph infection when I visited Hawai'i and used a topical poultice of *noni* to successfully treat it.

In contemporary Hawai'i, fermenting a *noni* beverage has become a widespread household practice, although whether or not it is traditional is a matter of some dispute.[21] "At present the most popular 'traditional' means of preparing *noni* in Hawai'i is fermentation," report a team of ethnobotanists. "Typically the fruit is sealed in a large glass jar, which is left out in the sun for hours, days, or weeks."[22]

Noni fruits are hard and white when first picked but rapidly transform into translucent fruits dripping with juice. This signifies that fermentation has begun! To do this yourself, simply place fruits into a jar. Seal the vessel to limit air circulation, but do release pressure occasionally. Gradually, the vessel will

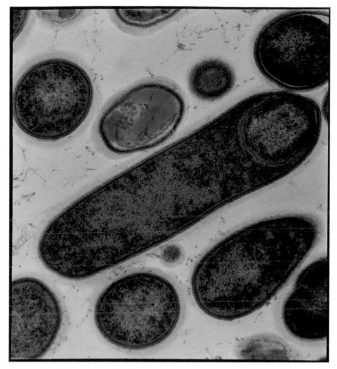

Scanning electron microscope image of *Clostridium botulinum*.
© Photo Researchers, Inc.

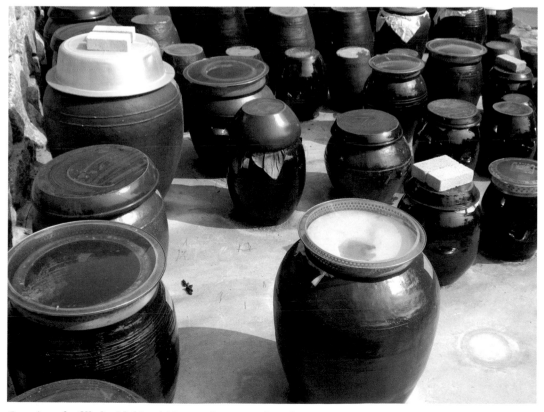

Onggi crocks filled with kimchi in Seoul, Korea. Photo by Jessieca Leo

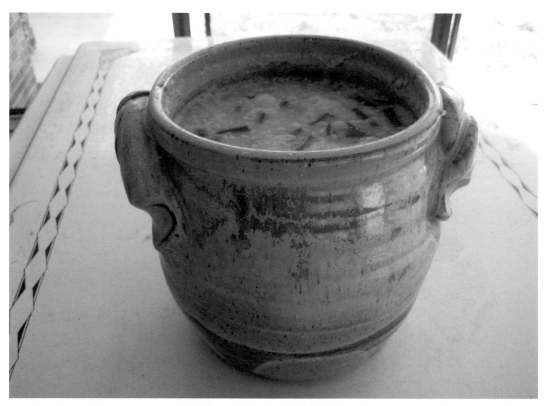

Handmade crock by Jeremy Ogusky, of Jamaica Plain, Massachusetts.

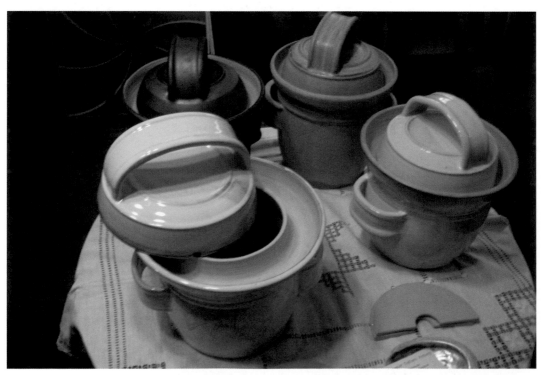

Handmade crocks by Sarah Kersten, of Berleley, California, in the style of the famous German Harsch crocks with moats that fill with water to create a water lock and prevent fresh air from entering the fermentation chamber, and semi-circular weights to keep contents submerged.

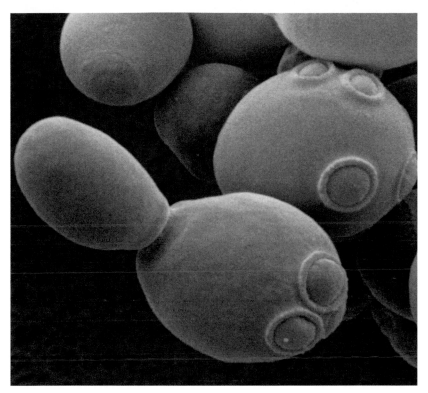

Scanning electron microscope image of *Saccharomyces cerevisiae*.
© Photo Researchers, Inc.

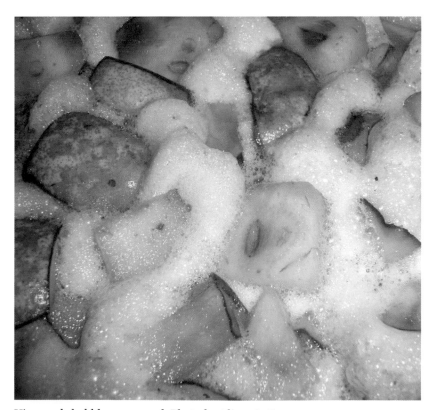

Vigorously bubbly pear mead. Photo by Alison LePage

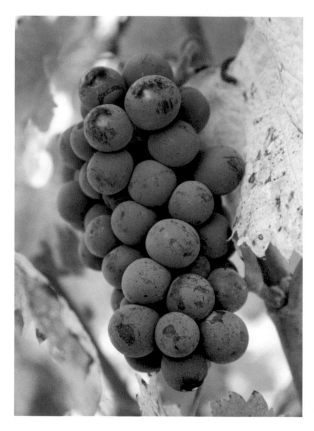

Frequently the yeast "blooms" on grapes and other fruits are visible as a white chalky film on the skins of the fruits. Photo by Timothy Bartling

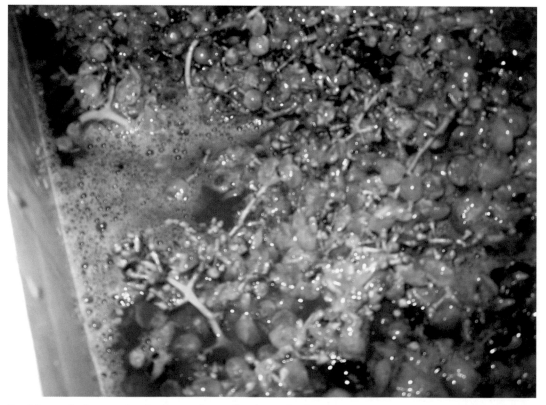

Freshly crushed grapes beginning to foam after just a few hours.

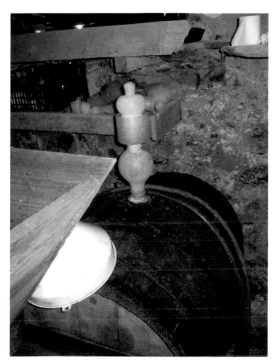

Wine fermenting in an air-locked barrel.

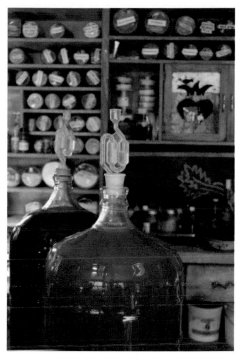

Country wines from blueberries (left) and peaches (right); ferments from different fruits yield a gorgeous rainbow of hues. Photo by Sean Minteh

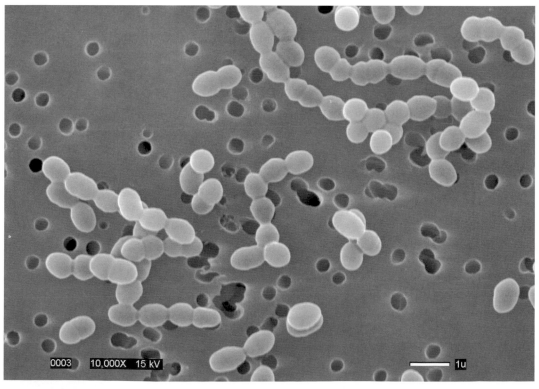

Scanning electron microscope image of *Leuconostoc mesenteroides*. Photo by USDA/ARS Food Science Research Unit at NC State University, Raleigh, NC

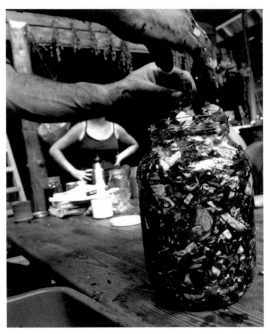

Stuffing shredded and salted vegetables into a jar. Keep stuffing until vegetables are submerged. Photo by Devitree

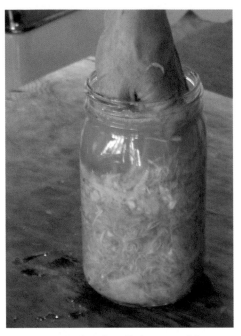

Keep pressing hard until the vegetables are submerged. Photo by Debbie Palmer

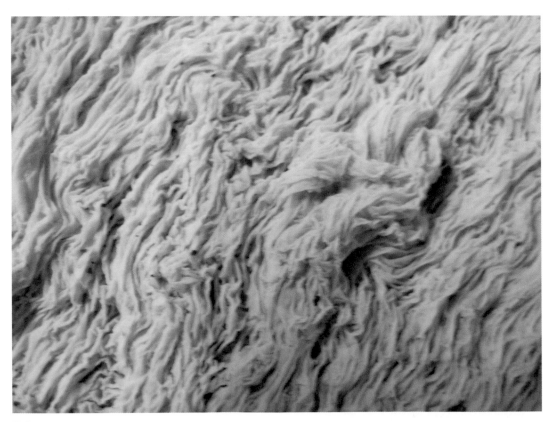

Kahm yeast.

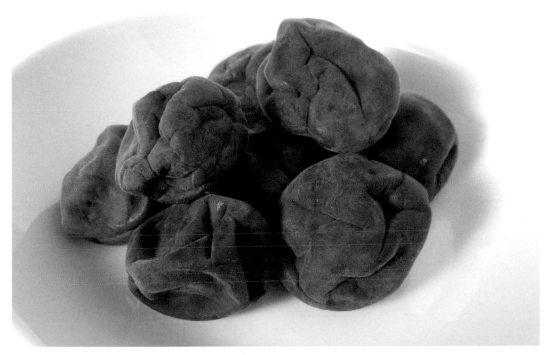

Umeboshi plums. Photo courtesy of Wikimedia Commons

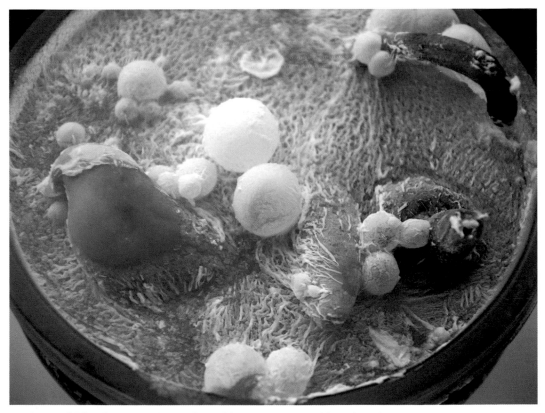

Surface mold developing on the surface of fermenting vegetables. Photo by Anoop Kapur

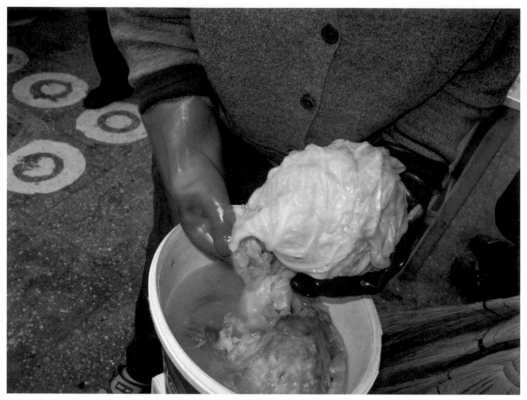

Whole cabbages fermented in brine, from a market in Romania. Photo by Luke Regalbuto and Maggie Levinger

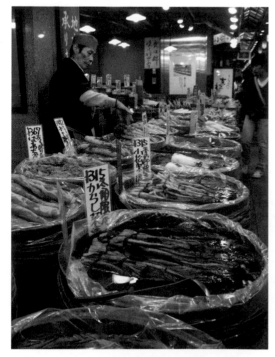

Different styles of fermented vegetables on display at a Japanese pickle market. Photo by Eric Haas

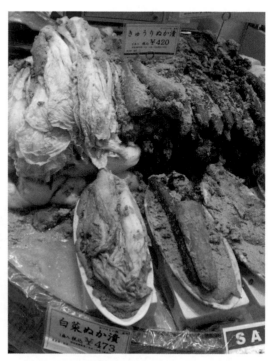

Nuka-pickled vegetables in a Japanese market. Photo by Eric Haas

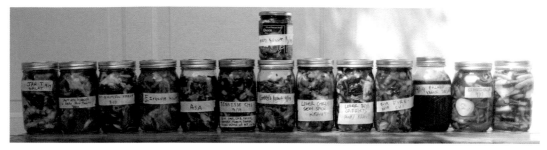

Jars of mixed vegetable kraut-chis produced by students at one of the author's workshops.

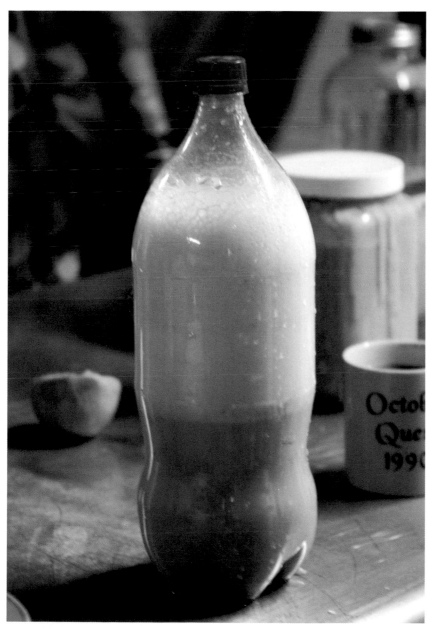

Lots of bubbles after opening a highly carbonated bottle of kvass. Photo by Timothy Bartling

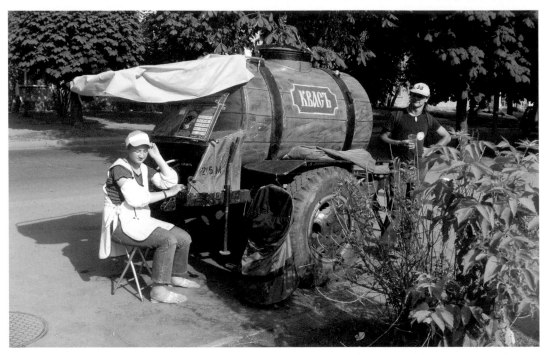

My friend Ellery, pictured at right, at a kvass wagon in Lithuania. "The cart was busy as hell, and people were filling up empty soda bottles, glass jars, and thin plastic cups. It was about five cents a cup."

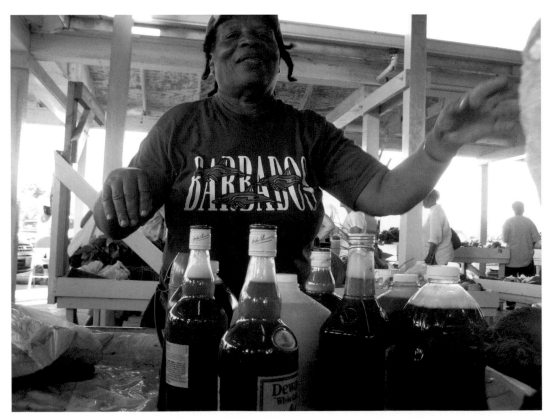

A mauby maker at a St. Croix (US Virgin Islands) market. The home-brewed ferment was sold in recycled juice and liquor bottles.

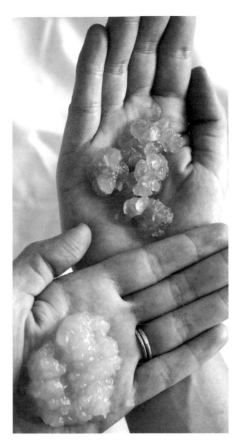

Tibicos (upper) and ginger beer plant (lower) side by side. Photo by Yemoos Nourishing Cultures, www.yemoos.com

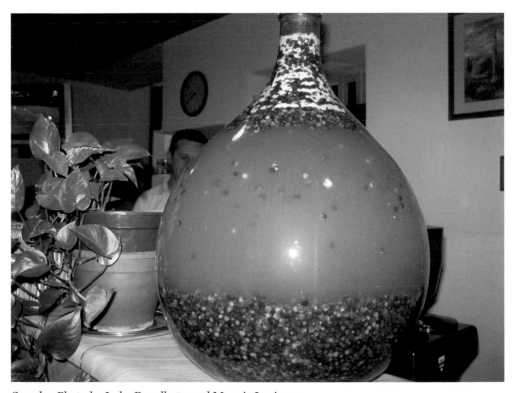

Smreka. Photo by Luke Regalbuto and Maggie Levinger

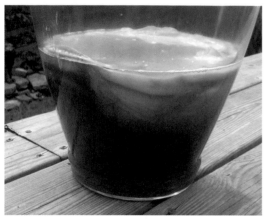

Kombucha mother floating in fermenting kombucha. Photo by Billy Kaufman

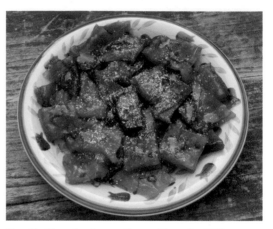

Candied kombucha mothers. Photo by Billy Kaufman

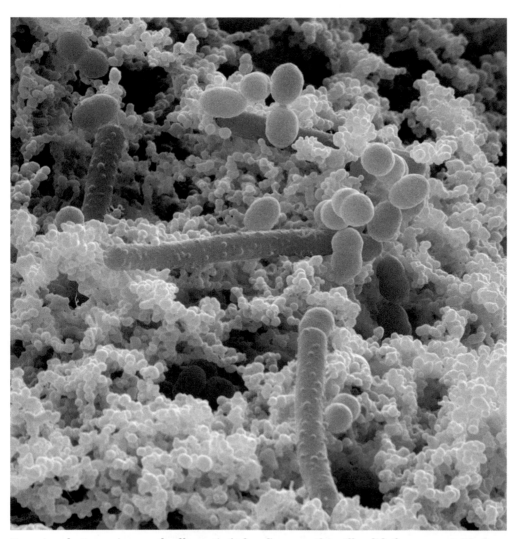

Scanning electron micrograph of bacteria (colored) among the milk solids from yogurt. The long rod-shaped bacteria are *Lactobacillus delbrueckii* subsp. *bulgaricus*; the shorter, rounder bacteria are *Streptococcus salivarius* subsp. *thermophilus*. Photo by Power & Syred

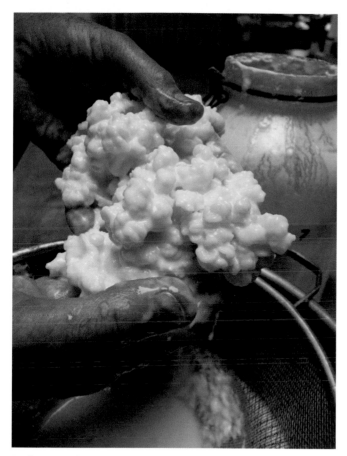

Kefir grown by vintner Lou Preston in California. Photo by
Lou Preston

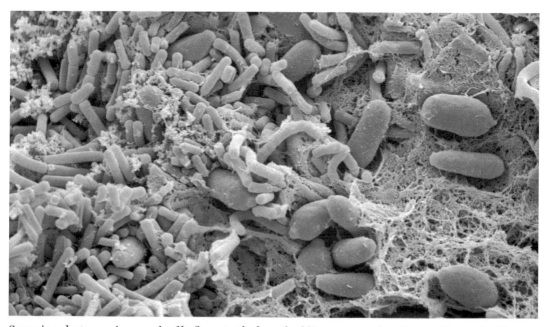

Scanning electron micrograph of kefir; note the large budding yeasts and various rod bacteria. Photo
by Milos Kalab

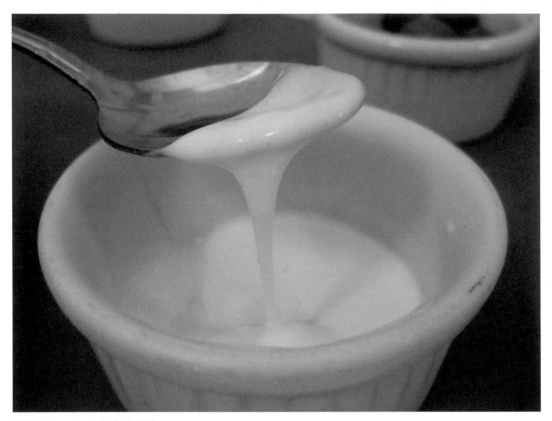

Viili. Photo by Rebekah Wilce

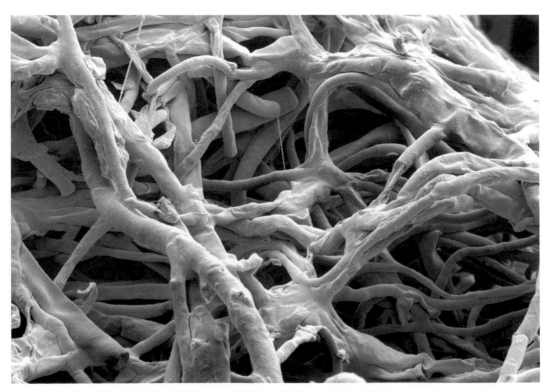

Brie cheese fungal hyphae (*Penicillium* spp.). Photo by Power & Syred

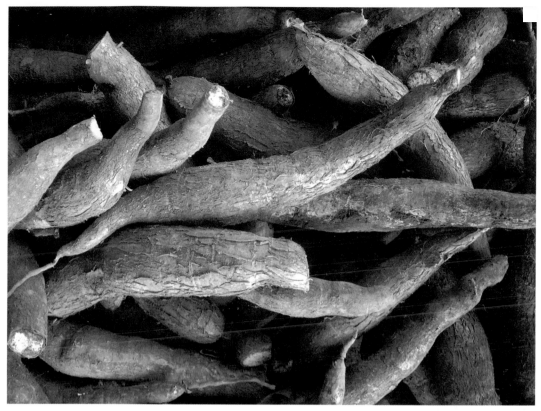

Cassava roots. Photo courtesy of Wikimedia Commons

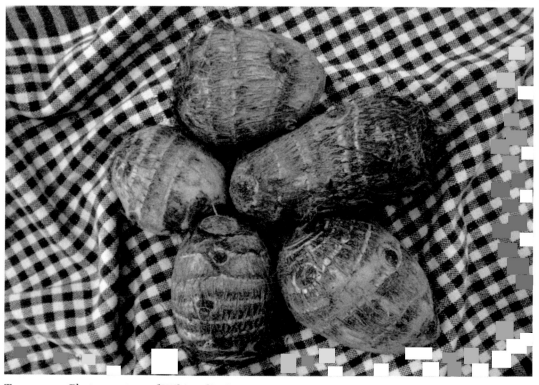

Taro corms. Photo courtesy of Wikimedia Commons

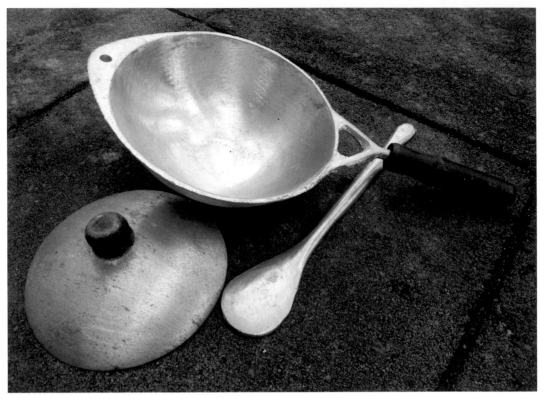

Woklike hopper pan, called a "China chatty." Photo by Jennifer Moragoda

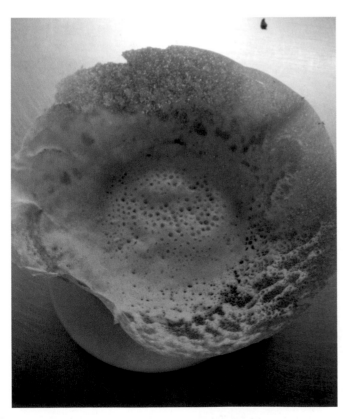

Hopper. Photo by
Jennifer Moragoda

contain more juice and less solid remnants of the fruits. "The juice appearance is initially an amber or golden colored liquid that gradually darkens with age," according to University of Hawai'i's *Noni* website. "*Noni* juice is produced under a wide range of temperature and light conditions in Hawai'i. For example, many backyard *noni* juicers place a large glass jar with *noni* fruits out in the direct sun for many months before consuming the juice."[23] Fermentation time varies from days to months. Fermented juice is drained from solids and enjoyed as a sour tonic. "The presence of fermenting vessels on countless *lanai* (porches) and rooftops across neighborhoods island-wide is taken as an affirmation of *noni*'s efficacy, at the same time that it evokes a sense of community—a key element in the success of complementary medicines."[24]

Kombucha: Panacea or Peril?

Kombucha is sugar-sweetened tea fermented by a community of organisms into a delicious sour tonic beverage, sometimes compared to sparkling apple cider. Kombucha is typically produced by a SCOBY, also known as a *mother*, that takes the form of a rubbery disk, which floats on the surface of the tea as it ferments. The community of organisms can also be transferred via the kombucha liquid itself, which can generate a new SCOBY. The kombucha mother closely resembles a vinegar-making by-product, mother-of-vinegar, and is composed of many of the same organisms; indeed, some analysts have come to the conclusion that they are exactly the same.[25]

No other ferment even approaches kombucha in terms of its sudden dramatic popularity (at least in the United States). Kombucha has enjoyed acclaim in many varied locales, widely promoted as beneficial to health, notably in Central and Eastern Europe over the course of the last century, and its use has been growing in the United States since at least the mid-1990s. I first tried kombucha around 1994, when a friend of mine with AIDS started making and drinking it as a health practice. It was touted as a general immune stimulant, though claims of kombucha's benefits have been extraordinarily varied and broad. In those days, kombucha was not commercially available in the United States, but it spread exclusively through grassroots channels as enthusiasts grew more and more mothers and sought to share them. Today there are dozens of commercial enterprises manufacturing and selling kombucha—ranging from small start-ups to multinational corporations. In 2009, a leading US brand, GT's Kombucha, sold more than a million bottles,[26] and *Newsweek* reports that between 2008 and 2009, US kombucha sales quadrupled, from $80 million to $324 million.[27]

Kombucha has inspired much polarized debate, with claims of dramatic curative properties matched by dire warnings of potential dangers. My own conclusion is that both sets of claims tend to be exaggerated. Kombucha is neither panacea nor peril. Like any ferment, it contains unique metabolic by-products and living bacterial cultures that may or may not agree with you. Try some, starting with small servings, and see how it tastes and feels to you.

Many enthusiasts regard kombucha as something of a miracle cure-all. Harald W. Tietze, an Australian promoter of kombucha, writes that he has received reports of kombucha being used to effectively treat disorders including arthritis, asthma, bladder stones, bronchitis, cancers, chronic fatigue syndrome, constipation, diabetes, diarrhea, edema, gout, hay fever, heartburn, high blood pressure, high cholesterol, kidney problems, multiple sclerosis, psoriasis, prostate disorders, rheumatism, sleeping disorders, and stomach and bowel disorders.[28] Herbalist Christopher Hobbs recorded the following additional claims from discussions on an Internet bulletin board: Kombucha is said to cure AIDS, eliminate wrinkles and remove liver spots, reduce hot flashes during menopause, and help muscle aches, joint pains, coughs, allergies, migraine headaches, and cataracts.[29] While people suffering from each of these conditions may indeed feel that their conditions improved by drinking kombucha, "there is no scientific data to back up any of these claims," writes Hobbs.[30] We cannot expect foods to be panaceas.

One common explanation for the healing power of kombucha is that it contains glucuronic acid, a compound produced in our livers, which binds with various toxins for elimination. Günther Frank, a German promoter of kombucha's health benefits, explains: "Kombucha does not target a specific body organ but, rather, influences the entire organism positively by . . . the detoxifying effect of its glucuronic acid."[31] Unfortunately, repeated laboratory analysis has found that glucuronic acid is not actually present in kombucha. Possibly it has been confused with a related compound that is a metabolic by-product of glucose, gluconic acid, which is commonly found in ferments and other foods. In 1995, a small group of kombucha enthusiasts began investigating kombucha chemistry through laboratory testing. One of them, Michael R. Roussin, explains: "Conflicting reports of the ferments' contents, along with a warning from the FDA, prompted me to take a closer look at what I was drinking."[32] After performing mass spectral analysis, specifically looking for glucuronic acid, on 887 different samples of kombucha, the group concluded that the compound was not present.[33]

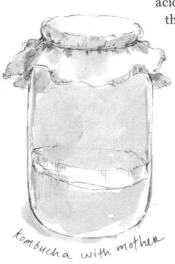

Kombucha with mother

As for kombucha's potential danger, in 1995 the US Centers for Disease Control (CDC) publication *Morbidity and Mortality Weekly Report* ran a story headlined, "Unexplained Severe Illness Possibly Associated with Consumption of Kombucha Tea," with *possibly* being the operative word. In two separate incidents, weeks apart, two women in Iowa had very different unexplained acute health episodes. One of them died. Both drank kombucha daily and made it from the same original SCOBY. The Iowa Department of Public Health immediately issued a warning to stop drinking kombucha "until the role of the tea in the two cases of illness has been evaluated fully." But they were never able to explain how kombucha may have been related to the illnesses, and 115 other people were identified who drank kombucha from the same mother without problems. When the mothers and the kombucha that possibly made the women sick were subjected to microbial analysis, "no known human pathogens or toxin-producing organisms were identified."[34]

Other medical reports have associated extremely varied symptoms with kombucha consumption, also without identifying any specific toxicity or causative factor.[35] Responding to a flurry of questions following the CDC report, the US Food and Drug Administration (FDA) issued a warning of sorts, cautioning that the acidity of kombucha could potentially leach lead or other toxins from vessels, and that "home-brewed versions of this tea manufactured under non-sterile conditions may be prone to microbiological contamination." However, like other investigations, FDA microbial analysis found "no evidence of contamination."[36]

Concern about kombucha's safety has not been limited to government regulators. Mycologist Paul Stamets published an article in 1995 called "My Adventures with 'The Blob.'" Because kombucha was mistakenly referred to as a mushroom, Stamets received frequent questions about it. As an expert in propagating and investigating isolated fungal species, a largely uninvestigated mixed culture worried him. "I personally believe it is morally reprehensible to pass on this colony to sick or healthy friends when, to date, so little is known about its proper use," he writes. "Making Kombucha under non-sterile conditions becomes, in a sense, a biological form of Russian Roulette."[37] While I have tremendous respect for Stamets's work with fungi, I reject the notion that making kombucha at home is random or dangerous. All of the ferments, kombucha included, involve creating selective environments to ensure success. The idea that kombucha (or any ferment) is safe only in the hands of technical experts denies the long lineages of home and village production that spawned them and plays right into the disempowering cult of specialization. Make sure you understand the parameters of the selective environment you need to create, and you are not playing Russian roulette. Basic information and awareness are important. Empowered with them, you may ferment without fear.

 ## Making Kombucha

Kombucha is usually just sugar-sweetened tea, fermented by a specific community of bacteria and yeasts. Increasingly, creative kombucha makers have been giving kombucha exciting new twists by adding herb, fruit, or vegetable flavors. Typically these flavorings are added to kombucha for a secondary fermentation following a primary fermentation of just tea and sugar.

By tea, I mean an infusion made from the tea plant (*Camellia sinensis*), not the infusions of other plants (such as chamomile or mint) that in the English language we also describe as teas. You may use black tea, green tea, white tea, kukicha, pu-er, or other styles of tea, but in general stay away from Earl Grey or other heavily flavored or scented teas, as the added essential oils may inhibit fermentation. You may use tea bags or loose tea, and brew the tea strong or weak, as you like. I typically brew a very strong concentrate, then dilute and cool it by adding water, so I can add the SCOBY without having to wait for the tea to cool.

To sweeten the tea, add sugar, meaning sucrose from sugarcane or sugar beets. Some people have reported excellent results making kombucha using honey, agave, maple syrup, barley malt, fruit juice, and other sweeteners; others have had their SCOBYs shrivel up and die. Similarly, some people report excellent results without any tea whatsoever, using herbal infusions or fruit juices as the sole flavorings. This leads me to the conclusion that there are divergences on the kombucha family tree. Just as some people, animals, and plants can adapt better than others to altered conditions, some kombucha mothers exhibit greater flexibility and resilience than others. I would encourage you to experiment with different sweeteners and flavorings if you like, but don't use your only mother. Use one layer of the SCOBY to experiment, while maintaining the other in the traditional sugar and tea medium. Try for a few generations, to make sure the mother grows and continues to thrive. The amount of sweetener may vary with your taste. Personally, I never measure the sugar, simply adding to taste. Try about ½ cup/125 ml (by weight 4 ounces/113 g) of sugar per quart/liter. Stir well to dissolve; this is easiest if the sugar is added to the tea while still hot. Taste and adjust the sweetness as desired.

Cool the sweetened tea to below body temperature. As described earlier, making a tea concentrate and diluting it with cold water is a fast way to do this. Place sweetened tea into a wide-mouth fermentation vessel, ideally glass or ceramic (with a non-lead glaze). Avoid metal vessels, even stainless steel, which may corrode in the prolonged presence of acids. Because kombucha is an aerobic process, in which fermentation occurs on the surface where oxygen is available, it is best to use a wide vessel only partially full, so as to maximize surface area in relation to volume.

To the cooled sweetened tea, add some mature kombucha, at a ratio of about 5 to 10 percent of the volume of the sweet tea. This both acidifies the tea and contributes kombucha organisms. Acidification is important for maintaining a selective environment that favors the kombucha organisms and prevents potential contaminants from developing. (If for some reason you do not have any mature kombucha to use as an acidifier, use vinegar of any kind, but in a much smaller proportion—about 2 tablespoons/30 ml per quart/liter.) Once you have combined cooled tea, sugar, and mature kombucha in the fermentation vessel, add the mother.

Ideally, the mother will float at the surface. Sometimes it will sink at first, then slowly float back up. Other times one edge of it will float to the surface and generate a new film over the surface. If your SCOBY fails to float or generate a new film after a few days, it is no longer viable. If your SCOBY is a different size or shape from the surface of the kombucha in your vessel, it will generate a new film that is exactly the size and shape of the surface. Always cover the vessel with a light porous cloth that allows air circulation while keeping flies and mold spores off the kombucha. Leave the vessel to ferment in a warm spot, away from direct sunlight.

You can purchase a mother, or obtain one from another home kombucha maker via online trading posts (see *Resources*), or grow one from commercially available live-culture kombucha. To grow one, simply pour a bottle of kombucha—preferably plain, without any particular flavoring—into a wide-mouth jar, cover with a cloth, and wait about a week (longer in cool temperatures) for a skin to form on the surface. This skin is a kombucha SCOBY.

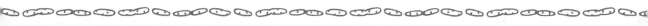

KOMBUCHA SYMBIOSIS

Molly Agy-Joyce, River Falls, Minnesota

I have been nurturing cuts of the same mother in my kombucha "farm" for nearly four years and find it to be a rewarding, symbiotic relationship. I harvest something she makes by just existing and it provides me with nutrition and a sense of connection to even the smallest life in my surroundings. In each new place I inhabit, she integrates me from the molecular level outward. I share pieces of her with friends and acquaintances, which brings me closer to other humans.

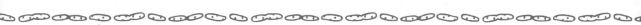

As you make more kombucha with your SCOBY, it will get thicker, generally growing in layers that you can peel off and use to start additional batches of kombucha, or share. I've seen kombucha mothers as thick as about 6 inches/ 15 cm. There is no particular benefit to a huge SCOBY, so most people peel away layers and share them. Other uses I have seen or heard of for extra SCOBYs include these:

- ◉ Blend them into a paste and use them for facials, spreading the paste on your face and leaving it to dry there.

- ◉ Brooke Gillon of Nashville, Tennessee, folds thin layers of kombucha SCOBYs into flower shapes and dries them in that shape. Gorgeous!

- ◉ Suzanne Lee, of the School of Fashion and Textiles in London, makes garments out of kombucha. According to a news report: "As the sheets dry out, overlapping edges 'felt' together to become fused seams. When all moisture has evaporated, the fibers develop a tight-knit, papyrus-like surface that can be bleached or stained with fruit and vegetable dyes such as turmeric, indigo, and beetroot."[38] (See photo in the color insert.)

- Several people have reported stretching kombucha SCOBYs and vinegar mothers onto frames and painting on them. They are composed of a cellulose, just like paper.

- *Nata*: In the Philippines, people grow a thick SCOBY, like the kombucha SCOBY, on coconut water, or pineapple juice mixed with sugar water, and then cook it into a candy. You can similarly transform a kombucha SCOBY into candy. See the next section for details.

Kombucha does best in a warm environment, from 75° to 85°F/24° to 30°C. The length of fermentation will vary depending upon specific temperature, and how acidic you like it. In warm weather, I typically ferment my kombucha about 10 days. Taste it every few days, and evaluate whether you want it to continue to ferment and acidify. In a cool space—say, 60°F/16°C—it takes a very long time; sometimes in winter I have left mine for months before it acidified to my liking.

Once kombucha has become as acidic as you like (only you can be the judge of that), remove the SCOBY, transfer the kombucha to bottles—reserving some to acidify the new batch—and brew more sweet tea to begin the process anew. Kombucha works best as an ongoing rhythm, because to remain alive, the SCOBY needs continual nourishment. If you go away, you can simply leave the SCOBY in kombucha for as long as several months, and then resume feeding it fresh sweetened tea upon your return.

When your kombucha is pleasingly acidified, you have several options. The simplest is to drink it. Bottle it as is and refrigerate. If you wish to further flavor, you can add fruit or vegetable juice, or a sweetened herbal infusion or decoction, for a secondary fermentation. The most exciting kombuchas I've tried have been made in this fashion. When I visited my friends at the Cultured Pickle Shop in Berkeley for a veritable tasting orgy, I was blown away by their incredible innovative kombucha flavors: Buddha's hand (a citrus fruit), mint, and bee pollen; turnip (oh, so good!); and beet. They do the primary fermentation with green tea and sugar with the kombucha mother; then decant kombucha and mix with fruit or vegetable juice for a secondary fermentation; and finally mix with a bit of honey at bottling for carbonation.

The secondary fermentation may be aerobic in an open wide-mouth vessel like the primary fermentation, or in a sealed or air-locked vessel. In an open vessel, the sweetened kombucha will likely develop a new mother on the surface, and growth will continue to be dominated by acetic acid organisms. In a sealed vessel (which could be the final bottle for serving, or not), the secondary ferment will yield more alcohol, as well as lactic acid.

Even if you don't care to incorporate additional ingredients in a secondary fermentation, you can carbonate kombucha in bottles. Simply decant it into sealable bottles while it is still a bit on the sweet side; seal the bottles; and allow it to continue to ferment in the sealed bottles for a few more days so carbonation can develop. Add a bit of fresh sweetener at bottling to speed or increase carbonation, but beware of excessive carbonation. I can't caution readers enough on this subject.

Questions continually arise as to whether sugar and caffeine persist in mature kombucha. The sugars do metabolize into acids, so you could ferment kombucha to the point that there is no sugar left. However, at that point, your kombucha would taste like vinegar, and most people prefer it when it is still somewhat sweet, and hence still with some of the sugar intact. As for caffeine, when herbalist Christopher Hobbs submitted a sample of kombucha to a laboratory for analysis, it was found to contain 3.42 mg/100 ml—much less than is typically found in a cup of tea, but most definitely present.[39] Michael Roussin reports that according to his laboratory analyses, caffeine levels remain constant throughout the kombucha fermentation period.[40] Specific caffeine levels will vary with type and amount of tea, length of steeping, and so forth. The notion that kombucha removes caffeine from tea is unsubstantiated; if you wish to avoid caffeine, make kombucha using weak or decaffeinated tea.

Another issue that has come up in relation to kombucha is its alcohol content. Kombucha probably always contains small traces of alcohol, as do nearly all fermented foods, including sauerkraut. Typically, the alcohol content of kombucha is somewhere below 0.5 percent by volume, which is considered a non-alcoholic beverage by law. (Traces of alcohol below 0.5 percent are typically found in fruit juices, sodas, "non-alcoholic" beers, and even breads and bread products.[41]) Sometimes, however—especially with anaerobic in-bottle secondary fermentation—kombucha's alcohol content can rise above the 0.5 percent legal limit. In June 2010, the US Alcohol and Tobacco Tax and Trade Bureau (TTB) tested off-the-shelf samples of various commercial kombucha products and found that, in some, alcohol levels exceeded the allowed 0.5 percent. TTB issued a "guidance document" declaring that "kombucha products containing at least 0.5 percent alcohol by volume are alcohol beverages."[42] Many retailers removed kombucha from their shelves until greater product control could be assured. Some manufacturers are taking measures to limit opportunities for in-bottle fermentation; others are switching from traditional kombucha to laboratory-derived defined starter cultures.

Finally, a word of caution about molds that sometimes develop on kombucha SCOBYs. I have experienced mold developing on kombucha, and I simply removed the SCOBY from the kombucha, scraped or peeled the mold away, rinsed the SCOBY, and proceeded to drink the kombucha and reuse the SCOBY, without incident. However, after reading Paul Stamets's article on kombucha, I would advise greater caution. "Of most concern are the species of *Aspergillus* I have found floating around with Kombucha," Stamets writes. (In contrast with *Aspergillus oryzae* and *A. sojae*, used for millennia to make rice beer, miso, soy sauce, and many other ferments, some *Aspergillus* species produce toxins.) "I fear that amateurs could think that by merely pulling out the *Aspergillus* colonies with a fork, that the culture would be de-contaminated, a dangerous, even deadly presupposition. The water-soluble toxins of *Aspergillus* can be highly carcinogenic."[43] Avoid molds by remembering to acidify each batch of kombucha with mature acidified kombucha from the previous batch. In the absence of mature kombucha, you can use some vinegar. If molds should form, however, discard the batch of kombucha, as well as the SCOBY, and begin anew with a new SCOBY.

Kombucha Candy: *Nata*

Nata is a candy made in the Philippines from the thick layer of cellulose that develops on the surface during vinegar fermentation of coconut water (*nata de coco*) or a pineapple juice infusion (*nata de pina*). I've used the *nata* method with a kombucha mother, and the result was a sweet, squishy candy, barely sour, with a hint of tea flavor, which almost everyone who tried it, kids included, liked. The process is extremely simple. A *jun* mother or mother-of-vinegar could be used with exactly the same process.

Take a kombucha mother, at least ½ inch/1 cm thick, rinse it, and cut it with a sharp knife into small bite-size pieces. Soak the kombucha pieces in cold water for 10 minutes. Drain, rinse, and soak again. Then transfer the kombucha pieces to a pot, cover with water, and boil for 10 minutes. Drain, rinse, and boil again for 10 more minutes. The reason for the repeated soaking and boiling is to remove as much acidity as possible from the kombucha mother. You may find that you prefer it more acidic, with fewer rinses and boilings. My friend Billy tried it after tasting mine and omitted the rinsing and boiling altogether. He preferred the flavor with the acidity intact. It reminded him of apple pie. "It's my new favorite way to enjoy the kombucha!" he announced. "It's better than drinking it."

The *nata* method of candying the kombucha pieces is to cover them with sugar, roughly as much sugar as kombucha cubes. Then heat this mixture and boil the kombucha pieces in the syrup that forms, for about 15 minutes, then remove from the heat, and allow to slowly cool. After cooling, drain off any remaining syrup, crisp up in the oven for a few minutes or air-dry, and enjoy kombucha candy.

wine vinegar

Billy loved it so much he invented his own method, without de-acidifying the kombucha and without cooking it, except at the end to dry it out. (For a live-culture kombucha candy you could air-dry, or use a dehydrator instead.) In a bowl, he alternated layers of sugar and still-acidified kombucha, then poured a cooled sugar syrup (also with butter and vanilla) over them and left it marinating overnight. In the morning he dried them, along with the extra sugar syrup, in a low oven. Finally, he sprinkled the crystallized sugar syrup on top "for a caramel flavor."

Jun

Jun is a culture similar to kombucha, made using honey rather than sugar, which gives it a lovely, distinctive flavor. *Jun* also seems to mature a little faster than kombucha, and to remain active at lower temperatures. Otherwise the process is exactly the same as kombucha, substituting honey for sugar. The lack of credible information on the history of *jun* leads me to the conclusion that it is a relatively recent divergence from the kombucha family tree. Some websites claim that it comes from Tibet, where it has been made for 1,000 years; unfortunately, books on Tibetan food, and even a specialized book on Himalayan ferments, contain no mention of it. Whether or not *jun* has a 1,000-year-old history, it is quite delicious. The culture is somewhat obscure and hard to find, but its epicenter seems to be the Pacific Northwest, where the Eugene, Oregon–based Herbal Junction Elixirs produces it commercially.

Vinegar

Many people have observed that the kombucha SCOBY is identical, or virtually so, to the mother-of-vinegar that often forms on the surface of fermenting vinegar. Some have even described kombucha as immature vinegar. Vinegar can be made from any fermented alcohol or solution of fermentable sugars. In chapter 4, vinegar was referred to as a possible undesirable outcome in the production of alcohol. Exposure of fermenting or fermented alcoholic beverages to oxygen allows for the growth of aerobic *Acetobacter* bacteria, which metabolize alcohol into acetic acid, commonly known as vinegar. Wine will yield wine vinegar; cider will yield cider vinegar; beer will yield malt vinegar; rice-based alcohols will yield rice vinegar.

If you wish to make vinegar, you do not need to have a mother-of-vinegar. "Historically, it was believed that vinegar could not be made without this mother," explains Lawrence Diggs, who calls himself "the Vinegar Man," wrote a book called *Vinegar*, and created a vinegar museum in Roslyn, South Dakota. "We now know that it is not necessary. As long as the *Acetobacter* are alive in the proper solution, under the proper conditions, vinegar will be produced."[44]

Generally, because *Acetobacter* is so omnipresent, exposing any preservative-free fermented alcoholic beverage to air will eventually result in vinegar. But vinegar production will be faster, more efficient, and more reliable if you add some *live* vinegar as a starter—about 1/4 the volume of fermented alcohol you are fermenting into vinegar. Understand that most commercially available vinegar is pasteurized, so the *Acetobacter* is no longer alive. A few brands, notably Bragg's, sell raw vinegar, and many people, going back to the Greek physician Hippocrates, consider raw vinegar to be a healthful tonic. Once you start making your own, you can simply use part of a previous batch as starter for the next.

For making vinegar, use a non-metallic vessel that enables you to expose a large surface area to air. One traditional setup is a wooden barrel, on its side, less than half full. A crock, wide-mouth jar, or bowl is also perfectly adequate. Fill the vessel no more than half full, in order to maximize the ratio between surface area and volume. Cover with a light cloth to keep flies out while allowing for good air circulation, and ferment in the temperature range of 59 to 94°F/15 to 35°C, out of the path of direct sunlight. The length of time required for fermentation will vary with temperature, starter, oxygenation, and proportions, typically from 2 to 4 weeks.

Once alcohol is fully converted into acetic acid, vinegar must be transferred to a sealed vessel, because if the vinegar continues to be exposed to oxygen, *Acetobacter* will metabolize acetic acid into water and carbon dioxide. "Whereas the presence of air was crucial in the acetification process, it is now, to the same degree, undesirable," explains Diggs. "The acid level will begin to fall after it has reached its peak. When it has fallen to 2 percent or lower, other microorganisms will now begin to take over."[45]

There are two methods for evaluating when the alcohol has been fully metabolized. The traditional method, perfectly adequate for the casual home vinegar-maker, is to smell and taste it to judge whether alcohol remains. The scientific method is chemical titration, for which inexpensive kits are easily available on the internet.

As soon as you determine that the alcohol has been converted into acetic acid, bottle the vinegar. If you wish to pasteurize it for greater stability, as many vinegar manufacturers do, the temperature at which *Acetobacter* is destroyed is 140°F/60°C; do not heat vinegar above 160°F/71°C or acetic acid will evaporate.[46] Bottle vinegar in small, narrow-neck bottles. Fill bottles completely and tightly seal them. As extra protection against further oxidation, many vinegar makers wax the seal of the bottles. Like wine, vinegar benefits from further aging after bottling. "The esters and ethers of the vinegars are allowed to mature, and many of the finer qualities emerge," writes Diggs, who recommends aging vinegar for a minimum of 6 months, ideally with chips of oak in the bottles.[47]

Although the most efficient way to make vinegar is from fully fermented alcohol, you can also make it directly from any sweet solution that could be made into alcohol. For instance, in *Wild Fermentation* I included recipes for fruit scrap and pineapple vinegars, which call for covering fruit peels and scraps with a sugar solution.[48] Mix the sugar solution at a proportion of roughly ½ cup/125 ml sugar per quart/liter of water. Use a bowl or wide-mouth vessel, and leave the mix to ferment open to the air, covered only with a cloth to keep flies away. It is important to stir the mix, especially in the early stages. If you do not stir frequently, not only will the process take longer, but surface molds are likely to develop. Once active bubbling is evident, strain out solid fruit residue and introduce live vinegar starter. Then proceed as described for vinegar from already fermented alcohol, although the process may take somewhat longer.

Shrub

Vinegar can be the basis for sour tonic beverages. A traditional name for a vinegar-soured fruit drink is a shrub. Perusing 19th-century cookbooks, the methods vary quite a bit, but a typical recipe calls for pouring vinegar over fresh berries (raspberries are most commonly referred to); leaving overnight for flavors to infuse; then straining out the berries and cooking the fruit-infused vinegar with sugar (often as much as a pound of sugar per pint of vinegar) into a syrup. The cooled sweet-and-sour syrup may be stored, diluted with water to taste as served, and enjoyed as a soft drink.

In addition to fruit, try infusing mint or other herbs into the vinegar. You can use honey or other sweeteners, and—especially if you are using raw homemade vinegar—you can omit the cooking step and simply stir to dissolve a more modest quantity of honey or sugar. For a bubbly shrub, dilute with carbonated water.

Troubleshooting

Doesn't start to ferment

It may be that your starter is not viable. It may be that the solution was too hot when culture was introduced and killed it. Maybe ambient temperatures where you placed your starter are too cold; try to find a warmer spot. Maybe chlorinated water is inhibiting fermentation. In the case of ginger bug, maybe the ginger was irradiated; try again with organic ginger. If there was no starter other than fruit: Stir, stir, stir. And be patient.

Gets too sour

This means you have fermented it too long. Try a shorter fermentation next time. Many beverages, however, notably kombucha, can be used as vinegar if they overly acidify. In addition, many overly soured beverages can be salvaged by diluting with some water or carbonated water, along with sweetener if desired.

Too weak

Next time, use more of the flavoring agent (ginger, tea, sweet potato, mauby bark, fruit, whatever) and/or sugar.

Surface molds develop

Acidifying kombucha with mature kombucha or vinegar helps prevent surface molding. With ferments other than kombucha, stirring or shaking daily while they are in open vessels prevents molds by disturbing them before they become visible. In making vinegar, stir the sugary solution at least daily until a mother forms. After that, increasing acidity will help protect the vinegar from molding, and stirring becomes impossible without disturbing the mother.

Kombucha mother sinks

Sometimes when you place a kombucha mother into a new batch of cooled, sweetened tea, the mother sinks to the bottom rather than floating on the surface. Be patient. Often within a few hours the mother will float to the top. If not, sometimes one edge of the mother will float to the top, causing a new mother to be generated, which at first looks like a thin film over the surface. If neither of these things happens, and your mother remains sunken in the sweet tea, it is no longer viable as a kombucha mother. Make it into *nata* candy and find another mother, or culture your kombucha with a high proportion (one-quarter to one-half) of mature kombucha, and it will generate a new mother on its surface.

Straining bread for kvass is difficult

The hardest part of making kvass is squeezing out all the liquid that absorbs into the bread. Strain the bread-water solution through a colander lined with a couple of layers of cheesecloth. Each time the colander fills with bread, gather the edges of the cheesecloth together, twist to wring out the liquid, and then knead the ball of cloth-encased soggy bread from different angles, trying to force out as much liquid as you can. Don't worry too much about forcing out every last bit.

Water kefir grains not growing

Water kefir grains typically grow pretty rapidly. Under ideal conditions, they can more than double with each feeding. If you find that yours are not growing, it probably means that they are no longer viable. Water kefir grains can become pickled if they are left more than a few days in an acidified solution without fresh sugar. When you find some more water kefir grains, feed them more frequently to avoid this.

Water kefir grains disappear

See above. If water kefir grains are left in an acidified solution without fresh sugar, they first become pickled, then may eventually disappear.

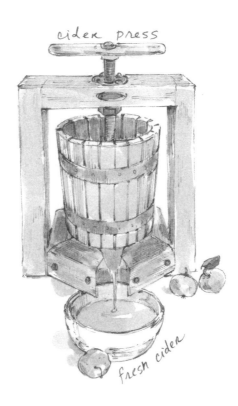

cider press

fresh cider

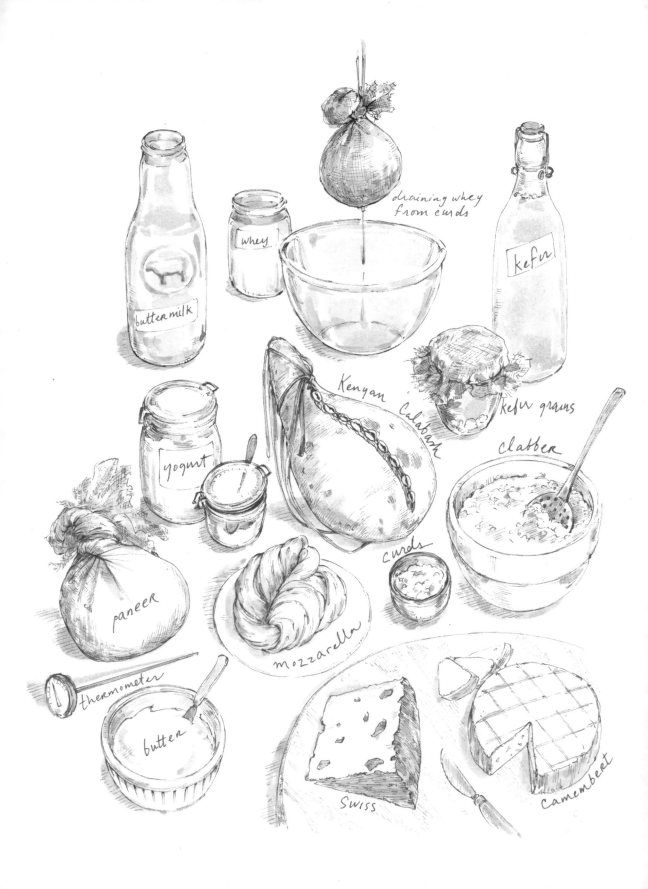

draining whey
from curds

buttermilk

whey

kefir

yogurt

Kenyan Calabash

kefir grains

clabber

paneer

curds

mozzarella

thermometer

butter

Swiss

Camembert

CHAPTER 7

Fermenting Milk

resh milk is largely a 20th-century phenomenon, made possible by the advent and spread of refrigeration technology (and the energy to run it). The people who milk cows, goats, and other ruminant mammals have always been able to enjoy fresh milk, but as a practical matter most other people have had access to milk primarily in fermented forms. Generally, fermentation stabilizes milk, transforming it from a highly perishable substance into much more stable forms. Milk can ferment in many different ways, depending upon methods, cultures and coagulants, environmental conditions, and manipulations.

All but the freshest of cheeses are fermented, often for months or even years. The harder the cheese is, which is to say, the more liquid (in the form of whey) has been removed from it, the longer it has the potential to ferment and preserve, generally speaking. Fluid milk and cream are also widely fermented, usually for only a few hours or days, rendering them stable for short-term storage, as well as protected from food poisoning organisms by their acidification.

The fermented milk best known in the United States is yogurt, with kefir a distant second. *Yogurt* is a Turkish name for a style of fermented milk from Southeastern Europe and around the Mediterranean. *Kefir* is also a Turkish name, for a very different style of fermented milk, from the Caucasus Mountains. Yogurt is typically a firm or semi-solid food, while kefir is a beverage. They also differ in flavor and chemical profiles, microbial cultures, their means of perpetuation, and methods of fermentation. But these are only two styles, and there's quite a bit of variation when it comes to milk. Indeed, around the world, everywhere humans have long traditions of domesticating animals for their milk, indigenous styles of fermented milk are found, with distinctive names, methods, and cultures.

For instance, in the West Pokot district in western Kenya, people ferment a milk known as *mala ya kienyeji* or *kamabele kambou*. When Slow Food designated this ferment as a Presidium, seeking to protect the practice, they could only describe it with reference to the number one global fermented milk superstar, as "ash yogurt in gourds." Yet it is not really yogurt at all. The milk that starts the ferment is its own particular fusion: It is a mixture of goat's milk with the milk of a local cross, cows bred with animals I had never heard of before, called zebus. Then:

> The milk is poured into a gourd or calabash. . . . No artificial starters are used and fermentation and acidification occurs spontaneously after a few days, either from the natural flora of the milk if raw, or from the bacteria found within the vessel. When the milk begins to coagulate some whey is removed and the vessel is topped up with fresh milk. This process is repeated and the vessel is shaken regularly for around one week.[1]

An English woman with whom I exchanged a few emails, Roberta Wedge, visited that region of Kenya many years ago and bought a milk-fermenting gourd. She recalls: "Every woman carries one, as every man carries a tiny stool and a herding stick." The gourd itself is the vehicle of perpetuation. The fermented milk then has ash mixed into it, which is made by burning a particular local tree, known as *cromwo*. The ash, according to a Slow Food website, "has antiseptic properties, adds an aromatic note to the flavor, and colors the yogurt a distinctive pale grey."[2]

Kenyan Calabash

Traditional forms of fermented milk like this evolved and spread wherever there was domestication of milking animals. A book I came across called *Application of Biotechnology to Traditional Fermented Foods* broadly defines "traditional" fermented milk products, in order to distinguish them from modern scientific ones: "Their production was a crude art . . . made with ill-defined, empirical cultures," meaning, "the inoculum is obtained from a previous production and its microbial identity is unknown."[3] The word in the technical literature for using the old batch to start the new batch is *backslopping*. The contrasting "non-traditional" milk ferments (like commercial yogurts and kefirs)—"based on known scientific principles"—were all developed in the 20th century, even though they are all based on traditional styles of fermentation.

For mass production, commerce, and marketing, consistency is critical. Traditional fermented milks vary by season, location, maker, and batch. In Zimbabwe, milk has traditionally been fermented by simply leaving it (raw) for a day or two at ambient temperatures in a clay pot. Thus it is fermented by bacteria present in the milk, the pot, and the air. In the 1980s, a mass-produced fermented milk product was developed and marketed with the name Lacto. In it, "Milk is standardized, pasteurized at 92°C [198°F] for 20 minutes, cooled to 22°C [72°F], and inoculated with 1.2 percent of an imported starter."[4] But in taste tests, the traditional ferment was "significantly more acceptable" than Lacto.[5] In addition, due to the diversity of the fermenting organisms, investigators found that samples of the traditional fermented milk contained higher levels of B vitamins thiamine, riboflavin, pyridoxine, and folic acid than did Lacto.[6]

Despite the superior nutritional profile of the traditional ferment, and the population's preference for its flavors, the researchers in this study seek to improve Lacto, "so as to entice rural populations to abandon traditional fermentation and adopt . . . a hygienically safer product."[7] In the name of public health, these traditions—evolved to sustain people with available food resources—are being intentionally eroded and replaced by products that can be mass-produced and generate profit for corporations. In fact, like languages, traditional fermented milk products are disappearing every year, and each silent extinction diminishes the diversity of culture and contributes to global homogenization. We must reject the notion that standardized cultures are superior to indigenous traditions, and confront the dogmas regarding hygiene and safety that justify this thinking. The diversity of fermented milk products reflects the glorious diversity of culture itself.

Raw Milk: Microbiology and Politics

Many traditional methods of fermenting milk have relied upon raw milk and its indigenous bacteria. Yogurt typically is made with milk that is heated past the point of pasteurization, then cultured after it cools. But while this technique results in a firmer, thicker yogurt than if you introduce the same culture into raw milk, it is not necessary in order to produce yogurt, and we have no idea how far back the practice of preheating the milk might go, nor how widespread it is or isn't, was or wasn't. But conceptually, the roots of yogurt and all other cultured foods must lie in spontaneous events that were noted, appreciated, and in some way perpetuated. Most likely these especially pleasing spontaneous events developed out of the lactic-acid-bacteria-rich environment of raw milk, rather than the microbial blank slate of cooked milk. Even if eventual refinement of the technique yields a process in which the historical culture (or a reasonable facsimile) is introduced into cooked milk, still the culture and the ferment develop out of such spontaneous events.

Raw milk is a very rich medium, and in the quantities that people milking animals have produced, accumulated in vessels, and stored—a phenomenon itself with no other precedent in nature—an extraordinary realm of specialized bacteria have evolved. According to geneticists Joel Schroeter and Todd Klaenhammer, humans "essentially domesticated these organisms over the last 5000 years through repeated transfer of LAB cultures for production of fermented dairy products."[8] Though the bacteria have evolved in various ways in these specialized ecological niches that human cultures and their domesticated partners have created, the bacteria grew out of the pool found in the milk itself.

The milk of healthy animals is generally wonderful and safe to drink. I first tasted raw milk when I visited the community I ended up living in for 17 years. Like the spring water and garden vegetables, the fresh milk was deeply compelling to me and was part of the allure of the change of life rural community living offered. Fresh raw milk is so much more delicious than the processed mass-market product that I am spoiled forever. After years of enjoying the sweet ambrosia of this milk, I got involved in the daily intimacy of hand milking the goats, which made the milk much richer and more meaningful. Now that I have moved down the road, I am no longer in the day-to-day milking grind and get my fresh goat's milk from a neighbor with a herd-share program.

When goats have adequate access to pastures and forests, they are typically healthy and produce healthy and safe milk. The indigenous lactic acid bacteria (LAB) in the milk protect it from other bacteria to which it may be exposed. Growing numbers of people concerned about health and nutrition are turning to raw milk as a nutrient-dense living food. And growing numbers of farmers are returning to small dairy herds on adequate pasture, then direct marketing raw milk as a more viable business plan than maximizing production and selling at a set price to the bulk processors. But healthy raw milk is dependent upon healthy animals, and healthy ruminant animals need land to graze. If the existing US milk supply were to suddenly cease to be pasteurized, it would be a terrible disaster. The milk industry as we know it excels at mass production of cheap milk. In order to accomplish this, land per animal is minimized, and extraordinary means are employed—such as giving cows artificial growth hormones—to boost milk production; unfortunately, these methods compromise the milk's quality and safety.

Animals in the large "farms" known as concentrated animal feeding operations (CAFO) do not enjoy the same health as animals allowed to roam and graze. Nor does their milk possess the same qualities. If we must drink the milk of these animals, it is safest pasteurized, due to high somatic cell (pus in the milk, from udder stress) and coliform bacteria counts. But let's not extrapolate from that unfortunate reality the simplistic notion that milk can only be safe with pasteurization. That is true only in the limited context of factory farming. Change the context, by providing animals with space to roam and graze, and raw milk can certainly be safe, not to mention delicious, nutritious, digestible, and rich in healthful and self-protective lactic acid bacteria. My previous book, *The Revolution Will Not Be Microwaved*, and many other books and websites, contain more information on the intense legal struggles over raw-milk distribution, as well as its nutritional aspects (see *Resources*). For now, suffice it to say that pasteurized and even "ultra-pasteurized" milk can

clabber

be successfully cultured, and you may think of this as a means of salvaging, enriching, and enlivening it. Raw milk too can be cultured; but only from raw milk will cultures emerge, and only with raw milk does it make sense to experiment with spontaneous fermentation.

Simple Clabbering

Clabber is a word that is rapidly fading into obsolescence. It is a surviving traditional English word for curdled fermented milk, deriving from the Gaelic *clabar*, meaning "mud." The metaphor is vivid. When milk clabbers (the word is a verb as well as a noun) it thickens, causing milk fats and solids to come together into something like sludge or mud. This mud is referred to as the *curd*. The thin liquid it separates from is *whey*.

My father's friend Ray Smith shared with me his aunt Helen's "recipe" for clabber, which he fondly remembered from childhood visits to his grandparents' home in North Carolina. "Back in the old days you simply set some milk aside and sooner or later it clabbered by itself," she wrote to him late in her life, after he inquired in a letter. "In this day of pasteurized milk, I guess you would need a starter." Here's Aunt Helen's "recipe":

> Put aside in a bowl the amount of milk that you want to clabber. Room temperature is what you want, and put it in a place where it will not be moved or shaken at all during the process. . . . It will probably take about 24 hours to set. You can check it by giving the bowl a slight wiggle, not enough to break the curd but enough to tell you whether it has set.

As the native lactic acid bacteria digest lactose (milk sugar) they create lactic acid. Harold McGee explains: "The increasingly acid conditions cause the normal bundled *micelles* of casein proteins to fall apart into separate casein molecules, and then rebond to each other. This general rebonding forms a continuous meshwork of protein molecules that traps the liquid and fat globules in small pockets, and turns the fluid milk into a fragile solid."[9] The speed at which this will occur depends upon temperature. At ambient temperatures in summer heat, it could take less than a day. In a cool environment, it could take a couple of days; in the refrigerator, it could take a couple of weeks. Despite our indoctrination that milk spoils easily and should not be consumed unless fresh—an unfortunate lesson of the age of pasteurization and refrigeration—the sour clabbered version of raw milk is still safe to consume curdled so long as the raw milk itself is safe to drink fresh. This is because the very bacteria that sour it protect it from pathogenic bacteria.

Please note that *stable* and *safe* do not necessarily equate with *delicious*. Milks from different animals in different locations will yield very different products when spontaneously fermented. Ambient temperatures during clabbering will strongly influence bacterial as well as enzymatic activity, and resulting clabber flavor. Most of my clabbering experiences came during summers milking five goats. At certain points, we ran out of space in the refrigerator and were not ready to make cheese. So milk would just sit on the counter, in Tennessee summer heat, with daily highs around 95°F/35°C, and clabber within 24 hours. We then skimmed the milk fats from the top. What spontaneously developed from the milk reminded me of sour cream. Maybe you will be so lucky and love what spontaneously develops on milk in your kitchen. But then, maybe you won't.

Because of the high degree of variability found in spontaneously fermented milks, people have frequently introduced a small bit of clabber from a batch they liked as a starter to guide the development of the new batch. It is this backslopping step that really distinguishes most of the different styles of fermented milks that people around the world enjoy. If you find yourself with a surplus of raw milk, try clabbering some spontaneously and see how you like what results. If milk is a scarce and precious resource for you, it probably makes more sense to culture it with a reliable starter that you know you will like.

 ## Yogurt

Yogurt is the most popular fermented milk in the world. It is distinctive for its thick and creamy semi-solid consistency, and its mildly tart flavor. The bacteria that ferment milk into yogurt are typically (there are exceptions) thermophilic bacteria, active at elevated temperatures. Therefore, to make nice thick yogurt you must incubate it, maintaining it in a temperature range between 110° and 115°F/43° and 46°C. Incubation strategies, the most challenging aspect of making yogurt (and some other ferments), are covered in chapter 3.

To make yogurt, you need a starter culture. If you can find or buy a traditional yogurt culture, and are good at maintaining a regular rhythm, you may be able to make yogurt from it for the rest of your life. If you want to try making yogurt without delay, you can use commercial yogurt for the starter, always live-culture, plain, and without additives. (A lengthier discussion of yogurt starters follows this description of how to make it.) The first step of the yogurt-making process is to remove your starter yogurt from the refrigerator and allow it time to warm to room temperature. Also, fill the jars in which you will make the yogurt, as well as your incubator if you are using an insulated cooler, with warm water, so they can pre-warm and will not later cool your yogurt mixture once it reaches target temperature.

As the starter and vessels warm, I heat the milk to at least 180°F/82°C. Heat milk slowly and gently, with frequent stirring to avoid scalding. "The faster you heat the milk, the more grainy bits of overheated congealed protein you'll find in your yogurt," warns Rosanna Nafzifer, co-author (with Ken Albala) of the excellent *Lost Art of Real Cooking*.[10] It is possible to omit this heating step and make raw yogurt, never heating the milk above 115°F/46°C. But raw yogurt will never be as thick as yogurt from milk that has been heat-treated.

What this heating accomplishes, aside from killing native bacteria that could compete with the introduced cultures, is to alter the structure of the milk protein, casein, a key to thick, firm yogurt.[11] Holding the milk at this high temperature, with constant stirring, will result in evaporation and concentration of milk, further contributing to a thicker end product. It is in simulation of this traditional evaporation step that many yogurt manufacturers and people making it at home add powdered milk or other thickening additives.

After heating the milk, you must allow it to cool before adding the starter culture. You may simply leave the pot of heated milk to slowly cool, monitoring it periodically so you can add cultures as soon as the temperature drops to 115°F/46°C. Or you can actively cool it, by filling a sink, tub, pot, or bowl with cold water and setting the pot of heated milk in the cold water. Stir the milk in the pot, as well as the water around it, for rapid cooling. Don't wait for the temperature to reach target before removing the pot of milk from the cold water, or it will cool further; remove it from the cooling bath as the temperature approaches 120°F/49°C. Once the temperature reaches 115°F/46°C, remove a cup of the milk into a cup or bowl, and stir in starter. I use 1 tablespoon of starter per quart/liter. Many recipes suggest using more starter, and in my early yogurt-making experiences I did, but based on the recommendation of *The Joy of Cooking* I tried a "less is more" approach and found that it made thicker yogurt. A tablespoon is just under 5 percent of a quart or liter. A dairy production reference book I consulted recommended using yogurt starter at a proportion of 2 to 5 percent, so you could use even less.[12] Thoroughly mix the starter with the cup of heated milk; once it is fully dissolved, mix it back into the full pot of heated milk. Then transfer cultured milk to preheated jars, seal, and place in the incubation chamber, leaving it to ferment undisturbed.

Incubated at 115°F/46°C, yogurt will coagulate within about three hours, but if left too long it can easily curdle. I prefer to ferment it a bit more slowly at a slightly lower temperature, four to eight hours at a more forgiving 110°F/43°C. Even longer fermentations can yield more tangy flavor and fuller digestion of lactose. I have heard of people fermenting yogurt for as long as 24 hours. At lower temperatures, coagulation will take longer, and the end result will probably not be quite as thick. If you should open your incubator and find your yogurt still runny, add hot-water bottles to heat it up, and leave it for a few more hours at warmer temperatures. If for some reason your yogurt fails to coagulate at all, which can happen, you do not need to discard the milk; you can easily turn it into a simple acid-curdled cheese.

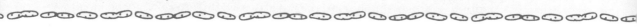

KAYMAKLI YOĞURT

Aylin Öney Tan, Istanbul, Turkey[13]

The basic method of making yogurt is pretty much the same all over, but there are a few tricks that make the whole difference. Boiling down the milk to a condensed state is one way to achieve thicker yogurt; constant stirring and airing with a spoon speeds the process and prevents burning the bottom of the pot. When transferring the milk to the setting vessels, pouring from a height forms a foamy froth, which will eventually turn into a thick clotted yogurt cream, a delicacy in itself. The skin or cream that forms on the surface of yogurt is called *kaymak*. The creamy crust is usually delicately removed from the surface of yogurt and eaten with a drizzle of honey at breakfast.

Yogurt is certainly wonderful as it is, plain. In the United States people typically sweeten it with jam, fruit, or sugar, but traditionally it has more often been used with savory flavors. With simple spicing yogurt becomes a sauce or condiment like Greek *tsatsiki* or Indian *raita*.[14] Hung over a bowl in fine cheesecloth or tea towel, whey drips out and it becomes *labneh*, yogurt cheese, popular in the Middle East.[15] Mixed with bulgur and further fermented, it becomes a soup flavoring and thickener known as *kishk* (see *Kishk and Keckek el Fouqara* in chapter 8). My friend Pardis once made me a Persian feast, accompanied by *doogh*, a yogurt-based savory soda, which I have come to love as a thirst-quenching refreshment in hot weather. (See the *doogh* sidebar.) In Turkey, where yogurt is incorporated into the cuisine in an extraordinary variety of ways, one way of preserving yogurt is to dry it into a hard (and very stable) block, known as *kurut*, which is then grated, crushed, or pounded into a powder.[16] In the cultures that have evolved using yogurt for thousands of years, it is integrated into all aspects of the cuisine.

Yogurt has become a ubiquitous food in Western supermarkets and kitchens. But it was not always so. A hundred years ago, yogurt was known primarily in Southeastern Europe, Turkey, and the Middle East. It was a regional food, known beyond that primarily among immigrant communities, but otherwise obscure. Pioneer microbiologist Elie (Ilya) Metchnikoff, who studied longevity in Bulgaria and attributed it to yogurt, popularized the idea that yogurt and other fermented milks could improve health and extend life, giving scientific credibility to a notion that was already part of the received culture in many traditions.

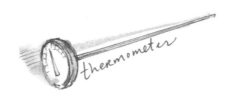

thermometer

Metchnikoff's research spurred popular interest in yogurt as a medicinal product. Dr. Isaac Carasso started a state-of-the-art yogurt factory in Barcelona, Spain, in 1919, using bacteria isolated and cultured by Metchnikoff's Pasteur Institute in Paris. Carasso, a Sephardic Jew, had recently moved his family to Barcelona from Thessaloniki (now part of Greece), where yogurt was an important food. He called his business Danone, a Catalan nickname for his son Daniel. Daniel learned the family business and set off for Paris in 1929 to establish Danone there. During World War II he left Europe for the United States and took Danone with him, establishing a yogurt factory in the Bronx in 1942. According to the website of the company, "He changed the name Danone to Dannon to make the brand sound more American."[17] Daniel Carasso died in 2009 at the age of 103. "My dream was to make Danone a worldwide brand," he said shortly before his death, at a celebration of the 90th anniversary of the company's founding.[18] He succeeded in making yogurt into a global staple.

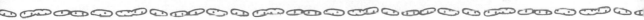

DOOGH: PERSIAN YOGURT SODA

To make *doogh*, stir plain yogurt, to break its structure, until it is smooth. Then stir in a little fresh or dried mint, salt, and fresh ground black pepper to taste. Once they are mixed into the yogurt, add either plain or carbonated water—at least as much as the yogurt you used, usually more—and mix to reach the desired consistency. Enjoy. You can also carbonate *doogh* the traditional way, mixing ingredients as directed above and leaving sealed in an airtight bottle for a day or two to continue fermenting so pressure will build.

But the yogurt that he made was different from traditional yogurt in at least one key respect: It was made using a blend of bacteria that had been isolated from Bulgarian yogurt at the Pasteur Institute, including the ones we now know as *Lactobacillus delbrueckii* subsp. *bulgaricus* and *Streptococcus salivarius* subsp. *thermophilus*. This was different from how yogurt had previously been cultured, which was simply to use yogurt from the last batch. All yogurt was made from a previous batch of yogurt, in long lineage.

In varied locations, the yogurt communities diverged. *Yogurt* is a Turkish word, yet yogurt-like ferments have been historically associated with not only Turkey but also Southeastern Europe and the Middle East. The cultures and techniques probably spread via nomadic herding peoples, and they evolved distinctively in different locations, as does any food that gets spread over a vast territory, especially a fermented one. And besides being regionally varied, traditional yogurt cultures also consisted of more complex communities, involving organisms beyond the two bacteria that the Pasteur Institute identified as the critical ones, and that legally define yogurt in our time. The traditional yogurt cultures were evolved communities, with a certain amount of inherent stability to them.

BULGARIAN-JAPANESE YOGURT CULTURE

Áron Boros, Boston, Massachusetts

I picked up a yogurt culture on a visit to Japan in 2001 and have been harvesting it ever since. (I'm sure if the customs officer at JFK had seen it, I wouldn't have it today!) I have a super-simple technique: I simply skim off any foul-looking stuff at the top, eat as much as I want, and leave about ½ inch in the bottom of the container. Then I fill it with whole milk and leave it on the counter for 24 hours, covered with cheesecloth. Every three or four times I make it, I move the whole thing to a clean container. No cooking, no stirring, no nothing—super easy, and it's lasted me nine years so far! It makes a somewhat runny yogurt (although sometimes it sets really nicely—I haven't spent much time thinking about what makes it set better, although I suspect it's timing when to put it in the fridge just right, and something about room temperature too).

I heard a rumor this is the famed "Bulgarian-Japanese yogurt culture" that will allow me to live forever, but that provenance is unverified. A few times I've neglected it for three or four weeks, and it gets a lot of yellow/brown/orange spoiled rind on the top, but if I can dig down and find a little bit of white yogurt underneath, I have always been able to use that to make successively larger batches to recover the whole thing.

Only in preparing to write this book did I finally get hold of a traditional yogurt culture. Actually, I purchased online and have been maintaining not one culture but two, which I have come to know as B & G, for Bulgarian and Greek.[19] The fact that I have made repeated batches for more than a year already sets these cultures apart from the store-bought yogurts I have used as starters until now. In my experience, the cultures in commercial yogurt never maintain their effectiveness as starters beyond a few generations. The problem with cultures derived from isolated laboratory strains, from a practical standpoint, is that they are inherently unstable. They cannot effectively perpetuate themselves.

Traditional yogurts can and do perpetuate themselves. Fourteen months after their arrival in my kitchen, B & G are making yogurt every bit as thick and delicious as the first batch. There is a century-old knish maker in New York City, Yonah Shimmel's, that serves yogurt they claim to still make from the original starter its founder migrated with to New York. After Eva Bakkeslett of Norway read about Yonah Shimmel's yogurt in *Wild Fermentation*, she bought some while visiting New York and brought a sample of it home with her. She has successfully perpetuated it for several years now, shared it widely, and established a blog[20] to chart the spread of this and other milk cultures.

Yogurt cultures need not be so fragile and lacking in resilience that starters require refreshing every second or third batch. For yogurt traditions to have been continuous, they had to be self-perpetuating beyond a few generations. I've asked a number of microbiologists and other "experts" how they explain why the traditional cultures remain so much more stable than the laboratory-derived cultures. Betty Stechmeyer, cofounder of GEM cultures, who commercially propagated numerous cultures for decades, views the microbial diversity of traditional yogurt cultures as the source of their greater stability and endurance. "An ecosystem (in a bowl) with less diversity can be more easily knocked 'off balance' than one with a whole host of players."

Microbiologist Jessica Lee concurs, making reference to bacteriophages, viruses that attack bacteria. With a single strain of bacteria, "a phage outbreak can quickly kill the entire bacterial population and end the fermentation process," she says. Yogurts made with two isolated strains are no more resilient. "Local bacteriophages eventually evolve to be able to infect the few strains that make up that starter and slowly kill them off." The difference with a traditional starter is that it is composed of more varied bacteria, "so that when one strain falls prey to phages, there will be others to take over and maintain fermentation. This is an elegant story to argue the practical value of biodiversity and traditional methods of fermentation."[21]

The New England Cheesemaking Supply Company sells several yogurt strains, some marketed as "re-culturable," some not. When I asked why, I received an email explaining that the reculturable cultures they sell are "undefined," while those that are defined are not typically regarded as reculturable. As for why: "When I ask the culture producer experts they are pretty vague on this."[22]

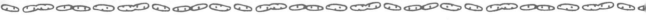

SOURCES OF HEIRLOOM YOGURT CULTURES

Although you can make yogurt from any live-culture yogurt, only traditional, heirloom cultures will be able to perpetuate themselves over time. Commercial sources of heirloom yogurt cultures are listed in *Resources*. If you are willing to do some searching, you may be able to find someone locally who has maintained a yogurt culture for years near where you live. Try posting notices on local computer bulletin boards, or contacting food advocacy groups and local chapters of groups like Slow Food and the Weston A. Price Foundation. Try contacting local food writers too; a brief write-up on your search in the local paper could easily catch the eyes of the right person.

I have no doubt that there are many practical benefits—especially in commercial production—to using defined strains rather than undefined or empirical cultures. The combination of *L. bulgaricus* and *S. thermophilus* does indeed render a lovely ferment with a pleasing texture and flavor. The laboratory-derived starters yield consistently good results, so long as you start with pure cultures in each batch.

But I can't help but wonder what has been lost of the diverse Old World milk cultures. It reminds me of the tragedy with vegetable seeds, where a handful of "improved" varieties led to widespread abandonment of localized varieties. The improved varieties outperformed under ideal conditions, but were not so well adapted to actual climatic and environmental conditions, thus demanding irrigation and pesticides. In addition, hybrid seeds—specific crosses that are not self-regenerating—breed dependence, by requiring the expertise of breeders, where previously the seeds had been self-perpetuating. Similarly with yogurt, where once it was always derived from the last batch of yogurt—like a seed, a living legacy from ancestors and their coevolutionary partners—without that living legacy we become dependent on technology that is beyond the scope of the generalist. Revive, reclaim, and reinvent living fermentation legacies. Find those surviving yogurt cultures, or more obscure ones. We cannot allow cultures that function as vibrant self-sustaining communities to be replaced by commodified pure cultures isolated and bred in laboratories, no matter what perceived improvements they may offer.

 ## Kefir

Kefir is another popular culture for fermenting milk. It produces a beverage, thicker than milk, that can be made from ever so mildly tart to super-sour, and best of all, if properly prepared, it is bubbly. The community of organisms that ferment milk into kefir includes yeasts, which produce alcohol at levels ranging from a few negligible tenths of a percentage to as high as 3 percent, depending upon length of fermentation and other factors. Because of its alcohol content and its effervescence, kefir is sometimes called "the champagne of milks."

Kefir is notable among milk cultures in that rather than using a bit of fermented milk to start the next batch, it relies upon a SCOBY, a rubbery mass of bacterial and fungal cells that has evolved an elaborate symbiotic arrangement, sharing nutrients, coordinating reproduction, and co-creating a shared form, which is not microscopic. I've seen extremely varied kefir forms. All of them are whitish and plump, with curvaceous undulating surfaces, something like a cross between cauliflower florets and little brains. Most of the kefir grains I have encountered grow into clumps measuring up to a few inches in any direction. Some have been smaller, so that as they grow there are more and more small clumps, but the clumps do not grow larger. On a few occasions I have seen extraordinarily large kefir clumps. In the color photo insert, the kefir depicted is a single connected mass of kefir so large that it fills both hands. The largest kefir I have ever seen was a clump that spread out like a sheet, more than a foot wide, with familiar kefir clumps connected by flatter sections. Again, we see that biological creations always exhibit diverging branches of the family tree.

The biology of kefir is quite fascinating. It is a symbiotic entity that self-reproduces; combining each of the individual bacterial and fungal members will not result in a new kefir grain. All kefir grains evolved from a spontaneous symbiosis—or a number of them—that has perpetuated itself. "Despite intensive research and many attempts to produce kefir grains from the pure or mixed cultures that are normally present in the grains, no successful results have been reported to date," reports the *Journal of Dairy Science*.[23] Biologist Lynn Margulis asserts: "Kefir can no more be made by the 'right mix' of chemicals or microbes than can oak trees or elephants."

Margulis, whose work in the field of symbiogenesis I referred to in chapter 1, has written about kefir as a vivid illustration of fundamental biological concepts, such as life, death, sex, and evolution. She points out that kefir grains do not possess "programmed death," as animals, plants, and certain other organisms do, and therefore may theoretically live forever, given adequate nutrition and tolerable environmental conditions. Margulis explains that kefir grains involve a community of 30 different types of microbes, including common food fermentation favorites, such as *Lactobacilli*, *Leuconostoc*, *Acetobacter*, and *Saccharomyces*, as well as others more obscure; in fact, according to Margulis, fewer than half the microbes involved are known or named. Nonetheless, "These specific yeasts and bacteria must reproduce together—by coordinated cell division that does not involve fertilization or any other aspect of sex—to maintain the integrity of the unusual microbial individual that is the kefir curd," she writes. The component organisms are "inextricably connected by chemical compounds, glycoproteins and carbohydrates, of their own making. . . . Kefir microbes are entirely integrated into the new being just as the former symbiotic bacteria that become components of nucleated cells are integrated. . . . Kefir is a sparkling demonstration that the integration processes by which our cells evolved from bacteria still occur."[24]

Despite their potential for immortality, forget to feed them too long, and kefir grains will die and decompose. I've had mine simply dissolve, from neglect for weeks at a time, into the acidic kefir they had created. Margulis observes: "Dead kefir curds teem with a kind of life that is something other than kefir: a smelly mush of irrelevant fungi and bacteria thriving and metabolizing, but no longer in integrated fashion, on corpses of what once were live individuals."[25] The moral of the story: Kefir grains require regular care and feeding.

Except for the challenge of getting into a rhythm, making kefir is extremely easy. No heating or temperature regulation is required (though kefir will ferment faster if you gently heat milk from refrigerator temperature to ambient room temperature). Simply add kefir grains to milk in a jar. Use about a heaping tablespoon of grains for 1 quart/liter of milk. Most of the literature concurs that kefir is best cultured at a ratio around 5 percent grains.[26] Do not fill the jar all the way, as carbon dioxide production can result in an increase in volume. You can either seal the jar, in which case pressure will build, or loosely cover it. Leave kefir to ferment at ambient temperatures, out of direct sunlight, and shake or stir periodically. Because microbial activity is concentrated on the surfaces of the grains, the agitation is important to move the grains around, circulate the milk, and thus spread microbial activity. Kefir is ready when you can see that it is has thickened, around 24 hours, or longer if you live in a cool environment (or prefer it sour). Shake the jar of kefir one last time before removing the grains. You can either fish the grains out with a spoon, especially if they're big, or strain through a strainer. To carbonate, transfer the strained kefir to a sealable vessel, allowing room for expansion, and leave to ferment sealed another few hours, or a few days in the refrigerator. When you open the sealed jar of kefir, it will froth and rise.

It's that easy. I always use whole milk, raw when available, though my friend Nina reports that she prefers making kefir from nonfat milk. I have had fine results with raw milk, pasteurized, and even ultra-pasteurized; goat's milk and cow's milk, both homogenized and not.

Some of the literature encourages not allowing kefir grains to come into contact with metal. I would certainly concur insofar as prolonged contact with metal can result in corrosion, as with any acidic ferment. But some kefir promoters are emphatic that even brief contact with metal (such as mesh strainers) can destroy kefir grains. I have never found this to be true; nor has the man I call the Internet King of Kefir, Dominic Anfiteatro of Australia, who in his typical comprehensive way conducted a small experiment: "We've used stainless steel strainers to strain kefir for months on end without any evidence to suggest that the grains or the microflora are impaired in any way," he writes on his website.[27]

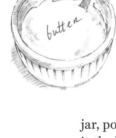

When you strain kefir from the kefir grains, transfer to a clean jar, pour fresh milk over the grains, and continue the rhythm. The rhythm is the hard part. Ideally, each time you strain a batch of mature kefir from the grains, you start another batch. Maintaining kefir grains, or any other SCOBY, ultimately is like having a pet; they require not constant but ongoing attention. If they are not adequately nourished, they will die. With all the traveling I do, I have lost my kefir grains on more than one occasion. At present I am making and drinking about 2 cups of kefir every other day. Every other morning I strain the kefir and pour fresh milk over the grains. The grains double every week or 10 days. You can store extras to share later, without having to keep feeding them, by drying them. Rinse them, drain on absorbent paper, and dry in the sun and/or a dehydrator at low temperature. You can slow kefir grains down in the refrigerator, but you still need to feed them after about a week. You can suspend them for a long while also by freezing them.[28] But kefir grains work best, and stay healthiest, with frequent engagement and regular feeding.

One characteristic of healthy kefir grains is that they grow and reproduce rapidly. As the proportion of grains to milk increases, your kefir will ferment faster and faster. It's best to remove excess grains, to maintain a grain:milk ratio of no more than about 10 percent. Thus, everyone who keeps kefir grains and makes kefir regularly ends up with more grains than they know what to do with. So if you can find those people, they will generally be thrilled to share grains with you. (See *Resources* for a listing of culture exchanges on the Internet where you can find people with grains to share, as well as commercial sources of kefir grains.)

One interesting aspect of kefir is that most of the products prepared commercially in the United States and much of the rest of the world are not made using traditional kefir grains. Instead they are made using starter cultures consisting of some of the known organisms that are part of the traditional kefir symbiosis, but not all of them, and without the complexity and resulting unity of kefir's evolved life-form. A few reasons for this are cited in the literature. One is the slow increase in the size of the kefir grains, resulting in limitations on expanding production. Another is the difficulty of producing a consistent product due to the complex microbiology of kefir grains. In addition, the alcohol present in kefir—which definitely has the potential to increase above the 0.5 percent maximum level for non-alcoholic beverages—can create regulatory and legal challenges, as we have seen with kombucha. And because the alcohol fermentation typically becomes dominant after the lactic acid fermentation, it "tends to occur at the distribution stage of the products, thereby resulting not only in substantial changes in flavor and taste due to the formation of ethanol and carbon dioxide gas but also in bulging of containers and leakage of the contents."[29]

For these reasons, much research has gone into the development of alternative starter cultures for kefir. "Several processes have been developed to produce a kefir-like beverage in which no grains are used," reports the *Journal of Dairy Science*.[30] That seems like the appropriate language to use: *kefir-like beverage*. Kefir is a specific product, created by a specific culture with a distinctive form. It hardly seems legitimate to call a cultured milk product "kefir" if it is fermented by anything other than the grains that have always defined kefir. The laboratory-produced starter cultures can produce beverages that may be very delicious and beneficial to health, but they are not kefir. "The quality of these kefir products is significantly different from that of kefir fermented with grains," concludes the *Journal of Dairy Science*.[31] "It is evident that the final product, as produced from kefir grains, will have a larger number and variety of microorganisms than kefir produced from a mixture of a small number of pure cultures," states the *Food Science and Technology Bulletin*.[32]

Powdered starters approximating kefir are not limited to large-scale manufacturing operations. Several powdered kefir starters are available for small-scale home production. I have never tried the powdered starters, but especially for people who do not want the commitment of maintaining live kefir grains and prefer to make kefir intermittently rather than in a regular rhythm, powdered starters could make sense, even if what they produce is not actually kefir.

Viili

Viili is a Finnish cultured milk, distinctive primarily for its extremely viscous, gluey consistency. People I've introduced to *viili* have likened its texture to rubber cement and marshmallow fluff. When my friend Johnni Greenwell was culturing *viili*, one night he filled his bowl of fermenting milk to the brim, not realizing that the fermentation would cause expansion. In the morning, not only had the *viili* spilled out of the bowl onto the table, but the bowl was empty. The mass of *viili* holds together so tenaciously that the bit that spilled pulled the rest of the *viili* mass from the bowl. Despite this "extreme" texture, *viili* has a delicate, mild flavor, barely sour.

Viili cultures are commercially available from GEM Cultures[33] and other sources. I got mine from GEM, and Betty Stechmeyer tells me that their *viili* came from Finland to Fort Bragg, California, via her late husband Gordon's family, the Kinnunens. Betty told me a poignant story concerning her husband's uncle Van, Waino Alexander Kinnunen, the last of 13 kids in that family, who was born after their arrival in the United States:

> Van lived alone in a 3 room cabin in the woods up the road from us and in his early 90's was still pretty independent. . . . After his 95th birthday, Van took a fall and his health began to fail. . . . One afternoon, watching TV by his bedside, he asked calmly, "Can you take care of the seed?" I assured him that he had shown me well how to do that and I would. The middle of the next night, I realized his light was on and I went in to find that he had died.

> The "seed" is one Finn way of expressing "the starter" or "culture" of the Finn dairy product *fiilia (viili)*. Though Van was born in Fort Bragg, the "seed" had come from Finland with the Kinnunen family and probably dozens of other families as well. The corner of a clean handkerchief had been spread with a bit of the cultured milk, dried, rolled up, and tucked carefully into personal belongings for the long trip to a new life. Seed or culture is the means for the continuation of life, a new life, in a new land, or phase of life.

For Uncle Van, knowing that the seed remained well cared for, the legacy that allows for cultural continuity, was reassurance that life would go on even as his own came to an end.

Making *viili* is very easy. Use a bowl or a jar as a vessel. Take a spoonful of mature *viili* and smear it around the interior surfaces of the vessel. Then fill it with milk, leaving a little room for expansion; lightly cover to keep flies and dust off but allow for limited airflow; and leave at ambient room temperatures for about 24 hours, until the *viili* thickens. Save a spoonful of each batch to start the next. Eat plain, with fruit and cereal, or as a base for dips and sauces. I've had trouble with *viili* in the Tennessee summers; it does not seem to like temperatures much above 80°F/27°C, or high humidity.

I received an email in 2008 from a Finn, Erol Schakir, who had listened to a podcast of a talk I gave, which included the story of Uncle Van's *viili*. "What was interesting is that they/he/the family still had the 'root' going after so many years. In my experience the 'root' or 'seed' weakens and eventually will no longer make milk into *viili*. How did he manage to keep the seed alive and strong? I personally just go to the shop to buy a new can of *viili* for a new 'seed.'" It sounds to me exactly like the situation with yogurt cultures: Erol is relying on commercial improved laboratory bred cultures, while Uncle Van and Betty kept an Old World coevolved community going.

I forwarded Erol's email to Betty to see what she thought. Here are excerpts of her response:

> I don't believe the commercial starters have the full spectrum of organisms needed for longevity. Most commercial entities need to meet a schedule and consistent end point production, so they pick the organisms that do that for them. . . . Erol, if you take commercial *viili* for seed, I think you're not getting all the players. . . . I suggest you advertise for seed from a traditional source, an old family that has had it going for quite a while.

As with yogurt and kefir, the starters used for mass production of *viili* evidently lack the stability of the traditional culture that was used continuously and passed from generation to generation.

Other Milk Cultures

Milk cultures are far too numerous for me to know them all or describe them comprehensively. Every region that domesticated animals for their milk, or where nomadic or migratory herding cultures passed through, has evolved cultures for fermenting milk. Here are a few more notable examples:

Koumiss is a fermented milk that developed in the Central Asian steppes, notable for its alcohol content. "The raw materials for a good fermented [alcoholic] beverage—fruit, cereal, and honey—were hard to come by on the grasslands," observes Patrick McGovern, the anthropologist who studies ancient alcoholic beverages (see chapter 4). "As ever, humans improvised by making a drink (Turkish *kimiz*; Kazakh *koumiss*) from mare's milk, which has a higher sugar (lactose) content than goat's or cow's milk and consequently yields a higher alcohol content (up to 2.5 percent)."[34] A 13th-century traveler to Mongolia described the process as follows:

> Take a large horse skin bag and a long bat that is hollow inside. Wash the bag clean and fill it with mare's milk. Add a little sour milk [mature koumiss, as a starter]. As soon as it begins to froth beat it with the bat and continue doing so until the fermentation stops. Every visitor to the tent is required to hit the bag several times when he enters the tent. The kumiss will be ready to drink in about three to four days.[35]

The 1953 edition of *The Joy of Cooking* contains a recipe for "American-style" *koumiss*, which calls for adding yeast to room-temperature milk, then transferring the mixture to sealable bottles, fermenting at room temperature for 10 hours, and finally refrigerating for 24 hours, shaking the bottles occasionally. "When opening the bottles beware of a 'spit in the eye,'" cautions *Joy*; concluding: "Koumiss is as effervescent as hope."[36]

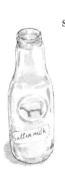

Buttermilk is a cultured milk product commonly available in supermarkets in the United States. You can use commercial buttermilk to add as a starter to fresh milk, leave it to ferment for a day at room temperature, and you will have more "buttermilk." I use quotes because what is sold as buttermilk in the United States is not the classic buttermilk. Buttermilk historically is the rich by-product that results from churning or agitating cream into butter. Buttermilk is to cream what whey is to milk. And because butter has historically been made from raw cream, both the butter and the buttermilk are teeming with indigenous (or added) bacteria.

Tara is a Tibetan milk culture embodied in a SCOBY, just like kefir. I was gifted with *tara* grains shortly before beginning work on *Wild Fermentation* and wrote about them there.[37] After I got my first kefir grains and started making kefir, I was unable to distinguish between the kefir and the *tara*, finished product or grains. So I regard them as closely related, if not the same thing. Unfortunately, my *tara* grains eventually died of neglect, and I have not been able to obtain more.

Skyr is a fermented milk from Iceland. A product called *skyr* is being marketed in the United States now as "Icelandic yogurt." When I asked Icelandic food writer Nanna Rögnvaldardóttir how similar traditional *skyr* is to yogurt, she responded "not very." She described the *skyr* she grew up on in the 1960s on a remote farm in the North as "thick, crumbly, and much more sour than the stuff they make now, which is more of a yogurt." She reports that homemade *skyr* is not widespread, but that Slow Food Iceland is seeking out people who still make *skyr* at home.

Gariss is a fermented camel's milk of the Sudan, prepared in goat skins (*si'ins*) hung from the saddle of a camel "under more or less continuous shaking," according to Hamid Dirar, who considers it one of four "truly indigenous fermented dairy products of the Sudan," alongside two other "quasi-indigenous" fermented milks introduced from Egypt.[38] "Fresh camel milk is added to the *si'in* whenever part of the fermented product has been consumed, so that the volume of the fermenting milk is more or less kept constant."[39]

This is just a cursory overview. Indigenous cultures around the world developed varied practices for fermenting milk that are rapidly fading into obscurity and disappearing, along with the cultures themselves, under the pressures of the globalizing economy, urbanization, and cultural homogenization.

Plant Origins of Milk Cultures

There are many stories about using plant and other natural sources as dairy fermentation starters. When making *gariss*, the Sudanese fermented camel's milk described in the previous section, in the absence of a starter from a previous batch, "fermentation is initiated by adding to the container a few seeds of black cumin and one onion bulb," reports Hamid Dirar.[40] A food blogger named Priya writes that where she grew up in India, "If the starter went bad or if we ran out of starter, families in my home town would use the stems of chili peppers to create a new one."[41] Turkish food writer Aylin Öney Tan cites varied recorded yogurt starters "ranging from fig sap to pine cones or acorns, or even more strangely from ant's eggs to morning dew collected from grass."[42] In Bulgaria too, writes ethnologist Lilija Radeva, "The oldest method of fermenting sheep's milk is by the addition of wood ants."[43] I've also heard of using figs—specifically the latex expressed from the stems of freshly picked figs—to start kefir. My friend Meka reported to me that he had heard it was possible to generate kefir grains by mixing a bit of raw goat's milk with fig latex, so I tried that, without success. (Meka thought there might be some other key to this magical creation: "Did you sing to them?" he emailed me.)

Tettemelk is a Scandinavian fermented milk, like most other fermented milks usually made using the last batch as starter. But enduring folklore also suggests that *tettemelk* can be cultured with leaves of a plant known in English as butterwort (*Pinguicula vulgaris*). Contemporary researchers tried this and reported that "experiments do not support this belief," although because butterwort is also used to curdle milk, and is known in Norwegian as *Tettegrasets*, they acknowledge that the plant may have been used with the milk in the past in a practice that has not endured. "The role of butterwort has probably been forgotten and misunderstood."[44] We cultural revivalists have our work cut out for us!

Many other plants have been associated with curdling milk, including stinging nettles (*Urtica dioica*), fig (*Ficus carica*), Indian fig (*Opuntia ficus-indica*), mallow (*Malva* spp.), creeping Charlie (*Glechoma bederacea*), lady's bedstraw (*Galium verum*), and several different thistles (including *Cynara cardunculus, C. humilis, Centáurea calcitrapa, Cirsium arietinum,* and *Carlina* spp.).[45] Herbalist Maud Grieve provides some guidance for using stinging nettles in this way: "The juice of the nettle, or a decoction formed by boiling the green herb in a strong solution of salt, will curdle milk, providing the cheese-maker with a good substitute for rennet."[46] Martha Washington's cookbook suggests a simpler method: Heat milk, pour it over nettles, and let it stand overnight to curdle.[47] When I tried Martha's method, the milk coagulated, but around the nettle leaves, and it was difficult to separate the curds from the plant material. But a small amount of a strong green nettles infusion (for ½ gallon/2 liters of milk about a cup/250 ml of boiling water poured over ½ ounce/14 g dried and crushed nettle leaves and left to infuse overnight) coagulates milk beautifully, although not nearly as fast as rennet; be prepared to wait up to 24 hours.

Another way that people have used plants in milk fermentation is using the smoke and ash from burning plants, as illustrated in the Kenyan fermented milk discussed in the opening of this chapter. The United Nations Food and Agriculture Organization reports, "The practice of smoking the vessels used for the storage of milk is a common feature of the various pastoral and agropastoral communities in the region. The treatment has the functions of passing the smoke flavour to the milk or milk product and disinfecting (sterilizing) the vessel." The FAO lists more than a dozen plants—including grasses, shrubs and hardwoods—used in this way by various communities in Ethiopia, Kenya, and Tanzania.[48]

Crème Fraîche, Butter, and Buttermilk

If you find yourself with access to raw cow's milk, skim off some of the cream to ferment. Cow's milk (unlike goat's and sheep's milk) naturally separates, with cream rising to the top. When you skim off the cream, what you have left is skim milk, the original low-fat dairy product. You can still drink that, or ferment it, or even make cheese from it. The milks of goats and sheep, on the other hand, are naturally homogenized, so the milk fats remain distributed throughout. But the cream that floats to the surface of cow's milk is rich and wonderful, and effortless to ferment.

Crème fraîche is simply cream fermented for a day or two. It's thick and rich and velvety. Most contemporary recipes call for adding a little buttermilk to the cream as a starter, which makes sense if you are working with pasteurized cream. But if your cream is raw, there is no need to add a culture to it. Ferment about 24 hours in a warm spot, until it thickens. Transfer to the refrigerator, where it will continue to thicken and develop flavor. Enjoy in sauces, soups, and desserts.

If you take the fermenting cream in process, as described above, and then churn or agitate it, it will solidify into butter—and not just butter but cultured butter. At a small scale, the easiest way to do this without special equipment is in a jar. Fill a jar no more than three-quarters full with cream and seal lid on tightly. Then shake the jar, or roll it back and forth, or vary agitation methods, for about 5 to 10 minutes, until all of a sudden the butterfats glob together and separate from the liquid buttermilk. When you notice that a big mass of butter is bobbing in the liquid in the jar, you can stop shaking. You can also do this in a food processor, or in a bowl with a spoon. Once butter forms, drain off the buttermilk. If you have a fridge, put the butter in it to harden it up a bit before finishing. Meanwhile, try the fresh buttermilk, so smooth and delicious! Once the butter hardens a bit, rinse it in cold water, and knead it to release any trapped pockets of buttermilk; rinse again after kneading, and repeat until the rinse water runs clear. Then let it dry, and store it, in or out of the fridge, to allow the fermented flavors to develop.

 ## Whey

As discussed previously, whey is the thin liquid that separates from the solid curd as milk acidifies or otherwise curdles. Sally Fallon Morell, in her book *Nourishing Traditions*, recommends whey as a starter for many other ferments (which I also advise in several chapters of this book), from vegetables to sodas. This has led to confusion for some people, who do not clearly understand what whey is or how to obtain it from fermented milk products. For instance, I have received emails from people who purchased whey protein powder and did not understand why it failed to initiate fermentation.

Whey contains much protein, with most of the milk fats removed. Thus, one use of it is drying for consumption by bodybuilders or others wishing to ingest concentrated protein foods. But in drying whey into a powder, whatever live cultures may have been present in the original whey are destroyed. Furthermore, because there are so many different ways of curdling milk, some of which involve heat, not all whey contains live cultures. For instance, simple heat- and acid-curdled cheeses such as farmer's cheese or paneer produce whey that does not contain live cultures.[49]

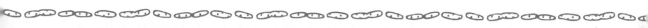

WHEY TO BRING CANNED FOODS BACK TO LIFE

Anna Rathbun, Mendocino, California

I have made a career of teaching healthy cooking to low-income families. One of the things we do on a regular basis is to "bring canned food back to life." Add a little whey and let it sit out for 12 hours and you can ferment beans, salsa, or just about anything. People who don't have refrigeration can add a bit of whey to just about anything and then it will last through the night and even a couple days, depending on the product.

In a perfect world, everyone would have a refrigerator and the means to buy fresh organic food on a daily basis. In this imperfect world, many depend on government rations of canned food with no means of preparation or storage. . . . We use whey to preserve food that may be going bad and to bring canned food back to life.

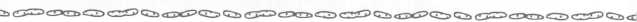

But the whey derived from fermented milks and raw or cultured cheeses is rich in live bacterial cultures. To obtain whey from yogurt, hang the yogurt, in a fine-mesh cheesecloth or tea towel, over a bowl. Whey will slowly drip from the yogurt and accumulate in the bowl. To obtain whey from kefir, simply leave the kefir in a jar at room temperature, until you can see a clear separation between curd and whey. Typically the curd will float above the whey. Gently and carefully scoop out the curd; what's left is whey. Note that the microbial differences between yogurt and kefir will be reflected in the whey they each produce. Because the kefir whey contains carbon-dioxide-producing yeasts, it is better than yogurt whey for starting sodas you intend to get bubbly (see *Whey as a Starter*, chapter 6).

Nanna Rögnvaldardóttir from Iceland reports that whey is in widespread use there. The fermented whey drained from *skyr* and other fermented dairy products is called *sýra*, and it is either drunk diluted with water or used as a medium for preserving other foods. Rögnvaldardóttir says that growing up, "We had whey-preserved food on the table almost every evening. Now, it is mostly consumed during the winter feasts." Foods preserved in *sýra* are called *súrmatur*, literally "soured food." For more on Icelandic ways of preserving meat in whey, see *Fermenting Fish and Meat in Whey* in chapter 12.

Cheese

Cheeses are condensed, solid forms of milk, requiring that much of the water content of the milk—the whey—be removed. Certain traditions and methods remove relatively small proportions of whey, resulting in soft cheeses; others remove more whey and make harder cheeses. The more whey you remove, the smaller your yield of cheese per unit of milk. Also, generally, the more whey you remove, the longer the cheese can ferment (more slowly) and be preserved.

I am in awe of the incredible diversity that exists in the realm of cheese. Different animals on different pastures in different climates and different seasons produce very different milks. Different culturing; different coagulation agents; different temperature treatment; different salting, spicing, and adjunct ingredients; different wrappings; different aging conditions, lengths, and methods; all these factors and more contribute to the unique qualities found in different cheeses. Cheese is testament to human inventiveness, in all the varied methods that people in different places use to turn perishable milk into products to store, sustain them through scarcity, and trade.

Making cheese is nothing short of a magical experience. Through a series of manipulations, you transform fluid milk into a solid block of concentrated flavor. You can make cheese in a home kitchen with just a bit of equipment: A double boiler (which you can improvise by nesting pots) is very helpful, as is an accurate thermometer, and for some cheeses, cheesecloth is essential. Beyond that you can improvise. As with many ferments, it is the sheer number of steps involved that makes cheesemaking a challenge; but each of the steps is fairly straightforward.

Culturing

It is necessary to introduce cultures for cheeses from pasteurized milk (do not attempt cheesemaking with ultra-pasteurized milk) or if you are attempting to replicate a specific style of cheese. Traditional raw-milk cheeses typically rely on bacteria indigenous to the milk, or in a vessel used repeatedly, or in yogurt or another cultured milk, or in some cases from a plant source.

Coagulation

Coagulation may be achieved via bacterial acidification, plant-source coagulants, or, most frequently, rennet. *Rennet* is a complex of enzymes (chymosin and others) originally derived from the fourth stomach, or abomasum, of infant ruminant animals. Once my friend Jordan slaughtered an infant goat and inside the stomach found a mass of cheese, coagulated as part of the digestion process. We made cheeses using rennet by simply soaking tiny strips of the dried stomach in warm water, which worked well, though it was difficult to regulate concentration. Commercial extracts, of standardized strength, are available. There is also a naturally occurring mold, *Mucor miehei*, that produces chymosin, sometimes marketed as "vegetable" rennet; and today most rennet is produced by genetically modified microorganisms, which have become the cheapest source of chymosin. Whatever type of rennet you use, when experimenting with cheesemaking, use rennet sparingly. A little goes a long way, and too much rennet can yield tough, rubbery curds, and a bitter flavor. For coagulation, whatever type of coagulant you use, leave milk undisturbed—movement can easily disrupt coagulation. Evaluate the progress of coagulation by examining the edges of the milk, which pull away from the vessel as the coagulated mass shrinks.

Cutting and Cooking

Once the milk coagulates, it solidifies into a gelatinous, custard-like mass. Typically at this point the curd is cut, to expose a greater surface area, enabling the rennet to act on many small masses, continuing to draw whey and tighten the curds. I use a sharp knife and cut slices at the desired interval in one direction; then I make another set of slices crossing the first set. Then I make a series of diagonal slices from different angles. As the curds shrink and I gently stir, I make further cuts as needed to reduce the size of any remaining large curds. The more uniform the size of your curds, the more uniform the texture of the resulting cheese. In many styles of cheese, the curds are further hardened by heating in whey, thereby hastening enzymatic activity. In almost every case, the literature emphasizes heating the curd slowly and gradually. A double boiler is the easiest way of accomplishing this. Don't heat the curds above 115°F/46°C or you will destroy the cultures that you want to continue to develop flavor in the cheese.

Swiss

Camembert

Draining, Salting, and Molding

When draining curds, save whey to drink, boil into ricotta ("recooked") cheese, soak grains, or use as a starter or pickling medium (as described earlier). Soft curds need to be handled gently or they can lose their cohesion and dissipate. Some cheeses are salted at draining; others only from the outside after the cheese has been formed in a mold. Typically, curds are drained in a mold that gives form to the cheese. The French word for cheese, *fromage*, and the Italian word, *formaggio*, come from the Latin *formaticum*, referring to the shape or form given to the cheese in a mold. I've heard of people fashioning molds from cans by drilling holes in them so they will drain, then lining them with cheese-cloth. Molds in different shapes are commercially available for less than the price of a gallon of raw milk. Most hard cheeses are pressed to force out more whey, with the amount of pressure and the length of pressing determining the hardness of the cheese.

Aging

Aging cheese can be very tricky, if you do not live next to a cave. I have met people who age homemade cheese in wine refrigerators, or use temperature controllers (see *Temperature Controllers* in chapter 3) to adapt regular refrigerators to roughly 55°F/13°C. Humidity is important too. A fairly humid environment permits slow drying. If the aging chamber is too dry, the outside of the cheese can dry, trapping moisture inside. Then the skin can become brittle and crack, exposing the cheese interior and making it vulnerable to molding. A critical part of aging cheese is rind development. Some cheeses are mold-ripened, in which case molds may be encouraged or even introduced via culturing. Other natural-rind cheeses may call for daily rinsing of the rind

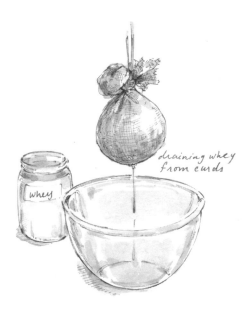

draining whey from curds

whey

with brine, wine, vinegar, or another mold inhibiter. Other cheeses may be encased in wax after sufficient drying, to protect the surfaces during a long aging period. There are many variables and possibilities.

To be honest, I have not made a lot of cheese in recent years. When I wrote *Wild Fermentation*, I was living in a community with a herd of goats and a handful of milkers; we were milking five goats, and when milk flow was heaviest, in the summers, we frequently *had* to make cheese as the milk rapidly accumulated beyond the capacity of our refrigerator. But a few years ago, we decided to scale down our milk production, and since then there has rarely been any excess. Meanwhile I've moved down the road and buy milk via a neighbor's goat herd-share program.

I miss the intimate interaction with the goats. And when it comes to cheese, I am an out-of-practice experimentalist. I made a few batches as I prepared to write this section, and I am reminded of how fickle cheesemaking can be, and how limited my experience and knowledge are. Rather than attempting to further guide you through a process at which I am not especially accomplished—certainly no more so than when I wrote the cheesemaking section of *Wild Fermentation*—I will guide you instead to the literature that I think covers the topic well, listed in *Resources*. If you are serious about learning cheesemaking, I would urge you to visit some farmstead cheesemakers to see how they do it, and consider some sort of apprenticeship, if possible.

Factory Versus Farmstead Cheesemaking

The complexity of cheesemaking tends to lead to specialization. Most professional cheesemakers I have visited attempt to master just a few styles, rather than a broad range. While the thrust of this work is on the simplicity of fermentation and encouraging people to experiment without fear, I also wish to acknowledge that many realms of fermentation, including (but not limited to) cheesemaking, are high arts to which people devote their careers and lives. Making good and consistent cheese is technically demanding. "The challenge for the farmstead cheesemaker is to strike the right balance between art and science," reflects Paul Kindstedt.[50] "It is time to abandon false pretenses about grizzled artisans and products that make themselves," write Bronwen Percival and Randolph Hodgson of Neal's Yard Dairy in London; "artisanship is truly about control."[51] In cheesemaking, there are a lot of variables to try to control.

Where specialization led, during the Industrial Revolution, was to the mass production of cheese. The world's first cheese factory appeared in New York State in 1851. In its first year, it produced more than 100,000 pounds of cheese, about five times the production of the largest farm operations of the time. "The resulting economies of scale, destined to drive future cheesemaking relentlessly toward larger and larger scales of manufacture, were immediately evident," writes Kindstedt.[52] "Farmstead cheesemaking all but disappeared. . . . Farmstead cheesemakers lost respect and even became the object of ridicule."

Kindstedt has a unique perspective on this, as someone who pursued a PhD in cheese science, with ambitions of working in the industry, just as the revival of artisanal cheesemaking was getting under way in the United States. His professor, Frank Kosikowski, was one of the founders of the American Cheese Society in 1983 and expected his graduate students to help him host its first meeting. Kindstedt recalls:

> Cheesemaking in my mind occurred in factories on a large scale. I had heard about farmstead cheesemakers, whom I glibly concluded were leftover hippies from the 1960s who had taken a shine to raising goats. I viewed farmstead cheesemaking as an anachronism, a naïve attempt to return to an era that had long since disappeared. With a degree of arrogance to which I now look back with shame, I asked myself why I should waste my precious time orchestrating a conference for these idiosyncratic nonconformists.[53]

Professor Kosikowski won over Kindstedt and his fellow graduate students. "He understood that traditional cheesemaking was not simply about food, or even about gastronomic delight, but rather carried with it the weight of the culture and local identity that are so essential for providing context and meaning to our lives." Indeed, all food exists in a broad context, and centralized mass-produced food diminishes that context.

The context for cheesemaking goes beyond the social to the biological. All the varied cheesemaking traditions developed out of particular environmental factors, specifically the varied climates and terrains favorable to different animals and producing very different milks, and the varied microorganisms present in the milk and aging environments in different places. "The names of these organisms are less important than the crucial role they play through history in giving specific places unique flavors and also in explaining why certain products can only be produced with specific environmental conditions with the right microbiota," writes historian Ken Albala, arguing that the notion of *terroir*—a term generally used to describe wines and the ways in which they express the unique environmental factors of the places in which they are produced—is equally applicable to cheese and other ferments.[54]

The initial microbial context for cheesemaking is the bacteria found in raw milk, and it is for this reason that raw-milk cheeses are so vastly superior to cheeses made from pasteurized milk with isolated, standardized cultures. Anthropologist Heather Paxson writes about the revival of raw-milk cheeses in the United States and identifies "the post-Pasteurian ethos of today's artisanal cheese cultures—recognizing microbes to be ubiquitous, necessary, and, indeed, tasty."[55] This contrasts with the dominant "Pasteurian" worldview—reflected in the US regulatory framework—that bacteria beyond specific strains chosen for utilitarian purposes pose a danger. But the real danger from milk and cheese is not so much bacteria as the conditions of factory farming, which produce unhealthy animals. In the context of healthy animals on pasture producing quality milk, microbes play a protective role and are key to our coevolutionary arrangement with the lactating animals we breed and keep. "From a microbiological standpoint, as cheese-making becomes more centralized with the use of commercial cultures of bacteria and fungi," predicts microbiologist and cheesemaker R. M. Noella Marcellino, "the biodiversity of indigenous microbial populations which developed in concert with each region's cheese is at risk."[56]

Homemade cheese and factory cheese are not the only options. There is a revival of farmstead cheesemaking in the United States, and we must encourage this to continue, by supporting it. Farmstead cheese is produced as an adjunct operation of a dairy farm, and this limits the scale of an operation. It is becoming increasingly difficult for commercial producers to exist at this scale. In the name of food safety, greater demands are being placed upon cheesemakers regardless of scale, making cheese production at the farmstead scale quite daunting (see chapter 13). Despite the regulatory hurdles, so far, farmstead cheesemaking is in revival. Support it and any small-scale food production you find in your midst.

Non-Dairy Milks, Yogurts, and Cheeses

Milk has come to refer to any creamy liquid of substance, such as coconut milk. In our time soymilk has become a ubiquitous alternative to cow milk, but any nut or seed can be extracted as milk (or turned into cheese). One great way to enjoy hickory nuts—plentiful in our region, tasty and nutritious, and, unfortunately, notoriously difficult and tedious to shell—is making them into milk. Extracting the oil and flavor of the nut into solution eliminates the need to separate out the shells, pith, and skins. Crack nuts between two large rocks. Remove the largest fragments of the shell, and grind or chop the nutmeat and whatever adheres to it into a coarse meal. Cover with fresh cold water and leave to soak overnight, stirring occasionally. Oils leach from the nuts into the water. Strain through a cloth, squeezing and pressing to remove as much liquid as possible. Less water in relation to chopped nuts will yield a thick, creamy milk, while more water makes a thinner product.

Any seed or nut can be similarly extracted into milk. Hemp seed milk is delicious, as is almond milk. To make almond milk, blanch almonds (add them to boiled water for about a minute, then rinse with cool water and easily squeeze off skins) before grinding, as skins can be very bitter. Experiment (in small batches) with different seeds and nuts and proportions.

Like mammalian milk, nut and seed milks can be fermented. But don't expect the result to be exactly like fermented milk. The seed milk ferment that most closely resembles its dairy analogue is soymilk fermented with yogurt cultures. You can ferment soymilk using the same procedure as dairy milk, and you can even buy commercial cultured soy "yogurt" to use as starter. But any *raw* nut or seed milk you can spontaneously ferment; or you can culture it with virtually any starter: dairy starters, sauerkraut juice, or water kefir (among others).

You do not necessarily have to discard the pulp (unless it is mixed with inedible shells, as in the case of the hickory nuts). I find seed and nut (as well as dairy) cheeses—thick, moldable, and spreadable, incorporating the ground nut or seed pulp—much more enticing than liquid milks. When I make a seed and/or nut cheese (often I mix them), I soak the seeds and/or nuts, then grind them (in a food processor or mortar) with just a little soaking water, sauerkraut juice or other live-culture starter, and fresh herbs. I add water slowly, as little as possible to achieve desired consistency, then age the seed/nut cheese a day or two, covered to keep flies away, and stir periodically. Hang in cheesecloth to thicken as necessary.

The best non-dairy "cheese" I've tried is *Keckek el Fouqara*, Lebanese fermented bulgur balls packed in olive oil, covered in chapter 8. Rather than thinking about foods that simulate or substitute for dairy products (or any other foods you cannot or choose not to eat), I would encourage you to focus instead on the foods you *do* wish to eat and all the wonderful ways you can ferment (and otherwise enjoy) them. In that regard, all the other chapters of this book are full of non-dairy ferments.

Troubleshooting

Yogurt did not set at all

Perhaps the starter was not viable. Perhaps the starter was added to milk that was warmer than 115°F/46°C. Perhaps incubation temperatures were too high (above 115°F/46°C) or too low (below about 100°F/38°C).

Yogurt is runny

Often the problem is that the yogurt lost heat during incubation. Try adding hot water to the incubator to bring it up to 110°F/43°C and gently heating the cultured milk to that temperature, then incubate a while longer. Other factors may be contributing as well. Goat's-milk yogurt is typically runnier than cow's-milk yogurt. Raw-milk yogurt is always runnier than yogurt in which milk has been heated to at least 180°F/82°C and then cooled. This heating denatures proteins and enables them to be restructured in the yogurt so it can take a solid form. For extra-thick yogurt, use cow's milk, heat it to at least 180°F/82°C, and hold it there for 15 minutes or so. Water will evaporate from the milk, concentrating it and resulting in even thicker yogurt.

Yogurt is grainy

Grainy yogurt is caused by heating the milk too quickly. Next time, heat the milk more slowly and gently.

Yogurt tastes burned

Heat the milk slowly and gently, and keep stirring to prevent it from burning.

Yogurt curdled

When whey separates from coagulated yogurt, it is called *syneresis*. To some extent this phenomenon is inevitable as yogurt ages, unless additional stabilizers such as gelatin are added to the yogurt. When it happens during the fermentation period, it suggests that fermentation proceeded for too long. I have had this problem when testing the limits of yogurt incubation temperatures. Yogurt incubated at 115°F/46°C for four hours was drowning in whey. At such a high temperature, the yogurt coagulates in a couple of hours; continued acidification causes a release of whey. If your fresh yogurt is covered with whey, try fermenting at a slightly lower temperature and/or for a shorter time.

Kefir is too sour

Try culturing for a shorter time and/or with a smaller ratio of kefir grains to milk.

Kefir curdles

Same as above. Kefir first thickens; then, as it further acidifies, it curdles. Shake vigorously to reintegrate.

Difficulty straining out grains

Sometimes when kefir is thick and gooey, it can be hard to strain. Kefir can clog the strainers and needs to be coaxed through. You can use a spoon and/or clean fingers to pick out the kefir grains, and stir, rubbing against the strainer itself and forcing the dense kefir through the strainer.

Kefir grains not growing

Sometimes, generally due to starvation, extreme temperatures, or other environmental stress, kefir grains can cease to grow, they can die altogether, and eventually they can even disintegrate into the acidic neglected kefir. I have killed many kefir grains and related cultures through neglect. Be good to your grains. Sometimes, for a while, kefir grains don't die but merely cease to grow. If the stunted grains are no longer producing kefir that is pleasing to you, discard them and try to find other grains. Sometimes even though they appear not to be growing, they continue to ferment milk that is tasty and consistent. Try to pamper the grains a bit, feeding them more frequently, giving them raw milk if you can access it, protecting them from extremes of heat or cold, and agitating them in the milk. Maybe they will start growing again.

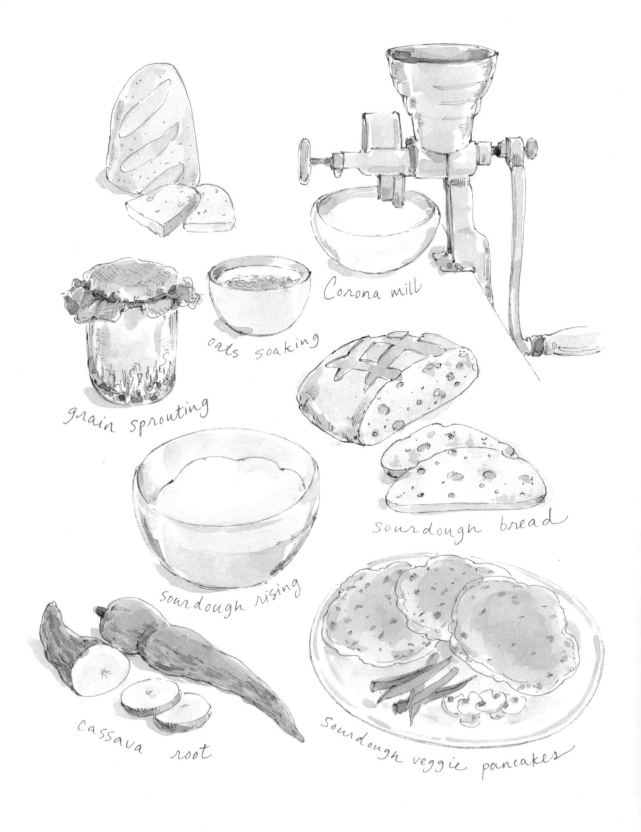

Corona mill

oats soaking

grain sprouting

sourdough bread

sourdough rising

cassava root

sourdough veggie pancakes

CHAPTER 8

Fermenting Grains and Starchy Tubers

$\mathcal{G}$rains and starchy tubers are the most basic daily staples that sustain most of humanity, filling our bellies and fulfilling our caloric requirements, embellished and supplemented when possible by vegetables, fruit, meat and fish, cheese, beans, and all the rest. According to the United Nations Food and Agriculture Organization (FAO), the most important cereal grains, in order of quantities grown and consumed globally (by both humans and our farm animals), are: corn (maize), wheat, rice, barley, sorghum, millet, oats, and rye. The most important starchy tubers are potatoes, cassava, sweet potatoes, yams, and taro.[1]

The emergence of grain agriculture gave rise to the earliest empires. The stability and storability of dry grains made possible unprecedented potential for accumulating wealth and building political power. "The emergence of complex societies, the need to keep written records, and the popularity of beer all followed from the surplus of grain," writes Tom Standage in *A History of the World in 6 Glasses.*[2] Grains continue to be of great economic, social, and political importance. Failures of grain crops have toppled governments and sparked revolutions.

The same dense, dry quality that makes grains so stable for storage also makes them difficult to digest. To nourish us well, they *need* the pre-digestion of fermentation. Grains contain several types of "anti-nutrients" that inhibit their digestion, including a form of phosphorous called phytic acid. According to an article in the *Journal of Agricultural and Food Chemistry,* "phytic acid and its derivatives can bind essential dietary minerals, thus making them unavailable or only partially available for absorption."[3] Phytic acid reduces the availability of minerals not only in the food that contains the phytic acid, but also in other foods being digested at the same time.[4]

Fermentation transforms phytic acid, as well as other toxic compounds found in grains, thereby neutralizing their harmful effects.[5] In grains, bacterial fermentation also increases the bioavailability of the amino acid lysine.[6] The pre-digestion power of fermentation is even more pronounced with cassava, a starchy tuber that is an important staple crop in many tropical regions. Cassava frequently contains a chemical precursor to cyanide (hydrocyanic acid), and can be quite poisonous if consumed unprocessed. As with phytic acid in the grains, fermentation reduces or eliminates the roots' toxicity. The miracle is that without knowing the chemistry of any of this, our ancestors intuitively understood or observed that grains and cassava roots need to be soaked (which initiates microbial activity) in order to be nutritious and easily digested.

Engrained Patterns

There is incredible variety in the particulars of regional styles of fermenting staple grains and starchy tubers around the world. And yet looking across cultures there are also recurring patterns of how different grains and tubers are fermented and prepared in different places. They are soaked. Often they are milled or pounded. Frequently grains are sprouted (also known as malted) prior to fermentation; this breaks down complex carbohydrates into simple sugars. In other traditions, molds are grown on grains, or sometimes the grains are chewed, in order to accomplish the same enzymatic transformation. Grains are cooked into stiff porridges and/or thin gruels. They are fried as flatbreads or pancakes; steamed; or baked as loaves.

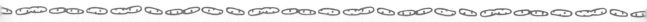

NIXTAMALIZATION

Nixtamalization is a process that emerged in the corn-centered cultures of Central America. The word is adapted from the Aztec Nahuatl language. In its vast geographic diffusion, there is considerable variation in the details of how this process is carried out. This is how I nixtamalize corn: I do it using hardwood ash, because that is a constant presence in my life. Most contemporary directions make use of hydrated lime (calcium hydroxide), widely available in Mexican markets as cal. For 2 pounds/1 kg of dried whole-kernel corn, use 1 cup/250 ml of sifted wood ash or 1 tablespoon/15 ml cal. Bring the water with corn to a boil. Add wood ash mixed with water, or cal dissolved in water, to the boiling corn. The corn will turn bright orange immediately. Gently simmer for about 15 minutes or until the skins begin to loosen from the kernels. (If you cook longer, the skins, and eventually the entire kernels, will dissolve; I've used too much ash, left the nixtamal boiling too long, and had the corn completely dissolve into the solution.) Once the skins are separating from the kernels, remove the pot from the heat, cover, and leave the corn to sit in the hot alkaline solution overnight or until cool. Rinse well. If the skins are still attached to corn, rub between the palms of your hands to remove. The corn is now *nixtamal*.

One grain with an impressive array of variations in its fermentation styles, exemplifying patterns found across cultures, is corn, known in much of the English-speaking world as maize. This grain is native to Mexico, where it is fermented into myriad foods and drinks. In ancient as well as contemporary Mexican ferments, in most cases—unless the corn is to be sprouted—corn is *nixtamalized*, an alkalinizing process in which whole corn kernels are cooked with wood ash or lime (see the sidebar). This process removes the hard outer layer of the kernel, alters the flavor, and improves the nutritional value of the corn.[7]

Descendants of the Mayan civilization that arose around corn ferment it by coarsely crushing the freshly nixtamalized corn into a stiff dough (*masa*), then forming it into balls (without any starter) and wrapping the corn dough balls in banana or other large leaves. (You can also wrap it in corn husks, like tamales.) These balls are fermented several days, or longer. Historian Sophie D. Coe cites reports on Mayan life by an early Spanish bishop of the Yucatán, Diego de Landa, "that great balls of this dough are given to travelers and that it lasts for months merely becoming sour."[8] This fermented dough is called *pozol*. Often molds develop on its surfaces as it ages. "It is possible that this surface mycoflora contributes to flavour and, hence, the traditional-style *pozol* dough might be viewed as a fungal-ripened, lactic-fermented product," observe a team of microbiologists,[9] which would make it analogous to cheeses, and the mixed mold grain cultures of China and elsewhere in Asia (see chapter 10).

The United Nations Food and Agriculture Organization reports that bits of *pozol*, "at various stages of the fermentation process," are mixed with water, at proportions ranging between 1:2 and 1:3. Salt, chili peppers, sugar, or honey is added "to produce a whitish porridge which is consumed in the uncooked state as a basic food in the daily diet of large communities." *Pozol* is convenient and easy, a restorative beverage in the field or on the road. *Pozol* is not to be confused with the whole-corn stew *posole* (though that too can be made with fermented corn). "*Pozol* is consumed by Indian and mestizo populations, mainly in the Southeastern states of Mexico."[10]

Atolli is another ancient corn-based beverage often fermented, known as *atole* in Spanish. *Atole* is corn cooked into a thin drinkable gruel. Diego de Landa describes its importance among the Maya at the time of the arrival of the Spanish:

From the most finely ground maize they extract a milk which they thicken over the fire to make into a kind of porridge, which they drink hot in the morning. They throw water on what is left over from the morning and drink it during the day because they are not accustomed to drink water on its own. They also toast and grind the maize and dilute it with a little pepper and cacao, which makes a most refreshing drink. From the ground maize and cacao they make a foaming drink with which they celebrate their feasts. They extract from cacao a grease which resembles butter, and from this and from the maize they make another drink which is both tasty and highly regarded.[11]

Atole is thought to be among the earliest cacao vehicles. Sophie Coe reports that the Aztecs often left *atole* to sour for four or five days—until it developed "an agreeable sourness"—into *xocoatolli*.[12] *Atole* could be soured "during many points in its preparation," writes Coe.

> One method was to soak the hard, ripe maize, without adding lime, for many days until it almost dissolved of its own accord. Alternatively it could be soaked, ground, and then left to sour before boiling. Souring could also take place after grinding and dilution. One recipe divides the ground maize dough mixed with water into two equal portions, one of which is boiled and then added to the unboiled portion and left to stand overnight. The next day the mixture is boiled again. . . . Even young maize atolli could be soured.[13]

In Spanish, *xocoatolli* is known as *atole agrio* (sour *atole*). (More on this ahead.)

A completely different microbial transformation of corn enjoyed in Mexico is *huitlacoche*, corn on which the fungus *Ustilago maydis* has grown, known in English as corn smut. The fungus appears in growing plants and is pathogenic to the plant. Kernels in infected ears of corn develop into enlarged and irregular spongy black masses known as "galls." Aztec and later Mexican cuisine came to celebrate the distinctive flavor of the fungus-blackened corn, so much so that the fungus is often deliberately introduced.

In parts of Mexico, especially among Huichol and Tarahumar peoples, corn is also fermented into a beer called *tesgüino*. To make *tesgüino*, corn is first sprouted (also known as malting, during which enzymes develop to digest complex carbohydrates into simple sugars). Then the sprouted corn is ground into a paste, which is simmered with water for about 12 hours or more, then cooled, before adding various botanical catalysts and fermenting. (See *Tesgüino* in chapter 9 for more details.) Malted corn is also fermented with hot chili peppers into a beer called *sendecho* by the Mazahua people of central Mexico.[14] A very different process of making beer from corn—called *chicha*—is practiced in the Andes Mountains of South America. The source of enzymes to break down complex carbohydrates into simple sugars is saliva; the corn is chewed to crush the kernels and saturate them with the salivary enzymes that initiate this conversion (see chapter 9). In Brazil, soaked whole corn kernels are ground, mixed with water, sugar, and sometimes fruit, ginger, or other spices, and fermented into a light beverage called *aluá*.[15]

Cherokee people ferment corn into a sour beverage called *gv-no-he-nv*, essentially like *tesgüino* only with the corn nixtamalized rather than sprouted.[16]

In *Zuni Breadstuff,* author Frank Hamilton Cushing, who lived among the Zuni people in the 1870s and 1880s, describes "the most prized leaven" as chewed corn "mixed with moderately fine meal and warm water and placed in little narrow-necked pots over or near the hearth until fermentation took place, when lime [treated corn] flour [*masa*] and a little salt were added," resulting in a yeast "in nowise inferior to some of our own."[17] Cushing describes a range of Zuni fermented corn products made with such yeasts, including dumplings, puddings, "batter-cakes," and "fire loaves."

In the southeastern US region of Appalachia, people pickle corn, on or off the cob, in brine. Ernest Parker of Gilmer County, Georgia, recalls that in his youth, "They'd brine-pickle barrels of whole ears of corn just like they pickled kraut and beans."[18] April McGreger, who makes and sells Appalachian Soured Corn (and many other ferments and preserves) as Farmer's Daughter Brand, is the one who first introduced me to this idea of brine-pickling corn. "I always thought that sour corn was the European tradition of sour cabbage brought over and applied to local ingredients," explains April. But after talking to a Cherokee folklorist, she came to understand "that sour corn was already a Native American tradition that Europeans raised on sour cabbage had a taste for." April recommends using fresh sweet corn, in 5 percent brine, roughly 3 tablespoons of salt per quart/liter of water (see *Brining* in chapter 5), spiced with peppercorns. For starchier field corn, she recommends boiling the corn for a minute, "in order to set the milk." Because sweet corn is so sugary, and it ripens in hot weather, it sours fast. Sour corn can be served still on the cob as a pickle, as a relish, mixed into salsas, or incorporated into a range of salads or cooked dishes.

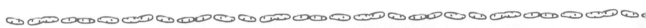

MAORI *KAANGA WAI*

Blogger Chef Tallyrand[20]

This literally translates as "corn water," but means a water cured corn dish. Maori food has its roots in their tradition, culture and also out of necessity; making use of foods readily available, in season or finding ways of preserving them for future use. *Kaanga wai* certainly comes under the latter, it is also known as "rotten corn." It has a very strong and unpleasant smell to it, which if you can get past (and most non Maori can't), is not a totally unpleasant flavour.

Originally the shelled white corn was placed in flour sacks and tied to stakes in running streams, but these days it is more often than not just placed into a drum of water and the water changed daily, for two months. By then the corn is really soft and mushy (not to mention smelling very ripe!) This is then cleaned, mashed or minced. Two parts corn to 6 parts water is then simmered on the stove until a porridge/grits/oatmeal type dish is produced (best done outdoors or with the windows open very wide!). This is then served with cream and sugar added to taste. A baked custard is also made with it by adding cream, eggs and sugar to the *Kaanga wai* and baking in the oven. If you are ever game to try it . . . *bon appétit!*

Corn, and styles of fermenting it, have migrated far from the cultivated grain's early range in the Americas. Maori people in New Zealand ferment corn in water in a process they call *kaanga wai* (see the sidebar). "Maize cobs can be kept in water for weeks for this ferment," writes Bill Mollison. "Kernels may be mixed with grated sweet potato, and steamed in muslin or corn leaves for about an hour (salt and pepper, or butter, sugar, and milk can be added to taste). The grains may be fried with salt and pork fat, or made into gruel."[19]

Across Africa, porridges and beverages made from corn have become subsistence staples. *Ogi* (Nigeria) and *uji* (Kenya) are sour porridges made of corn, millet, or other grains. The hot porridge is also known as *pap*, while the solidified form that results when the porridge is cooled is known as *agidi*.[21] *Kenkey* is a Ghanaian ferment, something like tamales, in which corn is soaked a day or two, ground into a paste, and fermented a few days. Then half of it is cooked into a porridge, which, after it cools, is mixed with the uncooked portion, formed into balls, wrapped in corn husks or plantain leaves, and steamed.[22] *Mahewu* is a sour fermented corn beverage widely enjoyed in southern Africa. Mix 1 part cornmeal with 9 parts boiling water, and cook the mixture about 10 minutes, until it begins to thicken. After it cools, mix in wheat flour (about 5 percent of the amount of cornmeal used), which functions as a live starter. Transfer to a fermentation vessel, and leave in a warm spot to ferment. Reportedly in southern Africa *mahewu* is typically fermented about 24 hours.[23] In Tennessee, I had to wait several days before mine developed some flavor, which was mild and pleasant. Stir and taste each day to gauge progress. Fermented corn has many other names and forms across Africa.

Of course, contemporary American corn dishes, such as corn bread and grits, can be fermented by simple soaking, as can Italian polenta. There is no food or drink made from corn or any other grain that cannot be fermented.

grain sprouting

One further form of corn fermentation worthy of mention is moonshine, also known as corn whiskey. Whiskey is distilled to concentrate alcohol, but distillation can only concentrate the alcohol that is formed by fermentation. Moonshine has been in the news in the rural county where I live in Tennessee, because voters just approved a referendum to legalize whiskey making here. What is most interesting to me is the history that has come to light: Before Prohibition, 18 distilleries were licensed to operate in our small county. They provided a market for local farmers' corn, and a non-perishable agricultural product to export out of the county to bring money in. After Prohibition and the locally imposed prohibition that has ensued, our county never found another viable economic foundation. Perhaps this fermentation-dependent value-adding activity will once again flourish here, sustaining farmers, creating jobs, and helping to revive the moribund local economy.

Wherever it has spread, corn has been of great importance, giving rise—or new expression—to elaborate cultural practices, different everywhere, and yet with recurrent patterns. All these ferments grow out of the same spirit of creative collaboration with life forces that give rise to the seed itself. "Seven thousand years of concentrated energy emanate from the seed," writes Marilou Awiakta in *SELU*, explaining the sacredness of corn and its powerful spirituality. We can feel that energy with our hands, and "take a quantum leap out of linear time and into a warm, wet place in Mexico where indigenous people are having a similar experience as, for the first time, they touch a certain wild grass." Beyond that mythical moment of original contact, Awiakta invites us to visualize the collaborative journey that has unfolded since between this plant and its human cultivators:

> Under their reverent, patient care, the wild seed gradually relinquishes its protective husk and entrusts its reproductive life to human hands, a process that the People interpret according to their sacred law and covenant with Mother Earth: Respectful care brings abundance. Lack of care brings nothing. If you take, you must give back—return the Gift.

> The people keep the covenant. From the seed they develop infinite varieties of what is now called the "supreme achievement in plant domestication of all time". . . . From the spirit—the nature of corn—the People learn survival wisdoms, common-sense ways of living in harmony with their environment and with each other. To revere the spirit and convey the wisdoms, each tribe, according to its customs, creates ceremonies, rituals, songs, art and stories. Each story is itself a seed, where the spirit of corn, as well as her basic teachings, is concentrated. Planted in a child's mind, the story matures along with the child, nourishing her or him to grow in wisdom and in stature. Story and life interweave.[24]

An important part of corn's story is not only how it has been cultivated, but also how it has been processed and fermented. Reclaiming our food involves investigating, learning, and ultimately retelling our stories.

Wheat has its own stories and continuum of traditional fermentation styles, as do rice, rye, and all the other grains. And every one of the styles of fermenting corn could be adapted to other grains. The results would be different, of course, because each of the grains is so distinctive in its nature, texture, biochemistry, and flavor. But the grain ferments all follow just a few basic patterns, all permutations and elaborations of the simple mixing of water with grains. Grains can be combined with water in so many different ways, and every one of them can be enhanced by fermentation.

Soaking Grains

The simplest way to ferment grains is to soak them. Water is the source of all life, and the dry seed is able to persist intact precisely because, in the absence of available water, the microbes inevitably present on the surface of it cannot function or grow. Yet they do remain, dormant until restored to life by water, much like the seed itself. When you soak the grain, it begins to swell, setting in motion a series of changes that, given the right conditions, will result in its sprouting into a new plant. At the same time, water also revives the bacteria and fungi that populate the grain's surfaces, and initiate fermentation.

Grains benefit from soaking whether whole or already milled. Here we are addressing whole and partially milled grains such as cracked wheat or rolled oats (flour will be addressed later). Use dechlorinated water, in whatever proportion you wish to use for cooking the grains. You can soak grains for just a few hours, if that's all you have; although pre-digestion will just be getting under way, it's better than not soaking at all. More pre-digestion will occur faster if you soak grains in warm (body-temperature) water and add some active live cultures—such as a little soaking liquid saved from a previous soak, whey, sourdough starter, buttermilk, or sauerkraut juice—or acids such as vinegar or lemon juice. Soak 8 to 12 hours for grains to fully swell, or you can soak for a day or several days to allow for a fuller pre-digestion and really develop flavor. If you get into a rhythm of this, I recommend saving a few cups of the soaking liquid each time to jump-start the next soak. Soaking is easy; it does not actually take any extra work, just a little planning.

There are different schools of thought as to whether to cook grains in their soaking water or discard the soaking water and replace it with fresh. I do not have a definitive answer to this question. In my own practice, I use the water from longer soakings; more nutrients have leached into this soaking water, and it has developed flavor. With shorter soaks, I often pour off unabsorbed soaking water and replace it with the same volume of fresh. Paul Pitchford, in *Healing with Whole Foods*, states clearly: "Discard soak water."[26] However, he gives no reason. Jessica Porter, author of *The Hip Chick's Guide to Macrobiotics*, and Aveline Kushi, author of the *Complete Guide to Macrobiotic Cooking*, both direct us in recipes to cook grains in soaking water, but neither includes any discussion of the issue. Sally Fallon Morell, who has gotten many people soaking their grains via her book *Nourishing Traditions*, does not specify in the book whether there is any reason not to use the soaking water. When I emailed her to ask, she replied, "Normally, I drain the grains, but with oatmeal, I do cook with the soaking water." Like me she is inconsistent, sometimes discarding soaking water, sometimes using it. There is not an ultimate answer to everything.

Sprouting

Although soaking is the first step in sprouting, grains or other seeds cannot sprout if left soaking. Germination, which is what sprouting is, requires water, but it also requires oxygen. Soaked seeds will swell and then ferment, but they will not germinate unless the water is drained from them. Therefore, to sprout whole grains or other seeds—only intact, unmilled seeds can generally germinate—soak them for 8 to 24 hours, then drain the water off. For sprouting, I typically soak seeds in a jar (no more than a quarter full) with a piece of vinyl window screening covering the top, held in place by a rubber band. After soaking, I simply pour the excess water off, then leave the jar inverted, sitting in the dish rack, or in a measuring cup or bowl, elevated so that the grains do not sit in the draining water. Fermenter Nancy Henderson suggests using nylon stockings for sprouting, "cheaper than jars, takes less room, easier to handle, and yields a better result. . . . Just soak overnight as usual, then pour into the stockings and drape over something like the kitchen faucet." Whichever system you use, keep grains moist by rinsing them at least twice a day (morning and night), or more frequently in summer heat, then draining well each time. The length of time required for sprouting will vary with the specific grain, as well as temperature and frequency of rinsing. Keep sprouting grains protected from sunlight, to prevent photosynthesis and the development of bitter flavor. As a general rule of thumb, grain sprouts are ready when the white tails grow to be about the length of the grain itself. Sprouted grains can be used fresh, in any kind of dough or batter, or beverages such as *rejuvelac* (see below) or *tesgüino* (see *Tesgüino* in chapter 9); or they may be dried in a dehydrator, under the sun, or in a low oven, for beer brewing (see chapter 9) or milling into flour.

Rejuvelac

Rejuvelac is a tonic beverage made by fermenting already-sprouted grains in water. To make *rejuvelac*, you need to first sprout your grains. After they have sprouted, cover them with water. Ferment them for a day or two, then strain off the liquid and enjoy. Store *rejuvelac* in the refrigerator. Cover grains with more water for a "second pressing," if desired. *Rejuvelac* was developed by Ann Wigmore, a raw food pioneer of the 1960s. Some people love its flavor; others find it unappealing. Many people have also reported success using *rejuvelac* as a starter for other types of ferments.

Porridges

Before anyone was making bread as we know it from cereal grains, they were making porridges and gruels. These are just simpler and more straightforward to make. Gruels are thin and runny, usually drunk. Porridges are thicker, typically eaten from a bowl with a spoon, or in some cases thick enough to pick up with fingers and dip into stews. But they both exist along a continuum, and it would be hard to say exactly where gruel ends and porridge begins. Porridge is my more common experience, but any porridge can be thinned into gruel by adding more water. Fermentation improves the flavor of porridges and gruels and enhances their digestibility and nutrient availability.

The porridge–gruel continuum is powerful comfort food. I lovingly recall my grandmother always making Cream of Wheat for my siblings and me whenever we were with her. Gruel is notable for being the first food most of humanity eats as infants transitioning from nursing. "All traditional weaning foods tend to be in the form of a gruel made from the local staple," states the *Journal of Tropical Pediatrics*.[27] Infants are at the peak of their vulnerability to illness and death during the weaning period, due to the potential for malnutrition and diarrheal infections. Fermentation of weaning gruels, traditional in many regions of the world, increases nutrient density of gruels, improves nutrient availability, protects gruels from bacterial contamination, and can help build the microbial ecology of the infants who eat them. These benefits have been shown to decrease illness and mortality in infants.[28]

In the United States, porridges have become a vehicle for sweetening with maple syrup, honey, sugar, or high-fructose corn syrup. I encourage readers to experiment with savory seasoning of porridges. I grew up eating porridge with butter, salt, and pepper, which my father, descended from Lithuanian Jews, described as the "*Litvak* way." Nowadays, I usually season porridges with butter, peanut butter, miso, and garlic (all together). If you are a condiment lover, as I am and as I believe most people are, let your porridge base serve as a vehicle for your favorite condiments, and don't be afraid of bold experimentation.

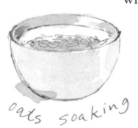

oats soaking

Fermenting Oatmeal

To ferment oatmeal, soak rolled or steel-cut oats in two to three times their volume of water. Two parts water will make thick oatmeal; 3 parts will result in a creamier and runnier product. Soak overnight, or for 24 hours, or a few days (stirring occasionally). Then gently bring the oats and soaking water, with a pinch of salt, to a boil and simmer, stirring, until all the water has absorbed into the oats and the oatmeal reaches a homogeneous consistency. If the oatmeal seems too thick, adjust by adding water, just a little at a time. If it seems too thin, add a little more oats. That's about how easy fermented porridge is. "In Brittany oat porridge was formerly eaten after one night of fermentation," writes Claude Aubert. "This overnight fermentation gives the traditional dish its characteristic taste, slightly acid, that one seeks in vain in modern porridges."[29] With soaking, you can even do this with whole oats, though they need to cook longer. Sometimes in winter, I've boiled soaked whole oats at night, then left them warming on a trivet atop the damped-down woodstove. The whole-groat oatmeal slow-cooked all night is incomparably creamy and delicious.

My friend Brett Guadagnino, a baker in New Orleans, uses sourdough starter to ferment oats and soaks them in milk rather than water. "I add a scant teaspoon of culture to a big mason jar of oats and milk," he writes. "The trick is to time it right so that it isn't too sour by breakfast time. Ideally, the mixture thickens and acquires a cheese-like consistency and flavor. It tastes great as a slightly sweetened or savory breakfast." Brett also uses this sourdough oatmeal in a novel way as a thickener for stews.

Dan Lepard, who writes about bread for the UK's *Guardian*, sent me a recipe for a porridge called *sowens* from a 1929 cookbook, *The Scots Kitchen: Its Traditions and Lore with Old-Time Recipes*. *Sowens* is made from *sids*, the inner husks of oat grains, which still have some starch attached after they are removed from the oats. First, the *sids* are soaked for four days or longer, then they are strained through a sieve. "Squeeze the *sids* to get all the goodness out of them, adding a little more cold water in the process," advises the author, F. Marian McNeill. The *sids* themselves are then discarded, and the soaking liquid is left to stand for another day, during which starch from the *sids* sinks and accumulates at the bottom. "When required for use the clear liquor is poured off, and some of the sediment is put into a pan with . . . water. . . . Add a little salt and boil it for ten minutes or more, stirring it briskly until it thickens."[30] Here, fermentation is a means of gleaning residual starch that would otherwise be discarded.

Grits/Polenta

Grits are the corn porridge of the contemporary southeastern United States. Growing up in New York, I knew grits only as an obscure cultural reference, as in Flo sassing to Mel on the 1970s television comedy *Alice*: "Kiss my grits!" But

I was familiar with polenta, the Italian corn porridge casserole, which I loved to eat and occasionally prepare. Once I moved to Tennessee, I was exposed to grits, and cheesy spicy grits with fried eggs became part of my breakfast repertoire. And as I made grits and polenta, I pondered the differences between them. Grits are usually, but not always, described as "hominy" grits. *Hominy* is an English word (adapted from the Algonquian) for corn that has been lime-processed, which I discussed briefly earlier as nixtamalization, an Anglicized version of an Aztec word. *Grits* just means a coarse grind, and hominy grits specifies that it be of hominy corn. In contrast, polenta is typically milled from corn that has not undergone this process, as the Europeans did not import the indigenous foodways along with the corn itself. But other than this distinction—whether or not the corn was nixtamalized—polenta and grits are exactly the same thing, coarse grinds of corn.

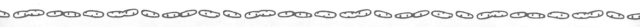

MILLET "POLENTA"

Lisa

My family grew up in the northern Italian Dolomites. In the cold winter months, we often ate polenta, which is coarsely ground cornmeal cooked into porridge. We served it with cheese and buttermilk made by our farmer neighbors. Since I do not eat as much dairy anymore, I have experimented with other grains that can mimic the flavor of those toppings. I have discovered that a delicious version of this dish can be made with millet. Try it out and enjoy the richness of this fermented cereal grain.

Pour ¼ cup/50 ml millet into a quart mason jar, then add 2 teaspoons/10 ml salt, and fill to the rim with water. Cover the jar with cheesecloth and let sit in a warm place for 24 hours to 2 days. Strain and rinse the millet, then pour into a cooking pot with 1½ cups/350 ml water. Bring to a boil; then reduce to a simmer. (Optional: Add 1 teaspoon/5 ml each: oregano, turmeric, cumin, paprika, salt.) Simmer until the millet begins to thicken (about 20 minutes). Begin to stir occasionally, as though you were cooking oatmeal. Add 3 tablespoons/45 ml olive oil and 1 tablespoon/15 ml lemon juice (optional). Cook on low heat and stir occasionally until the millet reaches a thick consistency. Pour into an 8-by-8-inch/20-by-20 cm container (or something similarly sized), and allow to cool. Finally, slice and serve toasted, grilled, or as it is.

Either can be fermented the same way: Soak it—with any kind of starter if you have one, or not—overnight, for a day or two, or even longer. This soak will make your grits or polenta creamier, more digestible, and more delicious. After soaking, cook with water and a pinch of salt, and keep stirring, to break up clumps and prevent burning on the bottom. I like to keep a kettle of hot water on hand to add hot water as needed.

Both grits and polenta can be served runny or set. Whatever consistency the dish has while hot, it thickens as it cools, like *ogi*, Nigerian fermented corn porridge, briefly touched upon earlier, which is called *pap* as a hot porridge and *agidi* after it has cooled and solidified. I usually make enough grits to enjoy some hot and thick but still stir-able, then spread leftover in a pie tin or baking pan to cool. After it sets, I slice and fry. Yum!

You can also make corn porridge directly from soaked whole corn kernels by pounding the kernels of dehulled, nixtamalized corn into a paste with a mortar and pestle, or grinding it in a food processor or grain grinder. (Note that if you mill wet grains in a grinder, it is imperative that you thoroughly clean and dry the grinder afterward to prevent rusting.) If you wish to ferment, let it ferment a day or two as a paste, with nutrients available to the microbes. Then bring the corn paste to a boil with a little salt and more water, stirring constantly, and cook until the desired consistency is reached, adding hot water as necessary.

Atole Agrio

Atole is a thin corn gruel, typically drunk as a beverage. According to Diana Kennedy, author of numerous books about Mexican cuisine, it is "a gruel of corn *masa* traditionally prepared with dried corn that has been barely cooked, without lime, and ground to a fine *masa*. It is served hot or cold, sweetened or seasoned, with a variety of ingredients, depending on the local custom."[31] One style of *atole* is *atole agrio*, which is soured *atole*.

Kennedy reports on the *atole agrio* process of Señora Blanca Flores in Huautla de Jiménez, who begins by soaking corn in water on a ceramic pot for four days, "which by then had begun to sour." Then the uncooked corn is rinsed, ground to a fine *masa*, and left to sour another day. Finally, the *masa* is diluted with water, strained to remove the coarsest pieces, cooked into *atole*, and served.[32]

I followed Señora Flores's process and loved the result, very smooth and satisfying in its unembellished simplicity, though it could be embellished in so many different ways, sweet, savory, and/or spicy. I ground the soaked corn kernels in my hand-cranked Corona mill (then cleaned and dried it thoroughly) and added enough water to make a workable paste. After another day's fermentation I added more water to produce a slurry and strained it through a wire strainer. Then I poured a little more water through the residue and pressed out as much starchy liquid as I could. I transferred this smooth starchy corn water to a pot and brought it to a gentle boil, stirring constantly to prevent burning. It firms right up as it cooks—just keep adding hot water. A pinch of salt brought out the flavor of the soured corn. Once I thought I had achieved the right thin gruel consistency, I removed the pot from the heat and let it cool, since I wanted to drink the *atole* cold in the summer heat. By the time it cooled, it solidified into a smooth corn pudding, which was lovely, but not the consistency I was going for. So I reheated the *atole*, adding more water, and stirred until it once again achieved a homogeneous consistency, this time thinner. Porridges and gruels are very versatile and can be cooked to a wide range of consistencies.

Millet Porridge

You can make porridge with any grain. Personally, I love to eat porridge of fermented millet. Millet itself has a very mild, sweet flavor, and fermentation contributes flavor complexity. To make millet porridge, coarsely grind millet and soak it for a day or two before cooking. (Alternatively, soak millet for a day or two, then grind it, then ferment another day or two as a paste.) Cook millet with water and salt into porridge, using a proportion of around 4 parts water to 1 part grain. Generally, I don't measure. I keep a kettle of hot water at the ready so I can add more hot water as the porridge thickens. People are often shocked at how creamy fermented millet porridge is; if they are familiar with millet at all, they think of it as dry and granular. Fermentation, grinding, and cooking it with a greater proportion of water all contribute toward its appealing creaminess.

Sorghum Porridge

Sorghum as a grain is even more obscure in the United States than millet. I bought some for sorghum beer making (see *Sorghum Beer* in chapter 9) and have fallen in love with it as porridge. To make *aceda*, I coarsely mill the sorghum into a bowl and ferment it in the Sudanese method, known as *ajin*. To do this, moisten the flour with a small amount of dechlorinated water. Add water to the flour just a bit at a time, mix, and add a little more water, until there are no more dry patches in the flour. Cover with a cloth and ferment one or two days, stirring periodically. When you are ready to make porridge, boil about three times as much water as your volume of *ajin*, add *ajin*, and stir. Keep stirring as it cooks and thickens. I usually cook it for about 15 minutes. "Experienced women have a simple test to check if the *aceda* is cooked," explains Dirar:

> A woman wets her finger and presses it on the mass of aceda. A well-done porridge bounces back on withdrawal of the finger, which comes off clean. An aceda that is not well cooked lacks resilience and sticks to the finger. A half-done aceda also falls apart and partly dissolves when water is added to it.[33]

I like to make a batch of *aceda* in the morning, eat some hot, and pour the rest onto a plate to cool and solidify, then eat it all day long with whatever else I prepare. Eating solidified porridge reminds me how similar porridge is to bread. In fact, in the Sudan, where sorghum is a daily staple, the word *kissra* was used to describe porridge; then, as flatbread spread as a way of eating sorghum, the flatbread became known as *kissra-rahifa*. By 1992, when Hamid Dirar published his *Indigenous Fermented Foods of the Sudan*, *kissra* had come to refer almost exclusively to sorghum flatbreads. "The influence of the city culture is spreading to the villages very rapidly and it is clearly seen that the stiff porridge is gradually being called *aceda* and the thin bread *kissra*."[34]

Rice *Congee*

The porridge of Chinese cuisine is called *congee*. Like other porridges, *congee* is creamier and more digestible if the grain is soaked beforehand. In addition to rice, *congee* can also be made from millet, spelt, and other grains. The best way to make *congee* is as I described making whole-groat oatmeal, earlier. Soak the grain. Then bring the water and grain to a boil and leave it gently cooking all night on a trivet atop a damped-down woodstove, radiator, or other gentle heat source. An alternative, practiced every day for decades by my recently departed friend Dr. Crazy Owl, and great for camping trips, is to combine grain and boiling water in a preheated thermos and leave it overnight. The rice *congee* is still hot in the morning, thoroughly cooked and ready to eat.

Crazy Owl sang the healing virtues of rice *congee*, especially for the infirm and frail. He was so devoted to a daily rice *congee* practice that when he abandoned it and started asking for fruit smoothies instead, it lent credence to his announcement that "I am ready to go." Two weeks later he was, indeed, gone. *Congee* is widely used as a healing food. According to Paul Pitchford, author of *Healing with Whole Foods*, *congee* "is easily digested and assimilated, tonifies the blood and the qi energy, harmonizes the digestion, and is demulcent, cooling, and nourishing."[35] Vegetables, beans, fruits, miso and other fermented condiments, meat stock, and medicinal herbs can be added for flavor and specific therapeutic effects.

Congee is sometimes referred to as a soup rather than as a porridge, and indeed it is typically soupy. Rather than a homogeneous texture, however, it is a starchy suspension with grains of rice floating in it. One part grain to 6 parts water is a rough proportion, but you could use less or more. "It is better to use too much water than too little," advises Paul Pitchford. "It is said that the longer *congee* cooks, the more 'powerful' it becomes."[36]

Old Bread Porridge

A great way to use old dry bread is to cook it into porridge. To do so, cut bread into cubes, and then soak them in water (or, if the bread is too hard to easily slice, soak it first). Cook in a little water (or milk), adding liquid as necessary to achieve the desired porridge consistency. Embellish with savory condiments (miso, *shoyu*, peanut butter, tahini, hot sauce) and/or sweet ones (jam, maple syrup, honey, sugar).

Potato Porridge

Finally we get to starchy tubers! The concept of potato porridge came to me from Jana and Vanda Fröberg, Swedish sisters who blog as "Porridgehunters Were Here" and have a book about porridge forthcoming.[37] Mashed potatoes *are* potato porridge! In the Porridgehunters recipe, they mash the potatoes in the water they were cooked in, then thicken that up with rye flour and cook a little while. But any creamy mashed potatoes can be thought of as porridge. And you can even pre-ferment the potatoes. Cut them into small cubes and cover with water and/or whey in a bowl or jar. Leave to sit, covered, for a day or two, then cook. I include this improvisational concept as a segue from grain porridges to the fermentation of starchy tubers, because frequently the starchy tubers are prepared in porridge-like ways. For more potato fermentation ideas, see *Fermenting Potatoes*.

Poi

Poi is a Hawaiian ferment of *taro* (*Colocasia esculenta*) mashed into a gluey purple paste. Taro is central and sacred to the native people of Hawai'i, who call it *kalo*. *Poi* made an impression on Captain James Cook, who described it in his earliest report from Hawai'i: "The only artificial dish we met with was a taro pudding; which, though a disagreeable mess from its sourness, was greed-ily devoured by the natives."[38] By 1933, a University of Hawai'i study reported that "other foods are taking the place of this ancient standby."[39] Nevertheless, *poi* has endured. "As Hawaiian culture and language continue their steady resurgence begun in the 1970s, an awareness of the importance of *kalo* is reemerging as well," reported *Maui Magazine* in 2007.[40]

The part of the taro plant processed into *poi* is the swollen underground base of the stem, known as the corm. The taro corm must be thoroughly cooked by steaming or boiling in order to neutralize calcium oxalate crystals, "which feel like eating fiberglass" if consumed uncooked, reports my friend Jay Bost. Once cooked, the corm's skin is scraped off and, while still warm, the starchy flesh is mashed into a paste, adding water as necessary. Traditionally, the cooked taro is mashed against a special wooden board using a heavy stone pounding tool, known as a *pohaku ku'i 'ai*. You can mash by hand, using either a mortar and pestle or a potato masher, or in a food processor. Try to find and crush any lumps, in order to get the paste as smooth as possible.

To ferment, simply pack the mashed taro into a ceramic or glass bowl or crock. Leave some room in the vessel for expansion, as the *poi* will expand as it ferments. Ferment it for a few days at room temperature. Typically no culture is introduced, unless you have mature *poi*, a little of which can be added to the fresh mashed taro. If white surface mold develops, mix it right in.

It remains a bit of a mystery to me how the ferment starts so quickly in a cooked substrate without adding any raw adjuncts to get it going; however, somehow it does. Two bacteriologists at the University of Hawai'i published a five-year study of *poi* fermentation in 1933. They performed bacterial cell counts on uncooked taro corms, on the skins immediately after cooking, on peeled cooked taro, and on fermented *poi*. "The organisms responsible for the fermentation were abundant on the steamed taro corms immediately follow-ing heating," they reported. "Grinding of the crushed corms aids in breaking the bacterial clumps or colonies on the corms, and therefore makes possible not only increase in numbers of organisms, but also their distribution rather homogeneously throughout the fresh *poi*."[41]

As with any ferment, some people prefer *poi* mild after just a day or two, while others prefer the more sour flavor that develops as more days pass. In Hawaiian temperatures, three to five days is the normal range; in cooler places, it may take longer. The color and texture of the *poi* also change as fermentation proceeds. Taste each day to evaluate.

Poi can be prepared thinner or thicker. The consistency of *poi* is usually described by the number of fingers it takes to eat. Most sources concur that two-finger *poi* is the ideal. Very thick *poi* is one-finger, while runny *poi* is three-finger. But ultimately, it's a question of what texture you like. Simply add water and mash until you reach that consistency. For slow fermentation and long storage, the *poi* is made as thick as possible and then thinned by adding water as needed.

Poi has its own unique healing properties. Pamela Day credits *poi* with saving the life of her daughter, who suffers from multiple food allergies and as an infant could not tolerate breast milk or soy formula, but did eat *poi*. "*Poi* shows promise for use in infants with allergies or failure-to-thrive," reports the journal *Nutrition in Clinical Care*.[42] In addition, research suggests that *poi* may have both anti-tumor and immune-stimulating effects.[43]

 ## Cassava

Like taro (only more so), cassava is a tropical tuber that is an important daily staple in many equatorial regions of the world. Cassava is known in the US mainstream primarily in the form of tapioca, used for puddings and in other thickening, binding roles. I was introduced to cassava, under the French name *manioc*, in West Africa, where I traveled for a few months in 1985. On our trip we mostly ate from outdoor market stalls, typically stews of vegetables with fish or meat, usually served with white fluffy starchy stuff called *fufu*, which, we were told, was made from *manioc*. What we learned, from watching other people eat, was to tear a bit of *fufu* (always with your right hand), form it into a ball, and squeeze it with your thumb into a sort of spoon with an indentation, then dip it into the stew to fill the indentation, scoop it into your mouth, and eat. I loved the weird gluey consistency of *fufu* and this sculpting and scooping ritual that goes along with it.

I wasn't familiar with *manioc*/cassava, but I eventually realized that this filling starchy stuff was made from the huge tubers sold at other market stalls. Sadly, I did not investigate then to learn the details of how the tubers were turned into *fufu*. But clearly it involved a lot of pounding, for the sound of women pounding *manioc*/cassava roots was a rhythmic beat frequently present in the background. After I returned to the United States, I searched for information on how to make *fufu*. Most available sources suggested substituting instant mashed potatoes for cassava, and simply mixing it up stiff, which was not very interesting. But eventually in my readings about fermentation, I learned that *fufu* is frequently made with cassava that has been fermented.

According to the *International Journal of Food Science and Technology*, "Fermentation is an important means of processing cassava to improve palatability, textural quality and to upgrade nutritive value by enrichment with proteins and for reduction of cyanogenic glucosides."[44] These cyanogenic glucosides can be highly toxic because they form hydrogen cyanide, familiarly known as cyanide. Different varieties of cassava, grown in different soils, produce varied levels of cyanide, in some cases extremely high. Various means are employed to reduce cassava's cyanide potential, including peeling, pressing grated cassava to express as much of the plant's juices as possible, thorough cooking, and fermentation. Many cassava traditions incorporate all of these methods. "Fatalities from cassava poisoning appear to be rare," writes food microbiologist Kofi Aidoo, "but long-term toxic effects (e.g. goiter and cretinism) in cassava-consuming populations may be more serious, especially in the Amazon where the pressed-out juices are used for making soups and stews."[45] Of the various cassava detoxification methods, the *International Journal of Food Science and Technology* reports that fermentation of peeled and chopped cassava roots submerged under water "is the most efficient process for reducing the levels of cyanogens in cassava, where reduction rates of 95–100 percent are often reported."[46] Microbiologist Mpoko Bokanga reports that in Zaire "whole roots are steeped in water and left to ferment naturally for 3 to 5 days." Not only are the cyanogens virtually eliminated, but roots are acidified and their texture goes "from hard and brittle to soft and mushy."[47]

As with any staple food (think of all the different names we have for concoctions of wheat and water), there are many distinct processes for fermenting and eating cassava, and many different names for them. In addition to *fufu*, in Africa there is *gari, lafun, attiéké, miondo, bobolo, bidia, chickwangue, agbelima, attieke, placali, kivunde*, and probably many more; many other fermented cassava foods are found in Asia, Central and South America, and the Caribbean.[48]

If you are starting from whole cassava roots, the first step is to peel them. The peels contain the highest concentration of toxic cyanogenic glucosides. In import markets in the United States, cassava is typically waxed, to slow its rapid decomposition. Following peeling, chop cassava into coarse chunks, and submerge in water. During the fermentation, in addition to the toxicity being virtually eliminated, the roots will soften and acidity will increase. Most sources report spontaneous fermentation of three to five days; according to an academic study comparing different lengths of cassava fermentation, "The preference of the panelists [Nigerian university students] for the characteristic texture and odour of cooked 'fufu' increased with the increasing period of fermentation."[49] Typically neither salt nor starters

cassava root

are added to the soaking water, but they can be. In some traditions, water is drained and replaced each day.

After fermentation, boil or steam the chunks of cassava root until soft, then pound them into a smooth paste using a large mortar and pestle. Pound (hard!) with one hand, while using the other (or a helper) to continually scrape cassava mush from the sides of the mortar into the center. Keep the hand doing this wet, and it will gradually add water to the mix. As the cassava is crushed and its exposed starch absorbs water, the pounded cassava will become gluey and cohesive. Keep pounding until you have a smooth ball of *fufu*.

A Jamaican student named Chad introduced me to his grandmother's method of grating the cassava roots, then placing the grated roots in a T-shirt and wringing it with great force in order to express as much as possible of the toxic cassava juice. Chad mixed the grated cassava with coconut and fried it into cakes he called "bammy," which were sweet, light, and delicious. I added some to sourdough and fermented it for a few days before making it into savory sourdough pancakes (see *Flatbreads/Pancakes*); the fermented cassava gave the pancakes a delicious cheesiness, and they were a big hit.

One popular form of cassava is called *gari*, from Nigeria. For *gari*, the cassava roots are grated after peeling. The grated cassava is often inoculated with a starter (from a previous batch), then placed in a bag and left with a heavy weight on it to press juice out of the grated roots. It is left under the weight for several days, during which it undergoes a solid-state fermentation, distinct from the submerged fermentation for *fufu*. After fermentation, the *gari* is dried and sometimes toasted. Dried *gari* in bags is exported from Nigeria and available in stores around the world catering to African expatriates. You can mix *gari* with water, cold or hot, and make thick or thin pastes with it. I like to cook it with hot water into a thick paste, stirring vigorously and using a spoon to crush any clumps that form. You can eat it with a spoon or form it into balls you can pick up and dip. *Gari* has a distinctive flavor, but it, like all forms of cassava, needs sauces to dip it in or scoop to make it enticing. It'll sure fill your belly.

South American Cassava Breads

One use of fermented cassava that is popular in South America is in breads, typically rich with eggs and cheese. In Brazil these breads are known as *pão de queijo*; in Colombia they are known as *pan de yuca* or *pan de bono*. The breads are usually prepared as small individual-serving balls. When the sour cassava starch is mixed into an eggy dough, it causes a dramatic rise, giving these cheese balls a lightness that reminds me of popovers. "The main characteristic of this product is its expansion properties during baking without using specific agents such as yeast or baking powder," reports the *International Journal of Food Science and Technology*.[50]

The fermented cassava starch that is the primary ingredient is called *polvilho amido azedo* in Portuguese and *almidón agrio de yuca* in Spanish. It can be found at Latin American groceries or online. One pound/500 g of flour will make about 50 small balls. Heat about 1¼ cups/300 ml milk with ½ cup/125 ml vegetable oil and 2 teaspoons/10 ml salt, to just below boiling. Pour the hot liquid mixture over sour cassava starch and mix together. When dough is cool enough to handle (but still warm) mix in two lightly beaten eggs and 1 cup shredded cheese. Knead the dough by hand about 10 to 15 minutes, until it is smooth. Heat the oven to 450°F/230°C. Oil a baking sheet, form the dough into small 1-inch/2–3 cm balls, space on the sheet with room for expansion, and bake about 15 minutes, until golden. Extra dough balls may be frozen uncooked and baked later. Serve warm.

Fermenting Potatoes

Potatoes too may be fermented. In the high altitudes of the Andes Mountains, where potato agriculture emerged, bitter varieties are fermented as *chuno*, in order both to remove toxic alkaloids and to preserve them. "The complex procedure enables potatoes to be 'freeze-dried' by means of extreme changes in temperature," states the Slow Food Presidium organized to promote *chuno*.[51] According to Bill Mollison, potatoes "are exposed to frost whole and uncooked; examined to make sure they have been fully frozen (when the cell walls separate and cell saps diffuse); they are then trampled to remove the skins and to squeeze out the cell water. Covered with straw by day to prevent blackening, they are then submerged in running water (straw-covered) for from 1–3 weeks to sweeten, and spread to dry in the sun."[52] The dehydrated potato "becomes white and very light, resembling pumice stone," notes the Slow Food Presidium. "In this condition the potato can keep for around 10 years."

I've often included cooked potatoes (mashed, steamed, or fried), among raw vegetables I was fermenting (see chapter 5). Jenny McGruther, a fermentation advocate and educator who created the website Nourished Kitchen,[53] ferments potatoes for frying. She slices potatoes into fries no more than ¼ inch/0.5 cm thick, covers them with water and a starter (she recommends whey or a commercial starter; I would expand the list to include sauerkraut juice, sourdough, or other active culture), and ferments at ambient temperature for one to three days. Potatoes will have a tendency to float, so if you're experimenting with this, use a plate or other modest weight to weigh down. After fermentation, potatoes will smell a little sour. Drain, rinse, and pat dry with a towel (so they will fry crisp). Deep- or oven-fry in the oil of your choice. Salt and season as desired, and enjoy the fries warm. Jenny makes the point that by reducing starch in the potatoes, fermentation results in reduced formation of acrylamide, a chemical by-product of frying starchy foods that the European Union and Canada are investigating as a possible carcinogen.

Sourdough: Starting One and Maintaining It

Sourdough is the most common English-language word to describe a mixed culture starter for rising bread (as well as many other culinary applications). Essentially it is backslopping, simply using a bit of the previous batch to start the next one. This is how virtually all bread was made until two centuries ago, when purer forms of yeast began to become commercially available. Even before Louis Pasteur isolated yeast organisms, in 1780 Dutch distillers started marketing yeast foam to bakers, skimmed from the top of fermenting alcohol. In 1867, a Vienna factory refined this process, taking the yeasty foam, skimming it off, filtering and washing it, and compressing the yeast into cakes. This became known as the Viennese process, still in use today.[54] In 1872, Charles Fleischmann patented an improved manufacturing process for compressed yeast and built an industrial empire upon its production. Today, the vast majority of baking is done using isolated yeasts, and sourdough persists almost as a novelty, except in artisan bakeries. Isolated yeasts certainly offer some advantages for bakers, in terms of speed and uniformity. But these benefits come with the sacrifice of other positive attributes of traditional mixed-culture leavens, such as flavor complexity, moist texture, superior keeping properties, and fuller pre-digestion. With wheat flour, researchers have found that mixed-culture sourdough pre-digestion results in "highly significant" increased available lysine content[55] and diminished presence of gluten.[56]

The simplest way of starting a sourdough from scratch is to mix a small amount of flour and water in a bowl, a little more flour than water, and stir until smooth. Add a little more water or flour as necessary to obtain a batter that is liquid and pourable, yet thick enough to cling to the spoon. Rye flour seems to work fastest, but you can make sourdough with the flour of any grain. Be sure the water is un- or dechlorinated. Press out any lumps of flour so the batter is smooth. It should be thick enough to cling to the spoon (or your hands), and to (soon) hold foamy bubbles. Stir at least once a day for a few days, until you see bubbles on the surface. Then feed it a high proportion of fresh flour, adding roughly three to four times as much fresh flour and water to the remaining starter. High-proportion feedings like this reduce the acidity of the sourdough environment and give yeasts a competitive advantage. It's a good way to build sourdough vigor.

There are many other techniques people use to start sourdoughs. Some people like to use water from boiling potatoes (cool to body temperature before adding), or starchy water from rinsing or soaking grains, or fruit, or fruit or vegetable skins. People sometimes use another starter to start sourdough. I've heard about people using foam off fermenting beer in bread starters, as well as yogurt, kefir, sour milk, water kefir, kombucha, *rejuvelac*, and fermented nut milks. Many people start a sourdough with a packet of yeast and let it naturally diversify from that. Some people start with established starters they are given, or purchase them online. Some people advocate stirring with your clean hands as a means of culturing. But really all you need is flour and water. Beyond that, all sourdough requires is a little patience and persistence.

I've started sourdough from flour and water many times. There is abundant microbial life present on grains. "Cereals and flours prepared from cereals are always heavily seeded with microorganisms," writes microbiologist Carl Pederson. "One cannot prepare a dough without incorporating these organisms."[57] This indigenous microflora is dormant in dried grains and flour, but when the flour is moistened by water, microbial activity resumes. Stirring stimulates and distributes microbial activity, encourages yeast growth via oxygenation, and prevents surface mold growth. If you keep feeding it and maintaining a hospitable environment, the culture—a complex community of organisms that microbiologist Jessica Lee calls "the interlocking metabolic relationships in yeast and bacterial consortia"[58]—can persist for generations. A crucial aspect of the microbial community's stability is its acidic environment, "a powerful weapon to keep other organisms at bay," writes Lee. Even using high-proportion feedings to limit the levels of acidity, sourdough's acidity protects its microbial community, then after baking continues to protect the bread from mold and bacterial growths. Sourdough breads generally age more gracefully, and in certain instances actually improve over time. (To maximize your bread's shelf life, wrap your loaves in breathable paper rather than plastic.) Even if the crust dries out, molds will not develop, and the interior will remain moist and delicious.

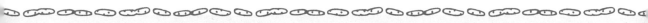

TASSAJARA REMINISCENCES

William Shurtleff is best known as the co-author, with his wife, Akiko Aoyagi, of The Book of Miso, The Book of Tempeh, *and many other books. Prior to that, he spent two years, from 1968 to 1970, at the Tassajara Zen center in Northern California. He shared the following reminiscence:*

To catch wild yeasts for sourdough at Tassajara we would prepare a sponge (a bit sweeter than usual) in a large pottery bowl (about 18 inches diameter), then mash and stir in 2–4 overripe bananas (which we thought was essential). We always ground our own flour freshly using a hand-turned Corona mill. Then we placed the sponge, uncovered, in a screened-in outdoor area, near the kitchen, where staple foods were kept. As I recall we stirred it once a day and left it for 3–4 days, usually in warm weather, until it started to show signs of life/activity/fermentation. We never saved any of it as sourdough. We started anew with each batch.

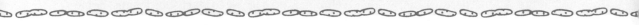

Sourdoughs cultivated by people in different places, using different flours and methods, can be very distinctive. People lavish their sourdough starters with care and attention and love to share them. Artist and baker Rebecca Beinart was inspired to give away samples of her starter, along with instructions, to strangers; she created an interactive map of her sourdough culture's spread on her website, www.exponentialgrowth.org. Some people seek out specialized sourdough starters from different parts of the world, and some enterprises, such as Sourdoughs International,[59] provide them.

Over the years, I have been gifted with sourdough starters by many wonderful people. One great starter was from the Bread and Puppet Theatre Company, which incorporates the baking and sharing of sourdough bread into its performances. Their sourdough came from Germany via company founder Peter Schumann. Another very different sourdough came from my friend Merril Mushroom, who has maintained it for decades, and originally got it from a friend. Merril's starter is very distinctive due to the fact that she replenishes it not with water, but rather milk. Readers and students have also shared their sourdoughs with me. Unable to maintain so many different starters over time, my current sourdough is one I started from flour and water years ago, to which I have added all the starters I have received. Let us celebrate mixed cultures and give up the futile quest for cultural purity.

No matter what they start as, sourdough starters are not static microbial entities. They become their environment and, to a lesser degree, what they are fed. "You can't pick and choose your wild yeast," writes baker Daniel Leader in his book *Local Breads*.

> Your culture will get its unique flavor characteristics from whatever yeast is present in your flour and your air. Say you obtain a sourdough culture from a baker in San Francisco. Once you bring it home and refresh it several times, it will adapt to its new environment. New yeast from your flour and air will begin to grow in the culture. A different mix of bacteria will emerge.[60]

To demonstrate this, Leader took a sourdough starter from a California baker. He sent part of it to a laboratory for microbial analysis and took the rest home with him to New York State. Four days, a cross-country flight, and several replenishments later, he sent another sample to the lab:

> New lab tests confirmed that the yeast now growing in the culture was different from the yeast living in it on the West Coast. It's possible that particularly strong strains of yeast may survive a journey to a new location and continue to thrive in a culture fed with local flour and air and water. But it's been my experience that local yeast predominates, making every loaf of sourdough bread a local product.[61]

There has been some fascinating research by microbiologists into the community dynamics of sourdough cultures. It turns out that in most sourdoughs, lactic acid bacteria are far more plentiful in number than yeasts; the consortia they form coexist as communities with great stability over time. Ilse Scheirlinck and colleagues in Belgium analyzed sourdough samples from different bakeries around the country; in some cases, several samples came from the same bakery, of different sourdoughs made from different starters and different grains. The analysis found that the microbial "community structure" of different sourdoughs "is influenced by the bakery environment, rather than the type of flour used to produce the sourdough."[62] A year later, the team repeated the experiment, this time sampling even more different sourdoughs at the same 11 bakeries. They found that the sourdoughs "varied little over time," and confirmed "only limited variation among the different sourdoughs from a single bakery."[63]

Bear in mind that your home is not (necessarily) as microbe-rich as a bakery. While the study cited above found that the specific bakery environment was of greater importance than the flour used, still, flour is rich in microbes to get things started. You do not need to be in a bakery, or in San Francisco (or Belgium) to start a sourdough. Lactic acid bacteria and yeasts are everywhere and just need gentle coaxing and periodic attention. "Only a handful of genera of yeast and bacteria have ever been found in any sourdoughs anywhere," reports Jessica Lee.[64] "The remarkable similarities in the microbial populations of leaven from widely separated places demonstrate the effectiveness of the selection process," concludes Keith Steinkraus.[65]

The way to encourage yeast in the mixed sourdough community is to repeatedly feed the bubbly starter a high proportion of fresh flour and water. This means using (or discarding) most of it (75 to 95 percent) and adding the small amount of remaining starter to fresh flour and water, in roughly the amount of what you have removed. Similarly, when using sourdough starter in breads, use a small proportion of starter, no more than 25 percent of the overall dough, unless you wish to accentuate the sour flavor, which I sometimes enjoy, but sometimes I enjoy breads with subtler flavor or other accents. Perpetuating and using sourdough starter in limited proportions such as these is the key to making sourdough breads in which sourness is a subtle note rather than an exclamation point.

I saw instructions years ago that advised developing and maintaining a sourdough like this, discarding most of the starter with each feeding, and the thought of discarding so much food horrified me, so I completely ignored it. Now I have experienced the benefits of this technique, in terms of better, faster, lighter breads; and I have found a good use for the excess starter: savory pancakes, detailed in the following section.

I typically maintain my sourdough in a liquid state, thick but not solid. Some people prefer to maintain sourdough starters in a solid state, as a firm dough. Experiment and find the style you prefer. If you are traveling with a sourdough, or wish to leave your sourdough behind while you travel, I would recommend thickening it up into a solid state. The higher density of a solid dough slows down microbial activity. People also freeze their starters, which maintain greater viability if the dough is in a drier solid form. Drying is also used to transmit or preserve sourdough. Legend has it that many immigrants brought their sourdoughs and other cultures dried on handkerchiefs.

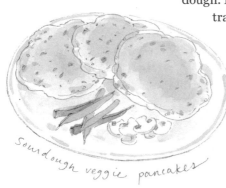

Sourdough veggie pancakes

Feeding your sourdough daily is ideal, although every two or three days is generally adequate. Be prepared to feed it more often in a warm kitchen than in a cool one. If you use your starter only occasionally, keep it in the fridge. Take it out of the fridge once a week, let it warm up to ambient temperatures, feed, and let it sit and ferment at ambient temperature before returning to the refrigerator. When you are ready to use your refrigerated starter, let it warm up, then give it a couple of high-proportion feedings before baking with it. Similarly, with a starter "backed up" in the freezer, thaw and allow it to slowly come to ambient temperatures, then feed it, repeatedly if necessary, until it becomes vigorously active.

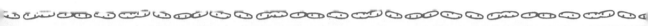

SOURDOUGH CULTURE

Lynn Harris; excerpted with permission from Gastronomica: The Journal of Food and Culture[66]

With experimentation and quasi-obsession—and the Internet—also come fierce debates or, at least, macro levels of minutiae. Sourdough folks divide the world into two kinds of people, those who cultivate "sour" and those who dump it, but they do not stop there. Consider the following subdivisions:

1. Those who permit vs. revile the use of commercial yeast to jumpstart a culture. ("When is a sourdough [starter] not a sourdough? When any ingredients other than grain and water are added! End of debate.")

2. Users of bells and whistles such as grapes and milk in their starter vs. flour-and-water minimalists. (Lest you reflexively award moral victory to the purists, note that the grapes side includes such heavy hitters as Nancy Silverton and the man Anthony Bourdain describes as "[God's] personal bread baker.")

3. Protective vs. permissive starter parents. ("The California gold rush prospectors made sourdough from whatever they had at hand. River water and whole grain flour. Maybe some old coffee. Hell, throw in some grapes. They fed it whatever they had, however often they could. None of this coddling the sourdough, giving it regular feedings, just the right amount of pablum. You ruin a good sour that way. Turns out to be weak and citified. Doesn't have the gumption to properly raise a little pancake much less a loaf of bread. Nope.") . . .

New sourdough questions continue to arise, along with their myriad answers. From the bakers of Giza to Great-Grandma Griffith to Internet newsgroups, the culture of sourdough enthusiasts today is reminiscent of the very starters they share, feed, coddle, or neglect. What has emerged is a macrocosm of its own beloved microbiological charges: elements both tart and light, old-time settlers guarding their land, wild newbies sparking fresh growth, active cells hungry for more spores of data and discussion. Like thousands of Carl's [retired air force colonel Carl T. Griffith, famous for the sourdough he spread] closest friends, these progenitors will surely keep sourdough culture alive and bubbling.

Flatbreads/Pancakes

I have found that since I bake bread so sporadically, the way I use my sourdough most frequently—and thereby keep it fresh and vigorous—is by making pancakes. You can make sourdough pancakes sweet, if you like. Prepare batter using a small proportion of starter, and let it ferment overnight. If you use a high proportion of starter, or your batter tastes more sour than you like, add *a little* baking soda (about 1 teaspoon/5 ml per 2 cups/500 ml of batter), just before you make the pancakes, which will make your pancakes extra fluffy and sweeten them by reacting with (and thus neutralizing) the lactic acid of the sourdough.

The pancakes I typically make are not the kind you cover with sweet syrup, but rather savory pancakes, which I find are enhanced by sour flavor, and so I omit baking soda. If I'm trying to use excess starter, sometimes I make the pancakes with pure starter; other times I combine water, flour, and a smaller proportion of starter in a bowl, mix vigorously, and leave overnight, or for a few hours to ferment. If I have leftover grains, I'll add them in place of some of the flour. I usually grate vegetables, such as radishes, turnips, sweet potatoes, summer squash, potatoes, or really anything, into the batter raw. When I'm ready to make my pancakes, I fry some onion, garlic, and sometimes other vegetables, such as sweet peppers and okra. While these veggies are frying, I add a beaten egg or two to the batter, salt, and grated cheese. Then I add the fried vegetables and mix. If the mixture seems too thick, I add a little more water; if it seems too thin, I add flour, just a little at a time. I fry this batter into pancakes on an oiled, well-seasoned pan, and eat with yogurt or sour cream, hot sauce, *ajvar*, and/or other condiments.

The world is full of flatbreads and fry breads. You can make them from any grain, as well as starchy tubers. *Injera* is an Ethiopian sourdough pancake traditionally made from *teff* flour.[67] Deanne Bednar of Oxford, Michigan, wrote to tell me how she uses her injera batter, very similar to how I use my sourdough for pancakes:

> I like to keep an injera style batter going most of the time. I can just make it up into a few "wraps" whenever I want . . . from the bowl of it on the counter, or the jar I keep in the fridge. Just before I use a portion I usually add a touch of baking soda (because it is so cool to see it froth up), some salt, and maybe chopped veggies, garlic, or even an egg and make an amazing wrap.

Funkaso is a sourdough pancake made from millet in West Africa.[68] *Kissra* is a paper-thin Sudanese sourdough pancake made from sorghum flour. The thin batter is poured along one edge of the pan then spread with a tool known as a *gergeriba*, simply a rectangular piece of a palm leaf, which sits in water between uses. "The *gergeriba* is held in the middle by the fingers of the right hand and held upright, on its long edge, on the right-hand end of the batter line at an angle," writes Hamid Dirar, the author of *The Indigenous Fermented Foods of the Sudan*:

The batter is next scraped in one stroke with the small tool from right to left and forward. Only the thin, baked layer sticking to the surface of the hot plate is left behind as the gergeriba moves. When the other end of the batter line is reached, the angle of the gergeriba and the direction of motion are changed with a twist of the hand, so that the batter is scraped, this time, in a left-to-right direction and slightly forward, i.e. towards the baker. The process is repeated until practically all the batter has been spread. . . . This "shuttle effect" of the gergeriba takes place so fast that the kissra sheet is spread thin in a matter of seconds.[69]

That is a detailed description! Technique is obviously best learned by direct observation; however, with trial and error guided by thorough descriptions such as this, cultural revivalists may learn and use techniques that other clever people have developed.

 ## Sourdough Bread

I love baking bread. It requires rhythm and tactile involvement, and delivers its rewards slowly, with great buildup. First come the relatively subtle aromas of the dough, the cohesion of the developing loaves, and the visual gratification of the rising. After the bread is baking in the oven, the smell of fresh-baking bread asserts itself more strongly, filling the house with palpable anticipation. After the bread is ready and removed from the oven, it's difficult to resist the temptation to slice into it and taste it steaming hot. But baking continues in the center of the loaf as it cools, so if you can resist temptation and enjoy the aroma and anticipation, the center of the loaf will have the opportunity to finish cooking. Half an hour later, the loaf is still warm, fully cooked in the center, and well worth the wait. Few things are as delicious as fresh bread, still warm.

It is definitely easier and faster to bake bread using a packet of yeast, but it is a more magical experience to make bread by harnessing the power of wild yeasts and bacteria, and the bread itself—in terms of flavor, crumb, storage potential, and nutrient availability—is far superior. The most important single ingredient for baking sourdough bread is a vigorous starter. It need not be an ancient pedigree, but it must be vigorous, meaning that it must be actively kinetic, visibly bubbling and rising. Do not build your dough with a flat or barely active starter. Feed and stir your starter frequently, as described previously, until you have a vigorous starter that froths at the surface and rises the thick starter batter. Only then is it primed to rise the denser bread dough.

Sourdough bread does not have to be sour. The breads I was making when I wrote *Wild Fermentation* accentuated the sour flavor by slowly thickening a sponge via repeatedly feeding it a small proportion of fresh flour, thus maintaining and accentuating its high acidity. Making dough, and maintaining your sourdough, by adding a small proportion of starter (25 percent or less) to a high proportion of fresh water and flour diminishes acidity, improves and speeds the rising, and results in loaves with much less pronounced sour flavor.

I will not dwell on bread baking here because there is such an extensive literature covering the topic so well. I love to read bread books and have been inspired by many of them (see *Resources*). I have found even greater inspiration watching gifted artisans in their baking routines, turning out dozens or hundreds of loaves in a baking, and doing so with such grace that it appears as an elaborate rhythmic dance. If you want to learn to bake great bread and you have the time, volunteer to help an artisan baker clean up so you can see how they bake and ask them questions. Read books. Nothing can replace experiential learning when it comes to baking bread. Definitely experiment with different methods and styles. There are many excellent books, web resources, and potential mentors to serve as sources of information and inspiration.

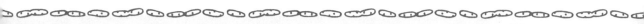

BRING SOURDOUGH BAKING TO THE NEXT LEVEL

Tips from Liz Tree, Williams, Oregon

- Really pay attention to the starter!!! Feed it like a pet. I bake a lot so I feed it every day. I keep a 100 percent hydration starter [equal weights of flour and water] and weigh the water and flour I add to keep it the same.

- Pay attention to temperature. Best for bread is 74–78°F/23–26°C. So I take the temperature of the flour and the starter and then adjust the water temperature as needed.

- I bought a kitchen scale, about $30, and I measure everything in grams. . . . This keeps my measuring consistent from batch to batch.

- Use bakers' percentages [flour is 100 percent; everything else based on percentages of that]; important if you want to go to the next level. Creating bread is all about the percentage of flour to water.

- I also take notes on the small changes I make from batch to batch. (I have been making the same bread over and over!)

So with the temperature regulation, the note taking, and the baker's percentage, I am adding a method or a science to the art, which I have been resistant to in the past, but the results are so worth it!!!

Sour Rye Porridge Soup (*Zur*)

Sourdough starters have many other applications beyond bread and pancakes. Polish cuisine features a soup called *zur*, the base of which is sourdough, cooked into what could be described as thin rye porridge. "In every urban or village household there was a clay pot for the fermenting of *zur*," writes Polish ethnographer Anna Kowalska-Lewicka. "This pot was not generally washed after each use so that a little of the solution was left to facilitate the fermentation."[70] With this soup (and its close relative *kisiel*, "prepared in the same way as *zur* but with a larger proportion of flour"[71]), we get a glimpse into the continuum of ways in which fermented rye is incorporated into Slavic cuisine, as the beverage kvass, loaves of rye bread, and this intermediate form, a savory rye porridge soup. The base for *zur* is *zakwas*, or rye sourdough. The Russian sour beverage kvass, made from old bread, was addressed in chapter 6. The Russian word for "sourdough," *zakvaska*, derives from *kvass*, as does the Polish *zakwas*. For enough *zur* to feed four, you'll need roughly 2 cups/500 ml of rye sourdough starter. Let the starter sit a few days without feeding to get good and sour. If you like, add garlic to the sourdough so the garlic flavor can infuse into the sourdough. In southern Poland, oats are sometimes used instead of rye; in eastern Poland buckwheat is sometimes used.[72] To make *zur*, fry onion, garlic, and (if desired) bacon, sausage, or other meat; then add boiling water, bay leaf, black pepper, marjoram, and allspice. Cook for a little while, then add *zakwas*. Bring to a boil, stirring frequently. Add chopped, cooked potatoes, chopped hard-boiled egg, or other ingredients as desired. This soup is substantial, especially delicious in cold weather. Serve with sour cream or yogurt.

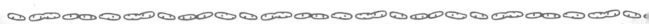

SOURDOUGH CHOCOLATE DEVASTATION CAKE

Bloodroot Collective

A very easy and delicious vegan cake. You will need good-quality unsweetened cocoa and sourdough starter to make it. Recipe makes a two-layer 9-inch/22-cm cake.

1. Lightly oil and line two 9-inch/22-cm pans with waxed paper. Preheat oven to 330°F/165°C.

2. Combine dry ingredients in a bowl:
   ¾ cup/180 ml unsweetened cocoa
   2 cups/500 ml sugar
   3 cups/750 ml unbleached white flour
   2 teaspoons/10 ml baking soda
   ¾ teaspoon/3 ml salt
   2 tablespoons/30 ml grain coffee (such as Cafix)
   ½ teaspoon/2 ml cinnamon

   Stir together with a dry whisk.

3. Combine wet ingredients in another bowl:
   1 cup/250 ml sourdough starter
   2¼ cups/550 ml water
   2 tablespoons/30 ml vinegar
   ¾ cup/180 ml grape seed oil

1½ teaspoons/7 ml vanilla

Stir well with a whisk.

4. Combine wet and dry with as few strokes as possible. Turn into pans immediately and bake 25–30 minutes, or until cakes test dry in center. Remove and cool on racks.

5. For frosting, chop
good-quality semisweet chocolate to measure 1 cup/250 ml
Turn into pot. Add
1 teaspoon/5 ml vanilla
3 tablespoons/45 ml maple syrup
¼ cup/60 ml grape seed oil
3 tablespoons/45 ml cocoa powder

Stir over lowest heat (or in double boiler) to melt. Set aside.

6. When cake and frosting are cool, spread frosting between layers and over cake.

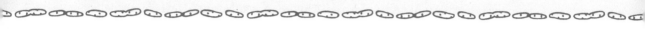

Sierra Rice

Sierra rice, also known as *arroz fermentado* or *arroz requemado*, is a style of fermented rice eaten in the high Andes regions of Ecuador. "Inasmuch as the fermentation subjects the rice to 50° to 80° C [122–176°F], Sierra rice requires less cooking, which is very important in the Andean altitudes where water boils below 100°C [212°F]," point out Andre G. van Veen and Keith Steinkraus in the *Journal of Agricultural and Food Chemistry*.[73] "Fermentation is induced by dumping moist rice on large cement or cane floors out in the open, and covering it with tarpaulins," reports Herbert Herzfeld in the journal *Economic Botany*. "This produces a rather pungent, unpleasant odor which permeates the grain. While this aroma appears to diminish once the rice is dried and milled, it seems to return to some degree when the rice is being cooked."[74]

Typically freshly harvested rice is fermented prior to drying or milling. Covering the moist rice prevents it from drying out and creates a hospitable humid environment for spontaneous microbial growth, including *Aspergillus flavus* and *Bacillus subtilis*.[75] According to the *Economic Botany* account, it takes from 3 to 10 days for fermentation to initiate, as indicated by rising temperatures. Moister rice ferments faster; if rice is dry, it is sometimes moistened. Four or five days after fermentation begins, the mound is turned, like a compost pile, to release heat and distribute microbial activity. "At a decreasing rate, the rice continues to ferment; six to fifteen days elapse, depending on relative humidity and temperature, before the rice is turned once more and left to dry in the open."[76] The progress of the fermentation is gauged by color:

> The hulls turn a cinnamon color, the shade becoming darker the longer fermentation proceeds. Individual kernels of fermented milled rice, on the other hand, range in color from golden to deep cinnamon brown. The most acceptable color to the trade is golden or light cinnamon. Excessive or spotty fermentation produces black rice unfit for sale.[77]

Fermented Sierra rice is then cooked in water just as you would cook unfermented rice, only it cooks much more quickly.

Hoppers/*Appam*

Hopper (sometimes spelled *appa*) is a Sri Lankan name and *appam* is a South Indian name for fermented rice and coconut pancakes. Jennifer Moragoda from Sri Lanka introduced me to hoppers (via email), then proceeded to send directions in exceptional detail, with accompanying photographs. When I finally got around to making them, I was not disappointed. Although Jennifer cautions that "they are not usually made successfully abroad for some reason," I loved the ones I made. The starchy rice fuses with the sweet, oily coconut, both lifted by a vigorous fermentation; the bowl-shaped pancakes are made with thin edges, which bubbling turns into a crispy fried lattice. Yum!

One pound/500 g of rice and one coconut makes enough batter for at least eight large hoppers or more small ones. Soak the rice overnight. Jennifer specifies using a non-sticky variety. I used short-grain brown rice, which worked great. To make hoppers by Jennifer's method, you need both coconut water and coconut milk, which you can extract from the same mature brown coconut.

Coconut water is the liquid at the center of the coconut, which you can hear and feel as you shake the intact coconut. Take the coconut to a hard surface you can hit against with force, along with a hammer, a big nail, and a bowl. Find the end of the coconut where there are three eyes. Steady the coconut with the eyes up, place the nail on one of the eyes, and puncture the eye of the coconut with the nail. Then puncture a second eye. Wiggle the nail in the holes to clear and enlarge them, and pour the coconut water out into the bowl or a cup.

Once you have collected the coconut water, hit the coconut directly with the hammer until the shell breaks into two or more pieces. Then bring the pieces of coconut back inside and use a spoon to pry the white flesh from the brown shell. Grate the flesh into a bowl and cover with about 2 cups/500 ml of boiling water. Once the water cools enough to handle, squeeze the coconut in the water using your hands to draw out the milk. This coconut-infused water is the coconut milk. Strain the milk through a cheesecloth-lined strainer. Then use all your strength to force as much milk out of the coconut as possible. Gather the pulp in the cheesecloth, twist, squeeze, and press it against a hard surface. Return the grated coconut and cover again with boiling water, this time less, for a second pressing.

Back to the rice, which has been soaking. Drain the soaked rice and grind finely using a blender, food processor, mill, or mortar and pestle. Next, make a well in the center of the ground rice and add a starter. In Sri Lanka, *toddy* (fermented coconut sap) is typically used as a starter. Jennifer's directions called for adding yeast and a little sugar to the coconut water and using that. Adding a little sourdough starter to the coconut water is another possibility. I used the coconut water plus a little rice beer I had fermenting. Mix coconut water and starter with the ground rice to make a soft dough. Add a little more coconut water (or water) if necessary. Cover the dough and leave in a warm place to rise until roughly doubled, several hours.

After the dough rises, you can refrigerate and continue the next day. (If you refrigerate, when you remove from the fridge allow a couple of hours for the dough to warm to room temperature before proceeding further.) Add salt to taste, and coconut milk, a little at a time, until the dough thins into a batter that can be spread very thinly. Let the batter ferment and rise about three more hours.

Then heat the hopper pan. In Sri Lanka, hoppers are typically made in a special pan called a *tachhchi* or "China Chatty," something like a wok only smaller and with more sharply rising slopes. A well-seasoned wok makes a reasonable facsimile. Oil the pan lightly with coconut oil. Pour a little batter into the pan and rapidly swirl it so as to coat the sides most of the way up. The sides should have just a thin coating of batter to form crispy edges, while the center should be thicker and spongy. Cover the pan so the center can steam. Cook over gentle heat until edges turn a golden color.

I did some in my well-seasoned flat crepe pan, which worked great. When I emailed Jennifer about my experience, she promptly responded: "I would strongly suggest you use the wok instead of a pancake pan because if you make them in the pancake pan, they are not really hoppers, as hoppers should have a lacey thin crisp ring around a spongy steamed centre and they should be '3-D'—not flat." Point taken—the form is essential to the food, as with a tortilla, nori roll, cheese, or salami. But even with my usual pan, I was able to achieve a "lacey thin crisp ring around a spongy steamed centre" by pouring batter into the center of the pan and slowly swirling, allowing batter to drip, so the edges were much thinner than the center, and covering so it could steam.

One popular way to prepare hoppers is egg hoppers. Simply crack an egg in the center of the hopper after spreading the batter and before covering. The steam from the frying hopper cooks the egg. Then you dip the hopper in the still-runny egg yolk as you eat. Hoppers are also served with various curries and/or *sambols*. Many different condiments could accent them, yet they are tasty enough to stand on their own. Recipes vary. Some use rice flour rather than rice, or canned coconut milk. *Appam* from Kerala in southern India

sourdough bread

is essentially similar, though recipes vary quite a bit and sometimes incorporate cooked as well as raw rice into the batter.

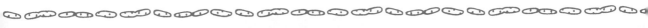

SAUER SEITAN

Alan Hardy, San Antonio, Texas

I would like to share what may be my own discovery. For years I have liked to make seitan—the Japanese wheat "meat." It is delicious and very nutritious but like most protein can be difficult to digest. I began making sourdough bread with a starter made from *rejuvelac*. . . . I got the idea that it might help to make the seitan a bit more digestible if it were fermented the same way as the sourdough bread. So . . . I mix the gluten in a flour form—called Vital Wheat Gluten in the stores—with *rejuvelac* instead of water, make a dough ball out of it, and let it sit for a day and a night and then either pressure-cook it or boil it for one hour. It makes a wonderfully tangy seitan with a bit of a different texture than regular seitan and of course a different flavor. [Author's note: I tried this with my sourdough starter and it worked great!]

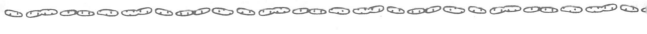

Kishk and *Keckek el Fouqara*

Kishk is bulgur (cooked, dried, cracked wheat) and yogurt, mixed together with a little salt into a dough, and fermented. The fermented dough is then dried into a crumble and used to flavor and thicken soups.[78] Maria Tarantino, an Italian fermentation experimentalist who lives in Brussels, reports that she sometimes makes *kishk* with couscous instead of bulgur. And rather than drying the *kishk* into a crumble, "I do not dry out the mix completely so I am able to form the *kishk* into little balls, add some dry herbs to them and keep them in olive oil like you would do with goat cheese." Yum!

At Terra Madre, the international Slow Food Event where I met Maria, we both tasted a food called *Keckek el Fouqara*, poor man's cheese, an adaptation of the *kishk* method by those without access to milk, and a rich taste sensation far cheesier in flavor than any other non-dairy cheese I've ever tried. According to its Slow Food Presidium designation, *Keckek el Fouqara* is made by adding water and salt to bulgur and fermenting three to five weeks (depending on temperature), then

worked by hand until a homogeneous, elastic mass is obtained. The product can have a plain taste or flavors are added, such as thyme, cumin, nigel seeds, sesame seed, red, green or black pepper. When the mass is still moist it is shaped into small balls. They are then stacked compactly in glass jars, local extra virgin olive oil will then be poured to cover entirely the vegan cheese for preservation and taste. Poor man's cheese can then be kept for a year or longer. This product is one of what are called mune products, from the verb mana, which means "to lay in supplies." These are food reserves which every family had to obtain in order to cope with the continuous alternation of periods of plenty and scarcity.[79]

I've made a couple of batches of *Keckek el Fouqara*, and they've been very popular. To start, mix bulgur with just a little more than its volume of water. Stir daily. After about a week, it develops a sharp flavor, which keeps getting better as the days pass. After two to three weeks, add spices. My best batch included garlic, caraway, cumin, and sage, crushed together with salt with a mortar and pestle. Mix spices into the bulgur mix, adjust as necessary, and form into balls about 1½ inches/4 cm in diameter. Pack spiced fermented bulgur balls into jars, cover with olive oil, and age at least a few weeks, or up to about six months. Serve with crackers as a cheese alternative.

Fermenting Grains with Other Kinds of Foods

Grains are fermented with just about every other conceivable type of food. *Kishk*, described previously, mixes wheat with yogurt for them to ferment together. My friend Merril mixes wheat flour with milk to feed her sourdough starter, and I've heard of other people doing the same thing. Grains can be essential to support lactic acid development in foods with little carbohydrate content, such as fish or meat. In chapter 12, I describe Filipino *burong isda* and Japanese *nare zushi*—fish fermented with rice. Chapter 5 refers to fermenting vegetables with rice and potatoes, and other grains and starchy tubers could be similarly incorporated. Grain-based beers, covered in chapter 9, were in some of their earliest documented forms mixed with fruits, saps, or other sugars. *Idli*, in chapter 11, ferments dal with rice; as does miso, which is made from not only beans but also grains grown with the mold *Aspergillus oryzae* into *koji*, covered in chapter 10.

Fermenting Leftover Grains (and Starchy Tubers)

Fermentation is a great way to make use of leftover grains and starchy tubers. I most often use leftover grains by incorporating them into sourdough breads and pancakes, as described earlier in this chapter. I also love *zur*, the Polish sour rye soup, and I make something like it with leftover grains. Cover cooked grains with water, break up clumps into a sort of slurry, add a little rye flour to thicken, and add sourdough starter. Ferment a few days, then cook into soup. Leftover grains, as well as leftover starchy tubers, may also be used in krauts and kimchis.

Troubleshooting

Sourdough never started bubbling

Did you dechlorinate your water? Chlorine or chloramine, used to kill waterborne bacteria, can inhibit fermentation. Also, stir, stir, stir, as aeration stimulates yeast growth. Move your starter to a warmer spot in your house. (Cool temperatures can slow fermentation.) Finally, if all else fails, try adding organic rye flour, which gets sourdoughs bubbling.

Sourdough got bubbly, then went flat and never came back

A sourdough that got bubbly and then went flat probably just needs a good high-proportion feeding. That means discarding roughly 75 percent of it (or making pancakes out of it) and feeding the remaining 25 percent a high proportion of fresh flour, adding roughly three or four times as much fresh flour and water to the remaining starter.

Sourdough smells awful

A sourdough is a complex community of microorganisms. When it receives a fresh high-proportion feeding, yeast activity is most vigorous and the sourdough develops a yeasty smell. Then, as lactic acid bacteria follow yeasts into dominance in the sourdough environment, it becomes increasingly acidic. But if you neglect feeding your sourdough and the lactic acid bacteria exhaust their nutrients, the putrefying bacteria, also part of the community, can rise to dominance. This is what it means when your starter smells awful. Rather than discarding it all, retain a small amount from the very bottom of the jar. Give it a high-proportion feeding to reawaken the dormant yeasts and lactic acid bacteria. Pamper it: Stir daily, keep it warm, and feed it every day or two, even if it doesn't bubble right away. Sourdoughs are very resilient and can come back from even extreme neglect.

Confused by conflicting information on how to start a sourdough

Like most things, there is more than one way to start a sourdough. Don't get stuck on the seeming contradictions among methods. They all work, if you stick with them. I advocate simply flour and water and stir, stir, stir. But many other methods (some quite elaborate) can yield great sourdough starters. Regardless of method, regular feeding is the key to a vigorous sourdough starter.

Surface mold and molding in jar above waterline

The best way to avoid surface molding is to stir frequently. Molds cannot easily grow on surfaces that are constantly being disturbed. If you notice a mold beginning to develop, skim it off and try to be more conscientious about daily stirring. The bowl or jar in which you maintain your sourdough may mold, as well, especially where residue of the sourdough dries as a crust stuck to the side. If you notice such molding, transfer the sourdough to another vessel and clean the original one before returning the sourdough to it.

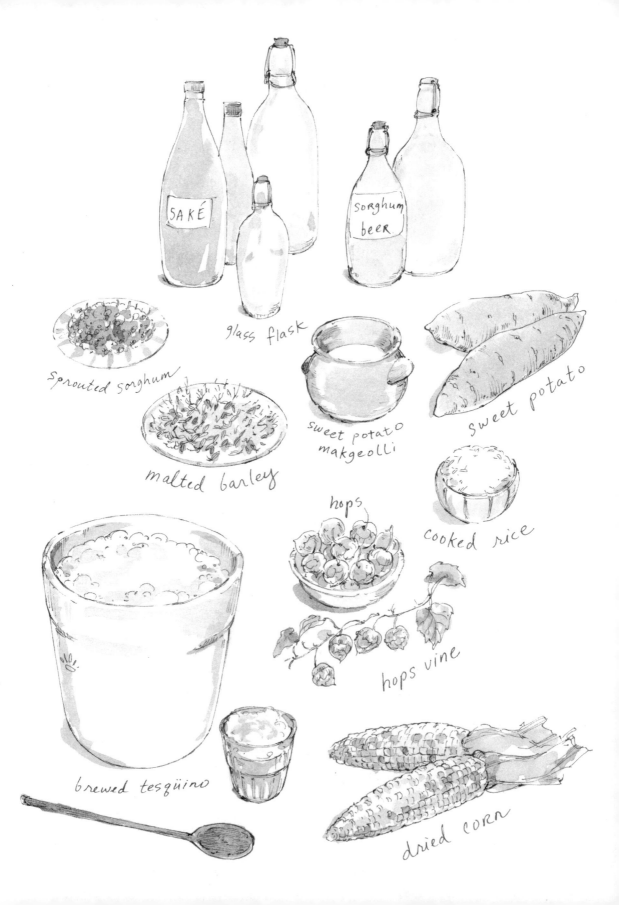

SAKÉ

sorghum beer

glass flask

sprouted sorghum

malted barley

sweet potato makgeolli

sweet potato

cooked rice

hops

hops vine

brewed tesgüino

dried corn

CHAPTER 9

Fermenting Beers and Other Grain-Based Alcoholic Beverages

*B*eer is the first thing many people think of when they hear the word *fermentation*, as I have learned, having had brief conversations on this broad topic with many people. I too love the beer they are usually thinking of, brewed from malted barley with hops. However, I define *beer* much more broadly than the famous 1516 Bavarian beer purity law (*Reinheitsgebot*), and other laws that have codified those or some others as beer's sole legitimate ingredients. I define *beer* as a fermented alcoholic beverage in which the alcohol derives primarily from the complex carbohydrates of grains (or starchy tubers).

As we have just seen in the last chapter, spontaneous fermentations of grains generally result in sour rather than alcoholic products. Whereas honey, sugar, fruit juices, plant saps, and other simple sugars ferment into alcohol spontaneously, grains require conversion of complex carbohydrates into simple sugars, via enzyme activity, before they can ferment into any significant amount of alcohol.

The enzymes that do this in the Western beer-making tradition come from malting grains, more commonly known as sprouting or germinating. "The embryo restarts its biochemical machinery and produces various enzymes, including some that break down the barley cell walls, and others that break down the starch and proteins inside the cells of the food storage tissue, the endosperm," explains Harold McGee. "These enzymes then diffuse through the embryo into the endosperm, where they work together to dissolve away the cell walls, penetrate the cells, and digest some of the starch granules and protein bodies inside."[1]

Malting is not the only method of enzymatic transformation for fermenting grains and starchy tubers into alcohol; the enzymes most often used in the Asian traditions of making alcohol from rice, millet, and other grains come from molds. In parts of South America, Africa, and Asia, a third source of enzymes used to break down grains (and starchy tubers) for making alcohol—possibly the most ancient—is the use of human saliva by simply chewing them.[2] Each of these methods is explored ahead.

Though making alcohol from grain requires more extensive processing than making it from grapes or other sources of sugars, grains offer certain inherent advantages, primarily related to availability of raw materials. McGee summarizes that grains are "quicker and easier to grow than the grapevine, much more productive in a given acreage, can be stored for many months before being fermented, and . . . can be made into beer any day of the year, not just at harvest time."[3]

There are an intimidating number of steps involved in making beer from raw grain. Virtually all contemporary brewers—homebrew hobbyists, craft and microbrewers, regional brands, and industry giants alike—rely upon already prepared malt, or malt extracts. There is a section ahead covering malting barley, for those like myself who are obsessed with directly experiencing all these different transformational processes. Most of the beer brewing that I have done has been the full process from grain to beer. But with an eye toward simplicity and technical ease, I have experimented more in the realm of thicker, starchier, more nutritive "opaque" beers than with refined styles, filtered and clarified, with most of the starch removed. The sections that follow focus on some opaque beers that I've learned to make. I have not experienced most of these in their indigenous contexts; the processes I followed were experimental, based upon written information, sometimes conflicting, varying in details. The processes I describe are my interpretations and improvisations.

Wild Yeast Beers

Another quirk of my beer-brewing practice is that it has mostly relied upon wild fermentation. The ingredients for wine, cider, and mead—fruit, honey, and other simple sugars—are always populated by fermenting yeasts, provided that they are raw and not cooked, or heated in their processing, as with sugar. In contrast, beer is almost always cooked before it is fermented, so the grains in the mash are not a reliable source for populating it with fermenting microbes. "Far more than a haphazard process, spontaneous fermentation requires a source of wild yeast and favorable circumstances," writes Jeff Sparrow, author of the book *Wild Brews: Beer Beyond the Influence of Brewer's Yeast*.[4] Sometimes mixed cultures are obtained from the air (as in the famed Belgian wild yeast brews), or from raw malted grains or other plant material, or starters from a previous batch, including in some cases simply residue left in a vessel or on a ritual stirring branch. Stephen Harrod Buhner, author of

Sacred and Herbal Healing Beers, encourages his readers to call upon spirits as well as use practical methods to help initiate wild yeast fermentation:

> When the wort [pre-fermented barley malt brew, filtered and ready to ferment] is ready, you might leave it out, uncovered, in a container with a wide opening. Then sit near it and begin to talk with the spirit of the yeast—to call on the bryggjemann or kveik to come—and see what it is like. To do so means reconnecting to the ancient tradition of fermentation—to connect to the thousands of wise women and wise men standing over their brewing vessels in small villages around the world calling on the spirits of fermentation to come to the wort and kindle the fire in it. Once you have brought a wild yeast to live at your home, place a carved stick in the fermenter and allow the yeast to fall deeply within its carvings. When the beer is finished, take the stick out and hang it up to dry somewhere out of the way. At your next fermentation, take it down and place it in the fermenter and call on it once again to awaken to life.[5]

As I was writing this book, I visited Brussels, the capital of Belgium, and Yvan De Baets, my brewer friend there, sent me to see the Brewery Cantillon, a small-scale producer of the region's distinctive wild-fermented *lambic* beer offering tours and public brewing sessions. There I met the owner and master brewer, Jean Van Roy, who is continuing a family enterprise going back four generations. When his great-grandfather founded the brewery in 1900, there were hundreds of breweries in Brussels. Today Cantillon is the last traditional brewery left in the city.

The beer brewed at Cantillon is fermented by wild yeast and bacteria, spontaneously drawn to it via the air. Cool weather favors the microbial mix that produces the best beer, so the brewery brews only in cool seasons. After brewing, the hot wort is cooled in a big open tank called a *coolship*, with a broad surface area, something like a shallow copper wading pool, under vented rafters. As the wort cools to temperatures yeasts and lactic acid bacteria can tolerate, it becomes populated by these organisms, present in the environment. "According to legend, such fermentation is only possible in the region of Brussels and more specifically in the Senne valley (the river which flows through Brussels)," states Cantillon's brochure. One explanation I've encountered for the quality of the Senne valley yeast is the historic concentration of cherry trees and other fruit-bearers there, which, unfortunately, has declined sharply over the past century.[6] When I ask Jean whether the concentration of yeasts in the valley meant he could relocate his brewery to any building there, he said definitely not. He was emphatic that he thought the characteristic wild organisms had become established in the building itself. "Considering the loss of the Schaarbeek cherry orchards surrounding Brussels as a continuing source of fresh wild yeast, the buildings now play a greater role than ever before," notes Jeff Sparrow.[7]

In the past, all beer relied upon wild yeasts. There is at least one brewery starting up in the United States brewing beer using local wild yeasts, called Mystic Brewery in Boston. "We aren't afraid of no stinking microbes (quite literally)," states the Mystic website. "Our way is to brew new beers in the old tradition. Our way is to make living beer."[8]

Wild yeast beers tend to have a sour edge to them. "At one time, all beers exhibited some level of tart, sour, acidic character," writes Jeff Sparrow. "Modern brewing methods helped to virtually eliminate these characteristics in beer."[9] Beer blogger Michael Agnew[10] enthuses that "sour beers are among the most mind-blowing, uniquely complex, and delicious beers in the world. These are beers that will forever shatter your notions of what beer is."[11] Yet we all have preconceived notions. "I think the most important thing for brewers to prepare is their own pallet," offers fermentation experimentalist Luke Regalbuto:

> Wild fermented beers are not going to taste like you expect, if you drink commercial beer in the US. Wild fermented beverages are often very sour, and different, they take a little getting used to. When we traveled to Europe, I was very surprised that the traditional wild fermented brews and ciders were very sour . . . so much so that I realized that I had tossed wild fermented brews thinking they had gone to vinegar when they were actually still good.

Our expectations are shaped by experience, and just a few isolated species of yeast are used in almost all brewing. "The use of different microorganisms is one of the least studied and (currently) least practiced fields of brewing," states brewmaster Peter Bouckaert of Colorado's New Belgium Brewing Company.[12] "There are not one or two varieties of beer-souring microorganisms but dozens and sometimes hundreds of different strains," according to Jeff Sparrow. "Scientists have isolated more than two hundred different organisms at work in the fermentation of a lambic."[13]

For most of the beers described in this chapter, rather than relying upon the air as the source of yeast exposure, we will introduce raw malted grains. This is an easy method used in some indigenous brewing traditions. But try the air, especially if you are near lots of fruit trees. You could also try using fresh organic fruit as a source of yeasts, or the foam from another active yeasty ferment, or try your hand at catching yeast from the air by frequently stirring (keep using the same tool without washing it); or skip all this wild experimentation and add a packet of yeast.

Tesgüino

Tesgüino is a traditional beer of some of Mexico's indigenous peoples, made from malted corn. Like many traditional beers, it is thick and starchy enough to be a nutritive food as well an intoxicant. *Tesgüino* is delicious and easy to make. In a nutshell, sprout dry field corn until sprouts reach about an inch/2.5 cm in length, roughly five days to a week, then crush it into a fine paste. Boil this paste in water for 8 to 12 hours, or as long as 24 hours, adding more water as necessary. The sprouted-corn paste smells and tastes grassy, which is, after all, what corn and all grains are—grass. The long cooking caramelizes sugars, transforming that grassiness into a sweeter, deeper, and more distinctive corn-flavored sweet syrup. Then dilute this syrup with more water, cool, and ferment into *tesgüino* in just a few days. (The process is described in greater detail in the following sections.)

For the Tarahumara people of northern Mexico, *tesgüino* "is of primary functional importance in the social organization and culture," according to anthropologist John G. Kennedy. *Tesgüino* drinking events, known as *tesguinada*, are "the basic social activity of the people," and are frequent ceremonial events. *Tesguinada* also play an important economic role. Often they are work parties, in which *tesgüino* serves as the reward for helping.

> The procedure, when one needs to accomplish a major task such as weeding, harvesting, cutting fodder, spreading fertilizer, fence making, or house building, is to make an appropriate amount of tesguino, and then to invite men from the surrounding ranchos to come to work and drink. Tesguino is considered the pay one receives for the work and is a mandatory ingredient in the situation, though basic motivations are the reciprocal bonds, obligation, and privilege which hold between the men in the vicinity. When the "inviter" makes his rounds to the various households, he says, "Would you like to drink a little tesguino tomorrow?" He feels it unnecessary to first mention that work will be a part of the program, and stresses the social aspect of the tesguinada to follow. A man may choose to perform any task alone or to make tesguino, but the latter method is much preferred because of the time and effort saved, and because of the euphoria of group participation which is so lacking in the relative solitude of everyday life. This group camaraderie is of course considerably enhanced by the effects of the alcohol.[14]

The importance of the *tesguinada* extends far beyond labor. "It is the religious group, the economic group, the entertainment group, the group at which disputes are settled, marriages arranged, and deals completed."

Ethnobotanist William Litzinger described the Tarahumara methods of *tesgüino* preparation in some detail in his 1983 PhD dissertation. "Sprouting the kernels is the longest part of the process," writes Litzinger, describing a range of containers used to sprout the corn while protecting it from light, so it does not develop bitter chlorophyll:

> Many kinds of containers are used for sprouting maize kernels, including wooden boxes and tin cans. Earthen pits are also used. They are dug in a sunny, protected spot near the house. The pits are lined with grass

leaves or other green foliage, and covered with a layer of pine needles. During the winter months the kernels are sprouted in containers placed inside the house, close to the cooking fire where a good even level of heat is maintained.[15]

I use a gallon jar, but draped with a cloth to shield it from light. One pound/500 g of corn will yield about ½ gallon/2 liters of *tesgüino*. Soak corn kernels for about 24 hours, then drain well. Continue to rinse several times a day and drain well each time, for up to about a week (see *Sprouting* in chapter 8 for sprouting basics), until the sprouts reach a length of about an inch/2.5 cm.

Often people do not understand what dry whole field corn is, or where to find it. Dry field corn is not fresh sweet corn. It is typically starchier, drier varieties of corn, grown for feed or milling, dried, with kernels removed from the cob. It is not popcorn varieties. Often you can find it in natural foods stores or buying clubs. These days, with genetically modified corn so commonly grown, I would definitely recommend seeking out organic corn. And if you want to try growing corn, try "dent" varieties. You can also buy already malted corn, called *jora* in Spanish, available in many Mexican markets.

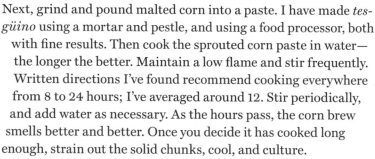

Next, grind and pound malted corn into a paste. I have made *tesgüino* using a mortar and pestle, and using a food processor, both with fine results. Then cook the sprouted corn paste in water— the longer the better. Maintain a low flame and stir frequently. Written directions I've found recommend cooking everywhere from 8 to 24 hours; I've averaged around 12. Stir periodically, and add water as necessary. As the hours pass, the corn brew smells better and better. Once you decide it has cooked long enough, strain out the solid chunks, cool, and culture.

The Tarahumara typically introduce yeast to the *tesgüino* by simply placing it into an *olla* (pot) dedicated to the purpose. "The Tarahumara never wash or rinse out their fermentation *ollas*," writes Litzinger. "Due to this the interior of the *ollas* become encrusted with a thick organic layer," which has been found to contain *Saccharomyces cerevisiae*.[16] According to W. C. Bennett and R. M. Zingg, who published a book on the tribe in 1935, the Tarahumara describe the *ollas* they use as having "learned to boil well."[17]

If you do not yet possess a vessel dedicated to *tesgüino*, you will have to culture it in some other way. You could simply add a packet of yeast at this point. My first batch I cultured with sourdough; the next I cultured with some raw sprouted corn paste that I put aside and did not cook. Both batches fermented vigorously and tasted great. If you get into a routine of doing this, you could save some of each batch of *tesgüino* in a jar in the fridge to start the next batch.

Litzinger writes that the Tarahumara gauge the progress of fermentation just as I do, by monitoring the rate of bubbling. "The cycle begins by a slow bubbling stage, followed by a fast bubbling stage. The end of the fast bubbling marks the point when the beverage is consumed." Once the bubbling starts to slow, drink up and enjoy. I like to bottle it while it is still fermenting—in plastic so I can gauge pressure (and avoid explosions!)—then drink or refrigerate as soon as a little pressure builds.

There are some contemporary recipes for *tesgüino* that call for fermenting a thin sweet porridge of *masa* flour with added sugar (*piloncillo*). Anthropologist Henry Bruman does not hide his disdain for this variation: "The post-Conquest vulgarization of the process is obvious."[18] Five hundred years into the post-Columbian experiment in globalization, no practices or traditions are unchanged. Culture is dynamic, and cross-cultural influence is a fact. "Methods of [*tesgüino*] preparation vary among different ethnic groups," notes Steinkraus.[19] Bennett and Zingg report: "We drank *tesguino* wherever we went, and it showed a great difference in taste."[20] Some groups consider various botanical additions to be important, while others do not. Practices with common roots often diverge over time, as each generation encounters different conditions and influences. For practices to remain relevant, they must be adapted.

Tesgüino is also made from the sap pressed from fresh, green cornstalks. Probably this is the "original" corn ferment, from which all others are adaptations; anthropologists have proposed that the use of corn as grain was preceded by the use of the stalks for fermentable juices. John Smalley and Michael Blake hypothesize that "maize was domesticated not for food but for drink," and that the earliest maize beverages came from the sweet stalks. "Initially, Early Archaic peoples in Mexico experimented with *Zea* by casually harvesting the sweet stalks and simply chewing them. Later they recognized that they could produce large quantities of sweet juice by mashing and squeezing the stalks. They then fermented the juice, probably using techniques and technologies already available for other plants." Only as a result of its cultivation for this purpose did larger ears and kernels emerge, according to this theory.[21]

We can never really know origins. But regardless of their origins, our cultural legacies disappear without continued use and adaptation.

 ## Sorghum Beer

Sorghum beer is the traditional beer of much of Africa. Homemade, it is fresh and appealing, with a complex sweet-alcoholic-sour flavor. The process is fun and educational. Like *tesgüino*, sorghum beer is a starchy suspension, sometimes referred to as "opaque beer." "Opaque beer is more a food than a beverage," states a report of the United Nations Food and Agriculture Organization. "It contains high proportions of starch and sugars, besides proteins, fats, vitamins and minerals."[22] Anthropologist Patrick McGovern reports that in the West African nation of Burkina Faso, sorghum beer "accounts for half of the caloric intake."[23]

Sorghum beers are now being commercially produced in the United States and marketed as gluten-free beers. These are made with sorghum, but in the style of barley beers, hopped and clarified, not opaque. "To most of the Western world opaque sorghum beer would hardly be recognized or considered as such," writes homebrew guru Charlie Papazian:

> I feel quite certain that these beers were among the first beers ever brewed. . . . Unlike the Mesopotamian and ancient Egyptian brews, these sorghum beers remain a living tradition, though no less historical. . . . In reality it has more tradition than any pils, bock, pale ale, or stout.[24]

Like any ancient tradition that has diffused widely, sorghum beers are made in different regions following "a bewildering variety of recipes under a confusing number of names."[25] Sometimes millet, corn (maize), or other grains are used in addition to or instead of sorghum.

This beer is essentially thin porridge fermented with malt, and it is prepared in at least as many varied ways as porridges are. Though the particulars can be somewhat quirky, the generic process is pretty straightforward: (1) Sprout sorghum; (2) dry it in the sun; (3) grind it; (4) make a porridge of unfermented grain, add some ground malt for saccharification and souring; (5) cook that in more water; and finally, (6) add more raw malt as a starter, and ferment.

Grain sorghum is not commonly available in the United States, except in African groceries and from seed suppliers. Millet works great and may be easier to find. Sorghum sprouts just like any other seed (see *Sprouting* in chapter 8). Soak seeds overnight, drain, and keep moist, well ventilated, and protected from sunlight for two to four days, until tails emerge from the sprouts about ¾ inch/2 cm long. Traditionally malt is dried in the sun, though dehydrators, fans, and other methods of low-heat drying can be used. After drying, the malted grain is stable for dry storage and is often aged for several months before use.[26] Prior to brewing into beer, grind malted grain using a mill, mortar and pestle, or other means. In addition, grind roughly the same quantity of *un*malted grain as you initially soaked for malting.

Sprouted sorghum

"To produce a variety of flavors and color in their beer, local village and homebrewers may roast all or a portion of their grains and malts," notes Charlie Papazian.[27]

Sorghum beer is made in (at least) two distinct fermentations. The first is primarily a lactic acid fermentation; the second primarily a yeast fermentation. If not consumed quickly, a third acetic acid fermentation follows. From reading I take it there is much regional and tribal variation in sorghum beer production; the method described here has worked well for me but is certainly not the last word. This method is followed by another very different sorghum beer method, for a Sudanese beer called *merissa*.

One pound/500 g of malted grain, plus another pound/500 g unmalted grain, yields about a gallon/4 liters of sorghum beer. The volume ratio of malted grain to unmalted grain to water is 1:1:3. Boil water. Stir in unmalted sorghum grits/flour and continue stirring to achieve a porridge-like consistency. Remove from the heat and allow to cool. Once the porridge cools to 140°F/60°C (or without using a thermometer, once it's cool enough to comfortably touch, but still quite warm), add half the malted sorghum grits/flour, reserving half to add later. Stir malt into the porridge thoroughly. The enzymes in the raw malt can act at peak efficiency at this temperature, digesting complex carbohydrates in simple sugars. Leave in a warm or insulated spot, protected from flies. After a few hours, when the mash cools to below 110°F/43°C, add half of the remaining malt (leave the other half for one more later addition) and stir well to distribute. Leave in a warm spot for 12 to 24 hours (depending upon temperature), during which time lactic acid bacteria proliferate, lowering pH and thus creating an advantageous selective environment.

The next step is to cook this soured mash, in more water, for several hours, to caramelize sugars, adding water as necessary to maintain a gruel-like starch suspension. Cool to around body temperature, then add the final portion of raw ground malted sorghum. Introduced into this soured and brewed mixture, the raw malt introduces yeasts for the final alcohol fermentation (or you could substitute a packet of yeast). Ferment in a warm spot protected from flies. In the tropics, fermentation time is measured in hours. In my temperate zone, I have typically fermented two or three days, then strained it through cheesecloth and bottled it in plastic soda bottles to ferment a few more hours to trap carbonation. Fresh sorghum beer is alive and pressurizes quickly, so always use caution not to overcarbonate.

Like all indigenous fermented beverages, sorghum beer exists in a shifting socioeconomic context, deeply embedded in community practices. It emerged in the context of gift exchange reciprocity and continues to exist as such in many places. But it also spread via trade routes and developed early as a cottage industry. "In Southern Africa, cash brewing initially took the form of women providing sorghum beer to men who had migrated to urban areas to work," writes economist Steven J. Haggblade in his doctoral dissertation on the shifting economic patterns reflected in sorghum beer in Botswana.[28] According to an International Labour Office report from 1972, brewing on a domestic scale "may well be the greatest single source of employment—particularly for single women—in some African countries."[29] The Botswana government reported in the 1970s that brewing "is the most widespread manufacturing activity in rural Botswana and is the most important source of female employment in the rural economy."[30] In Botswana and elsewhere in Southern Africa, the women who make and sell sorghum beer are called Shebeen Queens, their shops (typically their homes), shebeens.

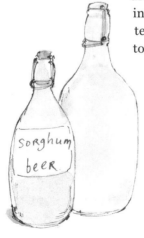

The first sorghum beer factories appeared in the region in the early 1900s. Haggblade reports that in Botswana, sorghum beer brewing was "the first modern manufacturing industry."[31] In the late 1930s, the South African government banned the sale of homebrew in urban areas and required municipal governments to supply sorghum beer. After that, explains Haggblade, "commercial brewing really took off."[32] Today the most popular brand of sorghum beer in southern Africa is Chibuku, sold in waxed cartons (how milk is sold); the beer is also known as Shake Shake, "because of its propensity to settle into its liquid and solid fractions," reports the BBC. "Shaking restores the beverage to its former grainy off-yoghurt consistency . . . [with] a zesty effervescence not unlike Lambrusco."[33]

Industrial brews have captured ever-growing market shares, but with economic repercussions. "Employment, incomes, and overall economic profit are all decreasing as a result of the rising importance of factory brewing," writes Haggblade, "leading to a large redistribution of income from poor and medium income groups to the rich."[34] That is part of the story everywhere, as the mass producers of food concentrate wealth, erase cultural difference, render vital cultural knowledge and skills obsolete, breed dependency, and decontextualize our food.

 ## *Merissa* (Sudanese Toasted Sorghum Beer)

One place where ancient beer traditions have endured, despite their official religious prohibition, is the Sudan, where sorghum beer is known mostly as *merissa*. "*Merissa* is one of the indelible features of the African heritage that resisted Islamic teachings, imposing itself prominently on the intricacies of the Sudanese way of life," wrote Hamid Dirar in 1993. "Its production and consumption in the Sudan is common to pagans, Christians, and Muslims alike."[35] *Merissa* is far from a standardized product. "The Sudan is a treasury of sorghum beers," according to Dirar. "It is impossible to enumerate all the kinds of beer found in the country. . . . These beers differ in ingredients and in the preparation procedures."[36] Yet because of the rule of Islamic law since the 1980s, Dirar reports that "the sale of *merissa* and its public consumption are illicit."[37] I tried emailing Dr. Dirar to confirm that *merissa* production is still widespread, but I was unable to reach him. Then I had the good fortune to meet Crazy Crow, a young Sudanese man now living in the United States, who reports that in Sudan, despite two decades of legal prohibition—with the threat of 40 lashes for violating that prohibition—the *merissa*-making tradition has persevered.

In honor of South Sudan's birth as an independent sovereign nation on July 9, 2011, freeing it from the constraints of Islamic law, I made a batch of *merissa*, guided by the incredibly detailed documentation of the process contained in Dirar's excellent book *The Indigenous Fermented Foods of the Sudan*. *Merissa* is simple in that the only ingredients are sorghum and water, yet these two ingredients are manipulated in many different ways. As with the sorghum beer above, 2 pounds/1 kg of sorghum will make about a gallon/4 liters of beer.

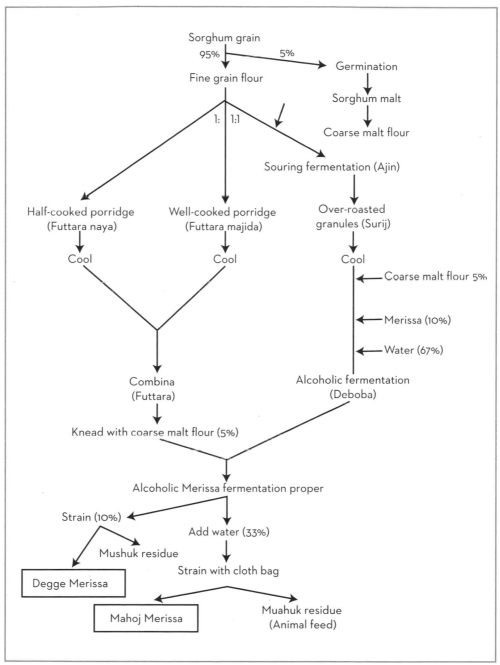

Flowchart from Hamid A. Dirar, *The Indigenous Fermented Foods of the Sudan: A Study in African Food and Nutrition*. (Wallingford, UK: CAB International, 1993).

Malting

Merissa requires only a small bit of malted sorghum, roughly 5 to 10 percent (by either weight or volume) of the total sorghum used in the beer. As in the sorghum beer described above, soak the grains overnight, drain, and keep moist, well ventilated, and protected from sunlight for two to four days, until tails emerge from the sprouts about ¾ inch/2 cm long. After sprouting, dry the malt in the sun, or using a dehydrator, fan, or other method of low-heat drying. The dried malted sorghum is stable for dry storage and is often aged for several months before use. To the small amount of malt, add 10 to 20 times as much unmalted grain; the rest of the process takes no more than 48 hours in Sudan, and a bit longer in more moderate climates.

Ajin Fermentation

Ajin is the sourdough at the heart of Sudanese sorghum culture. To make *ajin*, coarsely grind unmalted sorghum for the beer and divide it into three equal quantities, each of which will be processed separately. Take note of the volume of each of the three, as additions of water will be based upon that unit. One unit of the ground flour will be fermented into *ajin*. Place the ground sorghum in a non-metallic bowl or jar and dampen with minimal water. Add dechlorinated water, just a bit at a time, to the flour, then mix, and add a little more water, until there are no more dry patches in the flour. When I did this, it took about 50 percent as much water as flour I was dampening, by volume. Cover with a cloth. Dirar recommends fermenting this for 36 hours in the Sudan heat. I let mine go, stirring and smelling each day, for about three days, when it began to have a discernible sour aroma.

Surij Dry-Roasting

Surij is dry-roasted *ajin*. This is the step that gives *merissa* its characteristic flavor and color. Heat a cast-iron or other heavy skillet over medium heat. Add *ajin* and continuously flip, stir, and toss it in the pan to dry and toast evenly and prevent burning. Use a spatula or other tool with a hard edge that can get under the roasting sorghum meal; turn it over, so no surface stays in prolonged contact with the heat. Be sure to get into the corners of the pan. Break up clumps to facilitate drying. Feel the sorghum getting drier, and notice it darkening as it roasts. As water evaporates, "the colour of the fumes changes from the hue of steam to that of smoke," observes Dirar. This is a sign that the *surij* is done. "Charring of the *surij* is an integral part of the process."[38] It should just be beginning to char, not fully carbonized; like many roasted foods, the sorghum is enhanced by the slightly burned edge but could be ruined by outright burning. *Surij* can be stored dry or used right away.

"It seems that a major aim behind the harsh heat treatment given to *surij* is the destruction of acid-forming bacteria so only a very few of them gain access to the forthcoming yeast fermentation," explains Dirar.

> The major function of ajin fermentation is to provide the lactic acid necessary for lowering the pH to a level conducive to yeast growth and to provide

the slight sour flavour which is generally appreciated by Sudanese in many foods and beverages. However, production of too much lactic acid and, even worse, the production of acetic acid above certain limits are detrimental to the flavour of merissa. Hence the importance of the "sterilization" of ajin, which carries the microorganisms productive of these acids, to give surij.[39]

Deboba Fermentation

The next stage of the *merissa*-making process is to moisten the *surij* using a little water and a little mature *merissa*. Since I had no mother *merissa*, I made and used a batch of the more generic sorghum beer recipe (see the previous section), which uses no starter beyond the raw malt. You could try it with just raw malt as a starter, or add yeast, or another actively fermenting beer. Whatever starter you use, add it and the water only a very little at a time, and stir well. Add only as much liquid as the *surij* can absorb. The aim is to make the *surij* soggy, not submerge it. (When I tasted the soggy *surij*, it reminded me of the breakfast cereal Grape-Nuts.) Leave it to sit and ferment a few hours; four to five hours in Sudan, a few hours longer in a moderate temperature.

After this initial slightly soggy fermentation, mix in ground sorghum malt. Dirar's directions call for 5 percent malt, based on the unit of sorghum flour you started with for the *ajin*. I used twice that amount because I observed low germination of the sorghum during malting. Mix the sorghum malt into the soggy *surij* by hand. Then add water three times the volume of the sorghum meal unit—in other words, roughly equal to the total volume of unmalted sorghum used in the *merissa*. Once this water is added, active bubbly fermentation begins quickly. "Routinely, the brewer would follow the action of the malt on *surij* by tasting the mash, now and then, to see if it has turned sweet enough, adding more malt as required."[40] The resulting *deboba* "is a non-inviting, dark, thick sludge with a bitter taste," explains Dirar.[41]

Merissa Fermentation

The *deboba* ferments about seven hours like that before the next addition. At least an hour or two before that time has passed, the flour must be prepared to add to the brew. Each of the two thirds is cooked in a slightly different way. They are both cooked with water into porridge (*aceda*), but one is fully cooked, while the other is only half cooked. Then both *acedas* are cooled and mixed together into a dough called *futtara*. Dirar theorizes that perhaps the combining of fully cooked and undercooked porridges gives an optimal ratio of ungelatinized to gelatinized starches, though he reports that local brewers "explain the function of half-cooked *futtara* as providing the required, gritty feel on the palate of the consumer."[42] Start with the fully cooked porridge, as it takes longer to cool.

> To make porridge, fill a pot with fresh cold water, about triple the volume of the flour unit. Sprinkle a handful of flour on the surface of the cold water as it heats. Once the water comes to a boil, add the rest of the flour and stir vigorously; break up clumps of flour, and continually scrape the bottom of the pan so it does not begin to burn. As sorghum cooks, it absorbs all the water and thickens. Keep stirring. To test for doneness, press a wet finger briefly onto the aceda. Your finger should come away clean, and the porridge should bounce back. If necessary cook further, stirring continuously, and test again after a few minutes.

When *aceda* passes this test, it is spread out to cool. I pour it onto a cookie sheet, and it holds a cohesive perfectly rounded form as it cools.

> As the fully cooked *aceda* cools, start heating water for the half-cooked porridge. Start with less water, just equal to the volume of the flour unit. As above, sprinkle a handful of flour on the surface of the cold water while it heats. Once the water comes to a boil, add the rest of the flour and stir, breaking up clumps of flour and continually scraping the bottom of the pan so it does not begin to burn. In this case, stir until the porridge thickens, then cut off the heat, add another equal volume of cold water, and keep stirring until it reaches a homogeneous texture. Spread the half-cooked *aceda* to cool on a cookie sheet or in a big bowl.

cooked rice

> Once both the fully and half-cooked *acedas* are cool enough to comfortably handle, the two are "worked into each other by hand to give *futtara*." Then knead the malt into the *futtara*, roughly 5 to 10 percent malt based on the two units of flour now joined together. Transfer the resulting mass to the already fermenting *deboba*, "left as a solid mass overwhelmed by the thick *deboba* slurry"; do not even stir, "so the mass of *futtara* slowly dissolves."[43] This slows fermentation, desirable in the summer heat. In the winter months, when faster fermentation is desired, *futtara* is actively stirred into the *deboba*.[44]

> Finally, all the different sorghum and water combinations are fermenting together. But just for a short time. Dirar writes that the typical *merissa* fermentation time in the Sudan is about seven hours; then it is strained and drinking begins. "As the day wears on, *merissa* develops a sharp acid flavour and by the evening it would have spoiled."[45] In Tennessee's July heat, however, no step of the *merissa* process was quite as fast as Dirar describes. I strained some of my *merissa* after about 7 hours, and then some 24 hours later. The 24-hour-later batch was much stronger, without becoming excessively acidic at all.

> To strain, place a colander over a bowl and line the colander with a large finely woven cotton cloth. Fill with *merissa*. Carefully gather together the corners and edges of the cloth and use them to lift the *merissa* in the cloth out of the colander. Twist the contents enclosed in the cloth to force liquid through the cloth. Press it against the colander. Keep squeezing and pressing to force

liquid out; as the contents of the cloth become smaller and denser, wrap it more tightly and keep pressing. Press until it feels like there is no more liquid left. *Merissa* can be stored a few days in a full bottle in the refrigerator, but like most indigenous beers this is a gift to share and enjoy, not hold on to. As *merissa* sits in the fridge, the starch settles at the bottom of the bottle, leaving a clear, dark beer, not unlike a chocolate stout or other very dark beer, that can be carefully poured off and enjoyed. Delicious!

Dirar describes two grades of *merissa*. *Dagga* is pressed from about a quarter of the fermenting liquid. "The rest of the brew, comprising the bulk of *merissa*, is first diluted with an equal volume of water and then strained. The resultant weaker *merissa* is called *mahoj*, which is the usual form in which *merissa* is sold." I pressed all of my *merissa* into *dagga*, then covered the residue with a little more water, which yielded a very weak product. The solid residue from *merissa*, *mushuk*, is fed to animals, "a highly valued, fattening feed."[46]

I highly recommend *merissa*, as a delicious and unusual beer-making experience. Its rich layered flavor reflects the complexity of its preparation. May the culture of *merissa* once again flourish in the newly independent nation of South Sudan.

Asian Rice Brews

Japanese *saké* is the rice-based alcohol that is best known in the West. *Saké* is distinctive in certain ways but is also part of a much broader group of beverages produced throughout Asia using mold enzymes to saccharify rice and other grains. The next chapter covers the molds themselves, as well as concepts and simple methods for growing some of them. The discussion here, concerning basic techniques for fermenting grain-based alcoholic beverages using molds, presumes that you obtain mold cultures commercially or through gift exchange, or make them as described in the following chapter.

I've had great results fermenting with Chinese *qu* (see chapter 10), sold as "yeast" in the form of small balls about 1 inch/2.5 cm in diameter, available in many Asian groceries and on the Internet. Similar mixed culture starters, incorporating a variety of molds as well as yeasts and bacteria, are in use throughout Asia, and go by many different names, including *ragi* (Indonesia and Malaysia), *marcha* (India and Nepal), *nuruk* (Korea), *bubod* (Philippines), *loopang* (Thailand), and many others.[47] Japanese *koji* (see *Making* Koji in chapter 10) is derived from the same tradition, but in contemporary practice it is typically an isolated single mold (*Aspergillus oryzae*) cultured to the exclusion of yeast and bacteria.

Alcoholic beverages made from rice in these different places are produced by processes that vary in many details, but as a group they all share certain methods that distinguish them from beers made in the Western tradition. First of all, *saccharification*, the breakdown of complex carbohydrates into fermentable simple sugars, occurs simultaneously with the fermentation of those sugars into alcohol; in the Western tradition, saccharification (by way of malting and then holding the mash at high but controlled temperatures to optimize enzyme activity) always takes place prior to alcohol fermentation. Another distinguishing characteristic of these Asian grain ferments—which they share with sorghum beer, *tesgüino*, and most indigenous brews—is that the cooked grain itself is always fermented, rather than just a liquid extraction, as with contemporary Western malted grain beers, in which only the clear liquid wort extracted from the grain mash is fermented. As the rice saccharifies and ferments, it also liquefies. In ancient China, the liquid was extracted to drink via straws. (Actually, the practice of drinking beers with filtered straws is "a worldwide phenomenon," according to Patrick McGovern, used not only in ancient China but also the Fertile Crescent, the Pacific Islands, the Americas, and Africa, and "still widely practiced."[48] Nepali millet *tongba*, described in this chapter, is typically drunk through a straw.)

Basic Rice Beer

The generic process for rice beer is extremely simple. Cook rice. Cool. Add starter culture. Ferment. Strain. Drink. I love the simplicity of how I first tried it, even after surveying dozens of recipes and trying a handful of variations. I used short-grain brown rice, which I did not even pre-soak, and cooked as I typically do (though without salt). Figure about 2 pounds (4 cups)/1 kg (1 liter) of dry rice and one small *qu* yeast ball make about 3 quarts/liters of rice beer.

After cooking, allow the rice to cool to body temperature. As it cools, crush a yeast ball into powder. If you do not have a mortar and pestle, press with the back of a spoon against a sturdy bowl. Use one yeast ball per kilo/2 pounds of rice; some recipes use even less, and more can speed the process. As the rice cools, transfer it to a crock or other vessel. Once it reaches body temperature, add the powdered yeast ball. I clean my hands and get in there, squeezing clumps and getting it all thoroughly mixed. (I suppose you could also do it with a spoon.)

After the starter is well distributed in the rice, use a spoon to form a well in the center of the rice. As the fermentation proceeds and liquefaction occurs, this well fills with fluid—rice beer. Incubate in a warm spot. Most of the year, I use the oven (turned off) with the illumination light on; in summer, ambient temperatures are perfect. After liquefied rice fills the well, the bubbling liquid will cover the rice, but the bubbling will also lift the rice above the liquid. Stir several times a day at this stage.

Rice beer is quite delicious throughout its development, and strongly alcoholic after about a week. Strain off the liquid and enjoy cloudy, or allow the starch to settle and pour off the clarified beer. Refrigerate for short-term preservation or pasteurize for longer-term storage; otherwise lactic acid bacteria from the mixed culture will continue to acidify it.

Surveying recipes in books and online, there is much variation and cultural particularity in all the details of this process, as it is practiced by many of the billions of people sprawled across the vast continent of Asia in thousands of distinctive cultural lineages. "They may be clarified into liquid, or turbidly suspended liquid; even they may be semi-solid, unfiltered mash," explain Xu Gan Rong and Bao Tong Fa of Jiangnan University in Jiangsu Province, China, in their online *Grandiose Survey of Chinese Alcoholic Drinks and Beverages*.[49] Dr. S. Sekar of Bharathidasan University in Tamil Nadu, India, in his *Database on Microbial Traditional Knowledge of India*, details methods for 19 different rice beers, as well as the varied starters used to ferment them. Here's the process for one of them, called *ruhi*, from Nagaland, in India's northeastern hills:

> Boiled rice is spread on mat and allowed to cool. It is mixed with yeast grown on rice and hosan leaves. The inoculated rice is poured into cone shaped bamboo basket. An earthenware pot is placed under the cone to collect the fermented liquid. The liquid is transferred to new boiled rice successively for three or four times. The liquid finally collected becomes the first quality ruhi.[50]

Some recipes online are very specific as to type of rice. I think this is because so many different varieties of rice are important in different places, and these distinctive rices give beverages fermented from them distinctive qualities. But in my lackadaisical way, I have more often than not used the wrong type of rice in my rice brew experiments, and I've ended up using quite a few different varieties—sticky and not, brown and white and black—and somehow it's always good (though not necessarily authentic to any particular tradition). Some recipes say to boil rice, others say to steam it above water; I've tried both ways, and both work.

As for the starter, in some traditions the crushed dried yeast is soaked in water to bring it back to life and activate it. Other traditions mix crushed starter dry into rice, as I describe above. Also, in some traditions no water is added, so the microbial and enzymatic starters begin their activity in an aerobic environment, until the liquefaction they cause engulfs them. In others, fermentation takes place entirely in a liquid medium, with water added immediately to the cooked rice.

In some traditions, including Japanese *saké*, rice is introduced into the fermentation gradually, at repeated intervals, enabling yeasts to produce alcohol at unusually high concentrations, up to 20 percent, much stronger than any other type of fermented alcohol. In different traditions, different temperatures are deemed to be ideal. For *saké*, rice is fermented in a cool environment, around 60°F/15°C, for several weeks. In many other traditions, rice is fermented in a warm environment (around 90°F/32°C) for about a week, then sometimes finished in a cooler spot. Elsewhere people work with ambient temperatures.

Typically, rice brews are strained before drinking, to remove residual solids and yeast sediment. This sediment (equivalent to what the Japanese call *saké* lees) may be used as pickling medium (see *Tsukemono: Japanese Pickling*

Styles in chapter 5) or as an ingredient in pancakes and other concoctions, or fed to animals or compost. After straining, the liquid may be left to settle and be further clarified by gently pouring the clear liquor on top off the starchy suspension that sinks. But rice beer is not necessarily even strained. A fermentation enthusiast named Mick recounted:

> I was once walking through some farmland out in the middle of China somewhere with some friends and we stopped at a farmhouse where they served us food and bowls of alcoholic rice, not rice wine, but the actual fermented rice that would be strained for the wine. Very strong stuff.

The brew with rice still in it is often used as the basis of soups and other culinary creations. A blogger wrote that "in my family, we use rice wine most often to flavor soft poached eggs," also known as *jiu niang dan*.

> It is prepared by poaching eggs in simmering water until the whites are firm but the yolks are still somewhat runny. The eggs are placed into single serving bowls, with a small teaspoonful of sugar and a quantity of the hot water. Several tablespoonfuls of the jiu niang rice and wine are added to the bowl and stirred so that the rice warms up and the sugar melts.[51]

In another version I read about, water is boiled, rice wine and sugar are added, then scrambled eggs are mixed in, for more of an egg-drop-soup rather than poached-egg feel.[52] Either way it is very delicious (even without the sugar).

Below are further explorations of three specific variants on the basic rice beer theme: Korean *makgeolli*, in which the rice is supplemented by sweet potato as a fermentation substrate; Nepali *tongba* made from millet; and Japanese *saké*.

Sweet Potato *Makgeolli*

Makgeolli is a Korean rice beer. I first heard about it from Linda Kim, of New York City, who emailed me recounting her experience making some. "It's very simple, and only takes around 3–5 days to ferment." I liked the sound of that. Linda told me she had found the Korean starter culture, called *nuruk*, online. When I searched online for "*nuruk*," I found nothing; then Linda sent me a link to a Korean-owned grocery chain and website,[53] which sells *nuruk* as "powdered enzyme amylase," and I bought some for $5. My Internet searching turned up a number of *makgeolli* recipes, the most interesting being one from a blog called "Seoulful Cooking" that incorporates sweet potatoes, one of my favorite foods.[54] The *makgeolli* process described below is one in which I adapted elements from Linda Kim's emails, the Seoulful Cooking blog, and other online recipes.

To make *makgeolli*, rinse 2 pounds/1 kg sweet rice and soak overnight (or all day). Drain well, then steam the rice. I like to steam in stacking bamboo steamers, available in most Asian markets, lined with a cotton cloth to keep the grains from falling through the bottom. Once the rice is well cooked, spread it onto a tray or cookie sheet to cool. Meanwhile scrub ½ pound/250 g sweet potatoes, chop into big chunks with the skins on, steam until soft, and then cool. When the rice is cool enough to handle, transfer it to a crock, bowl, or jar with a capacity of at least 1 gallon/4 liters. Add about 2 quarts/liters of dechlorinated water. Use your hands to gently squeeze rice, separating individual grains. Add crushed *nuruk* and massage it into the mass. Add sweet potatoes, skins and all, and crush them with your hands as you mix them into the mass. Cover with a cloth and leave in a warm spot.

sweet potato
makgeolli

After a few hours, and at least twice a day thereafter, stir the rice–sweet potato–*nuruk* mass to help redistribute and spread enzyme and yeast activity. At first, all the water you added is absorbed by the rice, but as enzymatic digestion progresses, liquefaction occurs gradually and the mass is soon floating in liquid. After a couple of days replace the cloth covering vessel with a firmer, less permeable top that will restrict airflow. Ferment until most of the rice grains have sunk to the bottom. This may take just a few days in a warm environment, or as long as two weeks in a cool one. Strain and transfer to bottles. Leave bottles at ambient temperature for another day to carbonate, if desired. Store *makgeolli* in the fridge for a couple of weeks, but note that it will slowly acidify unless pasteurized. Many people add sugar to sweeten *makgeolli* when they drink it, but personally I don't think it's necessary.

Millet *Tongba*

Tongba is a millet beer, made in the style of rice beers, using a traditional mixed culture starter. I first heard about *tongba* from my friend Victory, who had fond memories of it from his travels in Nepal.

> The fermented grain was served in a tall glass with a thermos of hot water, and a straw on which the bottom was covered with a piece of cotton tied on to filter the grain. One tall glass was good for five or six water refills. After the second glass laughter seemed to follow all the imbibers for the rest of the evening until we all staggered home. It tasted like liquid bread.

Actually, it turns out that *tongba* (also transliterated as *toongbaa*) is the name of the bamboo vessel in which this beverage (*kodo ko jaanr*) is traditionally served. According to Jyoti Prakash Tamang's book *Himalayan Fermented Foods*, "a *toongbaa* is a vessel in which fermented millet seeds are placed and warm water is added. The extract is sipped through a narrow bamboo straw . . . with a hole on opposite sides at one end of the straw to avoid passing of grits during sipping."[55]

I love this strong and distinctive brew—warm and milky—and also the fun ritual that goes with it. To consume, fill a mug about halfway with fermented millet mush, then fill it the rest of the way with hot water. I let it sit for 10 minutes, then drink it warm, and repeat. For me two or three pours or pressings are plenty. I've mostly sipped the liquid off the grains without a straw, filtering with my teeth as needed, but it was fun to drink it through a *bombilla*, one of those steel straws used for drinking *yerba maté*. You can also filter it through a strainer.

The millet used in Nepal (kodo millet, *Paspalum scrobiculatum*) is somewhat different from the millet grown in the United States (pearl millet, *Pennisetum americanum*), but I love the *tongba* that the pearl millet produces. It so happened that my friend Justin Bullard, who lived in Nepal long ago and learned to make *tongba* and *chaang* there, was returning to Nepal to document methods for making the Nepali starter *marcha* (see *Plant Sources of Mold Cultures* in chapter 10), and he brought some *marcha* home for me, so I had a supply of the authentic starter. I have not been able to locate any Internet sources for purchasing *marcha*, but Chinese yeast balls can substitute for it with similar results.

First, prepare millet. I use a proportion of about 2½ volumes water to each volume millet. Bring to a boil, then gently simmer, covered, for about 15 minutes, until the seeds burst open; then remove from the heat. Justin instructed me to add a little cold water to the millet, so the water just covers the cooked millet. As soon as it is cool enough to handle, use your clean hands to massage the millet and break up clumps, so every grain is individual in the solution. When the millet is below body temperature, add crushed *marcha* or Chinese yeast balls and mix thoroughly to distribute. I followed Justin's recommendation of two cakes of *marcha* per pound of millet. With Chinese yeast balls, one per pound would be plenty; half that would probably suffice.

Justin writes: "Let it ferment, at least, until the mash stops bubbling. The mash will keep for about a season, but is best used, I think, after about a month of fermentation." Jyoti Prakash Tamang, author of *Himalayan Fermented Foods: Microbiology, Nutrition, and Ethnic Values*, describes a shorter process, 5 to 10 days altogether. I loved it at one week. It was strongly alcoholic, no longer sweet, and only subtly sour. What we didn't drink in the first episode remained in the crock for a few more days, then after I noticed that bubbling had ceased, I transferred it to a sealed jar, where I left it for another couple of weeks. When I tasted it again, the *tongba* had gotten stronger, both more alcoholic and more sour. Had I transferred it to a sealed jar earlier, as soon as bubbling slowed, I probably could have avoided some of the sourness.

Saké

As described earlier, Japanese *saké* is the fermented rice beverage that has become best known beyond its homeland. People who eat sushi or dine in Japanese restaurants often enjoy *saké*, smooth, strong, and often served warm.

Koji, the Japanese molded grain, covered at length in chapter 10, is the starter for *saké*. Or rather, it is part of the starter. *Koji* is the product of rice's inoculation with the spores of a single mold, *Aspergillus oryzae*. The enzymes in this mold accomplish the saccharification of the rice necessary to ferment it to alcohol (and many other fermentations); however, *koji* does not contain the yeast that actually accomplish the alcohol fermentation, as do Chinese yeast balls, *nuruk*, *marcha*, and all the other mixed culture starters that incorporate *Aspergillus* and other molds, as well as yeasts and bacteria. Most contemporary *saké* makers add specialized, commercially available, single-species yeast starters, a tradition going back more than 100 years in Japan.[56] There is also, of course, an older wild fermentation tradition.

One notable requirement of *saké* making is cool temperatures, as low as 45°F/7°C, and definitely below 60°F/15°C. My experiments have been in winter in a room that could be shut off from heat. You could use a wine refrigerator, or any fridge rigged up with an overriding temperature controller (see *Temperature Controllers* in chapter 3).

The first step of the *saké*-making process is making or purchasing *koji* (see *Making* Koji in chapter 10). A small amount of *koji* is mixed with water, freshly steamed rice, and, typically, a yeast starter. This is the *moto*, or *shubo*, and it bubbles for a few days in a warm environment, 70–73°F/21–23°C. This gets the yeast active before adding the bulk of the rice, but it also has traditionally served the purpose of allowing lactic acid to develop, which, when present in sufficient amounts, "prevents wild yeast and unwanted bacteria from proliferating and adversely affecting the flavor," according to John Gauntner, author of several books on *saké*. Early in the 20th century, it was determined that lactic acid could be added directly at the start of the process. "Adding lactic acid at the beginning speeds the process up" and "protects it from the start." This practice, by which most *saké* is now prepared, is known as *sokujo* (fast-developing) *moto*. The traditional process takes much longer, and "since the lactic acid comes into existence more slowly, a bit of funky bacteria and even wild yeast cells inevitably make it into the *moto* as it develops. This gives rise to gamier, more unabashed flavor profile in the end."[57] (I made a batch of *saké* using sourdough starter as the source of yeast and lactic acid bacteria and it had an unabashed flavor profile, for sure!)

Once the *moto* is mature, you make three successively larger additions of rice, *koji*, and water, roughly doubling the size of the batch with each addition. Each addition has its own name in this highly formalized process. The first is *hatsuzoe*. *Koji* and water are added in the evening, then the next morning more rice is added. For two days this is known as the *odori* (dancing) ferment, until you incorporate the second *nakazoe* addition of twice as much *koji*, twice as much water, and the following morning twice as much rice; then a day later twice as much of each element yet again for the final *tomezoe* addition. Once all the rice has been incorporated, the rice mash is known as *moromi*, and it ferments for two weeks. After this fermentation, *saké* is usually strained and pressed to separate the fermented liquid from the solid residue (lees). *Saké* can be enjoyed at this point, or transferred to an air-locked vessel until all bubbling ceases, a week or two later. At this point, *saké* may be filtered and clarified to remove its white cloudy suspended starches, if desired. Personally, I love it cloudy, with some body. *Saké* is typically pasteurized in the bottle so it will not continue to acidify. *Nama-zaké* is unpasteurized *saké*, which is very lovely, but must be stored under refrigeration or drunk quickly. Sour *saké* is not a bad thing to end up with. I love it as a steaming liquid in cooking and enjoy little shots of it as a tonic rich in lactic acid bacteria.

Saké in our time is generally made from polished rice, meaning rice that has been milled to remove the outer layers. The problem with this is the same as the problem with eating refined grains: The outer layers contain critical nutrients. Therefore, most *saké* recipes call for the addition of various minerals and yeast nutrients. "If you use brown rice, you don't have to add any other kinds of chemical foods for the yeast to grow," points out traveling fermentation experimentalist Eric Haas.

Eric wrote to me from Japan: "I found few people who make their own *saké*, but some people who make amazing stuff." He cited one *saké* maker in particular whose "*saké* was thick and cloudy (*nigori*), raw (*nama*), and dreamy like a cloud. The best I've ever had." According to Eric, the man grew his own rice, made it into *koji*, and never introduced any commercial yeasts, relying upon wild fermentation and using especially good batches as starters.

See *Resources* for books and websites with more detailed sake-making information.

Malting Barley

Finally, we arrive at our familiar beer, the beverage fermented from malted barley, with hops added for flavoring and preservation. Malting is the first step of this process. Beer makers have largely relegated the malting of barley to specialists. I have been able to find only one small-scale brewery that has an in-house malting operation (Rogue Brewery in Newport, Oregon), as well as a small handful of obsessed homebrewers who make beer from barley they malt themselves. Sprouting barley is no harder than sprouting any other grain, but malting has developed as an art and science, with much technique and technology to help achieve optimal enzyme development.

Although malting historically was regarded as part of the brewing process, as the scale of breweries grew, and specialization increased in every realm of industrial production, malting operations mostly split off from breweries, and local and regional malt houses supplied malt to multiple breweries. By the late 20th century, malting became highly centralized. A 1998 analysis found that in the United States and Canada, eight firms control 97 percent of malt production.[58] An otherwise informative book explaining the science behind brewing beer, *Brew Chem 101*, devotes exactly one sentence to malting:

"Since it's the rare homebrewer, indeed, who germinates his or her own grains, we won't say anything more about it."[59]

But malting is an integral part of the process of making beer, and malting your own grain will definitely enhance your understanding of the process by which grains become beer. Specialization may be warranted, given the technical challenges of malting; however, homemade malt can make perfectly fine beer, which does not require enzyme optimization, and even malting specialization does not have to result in centralized industry, just as grain itself need not be monocultured in remote regions. In the local-food revival of the past decade, a few regional relocalizing maltsters have started operations. Grain growing is also occurring as part of the revival of local food and agricultural diversification. These emerging movements promise to redefine our understanding of how local a beer can be.

To malt barley, be sure to start with whole *unhulled* barley, complete with outer husk. It is best to malt barley at a moderately cool temperature around 55–60°F/13–16°C. The barley should not be too freshly harvested; most sources recommend storing barley for a minimum of six weeks before germinating. Cover barley with water and stir. Chaff will float to the surface; you'll then want to pour off the chaff. Cover the barley with more water if necessary and soak about eight hours. After this soak, drain the water off and allow the barley to sit with air circulation for another eight-hour period. Then cover with water again and soak for another eight hours. This is "interrupted steeping," in which steeping is broken up by "air rests" to give the germinating grain access to oxygen.[60] After draining barley from the second soaking, you should start to see white bulges at one end of each grain; these are emergent roots. Give barley another longer air rest of 12 to 16 hours, then a third 8-hour steeping. Steeping schedules vary "depending on parameters such as variety, kernel size, protein content, and physiological status of the grain," explains Charles Bamforth, author of the definitive *Scientific Principles of Malting and Brewing*.[61]

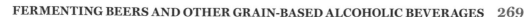

malted barley

The jar method I recommend for sprouting (see *Sprouting* in chapter 8) is not appropriate for quantities above a pound or two of grain. "Traditionally, steeped barley was spread out to a depth of up to 10 cm [4 inches] on the floors of long, low buildings and germinated for up to 10 days," writes Bamforth. "Workers would use rakes either to thin out the grain or pile it up, depending on whether the temperature of the batch needed to be lowered or raised."[62]

I've seen people malt barley for brewing in 5-gallon/20-liter buckets, with holes in the bottom for drainage and air circulation, and in tubs on the floor. German homebrewer Axel Gehlert, who wrote to me describing his malting experiments, used his *lauter tun* (a tool homebrewers use to filter solids from the wort) as a malting vessel. The key requirements are that the grains must have access to oxygen, but must also remain moist and not dry out. Turning the grain frequently so different grains are exposed to air helps keep germination even. Lightly misting the grain with dechlorinated water can prevent it from drying out.

As germination proceeds, the emerging roots grow, as does the sprout itself, although for most of the process, the sprout is hidden by the hulls. "The key factor is to stop germination when the main shoot (not the hair-like rootlets), called the *acrospire*, is three-fourths to one length of the grain," writes William Starr Moake in *Brew Your Own* magazine. "This produces fully modified barley malt."[63] From initial soaking, this takes about a week, though the exact time will vary with grain variety, temperature, humidity, and other conditions.

Once malt has germinated sufficiently, the process is halted by drying with heat, usually in a low-temperature oven or kiln. If germination were to continue, the developing embryo would consume the barley seed's newly available sugars. Kilning not only stops germination but also alters the flavor of the sprouts; in the words of Charles Bamforth, kilning is "a driving off of the undesirable raw flavors in the 'green' malt (notes reminiscent of bean sprouts and cucumber, nice in their own right but not as a component of beer) while introducing the pleasing malty flavors."[64]

Kilning temperatures vary greatly to produce different styles of malt with different purposes. High enzyme *diastatic* malts, for instance, are kilned at temperatures that typically do not exceed 131°F/55°C "to avoid destruction of the enzymes by heat," explains Bamforth. Other "specialty" malts can be kilned at temperatures as high as 428°F/220°C, "produced not for their enzyme content but rather for use by the brewer in relatively small quantities as a source of extra color and distinct types of flavor." Generally, kilning begins at temperatures around 120°F/50°C and slowly increases. For small quantities, you can work with your oven, with a light on, or the pilot light, or turning the very lowest setting on and off.

Simple Opaque Barley Beer

I decided to try barley beer in the style of indigenous porridge and malt beers, like sorghum beer. I malted a pound of unhulled barley. Then I coarsely ground some unmalted "pearled" barley and cooked it into a porridge. This I cooled to 140°F/60°C in an insulated "cooler," simultaneously warming the cooler to serve as an incubation chamber. When the porridge cooled, I added half of the malted barley (coarsely ground) and left it to incubate in the prewarmed cooler. After several hours, I removed the still-warm and now enzyme-sweetened porridge from the incubator and let it cool to about 110°F/43°C. Next, I added half the remaining malted barley and let it sit to sour for about 12 hours (this was the heat of summer; 24 hours would be the timing otherwise). Then I cooked the brew for a couple of hours, stirring periodically and adding water as necessary, and once again let it cool, this time to ambient temperatures. Finally, I added the last of the malt to introduce yeast and stirred the fermenting mash as it bubbled away.

I fermented it for about a week, stirring frequently. Fermentation bubbles kept lifting the barley solids, so stirring would mix them back into the fermenting solution, at least temporarily, until the vigorous bubbles lifted them again. After about a week, as bubbling activity slowed significantly, I strained the beer through cheesecloth, then poured a little more water through it, and finally wrung out the ball of spent grain in the cheesecloth, squeezing out as much liquid I could.

The beer was pretty strong. It was also somewhat sour, as is the intention and inevitability in this style of brew. I found this to be a worthwhile exercise that helped me see and taste the lineage between the indigenous brews with other grains and the beer with which we are more familiar. Interestingly, Hamid Dirar reports that *merissa*, the Sudanese sorghum beer, is also known as *bouza*,[65] which, according to food historian Priscilla Mary Işsin, is an ancient Turkish name for beer that "can be traced back to the Sumerians . . . has found its way into more than twenty languages in Central Asia, Eastern Europe, and North Africa," and probably gives us the English word *booze*.[66]

Cassava and Potato Beers

Cassava is made into beer in several different ways. In Amazon South America, as well as parts of Africa, women chew cassava as the saccharification step of a fermented beverage called *masato*. A team of anthropologists reported the preparation of *masato* as follows:

> First, cassava is boiled and allowed to cool in a wooden container. One woman continues beating the mass until it is smooth while other women chew to ensalivate it. Some families prefer to use sugar to effect fermentation thus avoiding the chewing. When reduced to a watery consistency, the mass is placed into clay jars to ferment. After three or four days, it is mixed with water and offered in cups to visitors.[67]

Interestingly, elsewhere in South America, in Guyana, people use molds to achieve the same goal of saccharification of cassava to ferment into alcohol, in this case a beverage called *parakari*. "*Parakari* is unique among New World beverages because it involves the use of an amylolytic mold (*Rhizopus*) followed by a solid substratum ethanol fermentation," according to mycologist Terry Henkel, who documented the method he saw used in Guyana, very similar to how molds are used and perpetuated throughout Asia (explored in chapter 10). "The domestication of *Rhizopus* in South America appears independent from, yet analogous to, ancient *Rhizopus* domestications in Asia," writes Henkel.[68]

As I pondered trying these with cassava (available in nearby cities, but imported from the tropics somewhere), just as I was harvesting potatoes, I decided to try these with the starchy tubers from my garden. Other than adding potatoes or potato starch as a minor ingredient in a barley-based beer (or sugar-based country wine), I have not been able to find any information on traditional potato-based fermented beverages.

Chewed Potato Beer

With the kind assistance of a workshop group, I made a chewed potato beer. I wouldn't say it was great, but it was definitely alcoholic (after just 24 hours' fermentation), with a flavor that was tolerable and interesting, though not altogether appealing. Lots of people enjoyed a taste; only one person, Hannah, drank a big mug full. This is the process I followed (I offer this not so much as a recipe as a point of departure for adventuring experimentalists).

First, boil whole potatoes until they are soft, then drain them and allow them to cool. The way to chew the potatoes is to take a bite and mash it thoroughly for a moment with your teeth and also between your tongue and the roof of your mouth. You want to form little mashed potato balls, pretty finely mashed, moistened by your saliva, but not too much. They have to be dry enough to hold together and not collapse into puddles. Do this in a group. You might be surprised how filling it can be chewing potatoes and then spitting them out—each person can only do so many! You can work with the mashed potato balls fresh, refrigerate, or dry in the sun or a dehydrator for longer-term storage.

In a pot, boil a little water with a few more (not chewed) potatoes, coarsely chopped. The enzyme-infused potatoes have enough salivary enzymes to convert starch in more potatoes. After the potatoes are soft, mash them up in the water; then add cold water, a little at a time, and mash it in, until the thin potato gruel cools to below 150°F/65°C. Then add the mashed potato spit balls to the gruel, and gently heat, stirring frequently, until the expanded mass of gruel heats to above 140°F/60°C. This very warm temperature stimulates the amylase enzymes in the saliva to be at their most vigorously active. Hold the temperature in this range for an hour or two. The lowest setting on a stove should work fine, with periodic stirring. Or you could use a prewarmed insulated cooler, or an incubator. After you hold the temperature a while, leave it to slowly cool.

Once the potato gruel has cooled to ambient temperatures, heat it again, this time to a boil, and gently boil it for a couple of hours. This stops enzyme activity, kills salivary bacteria that may be of concern, and caramelizes newly converted sugars. After boiling, remove the potato gruel from the heat and allow it to cool to ambient temperatures.

I wanted to ferment this quickly so the group that chewed it could taste it, so I added a packet of yeast. Alternatively, you could add a vigorous sourdough or berries as a starter at this point. I also added fresh leaves of sage as a flavoring. Once the fermentation began, it developed and peaked very quickly. I cooked the gruel in the evening; in the morning I pitched it with yeast; by midafternoon fermentation was highly active, with bubbles forcing the potato solids to float at the top, where they could easily be scooped off; and by the following morning fermentation had stopped and the liquid was still. I strained off the remaining potato solids and bottled the beer; left the bottles at ambient temperatures for another 24 hours to carbonate (being careful not to overcarbonate, as always); cooled in the refrigerator; and served the potato beer up that evening.

I also did an experiment fermenting potato beer using molds, employing Chinese "yeast" balls (see *Asian Rice Brews*). I steamed 2 pounds/1 kg potatoes, then mashed them with some of the steaming liquid, cooled them to body temperature, and mixed in two crushed Chinese yeast balls. At first it smelled sweet, and there was a bit of liquefaction, but then it developed a strong acetone aroma, which never left it, and I ended up aborting the experiment and discarding it. It was not my first failed experiment, and surely not my last.

Beyond Hops: Beers with Other Herbs and Botanical Additives

People in different places and times have incorporated many varying botanical ingredients into their beers. Or rather, the way I imagine it most likely unfolded, people began to incorporate grains into more ancient traditions of fermenting that already incorporated various plants. Brewing emerged as an extension of gathering and then cultivating plants and generating surpluses of grains; the people who brewed early beers were the plant gatherers—women—and in many cultures brewing still remains an exclusive domain of women.

In his book *Secret Life of Beer*, the late beer adventurer Alan Eames recounted an exchange he had with a group of Quechua women brewing *chicha*, after he asked them whether men ever brewed beer. "My question was met with gales of raucous laughter. The women howled. Bent over in hilarity, one replied, 'Men can't brew! Chicha made by men only makes gas in the belly. You are a funny man, beer is women's work.'"[69] The Quechua are hardly unique in this view. "Worldwide, women are recognized as the original brewers of fermented drinks," writes feminist theorist Judy Grahn. "The Brewster, or alewife, was a central figure from Africa to China, South America to northern Europe."[70] Alan Eames reports: "In hidden, remote places around the world . . . women still hold close the art of brewing. Praying to their ancient goddesses, the women of non-technological societies continue to pass down to their daughters the secrets of beer."[71] And the secrets of beer are among the many secrets of plants and their associated microbes.

Functionally, plant additives in beer have served as flavorings, preservatives, microbial inoculants, and yeast nutrients, as well as medicines and psychotropic agents. German archaeobotanist Karl-Ernst Behre lists more than 40 plant species used as beer additives in Europe alone, based on written historical records. This "resulted in a great variety of beers," writes Behre. "Each town and sometimes each brewer had their own specific beer in contrast to the rather uniform modern beers."[72] Herbalist Stephen Harrod Buhner, author of *Sacred and Healing Herbal Beers*, documents (and gives recipes for) beers made with heather, mugwort, sage, wild lettuce, nettles, ground ivy, sassafras, horehound, elder, various evergreens, and many plants other than hops.

In parts of Europe, local beer flavorings came to be known as *gruts* or *gruits*. Buhner explains that *gruit* typically contained "a combination of three mild to moderately narcotic herbs: sweet gale (*Myrica gale*), also called bog myrtle, yarrow (*Achillea millefolium*), and wild rosemary (*Ledum palustre*), also called marsh rosemary," along with "additional herbs to produce unique tastes, flavors, and effects," including juniper berries, ginger, caraway seed, coriander, aniseed, nutmeg, and cinnamon. "The exact formula for each *gruit* was, like that for Coca Cola, proprietary—a closely guarded secret."[73]

In the Holy Roman Empire, *gruits* became the means by which beer was taxed. "During the 11th century, the Holy Roman Emperor awarded local monopoly privileges in the production and sale of *grut*, the *Grutrecht*, to dioceses throughout the empire," writes economist Diana Weinert.[74] This was one step among many toward centralizing social control. Regulating beers and what could go into them across a vast territory effectively transferred power from the women who gathered herbs and brewed beer with it to the emergent institutions of empire. Locally distinctive *gruit* herb and spice mixes became exclusive franchises. In Weinert's analysis, "Uniqueness of flavor was essential for the clergy's ability to enforce their monopoly privilege and extract rents from beer producers and consumers."[75]

Hops (*Humulus lupulus*) was among the herbs used in some *gruits*. It was first referred to as a beer herb in writing in the 1150s by St. Hildegard of Bingen (*Physica Sacra*). Use of hops spread, in part because of the excellent preservative quality of beer brewed with it. And of course, the laws of the Holy Roman Empire did not extend everywhere. The north German Hanseatic cities were not bound by *gruit* regulation. Using new larger copper brewing kettles, brewers in Hamburg successfully scaled up beer production and began exporting beer made with hops. They pioneered the mass production and distant transport of beer.

"At one time the term *beer* referred only to barley drinks to which hops had been added, while ale might be flavored and preserved with any number of other plants," writes ethnobotanist Dale Pendell.[76] By the 1400s, beers brewed exclusively with hops were widely known and beginning to compete with *grut* brewed beer.[77] Hops, the bigger copper kettles, and the international beer trade they facilitated "effectively undermined the existing regulatory regime," concludes Weinert.[78] But another regulatory regime quickly followed. The earliest laws requiring the use of hops (1434) were broader edicts also regulating beer markets with price setting and entry restrictions. "Rather than protecting consumers, the law allowed brewers to collude and charge higher prices at the expense of the consumer."[79]

The *gruits* were controlled by the Holy Roman Empire, and the challenge to the *gruit*-centered regulatory regime coincided with the schism in that empire remembered in history as the Protestant Reformation. Stephen Harrod Buhner offers a compelling interpretation of how the use of botanical additives in beer came to be played out through this schism. "One of the arguments of the Protestants against the Catholic clergy (and indeed, against Catholicism) was their self-indulgence in food, drink, and lavish lifestyle," writes Buhner. "This behavior was felt to be very un-Christlike indeed."[80] According to Buhner, the three herbs at the core of most *gruits*—yarrow, sweet gale, and marsh rosemary—"are highly inebriating and stimulating when used in ale, far out of proportion to their individual effects outside of fermentation."[81] Of the bitter herbs besides hops used as "admixtures in fermented malt beverage," writes Pendell: "Many of them are psychoactive."[82]

In contrast, hops "cause the drinker to become drowsy and they diminish sexual desire," writes Buhner, arguing that hops' ascendancy was encouraged by Protestant judgments about the wild indulgences of the Catholic Church, fueled by aphrodisiac and psychotropic herbs that were commonly found in the church's *gruits*.[83] Hops beer still had alcohol but led to somewhat more subdued behavior and eventual torpor. "The result was, ultimately, the end of a many-thousands-years' tradition of herbal beer making in Europe and the narrowing of beer and ale into one limited expression of beer production—that of hopped ales or what we today call beer."[84]

Cultural revivalists are freeing themselves from the shackles of the hops beer monoculture, by reinventing herbal brews in a spirit of experimentalism and reclaiming our human legacy of alcoholic beverages as manifestations of plants occurring in infinite variety. Adrienne Jonquil, an herbalist and brewer, sent me a bottle of her incredibly delicious yarrow ale. Adrienne had written to me earlier, wondering about "the effects of ale made with plants other than hops to the mind, soul, and body." I think valuable cultural revivalist work asks to be done detailing exactly how fermentation may alter specific actions of various plants. Systematic or not, experiment! Any herb or spice, and for that matter any fruit, edible flower, bark, root, or other plant part that you could add to mead (see chapter 4) or consume in any other way, you can use to flavor grain-based alcoholic beverages.

 ## Distillation

Distillation is a process that concentrates alcohol (or other volatile substances). Only fermentation can create alcohol, and distillation can only concentrate alcohol that has already been fermented. Any type of fermented alcohol may be distilled. The process takes place in an apparatus known as a still. Distillation evaporates and then condenses the fermented alcohol, thanks to the different boiling temperatures of different substances. Alcohol boils at 173°F/78°C, while water, as we all know, boils at 212°F/100°C. So when fermented alcohol—a mixture of alcohol and water—is heated, the vapors contain proportionately more alcohol than the liquid, as does the resulting liquid when the vapors are cooled. With repeated runs through the still, a purer and purer product results.

Home distillation of alcohol is illegal in the United States and much of the rest of the world. The typical explanation for this prohibition is that distillation is potentially dangerous, since highly toxic methanol as well as ethanol concentrates in the distillation process. However, methanol has a lower boiling point than ethanol, so the first concentrated liquid that collects in the still—where methanol is concentrated, known to distillers as the "heads"—is generally discarded. The other explanation for the home distillation ban is that distilled spirits are an important source of tax revenues.

Aside from legal constraints, the other impediment to home distillation is the specialized apparatus required. You can buy a still, although in the United States the federal government's Alcohol and Tobacco Tax and Trade Bureau monitors their sale. I was very impressed by the ingenuity of a group of Bhutanese and Nepali immigrants I met in Oakland, California, who improvised a still from common household items, to carry on their tradition of distilling a liquor called *raksi* from *chang* they fermented from millet. The base of their still was an aluminum steaming pot on a portable burner, filled with the *chang* they were distilling. Into that pot, they suspended a simple ceramic flowerpot, with the drainage hole enlarged, to allow steam evaporating from the *chang* to rise. Then they suspended a small bowl with two handles in the flowerpot, so that steam could rise around it. Finally, they placed a second aluminum steaming pot, this one smaller and filled with cold water, so it fit snugly atop the flowerpot. This caused the steam hitting it to condense, and the condensation dripped into the small bowl suspended beneath it. To seal the crevices where the pots met, they wrapped wet handkerchiefs around them to prevent steam from escaping. We drank the smooth, delicious, and potent *raksi* still warm. (See photos of their still in the color insert.)

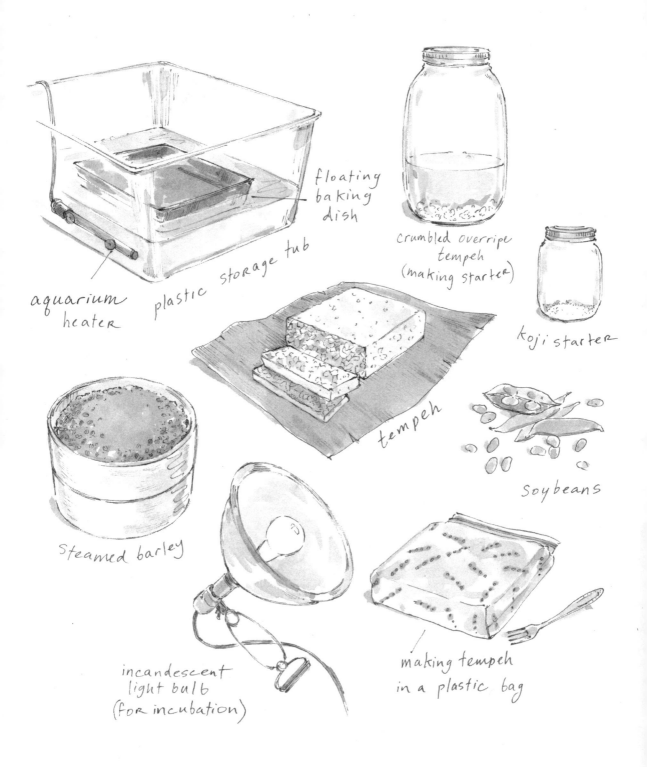

floating
baking
dish

crumbled overripe
tempeh
(making starter)

aquarium
heater

plastic storage tub

koji starter

tempeh

soybeans

Steamed barley

incandescent
light bulb
(for incubation)

making tempeh
in a plastic bag

CHAPTER 10

Growing Mold Cultures

*M*any people are disturbed by the notion of eating molds. Yet microscopic molds are inevitably present on much of our food, and certain molds have long traditions of use by people who grow them on foods as a means of processing. In the West, the most familiar mold ferments are cheeses, though molded cheeses do not seem to hold universal appeal. "Most Westerners still have a deep-seated prejudice against moldy products, and they generally associate the word 'mold' with food spoilage, as in 'moldy bread,'" observe William Shurtleff and Akiko Aoyagi.[1]

In Asia, molds are used much more widely and have greater acceptance. "The word 'mold' there has a rather positive connotation, something like 'yeast' in the West," write Shurtleff and Aoyagi. Mixed cultures including yeasts and bacteria but typically dominated by molds, grown on grains—transliterated from Chinese [麴] as *chhü* (or *qu* or *juiqu* or *da qu*)—have been used in Asia for thousands of years. "There is no exact English equivalent for *qu*," writes H. T. Huang.

> It has been translated variously as barm, leaven, yeast, and starter. None is entirely satisfactory but ferment is probably the best we can do since *chhü* contains both enzymes and live organisms. During incubation the enzymes hydrolyse the starch from the grain, the spores germinate, and the myceliae proliferate to produce more amylases. The yeasts grow in number and ferment the sugars generated *in situ* [in place] to alcohol. The procedure has been called Amylomyces, or simply Amylo process.[2]

Qu and related cultures typically contain some combination of molds (including *Aspergillus, Rhizopus, Mucor,* and/or *Monascus*), along with yeasts and bacteria,[3] traditionally derived from the environment, often via plant material. H. T. Huang points out that the form of *qu* as a solid cake or brick gives rise to different environmental niches in the cake itself that favor different molds. "Conditions in the interior of the cake tend to favour the growth of the *Rhizopus* species, while those on the surface, of the *Aspergillus* species."[4] The differing characteristics of these distinct mold populations were observed and noted long ago. Shurtleff and Aoyagi explain that by the 6th century CE, Chinese documents distinguish between two types of molds: "What we now call *Aspergillus* was then called 'yellow robe' and *Rhizopus* was called 'white robe.' These cultures were carefully distinguished and propagated from year to year."[5] Japanese *koji*, used to make *saké*, miso, soy sauce, and other ferments, consists of various substrates grown with a yellow robe mold, *Aspergillus oryzae*. Javanese tempeh, in contrast, is grown with a white robe mold, *Rhizopus oligosporus*.

From the fermentation of rice- and millet-based alcoholic beverages, *qu* use grew to incorporate wheat and other grains, vegetables, fish, meat, soybeans, and other substrates. "Although the mould ferment was developed originally for making wine, further exploitation of its activities soon paved the way to the production of an array of fermented foods which have helped to shape the character and flavour of the Chinese diet and cuisine," explains Huang.[6] *Qu* use also spread throughout Asia. With the advent of microbiology in the late 19th century, "microbiologists began to take note of the interesting preparations of mixed cultures," isolating individual molds and using them in new ways "the ancient Chinese could not have possibly dreamed of when they discovered a way to prepare a stable culture of grain moulds more than four thousand years ago."[7] In our time, enzymes from *chhü*-derived molds are used extensively in food processing (including the manufacture of high-fructose corn syrup), distilling, biofuels, and many other industries. "The genome sequence of *A. oryzae* has revealed striking mobility," according to the journal *Bioscience, Biotechnology, and Biochemistry*. "It is a treasure house of enzymes and metabolites."[8] According to Steinkraus, "more than 50 different enzymes have been found in *koji*."[9]

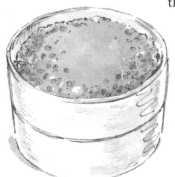

Steamed barley

This treasure house need not be the exclusive domain of professional biotechnologists. Molds can be extremely rewarding to work with, and they are simple and safe to grow at home. The environmental requirements of molds are somewhat different from most other ferments, however. In order to grow, molds need oxygen. This makes them aerobic. Most ferments—yeasts and lactic acid bacteria—are anaerobic; for biologists, this is a defining characteristic of fermentation. Aerobic fermentation is an oxymoron, strictly speaking. Or maybe more accurately a paradox, because *qu*, as well as tempeh, vinegar, kombucha, and countless other aerobic processes, are widely understood to be fermentations.

Molds need oxygen, but not too much of it; moisture, but not too much of it; and heat, but not too much of it. Compared with most other fermentations, they are rather persnickety. The people who discovered these processes long ago "found by chance, conditions favorable for the appropriate fungi to grow," writes C. W. Hesseltine.[10] With some basic insights into these conditions and a little creative ingenuity, anyone can create appropriate incubation conditions in a home kitchen.

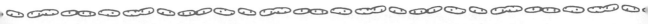

MICROORGANISMS IN MY BED

A poem by qilo, march 2008, urbana

> top drawer ferments
> incubate
> pearl barley
> dusty white.
> sweet earth rot
> under wrap
> in old linens off dinner tables everywhere
> 95 degrees fahrenheit
> constant
>
> soft skin curls around
> terry cloth
> plump heart packed tight
>
> i want rot
> to bloom audibly
> in star flung quiet nights
> eat the past
> digest
> act from now
> backed up by
> bacterial millions.

Incubation Chambers for Growing Molds

The biggest technical challenge to growing *koji*, *tempeh*, *qu*, or other Asian culinary molds—unless you are lucky enough to have a sustained ambient climate of roughly 80–90°F/27–32°C with high humidity—is to simulate those conditions in some sort of incubation chamber. Modestly warm temperatures like this hasten mold growth. Molds also require oxygen, so rather than relying solely on air-movement-blocking insulation to maintain temperatures, as described in chapter 3, it usually works best to incorporate into the incubation chamber greater airflow, along with a low-level heat source. But watch out—if temperatures get much warmer than the target range, the molds can be killed, and *Bacillus subtilis*, the slimy *natto* bacterium (see *Natto* in chapter 11), will typically be ready to develop.

Note that these conditions are required only for *growing* the molds, not for using them. You can use *qu* to make rice beer (see *Asian Rice Brews* in chapter 9), or use *koji* to make miso (see *Miso* in chapter 11), without such exacting requirements. But growing the molds that constitute these starters requires optimal temperature and humidity conditions. The following are several different improvisational incubation methods I have used or encountered.

Oven Method

Kitchen ovens are insulated chambers that can easily be adapted to this use. The oven is designed to maintain temperatures much higher than the mold-growing range, but the chamber itself can also be used to maintain more moderate heat. Most contemporary ovens have an illuminating light that can be switched on. In my oven, simply switching on the light heats the oven to a perfect 90°F/32°C. I use a thermometer in the oven to monitor the temperature and turn off the light or prop the door open a bit to adjust the temperature if it gets too warm.

Gas ovens with pilot lights can also be used as incubation chambers. Do not turn the oven on at all; rather, use the pilot light itself as the source of heat. Typically, with the door closed, an oven with a pilot light will maintain a temperature higher than 90°F/32°C; how high depends on the size of the flame, which can be adjusted easily on most ovens. Well before whatever you are preparing is ready for incubation, place a thermometer inside the oven. The ideal thermometers for this are those with remote readouts—some designed for cooking meat, others for reading outdoor temperatures—because you can read them without having to open the oven door and thereby alter the temperature. Still, you can also make do with whatever thermometer may be at hand.

Place the thermometer inside the closed oven, leave it for at least 15 minutes, and read the temperature. If it's higher than 90°F/32°C, turn down the pilot light if possible; otherwise, prop the oven door open with any small item (I like to use mason jar rings). Leave for another 15 minutes and check the temperature again. If it's still too high, the door needs to be propped open more, using something bigger. If the oven is now too cool (a temperature below 85°F/30°C), it needs less of an opening. Try propping the door with a wooden spoon, or a piece of cardboard. Adjust the oven opening until the temperature is just right and continue to monitor periodically during incubation.

If your oven has neither pilot nor interior light, or the light does not generate sufficient heat, you can place a bare low-wattage incandescent bulb in a simple fixture at the bottom of the oven. Place a ceramic trivet or a pan of water above the lightbulb to diffuse the heat and protect the ferment from a "hot spot" where the mold is killed by excessive heat. Check the temperature after it has heated up for a while, and prop the door open if the temperature climbs beyond the desired range.

With the oven method, the dry heat—whether its source is a pilot light or a lightbulb—can quickly dry out the substrate such that the mold cannot develop. Therefore it is imperative to take measures to prevent the ferment from drying out. The typical improvisation to accomplish this for tempeh is to contain the inoculated beans in a plastic bag dotted with tiny holes. The plastic keeps most of the humidity in, while the holes allow for needed air circulation. This simulates the banana leaves that are traditionally used in Indonesia to contain tempeh. Making *koji*, the grain is typically wrapped in breathable fabric that protects it from drying out quickly. Specific wrappings will be detailed as we cover each ferment.

One final note for incubating in the oven: Cover the oven controls with masking tape or a note, so that you or whomever you live with does not inadvertently turn on the oven and destroy your ferment with high heat.

Aquarium Heater Method

This method requires more in the way of special equipment, but it offers the advantage of being self-regulating. The equipment you need is: (1) a thermostatically controlled aquarium heater with heat settings up to about 88°F/31°C; (2) a hotel pan or other deep (at least 2 inches/5 cm) baking dish that can float in water; and (3) a plastic storage tub with a top, big enough to accommodate the pan, which floats on water inside it.

Fill the storage tub with water to 4 to 6 inches/10 to 15 cm deep. Place the heater at the bottom of the tub and plug into an electrical outlet. Set it at roughly 88°F/31°C. After the water has heated for a while, confirm the temperature with a thermometer and adjust the heater as necessary. Place the pan with inoculated substrate to float in water. The temperature of the water will maintain the temperature of the substrate floating in it. The top of the storage tub should have a towel wrapped around it, to absorb condensation before it drips onto developing mold. The top needs to be placed slightly askew; its presence prevents evaporation, but gaps at the edges guarantee good air circulation, which would be impeded by fitting the top tightly in place. I learned of this method from Santa Cruz, California, tempeh aficionado Manfred Warmuth, who has posted online a PowerPoint presentation on the method.[11]

floating baking dish

plastic storage tub

aquarium heater

Temperature Controller

With a temperature controller (see *Temperature Controllers* in chapter 3), an incandescent lightbulb incubation setup can be self-regulating. Using such a device, I plug the heat-source lightbulb into the temperature controller, set for 87°F/30°C, situated at the top of the incubation chamber. The light stays on until the thermostat reaches the target temperature; then the bulb switches off until the thermostat senses that the temperature has cooled, when it turns on again. A self-regulating system is convenient because it does not require as much monitoring as one that you must manually regulate.

Dedicated Incubator Designs

The incubator I use these days is a defunct commercial refrigerator, equipped with an incandescent lightbulb and a thermostat to regulate it. The only other modifications I made were to drill a few extra holes near the bottom of the fridge to encourage air circulation; the fridge was already vented on top. I have seen similar setups in Styrofoam-insulated boxes and insulated beverage coolers. If you grow large amounts of mold cultures in a small chamber, be sure to monitor it frequently during the second half of its process, when the mold growth begins to produce heat. If not adequately ventilated, heat can accumulate and kill the mold.

Some inventive tempeh makers have solved this problem by expanding their chambers, so the heat produced by a large mass of tempeh can eaily dissipate. Caylan Larson took the aquarium heater incubation system a step further, situating a rack inside a modified indoor greenhouse above the heated water, creating a much larger incubation space. Manfred (who first showed me the aquarium heater incubator design) also uses a thermostat with a space heater and a fan in a closet or bathroom to create a larger incubation chamber. "I can make huge amounts if I set up a rack in the closet," he writes. An Internet search of "tempeh incubator design" will yield many designs, schematic diagrams, and photographs for inspiration.

Bakers with rising or proofing chambers can usually use those. I have also heard of people using heating pads and hot-water bottles as heat sources. Favero Greenforest of Seattle, Washington, writes: "I have a radiant-heated floor which is a perfect place to incubate." No single incubation system or design is the best. They all have advantages and disadvantages. I would encourage experimentalists to work with resources at hand, and refine your system if you find yourself growing mold cultures frequently or in larger quantities.

Making Tempeh

The first mold I learned to make was tempeh (sometimes spelled *tempe*), from the Indonesian island of Java. Tempeh is made by growing molds, predominantly *Rhizopus oligosporus*, usually on soybeans; the mold pre-digests them, binds them together, and greatly reduces required cooking time. Fresh tempeh is truly delicious, vastly superior to what is typically available commercially. Although tempeh is best known as a soybean ferment, it can be made from any combination of legumes and/or grains (and other substrates as well). For years I thought that some legumes were necessary, but my friend and helper Spiky, an irrepressible experimentalist, insisted on trying a batch of all-grain millet oat tempeh, with no legume whatsoever, and it not only worked but was quite delicious, lighter than soy tempeh and almost nutty. I typically make tempeh that is half legumes and half grains.

My longtime familiarity with tempeh is due to its popularity in Western vegetarian subcultures. Forty years ago, in the early 1970s, the hippies at The Farm (a community in Tennessee) were trying to figure out how to feed themselves on a vegan diet. They grew soybeans and set up a soy dairy, making soymilk and tofu. In their quest to learn about how different traditions processed soybeans into food, they heard about tempeh, obtained cultures from the USDA culture collection,[12] and started not only making tempeh, but also writing and teaching about how to make it, producing spores, and retailing the spores with detailed directions. "A great deal of the credit for introducing tempeh to the American public goes to The Farm," write Shurtleff and Aoyagi.[13] And indeed, when I first attempted to make tempeh, the starter I used came from the Tempeh Lab at The Farm.

Tempeh starter is a culture of mold spores, the reproductive agents of fungi, akin to seeds from plants. You can overripen tempeh so that it matures to sporulation and propagate starter (see *Propagating Tempeh Spores*). Or you can purchase tempeh starter, usually in the form of mold spores mixed with a powdered grain substrate. There are a growing number of commercial sources of tempeh starter; those I know of are listed in the appendix.

It is possible to make tempeh without a starter, per se, but from a piece of fresh live tempeh. I emphasize that this method requires tempeh that is fresh, because most commercial tempeh is pasteurized and then often frozen, for greatest stability. But if you can obtain fresh live tempeh, mince it finely and mix about 10 percent mature tempeh into cooked, cooled, dried ingredients. "The mycelium continues its rapid growth without the use of spores," explain Shurtleff and Aoyagi.

> Tempeh made with this starter, however, generally has a slightly weaker mycelium and the incubation time is a little longer than for tempeh made with starter from the sporulation methods. . . . And remember that there are always some unwanted bacteria in the original tempeh. If you are careless and/or if the humidity is high, their numbers will increase with each generation until eventually they prevail, preventing the formation of good tempeh.[14]

Once you have some starter, you need to prepare the beans and/or grains that will serve as the substrate for the mold, which will bind the beans and grains into blocks of tempeh. If you are working with soybeans, the first step is to dehull them. Soybean hulls, like the hulls of some other beans such as chickpeas, are formidable barriers. If the beans remain encased in their thick hulls, the mold we are trying to grow on the beans cannot access their protein-rich flesh. Cracking the beans causes the hulls to fall off the beans. I usually crack the beans dry, before soaking, using a simple hand grinder set with the burrs about ¼ inch/½ cm apart, so that each bean gets broken in two or more pieces, but they do not get crushed into a powder. The traditional method is to pour boiling water over the beans and leave them to soak overnight in the cooling water. Once cool, the hulls fall off with gentle rubbing or kneading.

Generally, people actively seek to remove the fallen soybean hulls—either from the dry beans by shaking cracked beans and blowing away the husks that rise to the top, or by skimming them with a strainer or slotted spoon as they rise to the surface of the water—but this is not a functional necessity. Removed from the beans, the hulls do not impede development of the mold, and they add fiber and bulk to the tempeh.

Traditionally, beans for tempeh are always soaked prior to cooking. Although this step is not absolutely necessary, it is beneficial to the process and to the finished product. Steinkraus writes: "Under natural conditions in the tropics, tempeh production involves two distinct fermentations," the first being a 24-hour soak, which "is bacterial and results in acidification of the beans."[15] This acidification, to the range of pH 4.5 to 5.3, "does not affect the mold growth, but it does prevent the development of undesirable bacteria that might spoil the tempeh." A team of microbiologists studying the possible importance of tempeh soaking observed that previous research has "focused mostly on the stage of fungal fermentation by *Rhizopus oligosporus*," yet the acidifying preliminary fermentation "is emerging as an important event in the control of tempe quality."[16] Another group of researchers concluded that "mainly lactic acid bacteria are responsible for this acidification leading to better growth conditions for the mold and suppression of contamination or toxin production."[17] As in so many ferments, the bacterially produced acids protect against potentially pathogenic bacteria; in this case, even though cooking the beans kills the bacteria themselves, the acids they created continue to create an advantageous selective environment for growth of the desired molds.

In temperate climates, simple soaking will not lead to as rapid acidification as in tropical temperatures. The study quoted above found that sufficient acidic fermentation to lower the pH of the beans to 4.5 took three times as long at 68°F/20°C (36 hours) as it did at 98.6°F/37°C. Most of the Western approaches to making tempeh have substituted vinegar for the traditional pre-fermentation. William Shurtleff and Akiko Aoyagi, in *The Book of Tempeh*, recommend adding vinegar to cooking water (1½ tablespoons/25 ml vinegar to 10 cups/2.5 liters water for 1 pound/500 g beans). The Farm's tempeh recipe eliminates altogether the step of soaking beans and calls instead for acidifying them by adding vinegar (at a proportion of 2 tablespoons of vinegar per pound of dry soybeans) directly to cooked beans immediately prior to inoculation. (If you do that, be sure to distribute vinegar thoroughly before adding starter.) Betty Stechmeyer, cofounder of GEM Cultures decided to leave vinegar out of the process in the directions that accompanied the starter she made and sold. "My experimentation goes back almost 30 years when I was writing my original tempeh-making directions," recounts Betty:

> I was using *The Farm Vegetarian Cookbook* which uses added vinegar on the cooked beans before inoculation. Once I forgot it (the pre-measured vinegar was there on the counter after the tempeh was in the incubator) and found no difference in the tempeh. I repeated with less inoculum and no vinegar, still good.[18]

For years I made tempeh by Betty's method, without soaking or adding vinegar, with fine results. Only after reading Steinkraus's description of tempeh as two distinct fermentations did I realize that soaking could be significant. Sometimes soaking 36 to 48 hours is not a problem. You can also speed the water soak fermentation by doing it in the heat of the incubation chamber and/or by culturing it with sauerkraut juice, sourdough starter, whey, or other live lactic acid bacteria cultures.

A key to making tempeh is *under*cooking the beans. For soybeans, this means boiling them for about 45 minutes, until they are soft enough to bite through, but not as soft as you would want them for eating, when they begin to collapse and lose their shape. If beans are too well cooked, then the space between the beans—where oxygen circulates and the mold can develop—is eliminated. Therefore it is imperative to cook the beans only partially. Most beans require much shorter cooking times than soybeans. Many beans require only 5 to 10 minutes of boiling to prepare for tempeh. Red lentils take barely a minute. Monitor beans closely; drain as soon as they are soft enough to bite through and definitely before they begin to collapse and lose their shape.

Soybeans

Next the beans need to be dried and cooled. Cooked beans are coated with water, and this free water encourages bacterial growth rather than the desired molds. Keith Steinkraus summarizes various traditional methods of drying the beans to remove this excess water:

> The Malaysians surface-dry the beans by rolling them in a piece of cloth prior to inoculation. Some manufacturers also coat the beans with wheat flour, which absorbs any excess moisture. The Indonesians frequently spread the boiled beans on flat, woven bamboo trays. Excess water trickles through the bottom of the tray, and the surfaces of the bean cotyledons become dry as the beans cool.[19]

In *Wild Fermentation*, I recommended drying beans with a towel to absorb surface moisture, what Steinkraus identifies as the Malaysian method, which is fine if you are working at a small scale but becomes more cumbersome as you scale up production. An easier way to dry beans is with a fan. Aim the fan right at the beans, and stir while the fan blows air at the surface. This will dry and cool beans quickly.

One of the reasons that I have come to usually make mixed grain and bean tempeh is that by cooking the grain dry (using just one volume of water to each volume of grain) I can use the grain to dry the beans. To do this, add the cooked dry grains to the cooked beans and stir to mix thoroughly while everything is still piping hot. The surface moisture on the beans will absorb into the still-thirsty grains. I also often add a little seaweed, snipped with scissors into small dry strips that also absorb water from the beans.

It is essential that the tempeh mix be no warmer than body temperature when you culture, or heat may kill your starter. A fan, used in conjunction with stirring, will greatly speed cooling. So will spreading the beans and/or grains to expose more surface area. Once the mix reaches body temperature, add your starter. The amount of starter you need varies with the source of the starter. Most commercial sources recommend 1 teaspoon/5 ml of starter per pound (dry weight) of beans and/or grains, but if the source you use recommends a different proportion, follow that. If you use live tempeh rather than spores as a starter, use starter at a proportion of roughly 15 percent of substrate.

Stir starter in thoroughly. Be sure as you stir to scrape the edges of the bowl and mix everything together. I like to rotate the bowl with my left hand as I stir with my right hand. If you are low on starter you can compensate by putting extra time into stirring and maximizing beans and grain surfaces coming into contact with the starter. Don't mix so much that the beans overcool; they should still feel warm when you wrap them for incubation.

Once the starter is thoroughly mixed into the substrate, it is time to transfer it into wrappings that will contain the developing tempeh. Banana and other large leaves are the traditional wrappings in Java. If you have access to banana trees, or other large edible leaves, try making some tempeh in them. Gently fold leaves around the tempeh mix and secure with twine. Plastic bags perforated with tiny holes are the typical wrappings in tempeh production in the West. Use a needle, an ice pick, or a fork to make small holes every inch or so. If you make tempeh frequently, you may prefer to use Tupperware or other plastic food containers as tempeh forms by poking holes in them. I also frequently incubate tempeh in stainless-steel trays (sometimes trays with holes in the bottoms and sides), with the tops of the trays covered with perforated aluminum foil, waxed paper, or plastic wrap. People can be quite creative with tempeh forms. In his high-humidity incubator, Caylan made a gorgeous batch of tempeh in a basket. (See photo in the color insert.)

making tempeh in a plastic bag

SCULPTING WITH TEMPEH

Betty Stechmeyer

You can take young squares (¾-inch sandwich bag size) of tempeh, unwrap, slice, and build, Lincoln-log-style, with the slices. Return to the incubator and the overlap area will bind the basket or house together. I "built" a turkey once. You can also incubate the inoculated tempeh and stir it periodically to keep the mycelium from binding. At around 16 hours you can make forms from the loose fuzzy beans, such as a "bird's nest" in a bowl, or a protein pie shell, by lining a pie plate with partially done beans, with the next size smaller to press a form. The partially done tempeh also makes a good substrate to mix in robust seasonings that would otherwise inhibit mold growth, such as chorizo seasoning.

Incubation needs to be closely monitored. In the early period, the *Rhizopus* mold gains a strong competitive advantage over fungal and bacterial competitors from a relatively warm environment, and in fact has been shown to grow fastest at body temperature, 98.6°F/37°C.[20] It's good to encourage rapid mold growth because the mold creates substances that protect it against certain bacteria, specifically "gram-positive" and "anaerobic spore-formers," state Hesseltine and Wang.[21] But once the mold is vigorously growing, after about 8 to 14 hours (depending upon temperature), it begins to generate significant heat, and the potential exists for heat to accumulate to the point where it kills the mold (above body temperature). Therefore, tempeh is typically incubated at more moderate temperatures of 80–90°F/27–32°C. The fact that molds generate heat midway through their incubation is a critical concept for understanding the dynamics of growing mold cultures. It is helpful to monitor incubator heat at frequent intervals through the incubation period in order to make adjustments, such as propping the door open, turning off the heat source, or manually fanning, in order to avoid overheating.

Like most ferments, there is no objective moment when the fermentation is complete. Tempeh has been formed once the mycelium growth is dense enough to hold the beans and/or grains together in a cohesive mat. Fresh tempeh has a yeasty or slightly mushroomy aroma and flavor. Typically it is considered ripe when the first signs of sporulation—dark patches—begin to appear. In perforated containers, sporulation begins at the perforations, where airflow is greatest and the surface becomes driest. As sporulation proceeds, the tempeh develops a stronger aroma and flavor, tinged with ammonia, like a ripe cheese. The Javanese consider tempeh at various stages of sporulation to be distinct delicacies, and savor them. My French friend Luca loves to eat overripe tempeh raw; he says it reminds him of Camembert cheese.

At ambient temperatures, and even in the refrigerator, tempeh can continue to ferment, darkening with sporulation and developing an intensifying ammonia aroma and flavor. Traditionally, tempeh is eaten and sold fresh, and considered highly perishable. In other words, this ferment is definitely not a strategy for preservation. Much of the tempeh produced for resale in the West is frozen, and in many cases pasteurized by steaming prior to freezing. In my own practice, I always eat some tempeh fresh, as soon as I remove it from the incubation chamber. Then I store in the fridge only as much as I think will be eaten within a few days, taking care to not stack the tempeh (as that enables the mold to continue growing in the center of the stack where heat is retained) but rather spreading them around the refrigerator with maximum surfaces exposed to cool air. To store it beyond a few days, I freeze the remainder of each batch, again taking care to spread out rather than stack the tempeh pieces. Once the tempeh is frozen, it can be stacked for space-efficient storage. Well-wrapped tempeh can be stored in a freezer for at least six months.

Cooking with Tempeh

Many people have no idea what to do with tempeh. In Indonesia, it is typically cut into thin strips and fried, cubed and and incorporated into coconut milk curry stews, or barbecued in sweet sauces. Often the strips are soaked before frying, in a simple saltwater brine, sometimes spiced, sometimes with tamarind, or in other marinades. Some people like to steam the tempeh prior to marinating and frying, to make sure the tempeh cooks thoroughly. (I usually do not.)

I very much enjoy tempeh marinated in sweet-sour-salty sauces, mixing honey or another sweetener, vinegar and/or sauerkraut juice, miso and/or tamari, and sometimes hot sauce. I learned a new tempeh marinade I love from Ken Albala's *Beans: A History*. Mix salt, garlic, and coriander seeds and pound together into a paste in a mortar. Mix with water and marinate slices of tempeh in it. I usually fry tempeh in coconut oil or butter, though the one time I fried it in schmaltz (chicken fat) and called it chicken-fried tempeh it was a big hit. If I'm cooking tempeh for a crowd, I'll often marinate blocks of tempeh, oven-fry the whole blocks, and then slice after cooking, to make life easier.

As described earlier, when I've had batches of tempeh that don't bind well, usually due to overheating, I like to crumble it into chili or sloppy-joe-type concoctions. William Shurtleff and Akiko Aoyagi's *The Book of Tempeh*, the definitive English-language book on tempeh, is filled with recipes; vegetarian cookbooks and the Internet are other great sources.

ODE TO TEMPEH

Spiky

Tempeh, like a homegrown tomato, resembles its bland supermarket cousin in name only. Homemade, it is sublime. Freshly incubating tempeh fills the kitchen with its warm aroma, like bread baking in an oven. A hungry crowd will gather, salivating, waiting for it to be sliced up and served.

I love tempeh. When I am packaging up new tempeh for my friends, I sing the John Lennon song "Beautiful Boy," but I sing "tempeh" in the chorus instead of "boy." Tempeh seduces me and it always satisfies, no matter how it's cooked. My love affair with tempeh has, alas, left me equivocal about tofu, as if tofu were a regrettable high school crush I'd prefer to leave behind. Tempeh is so good that I crave it, I make gigantic batches of it, I want it for breakfast, lunch, and dinner. A kitchen with fresh tempeh is truly a blessed kitchen.

When Sandor and I started making tempeh together a few winters ago, we were experimenting with a new incubator, and thus making large batches on a regular basis. The resulting abundance allowed us, and our fellow cooks at Short Mountain, freedom to experiment. It being winter, I was cooking warm, thick, starchy foods, and I noticed that tempeh made a great companion to the meals I was already preparing. I laid butter-fried tempeh between my hash browns and runny eggs at breakfast. For lunch, I'd hash up some crumbly tempeh, spritz it with tamari, and sprinkle it inside a quesadilla. Potatoes brought out tempeh's nuttiness and sweet potatoes highlighted its savoriness. Creamy mashed potatoes were infinitely improved with tempeh mixed in, or laid on top; a slice of tempeh could be lowered into the buttery yawn of a baked sweet potato.

In Indonesian cuisine, tempeh is often fried or deep-fried, or simmered in a soup, with companions like hot peppers, coconut milk, lemongrass, and tamarind. Almost always it accompanies rice. One preparation calls for steaming mashed-up tempeh and coconut in banana leaves. Another marinates the tempeh overnight in a sweet sauce, then grills it in chunks on a shish kebab. Here in Tennessee, tempeh complements the full spectrum of our summer garden: yellow squash, green beans, basil, tomatoes, peppers, cabbage. I like to throw our summer harvest into a wok and stir-fry it with tempeh, coconut milk, and green curry paste.

In some vegetarian cookbooks, you'll find tempeh doctored up to replace bacon or steak. That is all well and good if you pine for meat, but homemade tempeh is so superb, so magnificent a food, so rich with its own flavors, that there is no reason to mock it up like something else. Liberate yourself from meat mockery. Experiment. Throw it into the mix of whatever you're already cooking.

Propagating Tempeh Spores

There are many different ways of propagating tempeh spores. As with all things tempeh, William Shurtleff and Akiko Aoyagi's books have the most comprehensive information on propagating tempeh.[22] In Indonesia, some tempeh is typically grown sandwiched between leaves of *waru* hibiscus trees (*Hibiscus tiliaceus Linn*). This tempeh is allowed to overripen, and the spores become bound in the hairy leaves, which are dried and used by mixing dehulled, cooked, and cooled beans by hand, holding a leaf, spore side out, in one hand. Any overripened sporulating tempeh can be used as a starter. But the more meticulous you can be, the purer the progeny. In the traditional context of mixed cultures, this wasn't an issue at all, because the tempeh community of fungi and bacteria had stability. "In Indonesia, good-quality mixed culture starter is prepared daily in thousands of neighborhood tempeh shops under extremely unsanitary conditions," point out Shurtleff and Aoyagi.[23] In the context of pure culture tempeh, which is what most of us outside of Indonesia know, each generation presents the possibility of contamination by bacteria and weakening of the mold. To maintain a pure culture requires scrupulous and methodical effort.

To be perfectly honest, I have had limited success in propagating tempeh starter. I have made a few good batches, using methods described here. But more often, after a few days of incubation, other molds have started developing, especially sweet-smelling yellow *Aspergillus* molds, which I have grown a lot in the same incubation space. Pure cultures are a challenge for a multi-cultural generalist.

Sporulation, the reproductive phase of mold growth, occurs after mycelial growth. In tempeh, sporulation is marked by darkening color. As discussed, the dark patches that often develop on tempeh near airholes are signs of first sporulation. Higher oxygenation and drier conditions both promote sporulation.

The easiest way to obtain spores is simply to overripen a batch of tempeh. To maximize spore production, expose as much surface area as possible. I do this by slicing myceliated bound tempeh into thin slices and leaving them in the incubator. Once they are bound, you can leave them with greater air exposure, thus encouraging both sporulation and drying. You can simply grind up your sporulated tempeh to use as starter, but then your next batch will have old, overripe soybean pieces mixed in with the fresh substrate, creating the potential for off flavors.

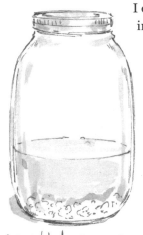

crumbled overripe tempeh (making starter)

The simplest way to extract spores from overripened tempeh is in water. Use non- or dechlorinated water. Crumble the sporulated tempeh into a jar, and cover with water. Seal the jar and shake hard for a minute or two; the water will turn black as spores release into it. After this vigorous shaking, strain out solids and discard them. Leave the dark spore-water still for about 15 minutes. The spores will sink to the bottom, appearing as a black sludge. Gently pour off the cloudy water, leaving just this sludge. This sludge is your new starter. The drawback of this method is that because the spores are wet, they are less stable than if dry, so you must use them within a few days. For longer storage, freeze the sporulated tempeh pieces and extract spores into water as needed.

The *best* way to produce a quantity of tempeh spores is to grow them on a substrate of rice, cooked on the dry side, with less water than rice (by volume): so it won't clump; so it can be effectively ground to a powder rather than a pulp; and so it will be more stable for storage. You get much less random bacterial presence in your starter if you sterilize your rice by steaming it under pressure. Random bacteria are not an issue when you make a batch of tempeh from starter, but if that level of contamination is perpetuated in successive generations, before too long the *Rhizopus* mold you are wishing to grow may no longer be dominant. For home or cottage industry production, scrupulous cleanliness and pressure-cooking the rice are adequate for making tempeh starter. Producing starter for broader distribution requires a higher level of protection—for instance, inoculating the rice inside a protected chamber—and microscopic inspection of each batch for quality control. These various levels of protection against contamination are thoroughly described in Shurtleff and Aoyagi's *Tempeh Production*. Here I will describe a method that has worked (with only moderate success) in my own modest-scale production.

The method in a nutshell is: (1) Soak rice in mason jars; (2) pressure-steam the rice, right in the jars, covered with a coffee filter secured by a jar ring or rubber band; (3) allow to cool slowly to body temperature; (4) inoculate the rice with starter; (5) incubate four to seven days, monitoring the temperature and shaking a couple of times a day to prevent clumping; and (6) grind into a powder in a blender that the mason jars can screw directly onto, or in a mortar with a pestle.

Most of the literature recommends using white rice for making tempeh starter. I cannot find any discussion of why white rice is typically used rather than brown. I assume it is because the mold grows more quickly on white rice, since protective outer membranes have been removed. Betty Stechmeyer recalls seeing a scanning electron microscopic image of brown rice grains showing "deeply convoluted surfaces. I imagine these grooves could harbor resistant bacterial and fungal spores leading to starter contamination." Nonetheless, in my own experiments I have had better results with brown rice, because white rice has a greater propensity for clumping, which makes it difficult to grow the mold to sporulation on each individual grain. If you follow the conventional wisdom and use white rice, definitely stay away from rice coated with talc (magnesium silicate); before you start, rinse the rice well, until the rinse water runs clear, to remove powdered starch from the surface.

The scientists at the US Department of Agriculture's Northern Regional Research Laboratory conducted experiments to determine viable spore counts of *Rhizopus* grown on different substrates at various moisture levels. This research determined that *Rhizopus* grown on rice produces higher spore counts than when grown on wheat, wheat bran, or soybeans. It also determined that with (white) rice, the highest spore production occurred if the substrate was prepared at a ratio of 10 parts rice to 6 parts water.[24] Shurtleff and Aoyagi report in *Tempeh Production* that a tempeh maker did further experiments and found that 10 parts rice to 5 parts water "gave more abundant sporulation and, more important, easier pulverization in a blender with less drying."[25] In terms of brown rice, Shurtleff and Aoyagi report that Australian investigator John McComb "found that whole brown rice worked better than white rice" and that it worked best "using 10 parts by weight of brown rice to 8 parts water."[26]

What these proportions translate to, in practical terms, is that ¼ cup/0.1 pound/50 g of rice (the quantity appropriate for a pint/16-ounce/500 ml jar) requires just under 3 tablespoons/40 ml of water for brown rice, or just under 2 tablespoons/25 ml for white rice. Note that at these proportions, the jar is mostly empty. This is necessary to be able to spread the rice in a fairly thin layer when the jar is laid on its side, so maximum surface area is exposed, encouraging maximum sporulation. If your pressure cooker is large enough to accommodate quart/liter jars elevated above the bottom of the pot, you can use those larger jars and double the quantity of all ingredients in each jar. I always do several jars at once.

Working with brown rice, soak the rice overnight directly in the jar with the recommended quantity of water. With white rice, rinse the rice well first, drain, then soak for just about an hour, shaking periodically. Cover the jar with a coffee filter and secure with a screw-on ring, or alternatively a rubber band or string. Add a couple of inches of water to the pressure cooker, then improvise a rack to hold the jars above the water. Steam under pressure (approximately 15 pounds/100 kPa if your pressure cooker has a gauge). For brown rice, maintain the pressure for 40 minutes; for white rice 20 minutes will suffice. After you remove the pressure cooker from the heat, leave it sealed and allow the pressure and temperature to reduce slowly.

Once it has depressurized and cooled to body temperature, open the pressure cooker, remove the jars, and shake them vigorously to break up any clumps of rice. If the clumps will not break up from shaking, use a spoon or other implement—sterilized in boiling water—to reach into the jar and break up clumps as best you can. When the rice reaches body temperature, inoculate with starter, again using a sterilized implement. For ¼ cup of rice, ⅛ teaspoon starter is sufficient; use ¼ teaspoon for ½ cup rice. Secure a coffee filter over the mouth of the jar, shake it in different directions to spread the starter in the rice, and lay the jars on their sides in the incubation chamber.

Incubate as for tempeh in the range of 80–90°F/27–32°C. Instead of just 24 hours, as for typical tempeh, however, the starter requires several days of incubation—as long as seven days with brown rice—to fully sporulate. Shake a few times each day to break up clumps. Once sporulated, grind rice using a blender, coffee grinder, or mortar and pestle. Whichever tool you use, sterilize it with boiling water, then allow it to dry and cool, to minimize contamination of your starter. Use starter at a proportion of approximately 1 teaspoon for each pound/500 g of dry beans or grains you make into tempeh.

With one exception, I have always worked with powdered tempeh starters commercially available in the United States (see *Resources*), all derived from spores of *Rhizopus oligosporus* from the USDA's Culture Collection, where it is listed as strain NRRL 2710, *Rhizopus oligosporus* Saito, with Keith Steinkraus credited as its source. Saito is the surname of the Japanese microbiologist who in 1905 first isolated *Rhizopus oligosporus* as the primary tempeh mold and named it.

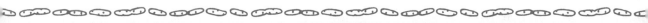

TEMPEH VARIATIONS

CHICKPEA TEMPEH
Lagusta Yearwood, New Paltz, New York

Chickpea tempeh is 100 percent chickpeas, you can get a batch in the incubator in under 2 hours because the chickpeas cook so fast, and it tastes so mellow—perfect for people who don't usually like tempeh.

FAVA BEAN TEMPEH
Greg Barker, Berkeley, California

An ingredient I really love and highly recommend for tempeh is hulled, dried fava beans. The flavor of favas is great. They compress down into an arrangement that makes for a good fungal mat. But the key is the time savings. I never had a mill/grinder or any way of getting the hulls off my soybeans. The hulled favas solve that (and they cook really quickly, too), making the transition from soaked beans to inoculated cakes brief and only 15 minutes of labor.

DRY-ROASTED SOYBEANS FOR TEMPEH
Betsy Shipley used to make tempeh commercially, then retired and posted this and many other innovative tempeh-making ideas online.[27]

The easiest way to make our tempeh is to start with dry-roasted, non-GMO or organic soybean halves (unsalted). This saves you all the work involved in dehulling and cooking regular soybeans. Pour 24 oz. of soybean halves into boiling water, remove from heat, and let them sit for 24–48 hrs. The beans will expand to twice the size—so use enough water. . . . After presoaking the soybean halves, drain and refill with clean water, about an inch higher than the beans, and bring to a boil.

The one exception was tempeh starter gifted to me some years ago by a fellow tempeh lover who had brought starter with him from Indonesia. This starter was a fine yellow powder, very different in appearance from the gray-black NRRL 2710 strain. The tempeh it made was also distinctive—sweeter and somehow more complex. I'm guessing the yellow starter was a more diverse mold mixture, incorporating *Aspergillus* as well as *Rhizopus* molds. After all, all traditional ferments are mixed cultures. I have read of other tempeh-like foods in which still other molds have been identified, such as Chinese *meitauza*, in which the substrate is the residual soybean solids (*okara*) from tofu manufacturing and the mold that has been isolated is *Actinomucor elegans*.[28]

The isolated pure cultures that microbiology has facilitated are not what people have traditionally used. Traditional ferments are *all* mixed-culture mutts, manifesting in varied and sometimes shifting forms. It's very exciting to see, taste, and work with different mixes. I welcome and encourage the informal spread of traditional cultures, as possible; unfortunately, casual importation of cultures is difficult and technically illegal, in the name of public health and safety. Perhaps someone will do whatever paperwork is required to start importing other tempeh strains. In the meantime, work with what is available, which makes wonderful tempeh.

Making *Koji*

The other mold fermentation I have a lot of experience with is *koji*, the Japanese manifestation of *qu*, also traditionally a mixed culture but today typically grown as a single strain of fungus, *Aspergillus oryzae*. Before I started growing *koji*, I would never have believed it possible to fall in love with a mold. But I have been seduced by fresh *koji*'s sweet fragrance, as rapid mycelial growth generates heat from enzyme digestion of complex carbohydrates. I am not alone in my passion for this mold. Missouri fermentation enthusiast Alyson Ewald writes: "I wish I had known that the aroma of rice inoculated with *koji* mold would put me under a spell from which I would never free myself and never wish to." Washington fermenter Favero Greenforest gushes: "The *koji* smelled so wonderful I just want to roll around in it. Few things have a more delicious fragrance." You'll never know what we're all so excited about unless you grow some *koji* yourself.

Koji itself is generally not eaten as a food (although it is delicious). *Koji* is the first step toward many elaborately processed foods and beverages. I have used *koji* to make miso, soy sauce, *amazaké*, *saké*, and pickles. At the point when I wrote *Wild Fermentation*, and until about 2005, I had only used *koji* obtained from others, first the American Miso Company and later South River Miso Company. *Koji* is not cheap, especially when I got to making 20 gallons/ 75 liters of miso (or more) a year. I knew spores of *Aspergillus oryzae* were readily available, but frankly, I was intimidated about maintaining incubation for as long as 48 hours. (Needlessly, as it turns out.)

Generally, to make *koji* you need a starter. At the end of this section I will describe how I was able to make *koji* from organisms spontaneously present on the husks of fresh corn, but I would certainly encourage you to try it at least once using a starter culture so you can experience the unique aroma of fresh growing *koji*, because recognizing that distinctive smell is the most straightforward way you have to gauge whether you have the right mold growing if you try starting *koji* spontaneously using corn husks.

The source I have used for *koji* starter is GEM Cultures,[29] which sells several different *koji* starters, for different substrates and, in the case of rice, different end products. Don't be overwhelmed by the choices. Just pick one to start with; later you can experiment with others. My favorite is barley *koji*, which I've used in miso, *amazaké*, and pickles, but the process I'll describe is similar no matter the substrate on which you grow the *koji*.

The basic process for *koji* is soak, steam, cool, inoculate, and incubate. The incubation is generally 36 to 48 hours. Soak the pearled barley overnight. Steam until cooked, about two hours; I use stacking Chinese bamboo steamers, lined with a cotton cloth to keep the grains from falling through the bottoms. The barley steams into a sticky mass. Release the steamed barley from the steamer into a big bowl or pot. Break up the clumps and allow the barley to cool to body temperature.

Meanwhile, heat an incubator to the 80–95°F/27–35°C temperature range. Line a baking pan or other wide, open vessel with a clean unscented cotton sheet or other smooth cloth, folded in a couple of layers. Once the barley approaches body temperature, inoculate it with starter (at whatever proportion is recommended by your source) and stir thoroughly. Place inoculated barley into the cloth, arranging it as a mound in the center. Put a thermometer into the center of the mound, and fold the sheet over the mound and around the thermometer, so you have a fabric-wrapped mound with a thermometer sticking out. Place the mound into the incubator and maintain the temperature in the range of 80–95°F/27–35°C. "In general, the higher the temperature of cultivation of the mold, the greater the amylolytic activity" (which converts starch to sugars), according to Keith Steinkraus. "Lower temperatures of incubation favor development of proteases," which digest proteins.[30] This suggests aiming for incubation temperatures at the top of the range for *amazaké* or rice beverages, and lower temperatures for *koji* for miso or *shoyu* production.

Monitor temperature periodically, and after about 16 hours start peeking at the barley. By about 24 hours, you should find that the barley has a sweet fragrance, appears dusted with a chalky white mold growth, and is starting to clump together. Once these developments have occurred, the mold begins to generate heat, and your objective switches from keeping it warm enough to preventing it from overheating. Spread the mound of barley out into an even layer no more than 2 inches/5 cm thick. This is important because if the *koji* mat is too thick, heat can accumulate in the center and kill the mold. If the pan holding your *koji* is too small, use a cookie sheet, or divide it into two baking pans. Improvise as necessary. To further modulate temperature, run your fingers over the *koji* like a rake and leave it with furrows, which increase surface area for releasing heat. Cover the *koji* with a cloth and return to the incubator.

Keep checking the *koji* every few hours. Stick your (clean!) hands right into it, find clumps and break them up, spread out barley from hot spots, relevel, refurrow, rewrap, and return to incubator. Enjoy the seductive aroma of the developing *koji* as you work with it. As *koji* develops, the white mold growth will increase and cover each grain. You can use your *koji* once grains appear to be covered with mold growth; definitely stop incubating *koji* if you begin to notice yellow-green patches on the surface, indicating that sporulation has begun. You can add fresh warm *koji* directly into your miso, *amazaké*, or *saké* project. Whatever you are not using right away, spread out in a thin layer to cool to room temperature, then wrap and refrigerate. For longer storage, dry *koji* briefly in the sun or a dehydrator before storing.

To grow *koji* on rice, at present GEM sells two different strains, which confuses some people. Their "light" rice *koji* is for making *amazaké*, *saké*, pickles, or some kinds of miso. Their "red" rice *koji*—not to be confused with Chinese red rice mold (*ang-kak*), similar to *koji* but with another mold, *Monascus purpureus*—is used for "red" misos. GEM's directions for both recommend using polished rice, which is white rice. I've also had fine results using brown rice. If you use white rice, be sure to avoid rice with talc added; and rinse the rice well to remove loose surface starch. In addition, after soaking and before steaming, let the rice drain in the colander for several minutes. The less surface water remains, the less the grains of rice will fuse together during cooking. You can even drain directly onto an absorbent towel for a few more minutes, or aim a fan at the rice and stir. "The added drying will aid in keeping the cooked rice lump-free," explains Betty Stechmeyer, whose step-by-step instructions that come with all the GEM cultures are clear and detailed. Brown rice does not fuse together like white rice does, so no need to be quite so meticulous.

Growing *koji* on soybeans is essentially the same as for barley. Steaming takes much longer, as long as six hours if not under pressure. Use a pressure cooker to steam soybeans, if you can, because it only requires about an hour and a half. Soybeans should be soft enough to easily crush between your fingers. Temperatures need to be monitored very carefully during fermentation, because the soybeans' high protein content makes them highly susceptible to *Bacillus subtilis* at temperatures above 95°F/35°C. The mold does not smell quite as sweet with soybeans. But it is still a pleasant aroma, especially when it's incubated with roasted wheat for *shoyu* (see *Soy Sauce* in chapter 11).

To propagate *koji* starter, or *tane koji*, literally "seed *koji*," use brown rice. "White rice is not used in making starter since it lacks the necessary nutrients to support optimal growth of the molds," explain Shurtleff and Aoyagi.[31] Soak rice, drain well, steam, and cool, as described earlier. When rice has cooled to body temperature, before inoculating, mix in sifted hardwood ashes, about 1.5 percent by weight of the quantity of dry rice you cooked. The ash provides potassium, magnesium, and other trace elements that promote healthy mold growth and sporulation. Inoculate with starter and incubate at a slightly cooler temperature than is typically used for growing *koji*, about 79°F/26°C. Mound the rice for the first 24 hours, then mix it and remound for another 24 hours. After about 48 hours, spread into an even layer wrapped in cotton, as described earlier. Leave the *koji* undisturbed, incubating at about 79°F/26°C, for another 48 hours. By now the *koji* should be covered with olive-green growth. Break up clumps and dry in the oven with the pilot or dehydrator at around 113°F/45°C. Store dry starter in a refrigerator or other cool, dark spot. Starter may be used as whole grains, or ground into meal; spores can also be extracted from grains by sifting, then mixing with flour. This process for making *koji* starter comes from Shurtleff and Aoyagi's book *Miso Production*, which devotes a chapter to the topic and explains it in considerably more detail.[32]

Amazaké

Amazaké is a Japanese sweet rice porridge, pudding, or beverage, made by fermenting rice (or other grains) with *koji*. *Amazaké* is essentially the first step of making *saké* or other rice-based alcoholic beverages. Shurtleff and Aoyagi translate *amazaké* as "sweet *saké*,"[33] and Elizabeth Andoh reports that it is also known as *hitoya-zaké*, or "one-night rice wine."[34]

I include *amazaké* here, rather than in the grain chapter, to draw attention to an important concept with *koji*, which is that it is typically used in ferments as a source of enzymes, rather than for the continued mycelial growth of the mold itself. As we have just seen, growing molds requires oxygen and is temperature-sensitive, with the mold prone to dying off at prolonged exposure to temperatures much above body temperature. The enzymes the mold produces, however, do not share the same environmental requirements. These enzymes do not require oxygen, and some actually work most efficiently at higher temperatures.

Amazaké uses the same ingredients as *koji*, almost exactly. They both are rice (or another grain) cooked and then inoculated with the mold *Aspergillus oryzae*. The only differences are the phase of life of the *A. oryzae* introduced, and how the environment is maintained. Making *koji*, you add the mold in its spore stage, and encourage it with moist but not wet conditions, moderately warm temperatures, and limited air circulation. To make *amazaké*, you use a mold that already has grown, mix it with freshly cooked rice that can be still quite hot (140°F/60°C) in a jar or crock, and try to keep it as warm as possible. With a good proportion of fresh *koji* and warm temperatures, the *koji* enzymes are vigorously active.

I was first introduced to making *amazaké* by Aveline Kushi, the wife of macrobiotics popularizer Michio Kushi, whose *Complete Guide to Macrobiotic Cooking* has a number of ferments in it and guided some of my earliest experiments. Kushi recommends ½ cup/125 ml of *koji* for 4 cups/1 liter (uncooked) rice, and for years I made occasional *amazaké*, which I liked, following these proportions. She recommends using sweet brown rice, overnight soaking, and pressure-cooking without salt.

> When cool enough to handle, mix the *koji* into the rice with your hands. Then transfer the mixture to a glass bowl (do not use metal), cover with a wet cloth or towel, and place near an oven, radiator, or any other warm place. Allow to ferment 4–8 hours. During the fermentation period, occasionally stir the mixture to melt the *koji*. After fermenting, put the amasaké in a pot and bring to a boil. When bubbles appear, turn off the heat.[35]

The proportions of *koji* to rice recommended by different sources vary dramatically. Kushi uses ½ cup *koji* for 4 cups (uncooked rice), a 1:8 ratio, while Shurtleff and Aoyagi suggest 2 cups of *koji* for each cup of rice (2:1),[36] as does Bill Mollison in his *Ferment and Human Nutrition*.[37]

Finally, after years of fretting about what proportions to use, I conducted a controlled experiment, with the help of intern Malory Foster. We cooked 6 cups of rice and placed equal portions of it in each of six jars. In two of the jars we mixed 2 cups of *koji* (2:1); in two of them 1 cup *koji* (1:1); and in two of them ½ cup *koji* (1:2). We took one jar of each proportion and incubated it at 90°F/32°C; the other jar of each proportion we incubated at about 140°F/60°C.

All the jars developed *amazaké*, but at very different rates. After 12 hours, all the jars incubated at 140°F/60°C were sweet. The 2:1 batch was vigorously bubbly, almost completely liquefied, and extremely sweet; the 1:1 batch was sweet and liquefied, but somewhat less so; and the 1:2 batch was still sweet and liquefied, only even less so. The jars incubated at 90°F/32°C, even at 2:1, were barely sweet.

After 15 hours, the 1:1 batch at 140°F/60°C was fully sweetened and liquefied, the 1:2 batch was "sweeter but still not there," and the jars incubating at the lower temperature were still barely sweet. At 21 hours, we judged all the warmer-incubation jars ready. Of the 90°F/32°C incubation batches, the 2:1 and 1:1 batches were good and sweet, with most of the rice liquefied, while the 1:2 batch was just starting to get sweet and its rice was still intact. The following day, that final batch had begun to sour.

The lesson of this exercise for me was that incubation temperature is more important than proportion of *koji*, but that more *koji* enables the process to go faster. This makes sense, because enzymes render their transformations repeatedly if not destroyed by excessive heat. If the process is too slow, through a combination of low incubation temperature and/or low proportion of *koji*, then maximum sweetness is never achieved, because souring begins before all the starch is converted to sugars. If you have enough *koji* to make *amazaké* at a 2:1 ratio, I would certainly recommend that. If *koji* is scarce and you wish to use it at lower proportions, then be sure to incubate as close as possible to 140°F/60°C.

When you judge your *amazaké* to be ready, stop fermentation or it will continue to ferment into acids and alcohol. (If you wish to ferment it into alcohol, see *Saké* in chapter 9.) Bring to a boil with a little water and a pinch of salt. Store *amazaké* in the refrigerator. To use as a beverage, add 1 part *amazaké* to 1 part water. Add ginger or other flavorings. Eric Haas recommends adding *saké* and/or *saké* lees to *amazaké*; "simmered for a little while, they make a great combination." Undiluted, enjoy *amazaké* as a pudding, or as a sweetener in baking. Shurtleff and Aoyagi recommend substituting 3½ units of *amazaké* for 2 units of sugar or 1 unit of honey.

Plant Sources of Mold Cultures

Obviously, people have not always had pure-culture spore powders available to them as starters. These traditional Asian mold cultures, like virtually all cultures used in fermentation, have their sources in plants. "Quality alcoholic beverages produced by the traditional indigenous flora will probably never be equalled by the use of pure cultures," write Xu Gan Rong and Bao Tong Fa of Jiangnan University in China, in their *Grandiose Survey of Chinese Alcoholic Drinks and Beverages*.[38] Botanical ingredients are used not exclusively to start the fermentation, but also to impart flavors and additional intoxicating qualities.

H. T. Huang includes several methods for making *qu* from ancient Chinese documents in his history of Chinese fermentation. From the *Qi Min Yao Shu*, or "Important Arts for the People's Welfare," written by Jia Sixie in the year 544, Huang translates the following description for "preparation of *Qin zhou* common ferment from wheat" using leaves of "artemesia," which could be mugwort, wormwood, or some other member of that large botanical genus:

> The process should start in the seventh moon [usually August]. . . . Take good, clean wheat free from insects and stir-roast it in a large pot. . . . The fire should be slow as the wheat is stirred rapidly with a rocking motion. The stirring should not be stopped even for a moment. Otherwise the grains will not be cooked evenly. The wheat is roasted until it turns yellow and has a fragrant smell; it should not be singed. When done, it is winnowed, and any extraneous matter removed. The wheat is then ground but not too fine or too coarse. . . . A few days before the start of the process, Artemisia plants are collected and cleaned. The weed free artemisia is dried in the sun

until the water content is low. The raw ferment is prepared by mixing the ground wheat evenly with water. It should be firm, dry and not sticky to the touch. When done, it is stored overnight and then kneaded further the next morning until the right consistency is achieved. A wooden mould is used to press the cakes. Each cake is one foot square and 2 inches thick. Strong young men are employed to press the cakes firmly. After pressing a hole is pierced through the center of each cake. Shelves of bamboo slats are set up on a wooden frame. Dried artemisia leaves are laid on top of the shelves. The raw ferment cakes are laid on top of the artemisia, and then covered with a layer of artemisia. The layer of Artemisia on the bottom should be thicker than that on top of the ferment cakes. The door and windows (of the hut) are then closed and sealed. . . . After the third seven-day period (total of twenty-one days) the ferment cakes should be fully cured. The door is opened and the ferment cakes examined. If there are fine coloured myceliae on the surface, the cakes are taken out and dried in the sun. If no myceliae are seen, the door is resealed and the cakes allowed to incubate for another three to five days. They are then dried in the sun. During drying the cakes are turned over several times. When fully dried, they are stacked on racks and stored until use. One tou of this type of ferment will digest seven tou of grain (after it is cooked).[39]

"In light of what we know today we can see that his directions are, on the whole, scientifically sound," concludes Huang, who reports that "it is now common practice to inoculate the cooked substrates with ferment powder before incubation"—in other words, backslopping.[40]

Across Asia, however, people continue to incorporate common local botanical ingredients into *qu*-like starters, so they tend to be somewhat geographically specific. *Ragi*, an Indonesian starter, is made by mixing rice flour with pieces of gingerroot, galangal roots, sugarcane, and other spices. "The exact additives vary with the manufacturer," notes Steinkraus.

The mixture is moistened with water or alternatively sugar cane juice . . . [and] inoculated with dry powdered ragi from previous batches. The cakes, which may be 3cm [1.2 inches] in diameter and 0.5 to 1 cm [less than ½ inch] thick when flattened, are placed on a bamboo tray and incubated for several days at ambient temperature followed by dehydration to preserve the cakes until needed. The air- or sun-dried ragi cakes preserve the essential microorganisms for several months at room temperature in the tropics.[41]

In Nepal, where *marcha* is the traditional starter, the plants are different, but the method is very similar. My friend Justin Bullard, who first told me about *marcha* after his return from a year living in Nepal a decade ago, traveled there again in 2011 to investigate *marcha* making. "I had the preconceived idea that the product was made from a single plant. So I was expecting Maila [who with his wife, Didi, was showing Justin the process] to show me that 'single plant,' but he ended up showing me two plants, and then later he and his wife began assembling 11 more plant ingredients to make the *marcha*!" The botanical ingredients included banana leaves and peels, sugarcane leaves, young pineapple leaves, gingerroot, hot pepper flakes and leaves, among others, as well as old *marcha* from a previous batch. "This particular recipe for *marcha* had been passed to Didi from her mother and grandmother, and may be considered to be Magar in origin," Justin writes. Yet,

> as with many homemade concoctions in Nepal, there are rarely precise measurements for ingredients. The individual making the concoction often just "eyeballs" or samples the mixture and determines, based on experience or exposure to the process, if a certain amount of a given ingredient needs to be added or subtracted. In other instances, some ingredients are omitted because of lack of availability.

Botanical ingredients are pulverized and mixed with millet flour and just enough water to bind the ingredients into a coarse dough.

> Cakes, a bit smaller than the size of the palm (about 3–4 ounces), are then shaped from the dough (if the cakes are too large, they will not dry properly). A marcha cake from a previous batch is broken up and then each new marcha cake is swathed in the powder of the old cake and laid out on a dried grass mat away from the sun, and covered with layers (this seems to keep the cakes warm and insulated). This is said to help facilitate the new marcha cakes to "flower" or "ripen." Day two, provided that the weather is hot and dry, the marcha cakes are uncovered and set in the sun to dry for a couple of hours on a flat woven basket. When asked how one knows when the cakes are ready to set out in the sun, or have ripened, I was told that they will have an "odor," and in fact, the cakes smelled yeasty, like bread dough. In addition, the cakes were covered in a very fine mildew (when Maila took the grass mat layers off the cakes, I could see they were covered in gossamer webs of must, and the odor was quite discernible), hence the term phool chha, or "flowered." After the cakes had set in the sun, they were replaced under the mats again under the porch. Day three, the cakes were placed out in the sun again to dry. It was explained that the drying process could proceed in this fashion up to 5 days or more, and that gradually the color of the cakes would whiten in sun. Then these would be stored and used at a later date.

Elsewhere in the Himalyas, in the Tons Valley, a starter for rice beverages called *keem* incorporates 42 (!) different plants, including cannabis, cinnamon, and datura. I learned about *keem* from the *Database on Microbial Traditional Knowledge of India* created by Dr. S. Sekar of Bharathidasan University in Tamil Nadu, India. According to Dr. Sekar: "Chopped fresh twigs of *Cannabis sativa* (8 kg), 5 kg leaves of *Sapindus mukorossi* [soap nut] and 10–15 kg in total of different plant species are dried in the shade and powdered. The powder prepared from the plants is mixed with about 50 kg of Barley flour." This dry mixture is moistened by an herbal infusion called *jayaras*; together they are mixed into dough and formed into small cakes.

> The cakes so formed are further processed by placing them on plant bed (locally called Sathar) made up of tender shoots of *Cannabis sativa* and *Pinus roxburghii* [pine] alternately between the cakes in a closed room. The whole set up is allowed to remain undisturbed for 24 days. On the 25th day, the room is opened and the cake is put upside down and allowed to remain there for another 12 days. The cakes are then taken out and allowed to dry in the sun or open air. When the cakes dry up, they are ready for use as starter.[42]

The investigators who collected the data on *keem* production report that "the plants used for this purpose vary slightly from place to place. During the course of this study the authors came across people who disclosed that their forefathers used several more plants for this process; however, nobody could identify or name all of them."[43] The botanical components of these starter cultures is important ethnobotanical information that is rapidly disappearing.

You can make *koji* without starter using appropriate plant material as the microbial source, in this case fresh corn husks. Steam rice, barley, or other grains as described earlier, only instead of inoculating and mounding in fabric, form into small (~2 inch/5 cm) balls, and wrap the balls individually in fresh corn husks. Bind the wrapped balls with cord and hang or place on a breathable rack. Maintain at incubation temperatures of 80–95°F/27–35°C. I've done this best in hot, humid summer weather outside under the eaves.

Of course, there are always exceptions, and some mixed-culture fermentation starters are made with neither botanical ingredients (beyond the grain substrate) nor backslopping from a mature batch, relying on organisms present on the substrate and/or in the aging environment. Korean *nuruk* is made from coarsely ground wheat, moistened, kneaded, and shaped into large cakes (roughly 4–12 inches/10–30 cm in diameter and 2 inches/5 cm thick). Traditionally no inoculum has been used, although in contemporary production, spores of *Aspergillus usamii* are often introduced. These cakes are then incubated for 10 days in the temperature range of 86–113°F/30–45°C, followed by 7 days in the narrower range of 95–104°F/35–40°C, then dried for two weeks at 86–95°F/30–35°C and aged for one or two more months at ambient temperatures.[44]

Troubleshooting

Mold not visible and beans not bound on tempeh

The mold failed to grow. Perhaps the starter was not viable. Perhaps the beans were still too hot when the starter was introduced. Perhaps the incubation chamber was too hot or too cool for the mold to develop.

Tempeh feels slimy

A slimy coating on the tempeh suggests that the tempeh overheated during incubation. Once the mold becomes established and starts to grow rapidly, it generates significant heat. It is possible for the heat that the mold growth generates to kill the mold, especially if the blocks of tempeh are thick, if there is limited ventilation in the incubation chamber, or if a large batch of tempeh is crowded in a small incubation chamber. Viable spores of the extremely heat-tolerant bacteria *Bacillus subtilis* are generally present on the tempeh substrates, even after cooking. While the tempeh mold is growing, it prevents *B. subtilis* from developing; however, if the tempeh mold is destroyed by excessive heat, the *B. subtilis* is at the ready, and starts to develop, with its telltale slimy coating and distinctive aroma. This does not make the tempeh dangerous, but it does result in poorly bound tempeh with a sharp flavor. When this has happened to me, I mark the tempeh "grade B" and crumble it into heavily seasoned chili and sloppy-joe-type dishes.

Tempeh turns black

When the tempeh mold first becomes visible, as its mycelia bind the beans and grains together, it is white. After about 24 hours of growth, the mold begins to develop darker patches of gray-black, indicating the beginning of sporulation. In a plastic bag with holes poked in it, sporulation begins near the holes, where the mold has the greatest access to oxygen. In an open-tray system, the entire surface can begin to darken. The early stages of sporulation are typically the sign that the tempeh has incubated long enough and is ready to eat. If the tempeh is not removed from the incubator, sporulation will continue, and with it stronger smell and flavor. In Java, this overripened tempeh, called tempeh *busuk*, is considered a delicacy in its own right.

Tempeh smells like ammonia

In the first 24 hours of mold growth, the tempeh smells fresh and earthy. When the mold continues to develop and overripens, as described above, tempeh develops an ammonia smell; or, in the appreciative words of William Shurtleff and Akiko Aoyagi, "a penetrating overripe aroma remarkably like that of a fine Camembert cheese, and its texture softens to a slightly creamy lusciousness that must be tasted to be understood."[45] Don't be afraid to try overripe tempeh.

Mold fails to grow on *koji*

Perhaps the starter was not viable. Perhaps the grains were still too hot when the starter was introduced. Perhaps the incubation chamber was too hot or too cool for the mold to develop.

Koji feels slimy

A slimy coating on the *koji* suggests that it overheated during incubation. Once the mold becomes established and starts to grow rapidly, it generates significant heat. It is possible for the heat that the mold growth generates to kill the mold, especially if the inoculated substrate is in a thick layer, if there is limited ventilation in the incubation chamber, or if a large batch of *koji* is crowded in a small incubation chamber. Viable spores of the extremely heat-tolerant bacteria *Bacillus subtilis* are generally present on the *koji* substrates, even after cooking. While the *koji* mold is growing, it prevents *B. subtilis* from developing; however, if the *koji* mold is destroyed by excessive heat, the *B. subtilis* is at the ready, and starts to develop, with its telltale slimy coating and distinctive aroma. If this happen, do not try to use the *koji* in further fermentation projects. Discard.

Koji turns yellow-green

When the *koji* mold first becomes visible, as its mycelia bind the substrate into clumps, it is white. After 36 to 48 hours of growth, the mold begins to develop patches of yellow-green, indicating the beginning of sporulation. For most applications, the earliest signs of sporulation are typically the cue that the *koji* has incubated long enough and is ready to use. If the *koji* is not removed from the incubator and cooled, sporulation will continue. For certain applications, such as *hamanatto* (see *Fermented Soy "Nuggets"* in chapter 11), yellow-green sporulated *koji* is preferred. Keep a close watch on your developing *koji* in the later part of the process so you can stop incubation at the appropriate time to obtain the type of *koji* you need.

Rice does not sweeten or liquefy in *amazaké*

Perhaps the *koji* you added was not viable. Perhaps the rice was hotter than 140°F/60°C when you introduced the *koji*, in which case the *koji* enzymes were destroyed by heat. Perhaps you didn't add enough *koji* or incubated it at too low a temperature. If this is the case, you can mix in more *koji* and create a warmer incubation chamber.

Amazaké sours

This suggests that the rice was left incubating too long. Once the *koji* enzymes sweeten the rice, lactic acid bacteria and yeasts start to ferment the sugars into acids and alcohol. *Amazaké* needs to be harvested after its fermentation. Typically it is then brought to a boil to kill the organisms poised to ferment it into something else.

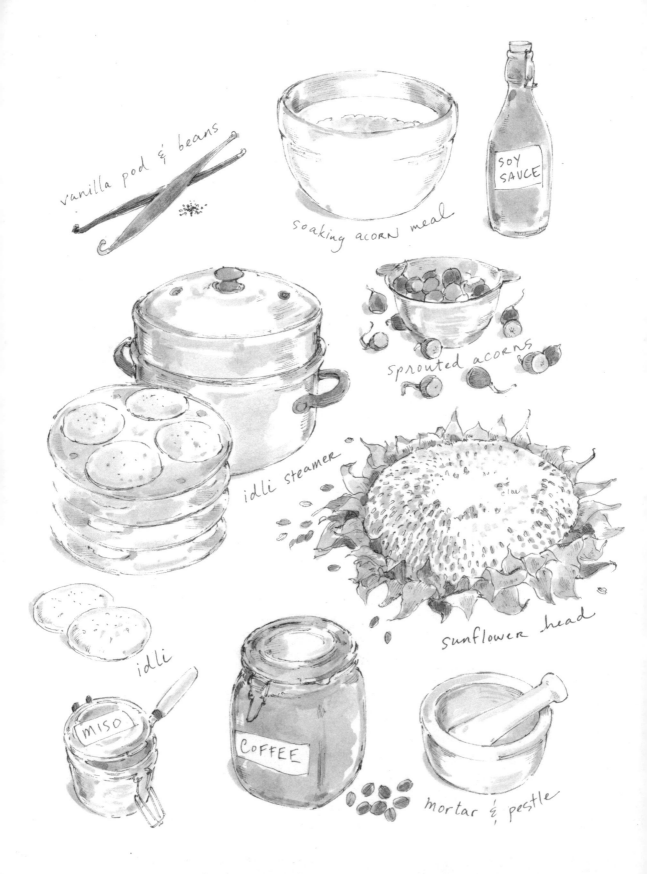

vanilla pod & beans

soaking acorn meal

SOY SAUCE

sprouted acorns

idli steamer

sunflower head

idli

MISO

COFFEE

mortar & pestle

CHAPTER 11

Fermenting Beans, Seeds, and Nuts

*B*eans are important elements of most agricultural food systems, if only for their "nitrogen-fixing" impact upon soil, actually the work of soil bacteria (*Rhizobium*) that thrive in legume root nodules, metabolizing atmospheric nitrogen into the soil. But legumes also provide critical nutrients, to both people and the animals we keep. "For many people, they have made the difference between life and death," writes historian Ken Albala in *Beans: A History*. "Beans are practically indestructible if thoroughly dried and well stored and thus have provided critical insurance against times of famine and death." Beans provide efficient nourishment, and many regions with high population densities depend upon them. "But in Europe and the so-called developed nations, only those people who could not afford meat depended on beans. Thus beans became a marker of class, the quintessential peasant food or 'poor man's meat.'"[1]

The same indestructibility that makes beans such important storage foods can also render them difficult to digest, as with grains, only perhaps more so. Soybeans in particular have enzyme inhibitors that render the bean's protein indigestible. Beans are notorious in folkloric humor in many cultures for the flatulence they cause. Along with soaking and often long cooking, fermentation has been used as a strategy to diminish anti-nutrients and toxins and thereby render the beans more digestible and their nutrients more available. Curiously, this strategy has been used extensively in Asia and to a lesser degree in Africa, but not at all in Western culinary traditions, despite the presence of both legumes and fermentation. No other edible bean necessitates fermentation for its effective digestion, as soybeans do, but the techniques used to ferment soybeans can be effectively applied to other beans.

Nuts and seeds also frequently have toxic anti-nutrient compounds that can be removed by fermentation. Certain seeds and nuts, such as acorns, require long soaking to leach toxins, which inevitably also initiates fermentation. Before delving into the fermentation of beans, I will briefly cover some ways of fermenting seeds and nuts, beyond tossing some in—raw, roasted, salted or not, whole or pieces, however you have them—with your fermenting vegetables, which can be quite lovely.

Cultured Seed and/or Nut Cheeses, Pâtés, and Milks

Nuts and edible seeds (such as sesame, sunflower, pumpkin, and flax) are rich and oily and can be ground or crushed, with (or without) other ingredients, into delicious cheeses, pâtés, and milks. These are creamier and tastier if the nuts and/or seeds are soaked before grinding and may be enjoyed fresh, or cultured and fermented.

I think of seed and nut cheeses and pâtés as existing along a continuum, depending upon texture and what is mixed in. Both *pâté* and *pesto* (as well as *pestle*) come from Latin *pestare*, to pound or crush. Typically what I know as pesto would contain a relatively low proportion of seeds and nuts, along with mostly basil or other greens, olive oil, and garlic. A seed or nut cheese, on the other hand, might be 95 percent seeds or nuts, with just a little liquid or oil, and just a few herbs, or none. A pâté could really be anywhere in between.[2] But the point here is that any of them may be cultured and fermented.

I have generally cultured seed and nut concoctions with sauerkraut juice, pickle brine, or miso. You could also try whey, raw soy sauce, sourdough (especially the liquid that separates at the top), *rejuvelac*, or other living cultures incorporating acid-producing bacteria. I have done these pâtés and cheeses as short-term ferments, overnight or a couple of days. Stir daily and taste. Like everything, they ferment faster in heat, slower in cool. When the taste is perfect, enjoy them fresh, or refrigerate for a few days to slow fermentation. If these go too long, they can become excessively sharp and to some unpleasant; eventually proteins will putrefy.

Nut or seed milks (see *Non-Dairy Milks, Yogurts, and Cheeses* in chapter 7) may also be fermented, although personally I have little experience with this. Linda Gardner Phillips reports on her experiences fermenting milk she makes from cashew nuts and dates.[3] "The first time it fermented was an accident, but I smelled it and realized it smelled very pleasantly sour, like buttermilk or sourdough starter, which I remembered my father making when I was a child." Linda uses her cashew and date milk as a sourdough starter. Another fermentation experimentalist, Shosh, writes that she uses sprouted sunflower seeds rather than sprouted grains to ferment *rejuvelac* (see Rejuvelac in chapter 8).

Acorns

Acorns, the nuts of oak trees, are edible and in fact have been a critical source of nutrients for many native peoples in North America and elsewhere. In mainstream culture, however, acorns are largely ignored as a food for human consumption. Meanwhile, ironically, the imminent threat of global food shortages is continually being used to justify deforestation and intensifying biotechnology. I'm not saying anyone should subsist on acorns alone, but let's tap into the abundant food resources we already have rather than acting based upon the myth of overall scarcity.

Gather acorns in the fall. Reject any with visible worm holes. Air-dry acorns before storing. It is not a problem if acorns have already begun to sprout. California acorn enthusiast Suellen Ocean writes:

> I like to gather sprouted acorns because the sprouting increases the acorn's nutritional value. It is no longer in a "starch" stage, but has changed to a "sugar" stage. The sprouting also helps split them from the shell. It is beneficial because if it has sprouted, it's a good acorn, and I haven't wasted time gathering wormy ones. I've found that an acorn with a two-inch-long sprout is fine, as long as the acorn nut meat hasn't turned green. I break off the sprout and continue.[4]

It is important to note that the acorns of many oak trees contain high levels of tannins and require leaching prior to consumption. To do this, remove acorns from their shells, grind, and soak in water. You can grind acorns dry using a mortar and pestle or mill, or mix acorns with water and grind in a blender or food processor. Acorns should be finely ground to expose lots of surface area, enabling the tannins to leach out.

Acorns can be leached in a fine mesh bag in a running stream (this is the fastest method), or in a series of soaks that can last for a few days. As acorn meal soaks, the meal will settle at the bottom of the vessel and the water will darken. Gently pour off the dark water at least daily and discard. Water will darken less with each soak, as tannin levels decrease. Keep rinsing with fresh water until it no longer darkens. If you wish to ferment acorn meal, leave it to soak a few more days in just a small amount of water after the tannins have been leached.

Acorns can be used to fortify and flavor many different foods. Once I made acorn gnocchi, which were excellent. Julia F. Parker, of the Miwok/Paiute people in California's Yosemite Valley, wrote a beautiful book about acorn preparation called *It Will Live Forever*, in which she describes traditional techniques for making a simple porridge (*nuppa*) using only leached acorn meal and water, which is delicious! And on a website devoted to the language of another California tribe, the Cahto, I came across reference to "fermented acorn/acorn cheese" (*ch'int'aan-noo'ool*).[5] I have not found further information on fermented acorn cheese, nor have I experimented, but I include this tidbit in the hope that other acorn-loving fermenters will experiment in this vein.

Coconut Oil

Fermentation can be used to extract coconut oil from coconuts. This simple process, brought to my attention by fermenter Keith Nicholson of Franklin, North Carolina, requires mature brown coconuts with hard flesh. The first step is to open the coconuts and remove the flesh. Then blend the coconut flesh with water to create a slurry, and strain out the solids, pressing to extract as much coconut milk as possible. Place the coconut milk in a jar, crock, or bowl in a warm spot and leave to ferment a day or two. As it begins to ferment and acidify, the coconut oil separates and rises to the top. Refrigerating solidifies the oil for easy removal.

Cacao, Coffee, and Vanilla Fermentation

These exotic tropical beans are everyday foods in affluent parts of our globalized world. Few people realize that they involve fermentation, which occurs post-harvest in the tropical places where these plants grow. I have no personal experience with them. The following descriptions are gleaned from the literature.

Cacao (*Theobroma cacao*)

Following harvest, pods are cut open and seeds "enmeshed in a white sweet pulp"[6] are removed. "The seeds are piled in heaps or vats, and covered with banana leaves, weighted with earth or sand, to ferment," writes Bill Mollison. "Fermentation takes place over 2, or even 10 days (the heap turned twice daily) when they rinse clean easily."[7] The turning is in order to release heat accumulating in the center and prevent overheating. "The microbes work like a symphony orchestra," offers Jeanette Farrell, with a vivid metaphor for community succession.[8] "Apparently, the fermentation depends to a considerable extent upon how tightly the pulpy beans are packed," writes microbiologist Carl Pederson. "Well-aerated beans would favor fermentation by yeasts and acetic acid bacteria while tightly-packed beans would favor a lactic acid fermentation." All three are typically present. "Chocolate precursors are formed immediately after the death of the seed," explains Pederson. "The death of the seed is caused by the acid and alcohol and the heat produced by the microbial fermentation."[9] Beans are ready when the "tree embryo within the seed is appropriately shriveled," according to Farrell. "If the beans are not dried, the organisms can begin to break down the embryo itself and fungi can begin to grow, adding their rich, but not necessarily desirable, flavors."[10]

Coffee (*Coffea* spp.)

Fruits the size of small cherries each contain two beans; each is wrapped in a membrane and embedded in yellow pulp. The fermentation digests this pulp, freeing the berries. "Fermentation involves placing the beans in plastic buckets or tanks and allowing them to sit, until the mucilage is broken down," according to the United Nations Food and Agriculture Organization.

> Natural enzymes in the mucilage and yeasts and bacteria in the environment work together to break down the mucilage. The coffee should be stirred occasionally and every so often a handful of beans should be tested by washing in water. If the mucilage can be washed off and the beans feel gritty rather than slippery, the beans are ready.[11]

Pederson reports: "The fermentation of coffee cherries is spontaneous and involves a variety of microorganisms. Underfermentation interferes with the normal drying process, while overfermentation results in adverse changes that affect the flavor and aroma."[12]

Vanilla (*Vanilla* spp.)

Vanilla is the fermented and dried seedpods of several species of orchids. Pods are harvested before they ripen, when the bottom of the pod begins to turn from green to yellow. If left on the vine to ripen, the pods split open, exposing the seeds and "making them practically worthless."[13] There are several different methods of curing, typically involving scalding the pods in hot water, then "sweating" them for several days. This process encourages dominance by heat-tolerant bacteria of the genus *Bacillus*.[14] Vanilla pods are fully cured when "fine needle-like crystals" develop on the surfaces.[15] Then the cured pods are typically extracted into alcohol for use as a flavoring.

Spontaneous Fermentation of Beans

The rest of this chapter will consider the fermentation of beans, meaning mature dried beans. Fresh beans are fermented as vegetables, sometimes raw, sometimes cooked (see chapter 5). Dried beans may also be sprouted and then fermented raw with vegetables. But other than that, at least by tradition, fermented beans are always cooked before and/or after fermentation. The microbial context for the fermentation is very different depending upon whether or not the beans have been cooked beforehand.

Raw beans are fermented spontaneously in a group of Indian ferments known as *idli* and *dosa* (along with many variations) and in an Afro-Brazilian preparation, *acarajé*. In each case, after fermentation, the raw fermented batter is cooked. When beans are cooked *before* fermentation, the kinds of organisms that spontaneously ferment beans are destroyed by heat, and the beans become a microbial blank slate, like pasteurized milk, prone to putrefaction.

Therefore, ferments of cooked beans are typically cultured with starters. Tempeh, covered in the last chapter, relies on molds, primarily *Rhizopus oligosporus*, while miso and soy sauce rely on different molds, of the genus *Aspergillus*, as well as mixed bacterial starters in the form of mature miso. Like many ferments around the world, the original sources of these common microbes were various plants in a raw state. The one bacterial spore that typically survives on beans after cooking is the hardy *Bacillus subtilis*, which transforms soybeans into the Japanese soybean delicacy known as *natto* and a range of similar bean ferments enjoyed elsewhere in Asia and Africa. If the *Rhizopus* or *Aspergillus* molds overheat and die while growing on beans, *B. subtilis* is present and will typically succeed them.

Idli/Dosa/Dhokla/Khaman

Idli are steamed cakes of fermented rice and lentils, popular in southern India. *Dosai* (the plural of *dosa*) are delicate, paper-thin crepes of a thinner version of exactly the same batter. Other variations on the theme include *dhokla* and *khaman*. To make *idli* or *dosai*, start by separately soaking rice and black gram dal, or other lentils, overnight. Proportions vary in different recipes; Steinkraus reports that "the proportions of rice to black gram vary from 4:1 to 1:4 depending upon the relative cost on the market."[16] I like 2–3 parts rice:1 part red lentils. Many recipes call for fenugreek seeds, as well, in much smaller proportion, which contribute microbes as well as flavor.

To make batter, blend or pound the soaked rice, lentils, and fenugreek seeds into a slurry, adding water as necessary. For *idli*, you need a fairly thick batter; for *dosai* add more water to thin. Add a little salt, and leave to ferment 12 to 48 hours, depending upon temperature. Typically no starter is added, and no starter is necessary, but you can add yogurt, kefir, a bit of mature batter, or other starters. You can also add other herbs or spices, if desired, though traditionally they are made simply and embellished via toppings (*dosa*), stews (*idli*), and chutneys. I like to ferment *idli/dosa* batter in glass (no more than two-thirds full) so I can see its dramatic rise.

Once the batter is visibly rising, you can cook it into *idli* or *dosa*. If you let it rise too long, it can exhaust its nutrients and lose its rising power, much like bread can. For *idli*, steam the batter in special forms designed for this purpose, or in any improvised steamer. One good improvisational technique is to wrap fermented batter in corn husks, like tamales, and steam them. Steam about 20 minutes until well set. *Idli* is frequently served with a spicy vegetable dal called *sambar*. For *dosa*, the batter must be much thinner and spread in as thin a layer as possible on a well-seasoned and oiled or stick-free pan.

Dhokla are similar to *idli*, only using different legumes and steamed in a different form. *Dhokla* are typically made with dehulled Bengal gram dal and rice. My friend Sean, who has visited family in India, reports that his favorite *dhokla* are made with chickpeas. The batter is steamed in larger forms (or greased pie tins); after steaming, *dhokla* are cut into small squares to be served. "The way I've experienced *dhokla*, once the cake has been steamed, mustard seeds are popped in oil with a pinch of *asafoetida* [a botanical flavoring used in Indian cooking]," explains Sean. "That mixture is spread on top of the dhokla, which is then sprinkled with unsweetened coconut shreds and coriander leaves." *Khaman* is exactly like *dhokla*, except that no rice is used; the batter is made of dehulled Bengal gram dal (or other legumes), mixed only with water and salt.[17]

idli steamer

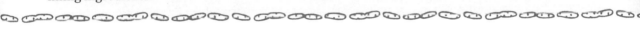

DOSA VARIATIONS

Orese Fahey, New Mexico

I have made dosa with Forbidden Rice (a black rice), which created a dark purple dosa; with red dal, which created a pink dosa; and with risotto rice, as well as yellow and white dal. As long as the ratio is 2 rice to 1 dal, all of these variations have been successful. Adding chopped green chile to the batter has been great (we live in New Mexico), and I have also added minced garlic and diced onion to the batter, and often add turmeric, as that creates a nice golden dosa. I make the dosai in a crepe pan, and I do not thin the batter to the degree that they do in Indian restaurants—we have had dosai in restaurants that are very thin and, in my opinion, quite tasteless. I make the dosai the thickness of a tortilla, so then they work very well as a wrapper for various fillings. I often take ground turkey or ground lamb and mix seasonings and diced onions, etc. into the meat, add a few tablespoons of coconut fiber and an egg to help hold things together, and shape the meat mixture into torpedo shapes so that they will fit nicely in a dosa. We also eat "dessert dosai" by wrapping a dosa around fresh fruit, whipped cream, homemade applesauce, and so on. We like the sourness of the dosa with the sweeter filling ingredients.

Acarajé (Afro-Brazilian Fritters of Fermented Black-Eyed Peas)

These Brazilian fry-breads made from fermented black-eyed peas are creamy, light, and delicious! My sister thought they tasted like latkes (potato pancakes). I learned about them from Selma Miriam of the Bloodroot Collective, which has operated a fermentation-friendly feminist vegetarian restaurant in Bridgeport, Connecticut, for more than 30 years. *Acarajé* comes from the Brazilian state of Bahia, and like black-eyed peas themselves, it is a transplant from West Africa, known as *acara* in Yoruba.

Making *acarajé* is pretty straightforward. Soak black-eyed peas overnight. One cup/½ pound)/250 ml/250 g) of peas will feed four to six people. After soaking, try to remove as many of the hulls from the beans as you can. While they are submerged, stick your hands in the water and roll the peas between the palms of your hands, pressing and moving your hands in circles in opposite directions, to try to remove the skins from the beans. You may need to reach in and squeeze the beans between your thumbs and index fingers, or pound the peas with a heavy blunt tool. Periodically rinse and swirl the water so the detached skins will float to the top. Remove them and discard. Add more water if necessary and repeat a few times. The more skins you get off, the smoother the batter will be, but you probably will not get them all. At least I never have. Then blend the soaked, dehulled peas with a coarsely chopped onion, a chili pepper, salt, and pepper. Blend well, or crush in a mortar and pestle, into a paste. Add just a little water if necessary to moisten and bind. Leave the paste/batter in a bowl to ferment. The Bloodroot recipe called for fermenting it for only one to four hours, but I have been experimenting with longer fermentation. I've gotten as far as about four days, and so far they just keep getting tastier. After several more days—exactly how many depends upon temperature, saltiness, and other factors—it ceases to get sharper and begins to develop more putrid flavor notes.

In Brazil, *acarajé* is usually cooked by deep-frying the batter in palm oil. It is indeed delicious deep-fried, though I have mostly pan-fried it in just a little oil as pancakes. Either way, use whatever oil you like. Just before cooking the batter, beat it for a good long while to make it smooth and stiff, adding water, just a little at a time, as necessary. This beating changes the batter dramatically, making it much, much creamier. As with cream or egg whites, the beating both develops the batter's capacity to hold air and whips air bubbles into it. Proteins have a tendency "to unfold and bond to each other when they're subjected to physical stress," explains Harold McGee (in a different context). "Thus disturbed and concentrated, they readily form bonds with each other. So a continuous, solid network of proteins pervades the bubble walls, holding both water and air in place."[18] Beat *acarajé* batter until it is stiff and maintains peaks. I've done it (in small quantities) with a hand whisk, beating about 10 minutes. You could use any tool you would use beating cream or egg whites, such as a mechanical or electrical mixer, or a food processor with a paddle. It never before occurred to me to beat legumes, but it's so light and fluffy! *Acarajé* is a common street food in Bahia, typically deep-fried, cut open, and served covered or stuffed with stew and/or sauce, often with shrimp. A quick online search will yield many enticing accompaniments.

In Nigeria, the same batter is also boiled or steamed in a banana leaf and called *abará*.[19] To steam as *abará*, leave the batter fairly thick, wrap in a corn husk (with a tasty morsel buried inside, if desired), tie with twine, and steam about 20 minutes, as for tamales.

Soybeans

Most of the rest of the traditional bean ferments I know developed in relation to soybeans in China, Japan, Korea, Indonesia, and other parts of Asia. Historian Ken Albala points out that China's rulers have been promoting soy agriculture for nearly three millennia, and that China's long stability as a civilization and empire has helped give rise to, spread, and perpetuate such elaborate transformations of the bean. Except for edamame, which are soybeans cooked while they are fresh, before they are dried, soybeans are rarely eaten merely cooked, because anti-nutrient factors the dried beans contain—including enzyme inhibitors and the highest phytate content of any legume or grain—make them difficult to digest.[20] In China and elsewhere in Asia, dried soybeans are almost always either fermented, or else processed into milk, curdled, and pressed into tofu (in a process similar to cheesemaking).

Because soybeans were not generally eaten intact, early accounts of European travelers to Asia "rarely recognized the connection between the bean and foods made from it," according to Albala.[21] The earliest interest in the plant in the United States was as a soil-building cover crop and animal forage rather than a food crop for humans.[22] Several unrelated events spurred a rapid growth of US soy agriculture in the early decades of the 20th century. World War I food shortages created demand for meat substitutes and cooking oil; the need for new sources of vegetable oil was compounded by a boll weevil infestation of US cotton crops in the 1920s. New developments in plant breeding led to soy varieties better suited to the midwestern United States, where farmers found the crop a good complement to corn.

In addition, improvements in agricultural technology, as well as government agricultural policy, favored soybean production. Decreased reliance on draft animals meant that millions of acres that had been pasture could be converted to crops, including soy; and as pigs, which eat soy meal, largely replaced horses on American farms, this further stimulated agricultural demand for soy. Bigger and better tractors and combines, which enabled greater labor efficiency, made US soy more competitive on the world market. Finally, US farm policies during the Depression, which aimed to maintain prices to support the farm economy by limiting production of corn and other crops, placed no restrictions on soybean acreage.[23]

Technology encouraged not only soy production but also innovations in how it was used. In 1934, the Archer Daniels Midland Company (ADM) derived lecithin from soybean oil, which quickly found numerous industrial applications. One important business leader who saw opportunity in soybeans was Henry Ford, who funded much research seeking ways to incorporate them into car manufacturing. Ford, who grew up on a farm, was eager to support farmers on a large scale and showcased a prototype automobile in 1941 with a body made of soy-based plastic.[24] Soy is now commonly found in cars as well as computers and is used in oils, paints, plastics, inks, cosmetics, and countless other industrial applications, including food processing. World War II shortages of butter and cooking oil introduced American consumers to margarine and shortening made from soy oil by means of a newly developed hydrogenation process. To meet wartime demand, US soy production increased rapidly, and during the war the United States became the world's largest grower, surpassing China.

Wartime necessity "became an agreeable and economical convenience during peacetime," writes Sidney Mintz. Today soy is among the top US cash crops; and not coincidentally 93 percent of that crop consists of a variety genetically modified for tolerance to the herbicide Round-Up. Given the nature of genetic drift, the engineered genes can be expected to show up in the other 7 percent, legal prohibitions against genetically modified ingredients in organic products notwithstanding.

Like genetic modification, soy is largely invisible to consumers, its oil "hardly ever marketed with the word 'soybean' on the front label," observes Mintz.[25] Oil, lecithin, proteins, and other forms of fragmented soy are present in nearly all processed foods but rarely receive any marketing prominence. And most of the soy Americans consume they eat indirectly through chicken and pork; if you count that, because we eat so much of these meats, US per-capita consumption of soy is considerably higher than Japan's.[26]

The only time soy gets talked about as food is as a meat alternative or for purported health benefits. Health food promoter John Harvey Kellogg wrote about soy as a high-protein meat alternative as early as 1921.[27] With the explosion of vegetarianism in Western countercultures in the 1970s, soymilk and tofu were embraced as substitutes for milk and meat. Paradoxically, this crop of prime importance to agriculture and industry became what historian Warren Belasco has termed the "icon of the countercuisine."[28]

The soy industry has sought to increase soy's appeal to the mainstream as a "functional food," by funding research to support its use as a therapy for menopausal women and to reduce risk of cancer, heart disease and atherosclerosis, and bone loss. But increasingly, health care practitioners and advocates are questioning these benefits and identifying problems that may be caused by consumption of unfermented soy. Nutritionist Kaayla Daniel, in her book *The Whole Soy Story: The Dark Side of America's Favorite Health Food*, presents evidence that high consumption of unfermented soy may play a role in many growing health problems, including irregular sexual development of fetuses, infants, and children; diminished cognitive ability, accelerated brain aging, and increased likelihood of Alzheimer's disease; infertility and suppressed reproductive functioning; heart arrhythmias, thyroid disorders, and increased risk of certain cancers; the list goes on and on.[29] Herbalist Susun Weed, veteran of decades of treating people who replaced milk and meat with soymilk and tofu, summarizes: "When unfermented soy is eaten frequently in a diet low or lacking in animal protein . . . the anti-nutritional factors can create havoc: brittle bones, thyroid problems, memory loss, vision impairment, irregular heartbeat, depression, and vulnerability to infections."[30]

Almost all of the critiques of soy that I have seen pertain to unfermented soy. If you want to eat soybeans, fermented is definitely the best way to do so. Use organic soybeans if you wish to try to avoid genetically modified foods. And almost anything you can do with a soybean, you can do with other beans, albeit with different results. Don't worry too much about it. Soy and other beans are improved in many ways by fermentation.

Miso

Miso is a Japanese form of fermented bean paste. It is made by mashing well-cooked beans with *koji* (grain grown with the mold *Aspergillus oryzae*; see *Making Koji* in chapter 10), salt, and often mature miso and/or other ingredients. Japanese tradition encompasses many different varieties and regional styles of miso. *The Book of Miso* by William Shurtleff and Akiko Aoyagi is the definitive English-language guide to miso, with much information on different traditional varieties. "Miso's range of flavors and colors, textures and aromas, is at least as varied as that of the world's fine wines or cheeses," write Shurtleff and Aoyagi, in another epic volume covering the history of miso.[31] My own experience has been more experimental; guided by Shurtleff and Aoyagi's presentation of the basic methods, I have incorporated every bean I could think of and over time used higher proportions of *koji* and eventually vegetables.

I started using more *koji* because I learned how to make my own, described in detail in the previous chapter. Once I experienced *koji*'s alluring aroma, and how potent it is fresh, and was unburdened from the considerable expense of buying it, my *koji* proportions increased. What I like about misos with high proportions of *koji* is that they generally use much lower proportions of salt and don't require cool cellar conditions for long aging.

This is the basic process for making miso. Proportions are addressed below. Before you can make miso, you need *koji*, which you can either make yourself as described in chapter 10 or obtain from commercial sources (see *Resources*). Soak beans for miso overnight, in enough water to keep them covered as they expand. In the morning, cook the beans in fresh water. As the beans come to a boil, skim off and discard any foam that accumulates at the surface, especially with soybeans. I usually add some kombu seaweed to the cooking beans. Cook until the beans are soft and easy to crush, how long varying with the type of bean, up to as much as six hours for soybeans. Overcooking is not a problem; just be sure to stir the bottom frequently so you don't burn the beans!

mortar & pestle

After cooking, drain the beans through a colander into a pot or bowl and reserve the cooking liquid. Pour a little hot bean cooking liquid (or boiling water) over the measured amount of salt to cover; stir to start dissolving the salt, and set aside. Next, mash the beans. Typically working in 5-gallon/20-liter batches, I like to place beans in a big pot on the floor and mash from above, with my super-size masher (also marketed as a cement mixer), adding bean cooking liquid and/or water as necessary to get a pasty consistency. You can mash the beans into a smooth homogeneous texture using any number of tools, or leave them somewhat chunky, as you prefer. It is my understanding that miso has traditionally been enjoyed chunky, and only in the context of relatively recent mass production has it been widely mashed and milled into the smooth product commercially available. You can strive for that, or enjoy a coarser texture, as I do.

Before adding *koji* to the bean mash, evaluate temperature. *Koji* enzymes can tolerate temperatures up to about 140°F/60°C, but be sure not to add it to beans hotter than that, or hotter than you can comfortably touch. If, after mashing, your beans are still too hot, leave them to cool longer, stirring frequently to release heat from the center. Once the beans are sufficiently cooled, add *koji* and stir and/or mash it in.

Now you can return to the salt you covered with hot water and/or bean cooking liquid earlier, which should have cooled to around body temperature by now. If you are making a long-aging, high-salt miso, add live unpasteurized mature miso to this, and stir to thoroughly distribute. The mature miso you add is sometimes called "seed miso" because it serves as a starter, introducing lactic acid bacteria and other organisms that develop in miso in addition to the *koji* mold. Any unpasteurized miso, including commercially available ones, may be used for this. Short-fermenting misos typically rely on the *koji* exclusively and do not incorporate seed miso, because that would hasten souring. Whether or not you add seed miso, add the salt mixture to the mashed beans and *koji*. Add vegetables (more on that soon) or any additional ingredients you desire. Add further bean liquid or water to achieve a paste that is moist and easily spreadable, but thick enough to hold its shape, and not runny. If miso is warm, it will continue to thicken as it cools; also, *koji* will absorb some of the water, especially if it is dry rather than fresh. If the miso seems too dry at any point, mix in more water in small increments.

Once the miso ingredients are well mixed, they need to be packed into a crock for aging. As you add miso to your crock, take care to pack down each addition, leaving no air pockets, which could result in internal mold growth and a musty flavor. After being packed into the crock, fermenting miso needs to be pressed down as it ages. In my experience, there is no avoiding this, as there is with vegetables, which you can ferment tightly packed into a jar. The initial *koji* fermentation of the miso is extremely active and expansive. I learned this once when I had some extra prepared miso left over after packing the rest of the batch into a 5-gallon crock. I packed the extra miso into a jar and left it, loosely capped, in the basement. When it caught my eye again about a week later, the miso had pushed off the cap and erupted up out of the jar, over the sides, and all around. Miso needs to be weighted down to hold it together in its vessel and prevent it from exploding or escaping. And it also needs to be able to release gas.

I always make miso in ceramic crocks, covered with plates or hardwood disks, usually weighted down by a 1-gallon/4-liter jug of water, with an old sheet or other cloth covering the top, tied tight around the crock with string, as a barrier to flies and dust. The setup is exactly as I use for sauerkraut, illustrated in *Crock Method*, chapter 3. You could also use a heavy or multiple-layer plastic bag filled with water as a cover and weight, especially useful in a jar or other vessel that is not cylindrical and has a mouth smaller than its internal size, as described in *Crock Lids*, chapter 3.

You need to think ahead about where to age your miso, as the options you have available have implications for what kinds of miso it makes sense for you to make. Sweet miso, which ferments for relatively short periods of time (roughly two to six weeks), can age in a variety of environments. Warmer temperatures will make them ferment faster; cooler, slower. Sweet miso uses a high proportion of *koji* and low proportion of salt. Longer-fermenting salty miso, which ferments for a minimum of about six months, and often for years, needs to be stored in an unheated space protected from temperature extremes, such as a cellar, especially if you age them beyond the minimum. These longer-fermenting misos generally use higher proportions of salt and lower proportions of *koji*. Only attempt these longer-fermenting misos if you have a suitable place to age them. If your living space is entirely heated, it's better for you to make a sweet miso. After a year or more in a heated space, miso can be shrunken and hard as a brick. I've seen it happen.

The simple proportions I work with are roughly equal amounts of beans and *koji* for sweet miso, with about 6 percent salt; and for salty longer-fermenting misos about twice as much beans as *koji*, with about 13 percent salt. These salt proportions are in relation to the weight of the dry ingredients. Here are hypothetical proportions for about 3 gallons/12 liters of sweet miso: Make *koji* from 5 pounds/2.25 kg (dry) of barley. Add that to the same dry weight of kidney beans. Then multiply the sum of those, in this case 10 pounds/4.5 kg, by 6 percent (0.06), to get 0.6 pound or 9.6 ounces/0.27 kg of salt, which roughly measures to 1¼ cups/300 ml. With a salty miso, the same 5 pounds/2.25 kg of barley *koji* could yield 5 gallons/20 liters of miso, because you mix it with twice as much beans, 10 pounds/4.5 kg. To calculate salt, multiply the total dry weight of grains and beans (15 pounds/6.75 kg) by 13 percent (0.13), to get 1.95 pounds/0.88 kg salt, which roughly measures to 4 cups of salt. These are simple calculations that are the same no matter what unit of measure you are familiar with. You can estimate dry grain or bean weight at 2 cups per pound, or 1 liter per kilo. A given weight of salt will vary in its volume depending upon fineness or coarseness, and density, so weight is the most accurate gauge. If you are without a kitchen scale, see *Salt* in chapter 3 for a rough translation of salt into volume measurements.

TABLE 11-1: MISO GENERIC PROPORTIONS

	SWEET MISO for 1 gallon/4 liters	SALTY MISO for 1 gallon/4 liters
BEANS	2 pounds/1 kg	2 pounds/1 kg
KOJI	2 pounds/1 kg	1 pound/500 g
SALT	~ 6 percent = 0.25 pound/120 g	~ 13 percent = 0.4 pound/200 g

There is no denying that miso is a salty food. Without heavy salting, beans rapidly putrefy. That said, you don't need to be a slave to these proportions. If you like, experiment with marginally smaller amounts of salt. I don't know exactly how little you can get away with. Salt in miso corresponds to the intended length of aging, so it's a question of how long it can beneficially age with a given proportion of salt.

MISO SOUP WITH WILLIAM SHURTLEFF

Co-author of The Book of Miso, The Book of Tempeh, *and others*

While I was writing this book I paid a visit to William Shurtleff at his home—also the SoyInfo Center—in Lafayette, California. From my first miso-making experience in 1994, his *Book of Miso* has been my guide. After years of email correspondence, I asked if I could come see him while I was visiting nearby San Francisco. I was thrilled when he invited me to come for a bowl of miso soup.

Shurtleff has devoted himself in recent years to scholarship and archiving information about all aspects of the history of soybeans. He has translated early Chinese documents into English, created a chronological bibliography of written references to soy, and documented early US commercial miso and tempeh makers. This is his life's work, and he is passionate not only about the subject but also about the idea that this information be freely available. Most of the books he and his wife, Akiko Aoyagi, have written are available in full for free on Google Books, and all of their recent books have been self-published digitally, free of charge, on both Google Books and their website.[32] Shurtleff loves what the Internet makes possible and wishes for the information and documentation he has compiled to aid and inspire people in far-flung locations to tap into the nutritional potential of soybeans.

Bill Shurtleff's devotion to scholarship and archiving has taken his focus away from the kitchen. I can relate, as writing books and teaching both have impinged upon the hours I used to devote to the garden and the kitchen. When I presented Bill with a jar of homemade miso, he marveled that it had been many years since he had made miso. And in fact, when lunchtime came, he made a perfectly lovely soup from dried instant miso packets, enhanced with fresh-grated ginger. In a way it was like finally meeting the Wizard of Oz, seeing that the guru of miso making eats a powdered instant version of this ultimate slow food. Bill was very matter-of-fact about the whole thing. He is clear and unapologetic about his priorities. He also happens to have consulted with the people who first developed the process of drying miso into a powder for instant soups, so indeed he had a role in making what we ate. Throughout our meandering conversations, Bill kept referring back to the Buddhist notion of the middle way, of not embracing extremes or dogmatic views, of always finding value in different approaches, of striving for both/and inclusion rather than either/or restriction. The instant miso Bill served me also has bonito (fish) flakes in it, though he has practiced vegetarianism for 40 years and that's how he became interested in miso in the first place. Again, he cited the middle way, the value of non-dogmatism. Bill seems quite at ease with seeming contradictions.

Long-fermenting salty misos are typically made in the cool part of the year, when airborne bacterial levels are relatively low. As a further guard against bacterial contamination, I usually sprinkle salt on the moist internal surfaces of the crock before filling it with miso. This is an idea, recommended by Shurtleff and Aoyagi, to increase the salt concentration at the edges. I do it unless I forget; and when I have forgotten, I have never had a problem with contamination. I think of it as a ritual of protection. More important, I also sprinkle salt, a little more heavily, on the surface before weighing down.

I will not dwell too long on miso, because Shurtleff and Aoyogi have not only covered the topic so comprehensively in *The Book of Miso*, but also have put that and many of their books online for all to freely access. Of the many traditional Japanese styles of miso Shurtleff and Aoyogi describe, my current favorites are two short-fermenting sweet misos. One, known as "finger lickin'" miso (a traditional name, not one I bestowed), incorporates vegetables. In addition to equal parts *koji* and beans and 6 percent salt, for finger lickin' miso you add already fermenting vegetables, in a proportion of roughly 10 to 25 percent of the rest, by volume. Finger lickin' miso is less a paste than a chunky chutney- or pickle-type condiment. It tastes sweet, salty, and sour all at once, with appealing textural variation. I usually start tasting it after about two weeks, and as time passes it gets increasingly sour.

Nattoh miso is another chunky sweet miso, distinguished by the fact that it maintains whole soybeans intact. One part whole cooked soybeans are mixed with roughly 2 parts barley *koji* and 1 part *shoyu* (make sure it does not contain preservatives), along with *kombu* seaweed, barley malt (or another sweetener), and slivers of ginger, all mixed together and fermented two to four weeks. The shiny whole soybeans in *nattoh* miso resemble the beans in *natto*, a very different soybean ferment (see *Natto*), hence the name, and a certain amount of confusion. For people interested in experimenting with miso but not wanting to wait a year or more, I recommend experimenting with finger lickin' miso, *nattoh* miso, or other short-fermenting sweet styles.

Using Miso

Anyone who has eaten in a Japanese restaurant is familiar with miso soup. Soup is indeed a wonderful use of miso, but miso is an extremely versatile flavoring with many other applications. Sweet miso and finger lickin' miso can be served as is for use as a table condiment, but generally saltier, longer-fermented misos are too strong for that. Here are a few ideas for using miso in cooking and other food preparation.

Miso Marinades

Miso makes a great base for marinades to flavor meats, vegetables, tofu or tempeh, or really anything you might barbecue, broil, roast, or stir-fry. Mix miso with vinegar, oil, hot sauce, honey or sugar, beer, wine, *saké* or mirin (sweet Japanese cooking wine), herbs—almost anything. Combine well, spread over the surfaces of the food being marinated, and marinate for several hours or several days, turning periodically and recovering surfaces as necessary. Leave residual marinade on the food, so when you cook it will caramelize.

Miso Dressings, Sauces, and Spreads

Fat-rich bases, such as seed and nut butters, yogurt, and sour cream, are ideal companions for miso's dense salty flavor. Miso-tahini is a vegetarian classic, but miso-peanut butter and miso-yogurt combinations are just as delicious. Start with a ratio of about 4 parts base to each part miso, and adjust the proportions to your liking. Thin this mixture with citrus juice, kraut or kimchi juice, pot "liquor" from cooking vegetables, or water. Add any other flavorings you like. Depending upon how thick or thin it is, the same mixture could be presented as a spread, sauce, or dressing.

Miso Pickles

Miso is a great pickling medium. See *Tsukemono: Japanese Pickling Styles* in chapter 5 for details.

Sweet Miso Porridge

Sweet miso, with its short fermentation, generally still has enzymes present that can digest complex carbohydrates into simple sugars. Christian Elwell, one of the founders of the South River Miso Company, first shared this technique with me. Cook porridge, without salt, in the evening. Cool to below 140°F/60°C and add sweet miso. Stir well to distribute the miso in the porridge, cover, and leave in a moderately warm spot overnight. By morning, the porridge will have liquefied somewhat and become much sweeter. Gently reheat and enjoy sweet porridge.

Miso Soup

Classic and wonderful. Miso is generally the last ingredient to be added. The idea is to avoid boiling the miso or subjecting it to unnecessary heat. "Overcooking spoils the miso's prized aroma while also destroying microorganisms and enzymes which aid digestion," note Shurtleff and Aoyagi.[33] Of course, hot soup temperatures even below boiling will destroy most of the organisms, but by avoiding boiling some enzymes may be preserved, and certainly volatile flavor compounds.

Typically miso soup is a simple broth or *dashi*, a stock made with *kombu* seaweed and sometimes bonito (fish) flakes. And as Bill Shurtleff taught me, you can enliven a simple miso broth with a little fresh grated ginger. Any soup or stew may be enriched by the addition of miso, including soups made from meat- or fish-based stocks. Before adding miso, remove the soup from the heat. Use a ladle or mug to scoop out a few ounces of soup. Mash the miso into that so it dissolves into a liquid. Figure about 1 tablespoon/15 ml miso per cup of soup, unless the soup already has a rich base, in which case use less. Stir the miso mixture back into the soup and taste. Repeat if necessary.

miso

Soy Sauce

The English word *soy* comes from the Japanese name for soy sauce, *shoyu*. Indeed, stable fermented soy sauce, an indispensable flavoring in Chinese, Japanese, and other East Asian cuisines, was the soy food that first found its way into Europe and is widely used today in Western kitchens. "Soy sauce is the most widespread fermented legume product on earth," states anthropologist Sidney Mintz.[34] The earliest soy sauces were simply the liquids that pooled at the top of vats of fermenting soybean pastes such as miso and its Chinese precursor, *jiang*. But over time, distinctive processes emerged for making soy sauce.[35]

The biggest difference between miso and soy sauce, in terms of process, is that in miso the *Aspergillus* molds are generally grown on grains (*koji*), and it is the *enzymes* produced by the mold that act upon the soybeans, rather than the mold itself. In soy sauce, the *Aspergillus* molds are grown not only on grains but also directly on the soybeans, leading to "the formation of more complicated metabolic compounds, a higher degree of protein hydrolysis and liquefaction, and the production of much sharper and stronger flavor in *shoyu* than in miso."[36]

From a microbial perspective, soy sauce is among the most complex of fermented foods, involving three distinct groups of organisms—*Aspergillus* molds, lactic acid bacteria, and yeasts—in two distinct fermentations. The United Nations Food and Agriculture Organization reports, "During these fermentations several intimate relationships take place between moulds, bacteria, and yeasts, resulting in the production of a host of different flavour and aroma compounds."[37] But beyond growing the molds on soybeans and generally with wheat, the rest of the microbial succession takes care of itself with the addition of a small amount of live-culture miso or soy sauce as starter. Across Asia, there are many distinctive forms of soy sauce, some incorporating fish, hot peppers, palm sugar, or other spices.

In our time, much soy sauce is being manufactured by acid hydrolysis of "defatted" soybeans, in other words the by-product after pressing out the oil. This method does not involve fermentation. "The acid hydrolyzed soy sauce is less attractive in aroma and flavor because of lack of aromatic substances such as esters, alcohols, and carbonyl compounds which are derived from the fermentation process," according to the *Journal of Industrial Microbiology*. "In some countries, a combination of fermentation and acid-hydrolysis procedures are used for making less expensive soy sauce. High quality soy sauce is made exclusively by the fermentation process."[38]

I have tried fermenting two Japanese styles of soy sauce: *shoyu* made from soybeans and roasted wheat, and *tamari* made from soybeans alone, with no wheat or other grain. I had much better results with the *shoyu* than the *tamari*, so it is the *shoyu* process I describe here. I assumed at first that soy sauce with wheat was an Americanized version, but I now understand that wheat has been used in China for thousands of years and has a long tradition of use in soy sauces, and in fact adds depth and complexity to soy sauce's flavor.

For shoyu, grow *Aspergillus* molds on a mix of soybeans and wheat. Three pounds of each will yield about a gallon of shoyu. Soak soybeans overnight, then steam until soft enough to crush easily, five to six hours over boiling water or an hour and a half in a pressure cooker. Meanwhile, dry-roast wheat berries (soft wheat is best) or bulgur in a cast-iron skillet, stirring frequently, until it is aromatic and beginning to brown. "Slight charring is desirable to develop flavor," says Betty Stechmeyer of GEM Cultures, whose detailed directions first guided me through the process. (Betty's excellent directions accompany all the GEM Cultures starters.) If you are using whole wheat berries, coarsely grind in a grain grinder, not into flour, but breaking each grain into several pieces. No need to grind if you are using bulgur.

Once soybeans are well cooked, drain them well, then, while still steaming hot, toss with roasted cracked wheat and allow to cool to body temperature. Once cooled, add starter—GEM recommends 2 teaspoons for this 1-gallon quantity—and incubate as described in *Making* Koji, chapter 10. After about 48 hours (but possibly shorter or longer), once your *koji* is covered with white mold and possibly beginning to show early signs of sporulation (yellow-green patches) developing, it's time to mix it with the other ingredients into the *moromi*, which will ferment for six months to two years into *shoyu*.

Based on the weight of the dry beans and wheat you started with, combine 40 percent salt (for 3 pounds/1.4 kg each, that would be 2.4 pounds/1.1 kg) with water equal in weight to the combined weight of the beans, wheat, and salt (in this case 8.4 pounds/3.8 kg, roughly a gallon/4 liters). Stir well to dissolve salt, then add *koji*. Also add a little *nama* (raw) *shoyu* or miso to introduce lactic acid bacteria and yeasts. Mix everything together and transfer to a crock or other fermentation vessel. Secure a cloth over the crock to keep flies out.

Stir daily for the first week, then once or twice a week (definitely twice a week in summer). Regular stirring should prevent mold, but if you encounter surface molds, skim off and discard. Keep the fermenting *shoyu* in a heated space. If the volume diminishes due to evaporation, add dechlorinated water as necessary to maintain the original volume. "Traditional fermentation continues for 1 to 3 years at ambient temperatures, as the color and flavor become more intense," according to Steinkraus. The mature *moromi* is a very dark rust color, with a thick consistency and pleasant aroma. It is not necessary to wait three years to try your *shoyu*. Give it at least a year. Then harvest a portion of it, and allow the rest to continue maturing.

The hardest part of the process (waiting aside) is physically pressing the liquid *shoyu* from the chunky *moromi*. Place *moromi* in a mesh, canvas, or other coarsely woven pressing sack, or a few layers of cheesecloth. Twist it and press to force out liquid. Use your body weight and all your might; press against a sturdy board, arranged so that liquid drains into a bowl. Get someone else to help you to double the force pressing liquid from the *moromi*. After you press as much as you think you can, open the sack, stir the contents, twist the bag as tight as you can, and press again. Use your engineering acumen to

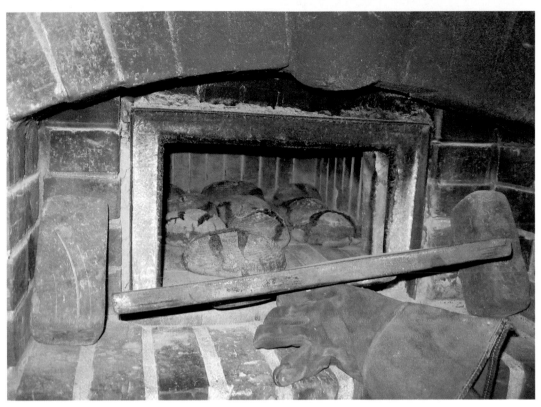

Freshly baked loaves of bread ready to come out of baker Brian Thomas's handbuilt wood-fired oven.

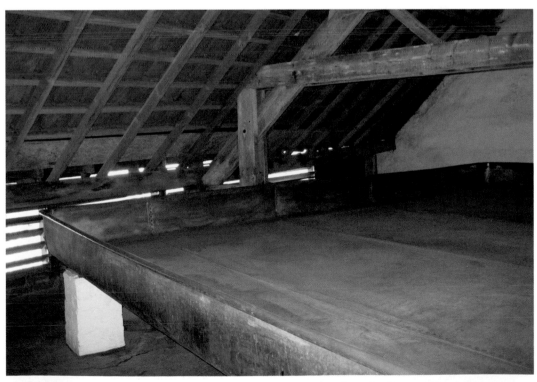

The *coolship* at Brewery Cantillon in Brussels, where the wort cools and collects wild yeast and bacteria from the air via its broad exposed surface.

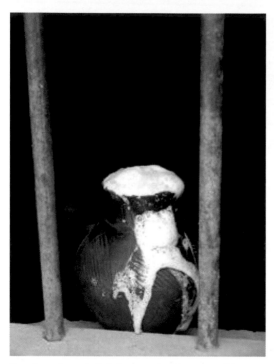

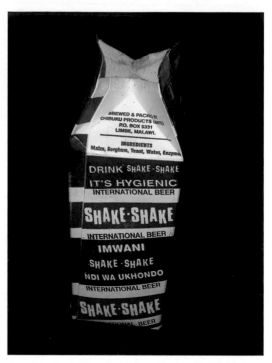

Sorghum beer (*pito*) fermenting in a gourd in Ghana. Photo courtesy of Fran Osseo-Asare, BETUMI www.betumi.com

Sorghum beer from a Malawi brewery, sold in waxed paper cartons, like milk. The name— Shake, Shake—is what you do to the beer before opening the carton to reintegrate starch that settles. Photo by Glenn Austerfield

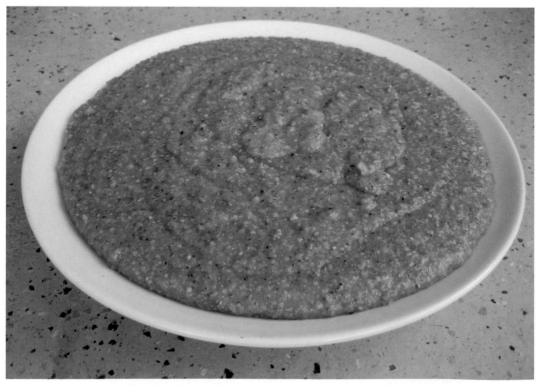

Aceda, Sudanese-style sorghum porridge.

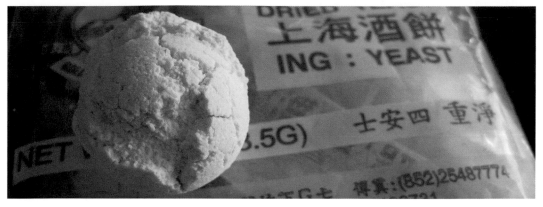

Chinese "yeast" balls, widely available in Asian markets.

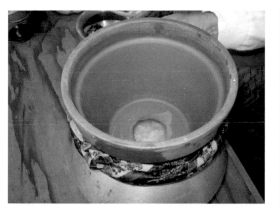
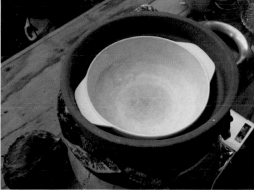

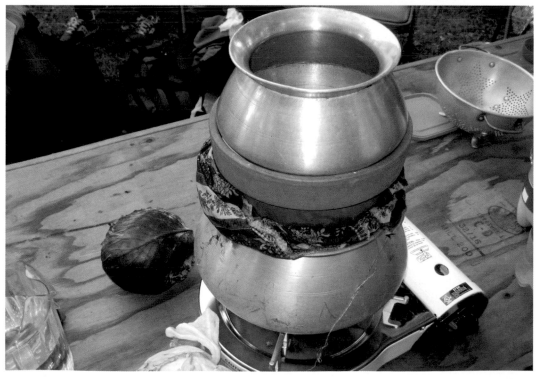

An improvised still constructed by Bhutanese and Nepali immigrants in Oakland, California, to make *raksi*.

19

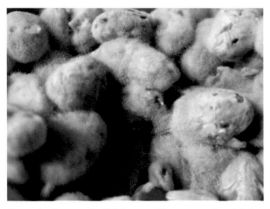

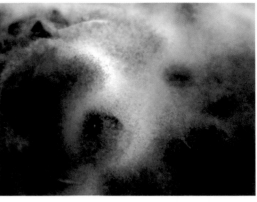

Sporulating soy *koji* (*Aspergillus oryzae*), with its "yellow robe." Photo by Lawrence Diggs

Sporulating tempeh (*Rhizopus oligosporus*), with its "white robe." Photo by Lawrence Diggs

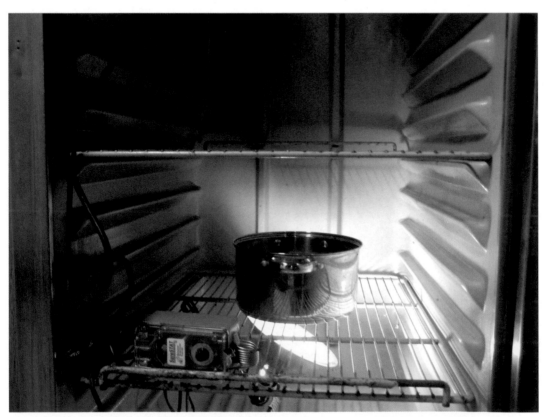

My incubator is a defunct commercial refrigerator, with an incandescent lightbulb as the source of heat. The light is under a pot of water, to diffuse heat and maintain humidity. The light is plugged into the temperature controller at lower left, which turns the light on when the temperature goes below 87°F/30°C and off when it goes above that. When the mold begins to generate heat and the temperature increases during the second half of a large batch, I prop the door open to release heat.

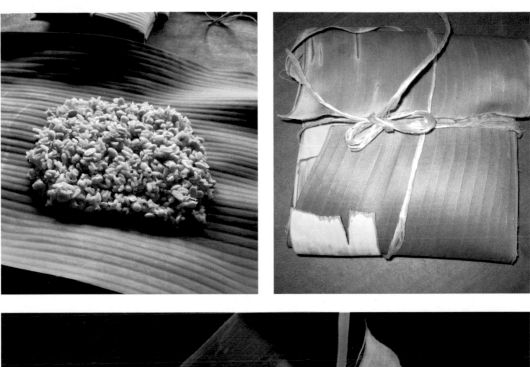

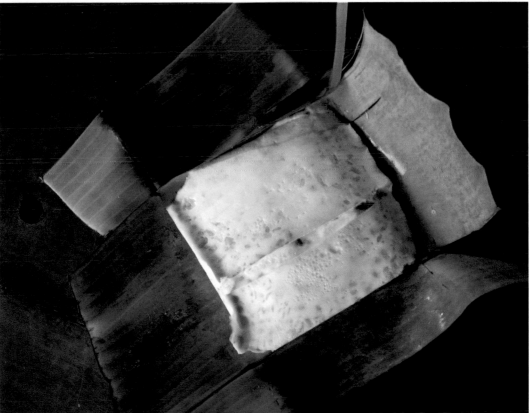

Making tempeh in banana leaves.

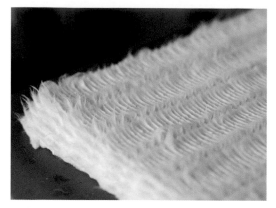

Making tempeh using a basket as a form in a high-humidity incubator. Photo by Caylan Larson

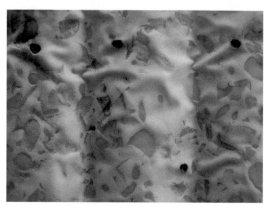

Tempeh made in a perforated plastic bag, beginning to sporulate; the dark spots, indicating sporulation, correspond with the airholes.

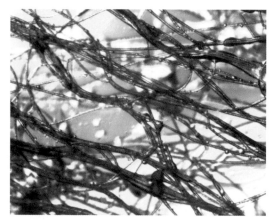

Mycelium of *Rhizopus oligosporus* on fresh tempeh. Photo courtesy of Erik Augustijns, www.tempeh.info

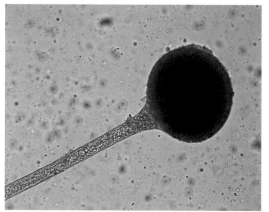

An *R. oligosporus* sporangium, ready to burst. Photo courtesy of Erik Augustijns, www.tempeh.info

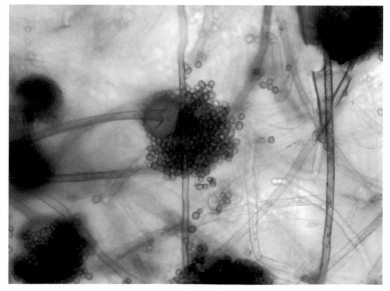

Spores release in sporulation. Photo courtesy of Erik Augustijns, www.tempeh.info

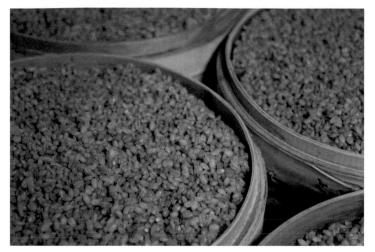
Steamed barley, in bamboo steamers, cooling. Photo by Timothy Bartling

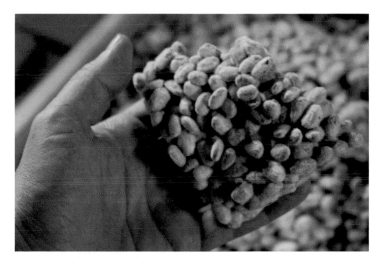
Soybean *koji*. Photo by Timothy Bartling

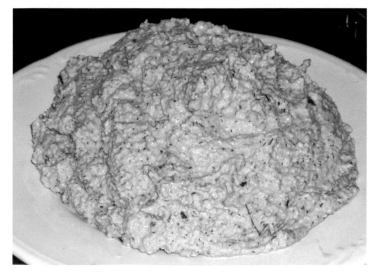
A sunflower seed cheese. Photo by Michelle Dick

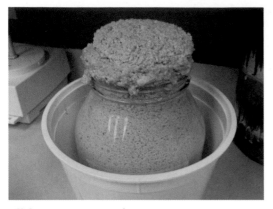

Idli batter rising out of a jar.

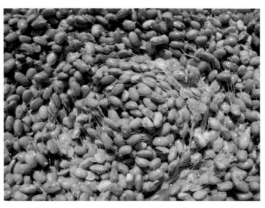

Natto is characterized by a stringy, mucilaginous coating on the beans.

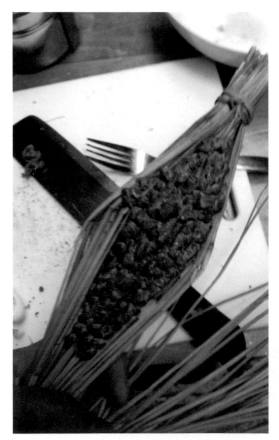

Wara natto is made and sold wrapped in straw. Photo by Sam Bett

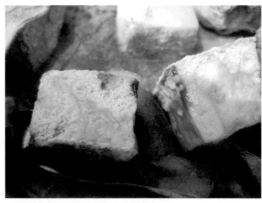

Bright-colored molds growing on tofu. Into the compost—a failed experiment.

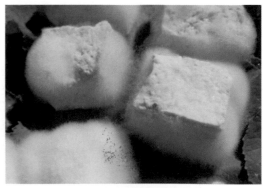

White, fluffy *Actinomucor elegans* growing on tofu.

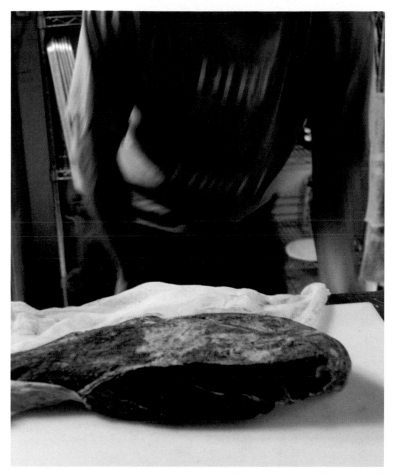

The author's first dry-curing experiment, a deer leg cured in the style of prosciutto. Photo by Timothy Bartling

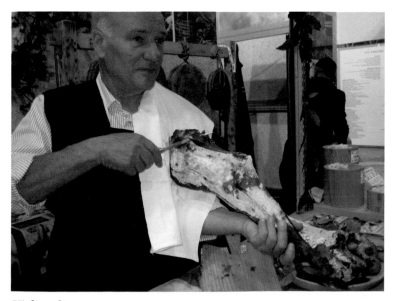

Violina di capra.

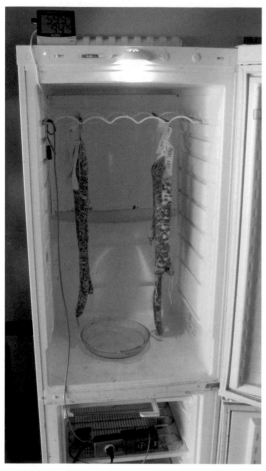

The author's salami-curing chamber, a refrigerator with an overriding temperature controller set for 57°F/14°C.

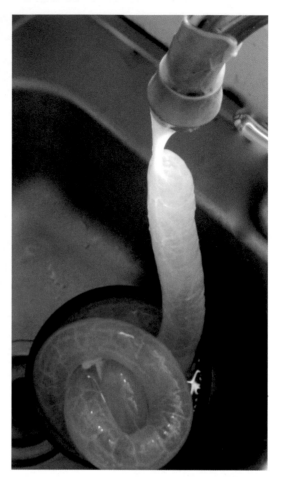

Rinsing casings prior to stuffing them.

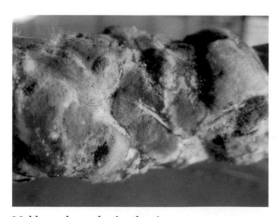

Molds on the author's salami.

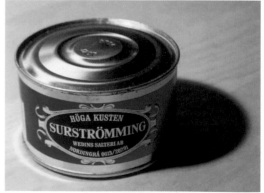

Bulging can of *surströmming*. Photo by Steffen Ramsaier

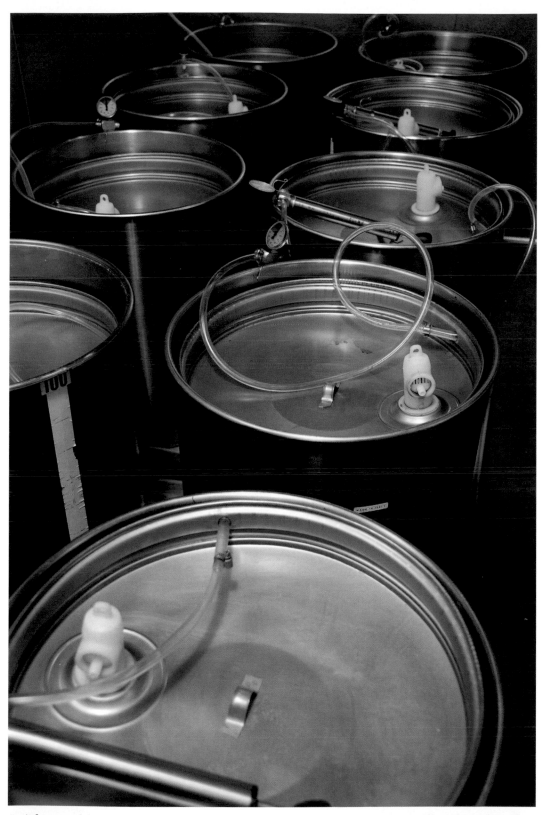

Stainless-steel fermentation vats at Cultured Pickle Shop in Berkeley, California. Photo by Cultured Pickle Shop

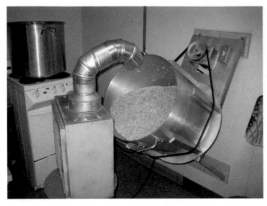

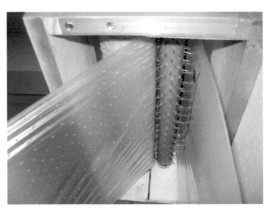

Tempeh drying device at The Tempeh Shop in Gainesville, Florida, created by the company's founder, Jose Caraballo.

The hole punch that Jose designed to perforate plastic bags for tempeh making.

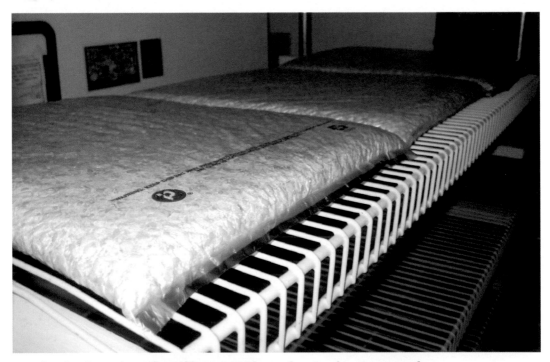

Inoculated soybeans in perforated bags, on racks, ready to incubate into tempeh.

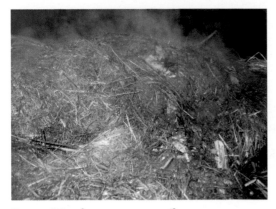

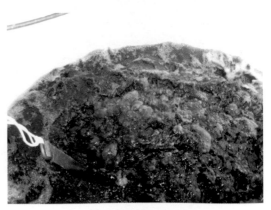

Steam rising from a compost pile.

Aerated compost tea bubbling away.

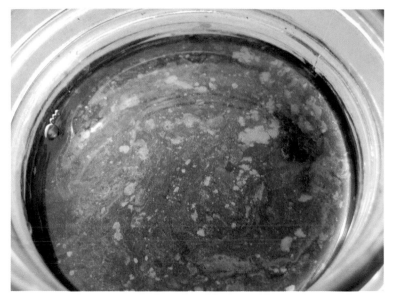

An indigo vat that has developed a coppery sheen following fermentation.

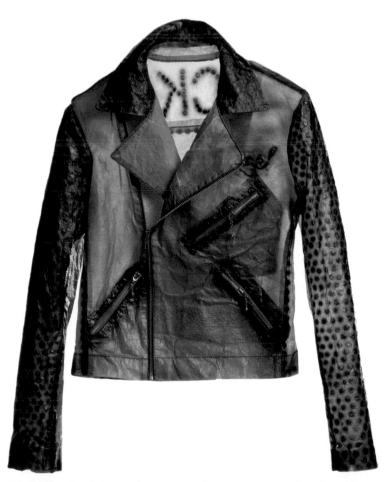

Kombucha fiber biker jacket designed by Suzanne Lee. Photo by BioCouture © 2011

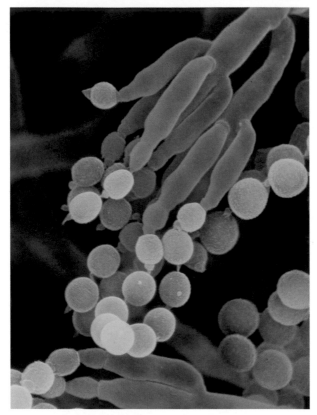

Penicillium mold. © Photo Researchers, Inc.

CULTURE

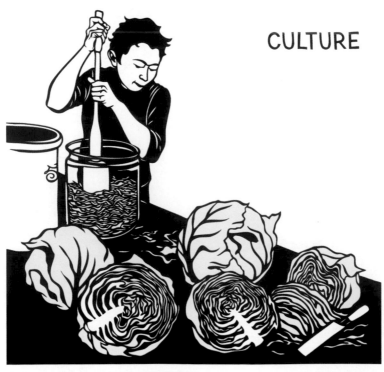

Culture, a papercut by Nikki McClure.

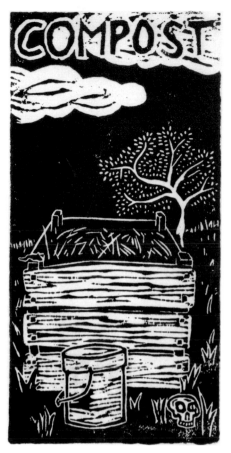

Compost woodblock print by David Bailey.

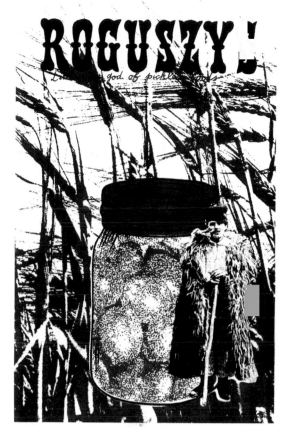

Roguszys: Lithuanian God of Pickled Foods, a silk-screen print by Caroline Paquita.

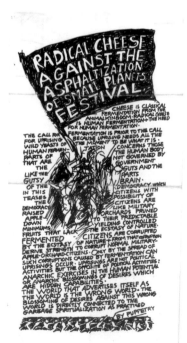

Radical Cheese Against the Asphaltization of Small Planets Festival, a print by Bread and Puppet Press.

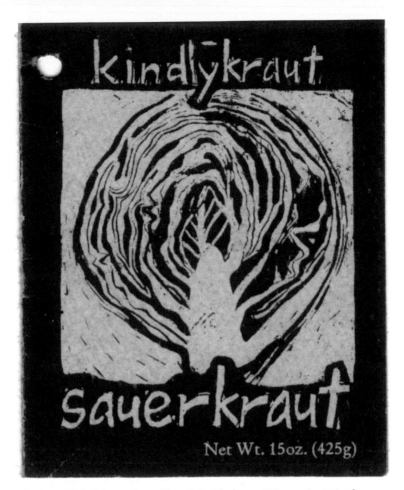

Artisanal label for artisanal kraut in Madison, Wisconsin. Print by Andy Hans

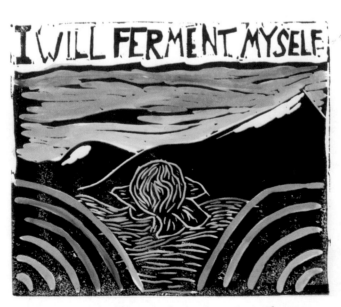

I Will Ferment Myself, a print by Modern Times Theater.

devise a makeshift press to express as much *shoyu* liquid as possible from the *moromi*.

Store *shoyu* in bottles in a refrigerator or cool spot. Mold may develop on the exposed surface of unpasteurized *shoyu*; if so, remove and discard the mold, and don't worry about it. Enjoy your rich, complex homemade *shoyu* as a seasoning, and save some to use as a starter for your next batch. The pressed *moromi* can be used as miso, or as a medium for pickling vegetables.

 ## Fermented Black Beans: *Hamanatto* and *Douchi*

Fermented black beans are whole fermented soybeans, known as *chi* or *ji* in China. They become black as a result of fermentation, but may be made from any soybeans. Fermented black beans are little known in the West but are considered to be the ancestor of all the more widely known fermented soybean pastes and sauces. "Ironically, this oldest of all fermented soyfoods is, today, the least widely known worldwide," write William Shurtleff and Akiko Aoyagi."[39]

The fermented black beans best known and most widely available in the West are the Chinese fermented black beans (*douchi*). A Japanese style, which I have made and describe below, is known as *hamanatto*. Note that *hamanatto* is completely different from the more widely known ferment called *natto* (described in the next section). I first became intrigued about *hamanatto* from a conversation with Cynthia Bates, a fermented soybean aficionado who has run the Tempeh Lab at The Farm in Tennessee for decades, who told me that the most delicious fermented soy she had ever tried was *hamanatto*. Indeed, the luscious, creamy, salty, sour, umami soybeans pack some dense and compelling flavor.

To make *hamanatto*, soak soybeans overnight and steam until soft. Drain the beans and allow them to cool to body temperature. Inoculate with soy *koji* (available from GEM Cultures). Incubate as described in *Making Koji*, chapter 10 at 80–90°F/27–32°C for 48 hours or longer. In this case, you want the mold to sporulate, so let it grow until it turns green. Once the mold sporulates on the soybeans, dry them in the sun or in a dehydrator. They need not be 100 percent crispy dry; an account by a USDA scientist investigating Japanese ferments notes that in commercial Japanese *hamanatto* production, beans are dried "until the moisture is reduced to 12 percent."[40] I have no means to gauge moisture content to that degree of precision, but the idea is that the beans should be mostly dry, but retain some moisture, and with it softness.

In the second stage of the fermentation, place these dried molded beans in a crock or other vessel that can be weighed down. Mix a 15 percent brine (15% salt based on the weight of the water) to cover it (that proportion is heavily diluted by the beans themselves). My pound-of-soybeans batch took less than 3 cups of brine to cover, and the brined beans filled just about a quart/liter of volume. Add thinly sliced ginger to the brined beans, stir well, weigh down, cover with a cloth to keep flies away, and ferment at ambient temperatures for six months to a year.

You can taste *hamanatto* beans as they ferment to sample their evolving flavor. When you deem them ready, dry them once again, in the sun or in a dehydrator. I dried mine after six months of fermentation. At first, while they were wet, it was difficult to separate out individual beans without crushing them. I just dumped the fermenting beans onto a baking sheet, broke them up into clumps, and put the tray outside under bright sun. Within a few hours, the clumps had dried enough that it was easier to crumble them into individual beans. As the beans dried, I was able to separate them into individual beans that looked like raisins. I also separated out the strips of ginger, which were super-tasty, and sliced them into slivers. After a few days of alternating between days in the sun and nights with a fan blowing on them, the black beans were dry. Don't overdry them. They shouldn't be hard or brittle, but still soft and supple, like raisins.

Hamanatto is so delicious! I enjoyed them as snacks, but they are too salty to eat more than a few. I used them mostly as a deeply flavored base for sauces and dressings, modeled loosely on the renowned Chinese black bean sauce. (The Chinese black beans are fermented in a nearly identical process, described below.) Cover a few tablespoonfuls of *hamanatto* with water. Let them soak in water a few minutes, then remove beans from water and mince them finely (save the soaking water). Heat oil and stir-fry garlic, shallots, and/or onions with the minced soy nuggets. Then add soaking water, stock, rice beer or vinegar, soy sauce, hot sauce, a little honey, sugar, or other sweetener, any other beloved condiments, and a little cornstarch, dissolved in water, to thicken. Keep stirring the sauce as it cooks for a few minutes, until it begins to thicken; enjoy this compelling fermented bean sauce on almost anything. You can also simply add them whole into sauces or braising liquids that will cook for a while.

Soybeans

Chinese black beans, *douchi*—the traditional basis for this sauce—are made in a process similar to *hamanatto*. Soybeans (yellow or black) are soaked, cooked until soft, cooled, inoculated with *Aspergillus* spores or mixed mold cultures, and incubated around 80–90°F/27–32°C for about 72 hours, until the mold on the beans turns green, indicating sporulation. In contrast to the *hamanatto* method described above, in the *douchi* method the beans are not dried at this stage but rather washed, to remove the spores, which would impart bitter flavor. For the second-stage fermentation, the beans are fermented in brine, sometimes with sugar and/or hot chili paste, for four to six months, then dried.[41]

Natto

Natto is a Japanese soy ferment that produces a slimy, mucilaginous coating on the beans, something like okra. In Japanese, this quality is called *neba*;

natto that is extra slimy is *neba-neba*. "High viscosity of the mucilage is the most important criterion of a good *natto*," according to the *Journal of Food Science*.[42] The flavor of natto carries notes of ammonia (like some cheeses or overripe tempeh), which gets stronger as it ferments longer. I have come to love *natto*, but many people not raised on it find it unappealing and even scary.

Natto is quite widely available in Japanese markets and restaurants, although in restaurants more often than not I have had waiters try to talk me out of ordering it, I suppose because the uninitiated so frequently dislike it. *Natto* is definitely not for everyone, but some people *really* like it, and if you are an adventurous eater, I would definitely recommend trying it. As with many foods, how it is prepared and presented can make all the difference.

Natto-like ferments are found in China (*tan-shih*), Thailand (*thua-nao*), Korea (*joenkuk-jang* and *damsue-jang*), Nepal (*kinema*), and elsewhere in East Asia.[43] A similar group of ferments, prepared from other seeds, are found across West Africa (see next section). *Natto* and its relations are different from all the other soy ferments in that no molds are involved in the fermentation, nor any lactic acid bacteria. *Bacillus subtilis* var. *natto* (formerly known as *Bacillus natto*), the bacteria that transform soybeans into *natto*, are alkaline-forming rather than acidifying. I have mostly made *natto* with a starter I purchased from GEM, imported from Japan. You can also start it from a commercially available *natto* or a previous homemade batch, use straw as a starter, as was traditionally practiced, or even let *natto* spontaneously develop on soybeans in the recommended temperature range, which it generally will, as it is typically present on beans and its spores are extremely heat-tolerant.

The only challenging aspect of making *natto* is finding or creating an appropriate incubation space. The ideal incubation temperature for fermenting *natto* is about 104°F/40°C, though it can tolerate a much wider range, from about body temperature to 113°F/45°C. I usually use the oven with pilot light for incubating *natto*. You can also use a prewarmed insulated cooler with hot-water bottles to help maintain temperature.

Natto is typically made with soybeans. I have tried to make it with other types of beans and always produced something edible, but in some cases without the characteristic slimy natto coating. To make *natto*, rinse beans and soak overnight in a generous amount of water, as soybeans more than double in size during soaking. Boil or steam the soaked soybeans until they are soft enough to easily crush between your thumb and index finger, about five hours. If you have a pressure cooker, steam under pressure for about 45 minutes; steaming soybeans is better than boiling them in a pressure cooker, as skins can slip off beans into the water, rise in the foam, and clog the release valve. Explosions have been known to occur.

Once soybeans are cooked soft, drain and begin to cool. If you are using spores to start your *natto*, inoculate the beans while they are still steaming hot, around 175°F/80°C. The literature suggests that the spores not only tolerate but benefit from "heat-shock" at temperatures as high as this.[44] Use whatever proportion of starter its source recommends. Such a minuscule amount of starter is required that it needs to be mixed with another more voluminous powdery medium—flour—in order to effectively distribute it. If your *natto* starter is a previous batch of *natto*, use starter at a ratio of roughly 5 percent. Mince starter *natto* finely, add a little incubation-temperature water to it, and add it to cooked soybeans only after they have cooled to incubation temperatures, since the growing bacteria do not possess the heat tolerance of the spores. Either way, mix starter into the soybeans thoroughly, taking care to scrape the edges to be sure to incorporate all the beans.

Spread cultured soybeans in an even layer, no deeper than 2 inches/5 cm, in a glass or stainless-steel baking pan. Cover them with plastic wrap, aluminum foil, or waxed paper, to maintain humidity. Place in the incubation chamber and ferment, for 6 to 24 hours, depending on the temperature and desired flavor. Monitor the incubation chamber and adjust the temperature as necessary, by propping open to cool, or adding bottles with hot water to heat. To test if the *natto* is ready, swirl the soybeans with chopsticks or a spoon and see if gooey strings form. Longer incubation will yield more pronounced stringiness and stronger flavor.

If you want to try making *natto* without a starter, follow all the steps described above, without inoculation. Do not pressure-cook the beans if you are attempting a spontaneous *natto* fermentation, because the higher temperatures of pressure-cooking would likely kill the spores that can survive boiling. Expect that the *natto* may take a little longer to develop, and may have a stronger flavor than *natto* made with a selected bacterial strain. You could also try the traditional method of using straw as a starter. According to Shurtleff and Aoyagi, "In the old days natto was generally made . . . by simply wrapping cooked soybeans in rice straw and putting them in a warm place overnight until they became sticky."[45] Fermentation enthusiast Sam Bett reports from Japan that he ate some *wara* [straw] *natto* that he bought at a grocery store. "It has an earthier flavor than the Styrofoam-packed varieties. It's also more pungent, far more sticky and stringy, and more delicious."

Natto is rarely eaten plain. If you want to experience *natto* in its full glory in a classic Japanese way, mix some with a raw egg yolk and a little *shoyu*, mustard, and rice vinegar. Stir with chopsticks in a circular motion to merge the liquid condiments with the slimy bean coating. Enjoy on warm rice, topped with chopped scallions and small pieces of nori seaweed. If you wish to avoid or downplay the sliminess of the beans, that can be minimized by incorporating the beans into nori rolls, salads, or savory pancakes, or mince them as an ingredient in sauces and dressings.

Natto has received considerable attention in recent years for the health benefits of a unique compound, called *nattokinase*, produced by the fermenting bacteria and found in the viscous goo. A 1987 report in the journal *Cellular and Molecular Life Sciences* announced that "strong fibrinolytic activity [meaning that it breaks down blood clots] was demonstrated" in what the investigators somewhat awkwardly described as "the vegetable cheese natto."[46] Fifteen years later, a review of the medical literature summarized: "All prior epidemiologic and clinical research points to *nattokinase's* effectiveness and safety for managing a wide range of diseases, including hypertension, atherosclerosis, coronary artery disease (such as angina), stroke, and peripheral vascular disease. Evidence from long-term use at high doses in Japanese people points to *nattokinase* as a safe nutrient that acts as a very powerful fibrinolytic agent."[47] The latest research is exploring whether in addition to breaking down fibrin, *nattokinase* may be effective in breaking down amyloid plaque characteristic of Alzheimer's disease.[48] Because medicine always seeks to isolate active compounds from the foods they come from, *nattokinase* is more widely available as an extract in vitamin supplement shops than in the whole-food form of *natto*.

Dawadawa and Related West African Fermented Seed Condiments

Across West Africa, cuisines feature a range of *natto*-like fermented condiments made from the seeds of a number of wild and cultivated plants, some inedible unless fermented. Plants whose seeds are used in such preparations include melons (*Citrullus vulgaris*), African locust beans (*Parkia biglobosa*), African oil beans (*Pentaclethra macrophylla*), mesquite (*Prosopis africana*), baobab (*Adansonia digitata*), Saman tree (*Albizia saman*), fluted pumpkin (*Telferia occidentalis*), castor beans (*Ricinus communis*), and others, including, increasingly, soybeans.[49] According to Nigerian microbiologist O. K. Achi, "The conventional substrates for condiment production are diverse and each can be produced from more than one raw material."[50]

Like *natto*, these ferments are alkaline, produced by the action of *Bacillus subtilis* and closely related bacteria, and used as condiments and flavorings. A few of the more commonly used names for the products of these fermentations include *dawadawa* and *ogiri* in Nigeria, *soumbala* in Burkina Faso, Mali, and Guinea, and *netetou* in Senegal. One Dakar survey "showed its use in almost all the main recipes of Senegalese cuisine."[51]

At the risk of overgeneralization, I am grouping these together to illustrate that the alkaline *Bacillus* fermentation of beans and seeds is fairly widespread, and not limited to a single geographic area. In my travels in West Africa in my youth, I undoubtedly ate stews flavored with some of these ferments, but unfortunately I was not aware of them and did not discern their flavors or inquire as to how they are produced. Yet when I finally experimented with making *dawadawa* and tried it as a seasoning in cooking, I realized how familiar its distinctive flavor was, a long-ago impression, barely conscious, of a deep umami undercurrent in the stews of West Africa.

From the literature I can see that the ferments making up this group are quite distinct, and specifics of preparations vary. However, they seem to exhibit some general patterns. Usually, beans or seeds are boiled, sometimes for a very long time, until they are soft enough to manually dehull. Then they are dehulled, and in some cases boiled again. In some traditions, seeds are fermented whole; in others, they are sliced or pounded. In some cases ashes are mixed in. Typically the preparation is wrapped in banana or other large leaves to maintain moisture. Usually no starter is used, although in some cases ferments are cultured by means of backslopping from a previous batch. Nonetheless, "there is a predominant development of *Bacillus* species during the various legume fermentation processes," according to Achi. "The consistency of the fermenting vegetable mash as fermentation progressed could be described as a thick cheesy pudding." Fermentation times vary with substrate, environment, and tradition. In most cases the completed ferments are sun-dried for storage because they "do not keep well if the fermentation is allowed to continue long uninhibited."[52]

The major limitation I faced in trying to experiment with these ferments was lack of access to the specific seeds described in the literature. I tried it with mesquite seeds from Southwest desert mesquite pods sent to me by my friend Brad Lancaster, in Tucson, Arizona, but the seeds were so tiny that after an hour of dehulling I had accumulated no more than about a teaspoonful of them. I wrapped these in an amaranth leaf, and they molded. I thought about trying it with castor beans, but my faith in the detoxifying powers of fermentation was challenged by my research, which found just 1 milligram of ricin, the most toxic compound in the beans, can kill an adult.[53] While the fermentation of the beans, as traditionally practiced, evidently detoxifies them, experimenting with a wild fermentation in a very different environment could potentially yield very different results. If I fermented a mash of castor beans, would I be prepared to taste it, knowing of the beans' potentially extreme toxicity? And would I want to encourage readers to do so? So, lacking access to any of the other African beans these condiments are made of, I followed the historical trend and tried the ferment with the number one global superstar legume, soybeans.

Charles Parkouda et al. summarize the process for *soydawadawa*: "Soybeans are sorted, washed, soaked in water for 12 hours and dehulled by hand. They are then cooked for 2 hours and incubated in calabashes lined with plantain leaves to ferment for 72 hours."[54] O. K. Achi describes a slightly different process:

> The cotyledons are spread in a raffia basket lined with banana leaves and then covered with several layers of the banana leaves. This is left to ferment for 2–3 days. Wood ash may be added. The fermented product is then sun dried for 1–2 days to yield a dark brown or black product.[55]

I soaked soybeans overnight and manually dehulled by rubbing beans between the palms of my hands. I boiled soybeans about four hours, until soft.

Then I placed them, with no added ingredients whatsoever, in a glass pie dish lined with corn husks (no banana or plantain leaves), and wrapped them in the husks to maintain moisture and support bacterial growth. I covered the wrapped soybeans with an inverted bowl and left it in my oven—with the heat off, the illuminating lamp on, and the door propped open slightly—to ferment. I left it about 36 hours, around 100°F/38°C. It was just like *natto*, when it's getting really strong.

What really distinguishes *soydawadawa* from *natto* is what you do next, which is to dry it. I dried mine as whole beans—although some of these condiment traditions grind it into a paste first. Sun-dry if possible, or use a dehydrator or a low oven. The dried fermented beans are shelf-stable. Grind them into a powder to use. Add to stews and other foods as a seasoning. No need to add a lot; just a dash of it adds a subtle yet dense layer of flavor. Senegalese food blogger Rama uses *netetou*, a condiment in this group, in one of her online recipes, with a blunt warning: "It has a VERY strong smell but adds such incredible flavor to stews."[56] I love it, and now that I know about it I intend to experiment more with using it. Yum!

Fermenting Tofu

Among the few traditional soy foods *not* fermented in their preparation is tofu. However, once it is tofu, it may be fermented. In fact, there are many different ways of fermenting tofu. Fermented tofu is known by various names, among them *sufu* and *doufu-ru*. Tofu being the ultimate in bland foods, the process of fermentation gives it a more pronounced flavor. Fermented tofu is "long renowned as one of those special gastronomic delectables that is often irresistible to the aficionado but obnoxious to the uninitiated," observes H. T. Huang.[57] Depending upon the process used and the length of fermentation, the resulting flavor can range from subtly sharp to overpoweringly acrid. The fermentation also improves tofu's digestibility. An 1861 Chinese food encyclopedia states: "Hardened tofu is [difficult to digest], and it is not healthful for children, elderly persons or ill persons. *Sufu*, which is prepared from tofu, is better because it is aged; it is very good for patients."[58]

The most comprehensive information on the subject that I've been able to find in English is yet another book by William Shurtleff and Akiko Aoyago, their *Book of Tofu*. The most straightforward method they describe for fermenting tofu is to cut it into slices or bite-size cubes and simply marinate them for a few days in miso, its Chinese equivalent *jiang*, or soy sauce. In China, this is known as *jiang-doufu*. You can eat *jiang-doufu* uncooked, prepare it any way you would tofu, or blend the fermented tofu and its marinade together into a sauce.

Most methods of fermenting tofu involve growing molds on the tofu and then aging the molded tofu in brine and/or rice wine with various spices. The molded tofu is known as *pehtze*. Microbial analysis has revealed that the molded *pehtze* is typically dominated by molds of the genera *Actinomucor*, *Rhizopus*, and *Mucor*. Among the traditional methods of inoculation are placing slices or cubes of tofu on rice straw[59] or pumpkin leaves[60] and/or coating them with fresh wood ash.[61] By some accounts, the cubes of tofu are partially dried and sterilized first in a minimally heated oven for 10 to 15 minutes.[62]

I've tried spontaneously growing molds on cubes of tofu packed in both straw (though not rice straw) and pumpkin leaves. The descriptions in the literature refer to white or gray mold growth. Shurtleff and Aoyagi describe a "dense mat of fragrant white mycelium,"[63] while Steinkraus refers to "grayish hairlike mycelium."[64] The molds that developed spontaneously on my two experiments were yellow with patches of bright red, nothing suitable for consumption. But when I tried it with a pure culture sample of *Actinomucor elegans* that I obtained from the US Department of Agriculture's Culture Collection,[65] I had great results. After the fluffy white mold developed, I mixed brine (see *Brining* in chapter 5), added rice beer (see *Asian Rice Brews* in chapter 9) and fresh chili peppers, and fermented the molded tofu in that. The molded and fermented tofu cubes developed a sublimely smooth texture and a compelling sharp flavor. They are extremely cheese-like and became more and more delicious with the passing weeks, until they went too far, after about three months.

I've also had great results fermenting tofu, without molds, using a method from the Chinese city of Shaoxing, called *chou dou fu*, or "stinking tofu," which I prepared following a description by food writer Fuchsia Dunlop. Prior to fermenting the tofu, you must ferment amaranth stalks in brine to prepare a *lu*, the medium in which the tofu is fermented. That process is described in *Chinese Pickling*, chapter 5. Then you simply add cubes of tofu to this brine and leave them to ferment submerged in the jar or crock. Like much information on fermentation, Dunlop's account gave no specifics as to the length of fermentation. In the early days and weeks, the fermenting tofu smelled and tasted wonderful. Nothing was stinky about it whatsoever. As late as six weeks into the fermentation, the tofu tasted delicious to me, sharp and pungent, but in no way off-putting or challenging.

However, when I went away for three weeks and tasted my fermenting tofu upon my return, it had developed the stinkiness suggested by its name. "Hydrogen sulphide produced during the breakdown of one or more sulphur-containing amino acids is the source of the finished product's disgusting smell," explains Dunlop. This is the same gas that gives rotten eggs their notorious odor. According to Dunlop, Shaoxing street vendors, who deep-fry the stinky tofu, "perfume their entire neighborhoods" with this odor, which "inspires incredible passion in its devotees."[66] At this stage of development I fed the stinking tofu to the compost, and the next batch I enjoyed while it was still fragrant and delicious.

Even without preparing special brine, tofu can be incorporated into vegetable ferments. "Usually I put it up with kimchi seasonings, but it's also good plain," writes fermentation enthusiast Anna Root. "It keeps well (unlike fresh tofu), and it's very easy to digest, even eaten raw. If you make it salty enough, it tastes like feta cheese."

 ## Troubleshooting

Surface mold on miso

You can be sure that a miso crock that sits fermenting, undisturbed for a year or longer, is likely to be covered with mold. Sometimes when a crock is first uncovered, the surface growth makes the miso look hideous. Sometimes it smells awful too. Do not be afraid. Scrape the moldy layer off, along with any miso that has been discolored by it, and discard. Below it, the miso protected from air always looks, smells, and tastes good.

Dry and shrunken miso

If long-fermenting miso is aged in a space that is heated, it will dry out and shrink over the course of its long fermentation. How to proceed depends upon how dry and shrunken it is. If it smells and looks fine (once you scrape away the mold), simply add a little water and stir it in evenly to restore the miso to a pasty, spreadable texture. If the miso has hardened and feels like a brick, there may be no way to moisten it into a paste. If that is the case, discard it. Long-fermenting misos really require an unheated cellar space or burying crocks in the earth. If you wish to make miso in a heated living space, I would recommend trying shorter-fermenting sweet misos that take only several weeks, ferment fine at ambient heated temperatures, and do not age long enough to be dehydrated by dry heat.

Moldy pockets throughout miso

Surface molds are easy to remove, because they are limited to the surface. However, if you make miso and fail to pack it firmly enough into its vessel, leaving large air pockets, it is possible for those pockets of air to develop molds that you encounter as you dig the miso out of the crock. If it is limited to one or two pockets, you may be able to isolate them and remove the mold. If there are pockets throughout, removal may prove to be impossible. To avoid this problem, be sure to press miso firmly downward as you pack it into its fermentation vessel to eliminate air pockets.

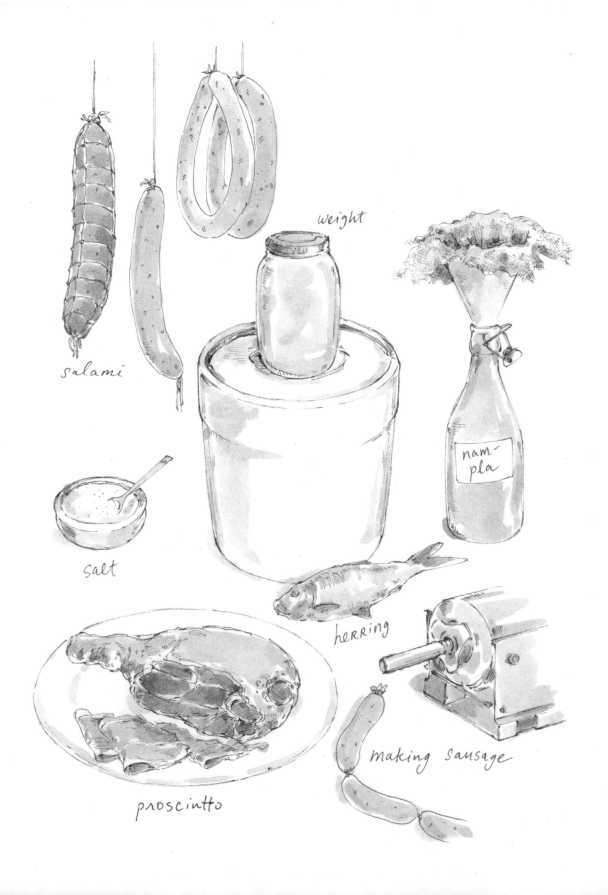

salami

weight

nam-pla

salt

herring

proscintto

making sausage

CHAPTER 12

Fermenting Meat, Fish, and Eggs

*A*ll around the world, wherever people have faced seasonal scarcity preceded by periods of abundant meat or fish, cultures developed means of preserving these critical food resources. From our vantage point—through the distorted lens of our historical bubble of refrigeration and freezing—it is almost impossible to conceive of how meat and fish can be stored, distributed, and used without these technologies. Flesh is the least stable of any food we eat. At typical ambient temperatures, it rapidly loses its freshness through the action of putrefying bacteria and enzymes. More than any other food, flesh is susceptible to bacterial contamination and regarded as a potentially dangerous vector of contagion. Refrigeration extends the edibility of meat and fish (as well as other foods) essentially by slowing fermentation and enzyme activity. Prior to the advent of refrigeration, people used various other lower-tech approaches to more modest cooling, such as burying, cellars, spring boxes, and iceboxes. Throughout history, people also developed a range of other techniques to stop, slow, or limit the enzymatic and bacterial degradation of meat and fish, including drying, salting, smoking, curing, and, of course, fermentation.

These methods have been used in many different combinations. Fish and meat may be dried with or without salting or curing, and with or without smoking, depending upon climate, available resources, and traditions. They may also be salted and/or smoked without being fully dried. The role of fermentation has not always been self-evident, though in many cases the means by which meat and fish are preserved also involve fermentation. In general, limited drying, salting, smoking, and/or curing are used, sometimes along with the addition of other substrates, to strategically create selective environments to inhibit growth of pathogenic bacteria and allow for more desirable forms of microbial growth.

Meat and fish, in particular, are fundamentally different from all the other food substances that people ferment. With only minor environmental manipulation, lactic acid bacteria and yeasts reliably dominate all raw plant substrates, as well as animal products such as milk and honey. To the extent that potentially dangerous microorganisms may be present on these foods, the rapid production of acids and/or alcohol destroys them. In contrast, meat and fish flesh comprises virtually no carbohydrates, the nutrients that support the usual fermentation organisms. Furthermore, interior flesh is sterile, and when it is exposed to a multitude of microbes during slaughtering and butchering, the microbes that typically develop can result in decay and putrefaction in addition to fermentation (a sometimes slippery boundary).

The most feared microorganism of them all, *Clostridium botulinum*, creates no visible decay or perceptible putrefaction, but rather the most toxic substance known to humans, the botulism neurotoxin, fatal at oral doses as small as a single one-millionth of a gram per kilogram of body weight.[1] Botulism is most widely known in association with low-acid canned foods, including vegetables. This is because *C. botulinum*—a common soil microorganism— produces spores that are tolerant to extremely high heat. So if insufficient heat treatment of the canned food succeeds at killing all other bacteria but leaves spores of *C. botulinum* intact in a low-acid medium, they can develop and produce the neurotoxin, facilitated by the perfectly anaerobic environment of a vacuum-sealed jar or can.

Before the invention of canning in the 19th century, botulism was associated with sausages. Ground meat stuffed into casings presents another potentially hospitable anaerobic environment for *C. botulinum*. The word *botulism* even derives from the Latin word for "sausage," *botulus*, and it was through people getting sick from uncooked dry-cured sausages that botulism was first observed and named. Today in North America, a high proportion of botulism cases are reported in Alaska, where some native people, who have traditionally fermented fish in grass-lined pits, are now making the mistake of using plastic to contain fish ferments, thereby creating a perfect anaerobic environment for *C. botulinum*. With this potential in mind, I encourage readers to be sure they understand the parameters for safe fermentation of fish and meat and heed them; in contrast with the realm of raw plant matter, where it is perfectly safe to experiment free from fear, meat and fish have greater potential to be dangerous. This is not intended to discourage you from trying your hand at fermenting meat or fish. Do experiment, but be aware of potential dangers and be smart about it.

herring

That said, flesh can be fermented with delicious results. Fermented meat and fish are crucial to survival in some regions of the world and make up some of the greatest culinary delights in many more. In some places, *fresh* meat and fish have even been regarded with suspicion.[2] To be perfectly honest, I have much more limited personal experience fermenting flesh as compared with plant matter or other animal products (such as honey and milk). My experimentation is ongoing. Despite the limits of my experience, I have extensively researched this realm of fermentation, exploring the literature and visiting, questioning, and corresponding with fellow experimentalists and artisan practitioners. Knowing well that there is a huge amount of interest in this topic and little clear information, I offer this chapter as an overview of meat and fish fermentation concepts and methods, and the broader range of preservation techniques with which it is practiced.

Drying, Salting, Smoking, and Curing

When fish or meat is dried, it is precisely in order to prevent microbial and enzymatic transformations. With drying, the objective is to deprive these organisms and processes of the water they need in order to function. *C. botulinum*, for example, cannot grow in an environment with a water activity (a_w) measurement below 0.94, while inhibiting *Listeria monocytogenes* requires a drier environment, below 0.83 a_w.[3]

Of course, flesh does not dry instantly, so there is always some level of incidental microbial activity along the way. Botulism is not a concern in this context, because the environment is far from anaerobic. In dried meats, such as jerky, biltong, and pemmican, and dried fish, such as stockfish and salt cod, microbial growth and enzyme activity that occurs during drying may indeed even contribute to the flavor and texture of the resulting product. However, fermentation is not what preserves the flesh; it is the drying that does.

Overlapping with drying, there is also salting and smoking. In a dry, cool, sunny climate, such as the coast of Norway, lean fish can be rapidly dried in the air without either salt or smoke. But in many climates, the sun cannot typically dry flesh before putrefaction sets in. Along the Pacific coast of North America, for instance, many native peoples relied upon smoke from smoldering fires to dry salmon. But smoke also transforms food in other ways as it dries. Wood smoke contains many chemical compounds. "The sugars in cellulose . . . break apart into many of the same molecules found in caramel, with sweet, fruity, flowery, bready aromas," explains Harold McGee. Wood smoke also produces "volatile phenolics and other fragments, which have the specific aromas of vanilla and clove as well as generic spiciness, sweetness, and pungency."[4] The chemicals in smoke include not only rich flavors, but also antimicrobial and anti-oxidant compounds that inhibit the growth of bacteria and fungi, and slow the oxidation of fats that results in rancidity.[5] Unfortunately, residual compounds from smoke in meat and fish may also be carcinogenic to people.

Salting has also played an important role in meat and fish preservation, in both products that are dried and those that are not. (And heavy salt consumption, too, has been associated with many health problems.) Through the physical process of osmosis, salting draws water out of flesh, while simultaneously making the water that remains less available for microbial growth, even without sun, heat, or smoke. In addition to reducing water activity in the flesh, salt itself inhibits certain microorganisms and enzymes; therefore the level of salinity is an important determinant of what types of organisms can grow. Ten percent salt content—extremely salty—inhibits the growth of *C. botulinum* at typical ambient temperatures and a neutral pH.[6] Much lower salt concentrations can inhibit *C. botulinum* and other pathogenic bacteria when used in combination with acidification, cool temperatures, and/or limited drying.

Curing is closely related to salting. In the preservation of meat and fish, the word *cure* is simultaneously vague and specific. Broadly it encompasses all forms of post-harvest ripening; tobacco, firewood, sweet potatoes, olives, and bacon are among the many plant and animal products that are routinely described as being cured. In the context of preserving meat and fish, curing often means simply the application of salt, often along with spice and sometimes sugar. For instance, the Scandinavian preparation *gravlax* is today prepared not by burying salmon underground (as its historical antecedents were), but rather by coating the fish with salt, sugar, dill, and other spices and thus curing it in the refrigerator for several days. The curing reduces the water content of the flesh, limits its microbial and enzymatic degradation, and causes chemical reactions that alter its texture and structure.

In some cases, *cure* has a much more specific meaning: the use of specific mineral salt compounds called curing salts—nitrite and sometimes nitrate—to cause chemical reactions that help preserve meat. Potassium nitrate (KNO_3), more commonly known as saltpeter, has long been used as a meat-curing agent (as well as an ingredient in gunpowder, and more recently in agricultural fertilizers). Historically, in meat curing, saltpeter was prized especially for its ability to enhance the red color of meat and was also recognized as improving the safety of the meat and the length of time it could be preserved. After the advent of microbiology, around the beginning of the 20th century, it was recognized that bacteria in the curing meat slowly break down nitrate (NO_3) into nitrite (NO_2), and that nitrite is actually the compound that preserves meat, rather than nitrate. By reacting with the meat protein myoglobin, nitrite prevents oxidation of fats and produces the bright pink color characteristic of cured meats. By reacting with proteins in some bacterial cells, nitrite deactivates enzymes critical to the growth of *C. botulinum* and certain other bacteria.

Nitrite is used for meat curing primarily in the salt form of sodium nitrite ($NaNO_2$). In longer-curing meats, where the slow breakdown of nitrates into nitrites is desirable, sodium nitrate ($NaNO_3$) is also used. Nitrite and nitrate are often described as curing salts, "insta-cure," or pink salt. These chemicals are used only in minute amounts, because in larger doses, nitrite is toxic. Just as it binds with myoglobin in meat, nitrite binds with hemoglobin in our blood to create methemoglobin, which decreases the capacity of the blood to transport oxygen.

Some nitrite and nitrate consumption is inevitable. Nitrate is an integral part of the nitrogen cycle and is so common in soil and plant tissue that we typically ingest it every day. Even cabbages and sauerkraut contain nitrate, kraut at slightly higher levels than raw cabbages.[7] Our saliva and digestive tracts break down some of the nitrate we eat into nitrite, and our bodies normally tolerate a limited ongoing level of methemoglobin in the blood. But excessive consumption of nitrite and nitrate causes excessive production of methemoglobin, which can be fatal. US law limits the level of sodium nitrate in cured meat products to 500 parts per million (ppm) and the amount of sodium nitrite to 200 ppm. In the European Union, permitted levels are even lower.

Toxicity due to methemoglobin production is not the only health concern about nitrate and nitrite in meat. Nitrite can react with amino acids to form compounds called nitrosamines, especially in the highly acidic environment of our stomachs, and the high-temperature environment of a frying pan. "Nitrosamines are known to be powerful DNA-damaging chemicals," states Harold McGee.[8] Yet epidemiological studies have been inconclusive at linking consumption of nitrite-cured meats with increased cancer risk. "Still, it's probably prudent to eat cured meats in moderation and cook them gently," concludes McGee.

Dry-Curing Basics

Dry-curing is simply the direct application of salt to meat (or fish). The salt simultaneously draws water out of the meat and absorbs into it. "The longer you cure meat in salt, the more stable, and salty, it will become," explains Hugh Fearnley-Whittingstall, whose *River Cottage Meat Book* has an excellent section on curing meat. "Almost any part of any animal will have been tossed or packed or rubbed in salt somewhere in the world."[9] For salt to be the primary means of preservation, typically the meat or fish must be saltier than is generally regarded as palatable. In this case, either meat is used to flavor and salt stews and sauces or soaked in order to remove salt before consumption.

Sometimes salted meats are cured only a short time and then cooked, as with bacon and some styles of ham. In other instances, when salted meats are hung for long aging after the salt has penetrated the meat and lowered water activity enough to make the meat stable and protect against putrefaction, the aged meats are typically eaten raw, as in "country hams" of the southeastern United States and Italian prosciutto.

There is some confusion and dispute as to what aged meat products are actually fermented. Most often, the word *fermented* is applied to dry-cured sausages rather than hams or other whole pieces of meat. In sausages, sugar (often in the form of dextrose) and/or other carbohydrate sources are often mixed with the meat and salt, giving lactic acid bacteria nutrients that enable them to play a more significant role. (More on salamis and other dry-cured sausages in the following sections.)

In hams and other dry-cured meats that are not ground, the internal flesh is never directly touched by tools, hands, or even air, "so essentially the internal ham is sterile from the beginning," points out Peter Zeuthen in the *Handbook of Fermented Meat and Poultry*.[10] Furthermore, carbohydrate ingredients cannot be intermixed with the flesh. As a result, microbial action "exerts only a minor role in ripening," according to a study published in the *Journal of Applied Microbiology*.[11] Yet without question microorganisms are present. "The typical microflora of these meat products is made up of *Micrococcaceae*, lactic acid bacteria, and moulds and yeasts, with the involvement of the *Micrococcaceae* being very important," explain a team of food scientists in a study of a traditional Spanish style of ham. "Their halotolerant [salt-tolerant] character allows them to be permanently present during the manufacturing of the product, and they play an important part in the formation of the colour, by reducing nitrate to nitrite, and in the proteolytic [protein-digesting] and lipolytic [fat-digesting] processes, which could contribute to the development of the characteristic flavour of these products."[12] Another study, in the *Journal of Agricultural and Food Chemistry*, is more emphatic: "Microorganisms are important for the development of flavor in Parma ham, as all of the correlating volatile compounds can be generated by secondary metabolism of microorganisms."[13]

My personal experience with dry-curing meat is pretty limited. My first time was with a deer thigh given to me by my hunter friend John Whittemore, which I cured in the style of prosciutto. The process is surprisingly simple. First, find a non-metallic container, large enough that the meat can lie flat in it. (I used a plastic dishwashing tub.) Glass or ceramic is fine, if you can find the right size, but metal can react with the salt.

Some recipes call for using curing salts, but in the case of whole slabs of meat like this, as opposed to dry-cured sausages that involve ground or chopped meat stuffed into a casing, the curing salts are for color and flavor rather than safety. Except when safety is at stake, in the case of dry-cured sausages, I personally avoid using curing salts and work instead with unrefined sea salt, which naturally contains traces of nitrate. But if you are after the bright color and distinctive flavor that curing salts impart, then by all means use them.

Salt the meat, using about 6 percent salt based on the weight of the meat you are curing. Four pounds/2 kg of meat would require ¼ pound/120 g salt, which measures to roughly ½ cup. With clean hands, massage the entire surface of the meat with salt, place it in the tub, and spread salt under and around the meat so that it is completely covered. If there is extra salt, keep it handy.

Cover the salted meat with parchment or plastic, and refrigerate, or leave in a cellar or other cool spot. In many climates, slaughter and curing were done only in cold weather, as warm temperatures can spoil meat quickly before salt penetrates.

Every couple of days, take the salting meat out of the refrigerator to check it. Pour off the liquid that will accumulate in the tub as the salt pulls it from the meat. Redistribute salt over the surface as needed, and turn the meat so that the surface that was facing down faces up. As necessary use any extra salt that was left over from the initial salting, and add further salt as needed to keep the surface salted. Notice how the meat changes, becoming firmer as it loses water. The initial salting will take approximately one to two days for each pound/500 g of meat. The best way to judge when it has been adequately salted is to weigh it. From water losses, the meat should lose about 15 percent of its initial weight.

Once you determine that your meat has completed the salting phase, rinse it in fresh water and dry the surface. Spread a layer of lard over the surface, to prevent it from drying and potentially cracking, and sprinkle cracked peppercorns onto the lard, which help keep insects away. Wrap the whole salted, larded, and peppered piece of meat in a few layers of cheesecloth. Then tie the whole mummified package with string, finishing off with a loop by which to hang it. Hang the meat to cure in a cool dry spot, such as an unheated cellar, for six months or longer. Water will continue to drain from the meat, so you will find some drip residue on the ground under it. The meat will feel firmer as time passes and is ready when it has lost at least one-third of its original weight. Wipe away the lard coating, slice thinly, and enjoy.

prosciutto

The deer thigh I cured in this way came out great. After six months of aging, it was tasty and tender and attractive. I got the idea to cure deer meat in this prosciutto style from tasting a wonderful cured goat thigh at Terra Madre, the International Slow Food event in Italy. The meat was called *violino di capra* (violin of goat), because it is shaped something like a violin. It is a specialty of Valchiavenna in northern Italy, and its Slow Food purveyor held it and sliced it as if it were one. This meat was not only incredibly rich and delicious but tender, no easy feat for the meat of an eight-year-old dairy goat. The conventional wisdom I had always heard was that the only goat meat worth eating (to the extent that goat meat is considered worth eating at all) is that of young kids just a few months old, for after that the musculature of these highly active creatures becomes extremely tough. Subsistence cultures, without the luxury of overabundance, pioneered strategies such as this for rendering foods not only stable for preservation but also tastier and tenderer, strategies that have largely been abandoned.

Most of the guidance I could find in books and online for my deer-sciutto experiment was geared toward curing pigs rather than goats or deer. For the most part the procedures for curing different meats are pretty similar. The only problem with my deer-sciutto was that it was way too salty, because I salted it for over a month, a length of time more appropriate for a pig's thigh than a deer's. Evaluating adequate salting time by weighing the meat regularly to gauge 15 percent water loss should avoid oversalting. For more detailed information on dry-curing meats, see the listing of books in *Resources*.

Brining: Corned Beef and Tongue

An even simpler way to salt meat is in brine. "Turning salt into liquid makes it an especially effective tool because it touches 100 percent of the food's surface in a uniform concentration," observes chef Michael Ruhlman.[14] In our time, people usually brine meat primarily to flavor and tenderize it, rather than to preserve it, but the original reason for the practice was preservation.

Possibly the best-known brined meat is corned beef. *Corn* is an archaic English word for any small, hard particle, whether of grain, sand, or salt. Thus, salted beef is corned beef. In ancient Ireland, beef was salted and buried in peat bogs;[15] over time this practice evolved into a brining process. Homemade corned beef, made from brisket, considered one of the toughest of beef cuts, is so tender it practically melts in your mouth. Much of that tenderness derives from brining the meat. Tongue, a luscious fatty meat, is brined in exactly the same way.

Start by mixing a brine of about 10 percent salt and 5 percent sugar, roughly 6 tablespoons salt and 3 tablespoons sugar per quart/liter of brine. Many recipes call for saltpeter or other curing salts. As with prosciutto or other dry-salted whole slabs of meat, the nitrate and nitrite are used purely to give the meat an extra-bright red color, rather than as a necessary botulism inhibitor, so I don't include them, and I've found the meat to remain plenty red nonetheless. (I'm willing to use these compounds where there is a safety imperative, but not for the sake of appearance alone.)

A 6-pound/2.5 kg brisket takes about 3 quarts/liters of brine. A 2-pound/one kg tongue takes about 1 quart/liter. I like to add cloves, garlic, peppercorns, and bay leaves to the brine. I've also seen juniper berries, thyme, cinnamon, allspice, and ginger used in published recipes. Spice the brine as desired. Add salt, sugar, and spices to dechlorinated water, stirring until the salt and sugar are completely dissolved.

Most contemporary corned beef recipes recommend brining in the refrigerator. If you have fridge space, use it. If not, you'll need a cool spot, like a root cellar. Typical ambient temperatures around 68°F/20°C will result in some really nasty meat after a few days. Unfortunately, I can't tell you exactly how high a temperature meat in brine can tolerate. There is a relationship between brine strength, temperature, and time. At warmer temperatures, use stronger brine and shorter brining time. And all meat curing has traditionally been a seasonal activity undertaken in relatively cool temperatures. I would advise against brining for more than overnight at temperatures above about earth temperature (55°F/13°C). At refrigerator temperatures, brine meat for about 10 days to two weeks. I think the easiest way is in a sealed ziplock bag in one of the crisper drawers, but you can improvise. Flip the brining meat over every few days.

When brining is complete, rinse the brisket under fresh water, then place it in a pot and cover it, by about an inch/2.5 cm, with water. Add an onion and a little more (fresh) of whatever spices you used in the brine. Bring to a boil, then reduce the heat and simmer for two to three hours, until the meat easily comes apart with a fork. Add chopped potato and wedges of cabbage, and cook about 15 minutes more, until the potatoes are tender. Remove the meat and veggies from the water, slice the meat, and enjoy your corned beef. (Instead of boiling corned beef, you can prepare your cured brisket as pastrami by rubbing lots of coarsely ground pepper, coriander, and other spices into it, and smoking it.)

For tongue, after brining I follow the directions in my trusty 1975 edition of *Joy of Cooking*: Place tongue in cold water, bring to a boil, and simmer for about 10 minutes. Remove the tongue from the hot water and immerse in cold water. Then place in a pot with fresh water, onion, and a little more (fresh) of whatever spices you used in the brine. Cook about 50 minutes per pound/500 g. Remove tongue from the cooking water and plunge briefly in cold water to cool it so you can handle it. The skin will have partially separated from the tongue. Peel it off entirely and discard. Remove any bones or gristle from the base of the tongue. Return the tongue to the cooking water to rewarm if serving hot. Slice on a diagonal. [16] Sliced tongue is also wonderful cold as a sandwich meat with mustard. Now that we've gotten this far, I will concede that brining meat like this, in the refrigerator, involves little, if any, significant fermentation. But it sure is good.

Dry-Cured Sausages

The meat products most frequently described as fermented are dry-cured sausages, widely known as salamis. Lactic acid production from fermentation—along with curing and air-drying—preserves the meat, and other bacteria, specifically of the genera *Staphylococcus* and *Kocuria* (formerly known as *Micrococcus*), facilitate the curing by metabolizing nitrate into nitrite. Yeasts and molds also contribute to the process. [17]

Two things are special about salamis that facilitate effective fermentation: First, the mincing or grinding of the meat exposes greater surface area, which results in increased contact with fermentation organisms (as well as spoilage organisms and potential pathogens) and more nutrients available to them. The mincing and mixing also enable a range of added ingredients—salt, curing salts, spices, carbohydrates to nourish lactic acid bacteria, and starter cultures—to be evenly distributed in the meat. The other feature of salamis that encourages healthy fermentation, drying, and aging is the protection afforded them by the casings—made from animal intestines—in which the meat is stuffed. "The special quality of these intestinal tubes is that they are robust enough to act as a barrier against airborne contaminants, yet permeable enough to 'breathe,'" explains Hugh Fearnley-Whittingstall:

> Natural molds bloom on the outside of the salami but can't penetrate and spoil the meat. A fly may even lay its eggs on one, but the tiny hatched maggots simply won't get through the skin. Given a reasonable circulation of cool air, these natural casings allow steady moisture loss and gradual dehydration, until the salami reach the required state of "ripeness"—firm, dense, and richly flavored with just a hint of residual moisture.[18]

Many contemporary fermented sausages are only briefly fermented, sometimes followed by cold-smoking, to flavor the sausages and improve their longevity under refrigeration; these are "fast-fermented" or "semi-dry" sausages and are often intended to be cooked before eating. These typically involve the use of starter cultures, to assure rapid acidification of the sausages during the brief and often warm fermentation period. However, most traditional fermented sausages, such as salamis, are cured, fermented, and dried at low temperatures and moderately high humidity for several months. Their safety and effective preservation is the result of a combination of interventions—together known as the 'hurdle effect'"[19]—each of which is applied in a moderate way, so that they are only effective when applied together. Though salt and curing salts, drying, or acidification could theoretically preserve the meat as a singular strategy, the result would be excessively salty, dry, or sour. By combining these methods, but applying each in moderation, the salami retains moisture, flavor, and appeal. Once sufficiently salted, cured, acidified, and dried, salamis and other fermented sausages are stable indefinitely if stored in a cool, dark spot and are generally eaten raw without any further processing.

salt

The process has traditionally been quite simple. To make salami, mince meat and fat. Mix it with salt, curing salts, and spices. Sometimes sugar (or, in the Thai tradition, rice) is added to contribute additional carbohydrates to support acidification. Stuff the mixture into casings; hang in a cool, moderately humid environment so it ferments slowly and doesn't dry out too fast. Historically this has been a seasonal activity, done only during cool weather in places with appropriate climate. As always, food traditions evolve in their particular geographic contexts. The only thing hard about dry-curing salamis at home is controlling heat and humidity to simulate these conditions.

Even though the process of dry-curing is not especially complex, "there is no topic treated by food writers with greater forewarning and trepidation than curing meats," observes food historian and fermentation enthusiast Ken Albala in his intrepid *The Lost Art of Real Cooking*. I've treated the topic with a certain amount of caution myself, with stern warnings earlier in this chapter about botulism standing in stark contrast with the "try anything and don't worry" attitude of the rest of the book, because there is a real potential for danger. Yet I agree absolutely with Ken when he writes, "With a few basic precautions, there is no reason not to cure your own meat, nor quake in fear at the prospect of poisoning yourself."[20]

I tried my hand at dry-curing sausages for the first time as I wrote this, so I am certainly no expert. Most of what I have to share I have learned from reading, as well as visits, tastings, conversations, and correspondences with meat-curing farmers, artisans, hobbyists, and other experimentalists. But the result of my first try was the most delicious salami I have ever eaten! My friend Vincent and I hand-minced the meat and fat, so it was chunky, and those big chunks just melted on my tongue. Yum!

The major challenge in dry-curing meat, especially as a novice without a dedicated setup, is how to maintain the environment at optimum temperature and humidity. Except for the initial few days of fermentation, which often take place at warmer temperature, salamis are best dry-cured in an environment with temperatures in the range of 54–59°F/13–15°C, and 80 to 85 percent humidity. The reason it's so important to maintain a humid environment, even though the objective is drying the sausages, is that if the environment is too dry, the outside of the sausages will dry fast, trapping moisture inside and leading to spoilage. If you observe that the casings of your sausages are drying out, slow down their drying by lightly misting them with water.

A friend of mine rigged up an old refrigerator so it plugs into a controllable external thermostat, which enables me to control temperature (see *Temperature Controllers* in chapter 3). Inside the fridge, I placed an open pan of heavily salted water to help maintain humidity (the salt discourages mold from forming on the surface of the water), as well as a hygrometer (humidity meter) sensor to monitor humidity. When the humidity got below 80 percent, I'd open the door for a moment to let humid summer air in and occasionally spray a light mist. Friends of mine have also used wine refrigerators, and an online search will yield many other clever improvisational ideas for dry-curing chambers. In the right climate, season, and cellar, this can be done very simply, in an unheated cellar.

Once I figured out my incubation chamber, the biggest dilemma I faced was whether to rely on wild fermentation or use a starter culture. Almost all of the mainstream literature, at least in the United States, will tell you to use starter cultures. And in contemporary salami making in the United States, use of starter cultures has become the norm. The oldest form of culturing in this context, practiced long before any specific organisms were ever isolated, is backslopping, which is simply introducing a small amount of already-fermented sausage stuffing into a fresh batch, just like culturing fresh milk with already-fermented yogurt. As with dairy cultures, microbiologists have isolated selected bacterial strains; these commercially available cultures are widely believed to produce more consistent results than traditional wild fermentation and to make sausage-making safer by starting fermentation faster and thus reducing the lag time before pH begins to fall. "In the latest production methods, huge numbers of lactic acid bacteria (starter cultures) are introduced into the meat right at the beginning of the process and that guarantees healthy and strong fermentation," write Stanley and Adam Marianski, co-authors of *The Art of Making Fermented Sausages*. "These armies of beneficial bacteria start competing for food with other undesirable bacteria types, decreasing their chances for growth and survival."[21]

Traditionally, fermented sausages have been made with organisms that find their way onto the meat during processing. "In most cases, sufficient numbers of the microorganisms necessary are present in the raw material," reports German microbiologist and food scientist Friedrich-Karl Lücke.[22] The 2007 *Handbook of Fermented Meat and Poultry* states that "Reliance on natural flora results in products with inconsistent quality" and advocates the use of starter cultures. Even so, the authors acknowledge a trade-off, as starter use "translates into a lot of very good and acceptable product. However, very little extremely excellent product is produced, because most starter cultures are a combination of just a few species of microorganisms and they cannot produce as balanced a flavor as sometimes can be obtained when many species are included."[23] This corroborates the analysis of food historian and cookbook author Ken Albala, who writes:

> In the name of food safety, predictability and product consistency these foods are routinely . . . inoculated with lab-tested, carefully controlled strains of microorganisms. The unique properties of local bacterial populations are thus obliterated through such seemingly benign processes as

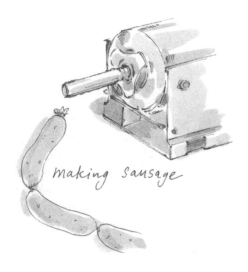

making sausage

pasteurization, or crowded out with super quick-acting starter cultures. The result is bland homogeneous food catering to the lowest common gastronomic denominator. Flavorless, characterless, sterile products no longer reflect place but the demands of the industrial marketplace which require long distance shipping, stable shelf-life and most importantly uniformity and consistency.[24]

Ken suggests that mixing the sausage ingredients together using your own clean but unprotected hands is an effective way to introduce fermenting bacteria. "The biggest concern most modern authorities have is how to get the bacteria to colonize the chopped meat. Since you are using your hands, this should be no problem. This is the way it has always been done until a few decades ago."[25]

Artisan salami makers using traditional methods are being forced by regulators to defend their practices. Because he did not have a "kill step" in his processing (heating, irradiating, or using chemical preservatives), and because he was not introducing selected cultures, New York salami maker Marc Buzzio, proprietor of Manhattan's Salumeria Biellese, had to prove to the US Department of Agriculture that the traditionally fermented salamis he produces were safe:

> Making cured sausages the same way your father did, the way others have for hundreds of years, doesn't constitute proof. Neither does the fact that no one ever gets sick on your product or that you use only heirloom pork and tend to your salamis like some people tend to their children. It isn't even proof if your product tests negative for bacteria. All the USDA cares about is the process. The traditional method—raw meat transformed into an edible product with nothing but a little salt and a lot of time—makes them very nervous.[26]

What Buzzio had to do to prove the safety of his process was commission a scientist who was frequently cited by the agency (for over $100,000) to study it.

> The scientist followed Salumeria Biellese's process to the letter, with one exception: He injected each product with pure *E. coli* and *L. monocytogenes*, producing much higher levels of bacteria than would normally be found in raw meat. Then he aged the products in the same way that they are aged at the salumeria. When the scientist tested the meats at the end of the aging period, he found that the very high levels of bacteria had been eliminated. Essentially, his study validated what centuries of practice had already demonstrated—that dry aging, when done knowledgably and with care, makes raw meat safe to eat.[27]

The USDA accepted the study as proof and Buzzio continues to be one of the most celebrated salami makers in the United States.

Fidel Toldrá, the Spanish author of several textbooks on dry-cured and fermented meats, characterizes the selective environment of the dry-cured sausage:

> The origin and composition of the microflora naturally present in the raw sausage mix is diverse. There are many factors that determine which microflora are present, such as the hygiene in meat manipulation, the environment and microorganisms present in the additives. However, the presence of salt and nitrite, oxygen depletion, pH drop, reduction in a_w, and accumulation of certain metabolites, like bacteriocins, during the processing will result in a kind of selectivity that favors the development of Kocuria, Staphylococcus, and lactic acid bacteria but will prevent the growth of undesirable microflora like pathogenic and spoilage microorganisms.[28]

As in most fermentations, the environment selects the bacteria. The hard part is creating the appropriate environment, not getting the bacteria there. Starters may speed things up and improve consistency, but they are not necessities, and most of what are considered the best artisan salamis, like the best artisan cheeses, are made with the broad spectrum of indigenous bacteria that are naturally occurring, rather than a mix of selected strains.

To try to evaluate the starter question experientially, I prepared two batches of salami otherwise identical in meat, grind, salting, curing salts, sugar, and spicing. Half I stuffed into the casings with no added starter, and to the other half I added a culture I bought, called T-SPX. The flavor of both salamis was wonderful. The thin slices just melted in my mouth. I could not discern any difference, really. I do not feel that the cultured ones were enhanced by their culturing; nor were the spontaneously cultured ones noticeably more complex or special. My experiment demonstrated to me that either approach can produce excellent salami. But of course, that is determined by many factors.

More than anything, good-quality salami requires good quality meat. I got pork and back fat from a farmer friend, Bill Keener, in Whitwell, Tennessee. Any type of meat may be used for sausages, typically with a good amount of minced fat mixed with lean meat to keep the sausages moist and rich. Meat may be ground with a mechanical grinder or chopped by hand; both the meat and fat may be chopped finely or coarsely for a more rustic appearance. (Note: Fat is much easier to mince when partially frozen.) Meat should be kept cold and not left at ambient room temperature for long periods, and tools and workspace should be as clean as possible. "Because of the warm, moist conditions involved with dry-curing foods, bacteria can multiply with abandon," explain Michael Ruhlman and Brian Polcyn in their book *Charcuterie*, "so sanitation is a much more salient concern than when working with food that will be cooked or eaten immediately."[29]

Natural casings need to be soaked in several changes of cold water and rinsed before stuffing, in order to remove salt and make them flexible. Larger casings like beef middles take much longer to dry (three to four months) than smaller casings (three to four weeks). "For novices, the best strategy is to start with skinny items, sausages that don't take long to dry, sausage stuffed into sheep casings or hog casings," advise Ruhlman and Polcyn. "The longer something takes to dry, the greater potential for problems."[30]

For curing salts, the long curing involved in dry-cured sausages requires both nitrite and nitrate, which bacteria metabolize into nitrite in a slow release. In the United States, this combination is sold as "cure #2." Actually cure #2 is mostly sodium chloride, with 6.25 percent sodium nitrite and 4 percent sodium nitrate. For safe dry-cured sausages, use 0.2 percent cure #2 in relation to meat, which translates to 1 level teaspoon per 5 pounds of meat, or 2 grams per kilogram. Cures available in other places may contain different proportions, so follow guidelines. But for dry-cured sausages, be sure to use curing salts with nitrate as well as nitrite! For salt, use 3 to 3.5 percent, based on the weight of the meat if you are relying on wild fermentation; with starter cultures you can use as little as 2 percent. Many recipes call for sugar, generally no more than 0.3 percent. Some specify dextrose, which is a name for glucose, because it is the most basic form of sugar used by cells as a source of energy, and as Stanley and Adam Marianski explain, only it "can be fermented directly into lactic acid by all lactic acid bacteria."[31] Add seasonings and spices as desired; some recipes call for a little wine.

I had access to a simple mechanical stuffer and stuffed some using that; some I stuffed manually, using a tube that came with the mechanical stuffer (a large funnel is often recommended for hand-stuffing). Both ways, I had to restuff the first sausages I did, as there is a tactile learning curve to seeing how full and how fast to stuff the casings. But I caught on quickly, and both ways produced firm, full, evenly stuffed sausages. I rather enjoyed the manual stuffing, and for small batches I think it works perfectly well. When you notice air pockets in the stuffed sausage—inevitable in home production—poke them with a flame-sterilized pin to release the trapped air and enable the casing to shrink around the meat.

Typically, molds develop on salamis as they dry-cure. The most commonly found molds are of the genera *Penicillium*, *Aspergillus*, *Mucor*, and *Cladosporium*.[32] "A thick layer of desirable molds on the surface serves as protection against the adverse effects of oxygen and light and prevents mycotoxigenic molds from becoming established," explains Fidel Toldrá.[33] In fact, in some commercial and home production, the surfaces of salamis are cultured with mold spores. Some of the literature suggests discarding salamis that develop

salami

molds that are green or any color except white. But many traditionalists dispute that advice. "A number of molds, ranging in color from gray-green to white and even orange, may form on the casings," explains Hugh Fearnley-Whittingstall. "None of these should worry you."[34]

"While modern processors employ science to maintain an aesthetically pleasing white mold, nature on its own will normally generate an artist's palette of colors," write John Piccetti, Francois Vecchio, and Joyce Goldstein in their book *Salumi*.[35] My salamis developed hues of white, grey, and blue-green as they dry-cured. My confidence in the moldy salamis was bolstered by the pleasant, alluring aroma that wafted from the curing chamber each time I inspected them.

As with any fermentation process, the big question is: How will I know when it's ready to eat? With dry-cured sausages, this is mostly a matter of the sausages losing enough water to be shelf-stable. The easiest way to gauge this is by weighing the sausages when they are first made, recording their weight, and then weighing them periodically as they cure to monitor dryness. Dry-cured sausages are usually ready when they have lost about one-third of their original weight. The length of time this takes will vary from a few weeks to a few months, depending above all on sausage diameter—thicker salamis take longer to dry than thin ones—as well as humidity, temperature, air movement, and other ripening conditions. I tried mine after a month, by which time they had lost about 40 percent of their weight. After that, I hung them in a dark corner of the basement, where they did fine despite the hot and humid summer weather.

Fish Sauce

Fish sauce is the mother of all condiments. Most prevalent today in Southeast Asian cuisines, 2,000 years ago it was the favorite condiment of classical Rome. Then and now, fish sauce is a strategy used in coastal areas to turn abundant small marine life into a nutritious, stable, and flavorful food resource. Fish sauce is essentially liquefied fish; the cells of the fish are transformed from solid to liquid state by enzymatic digestive processes described in the scientific literature as *autolysis* [self-digestion] and *hydrolysis* [digestion into water]. Reflecting on the fact that this process spontaneously begins in salted fish if not quickly dried, historian H. T. Huang writes that fish sauce "was an invention that was just waiting to happen."[36]

Use fresh whole small saltwater fish, mollusks, or crustaceans with their viscera (organs). "The enzyme or enzymes responsible for fish protein hydrolysis are chiefly located in the visceral organs," reports Keith Steinkraus.[37] According to a team of researchers investigating the production of Thai *nampla* fish sauce in the *Journal of Agricultural and Food Chemistry*, fish are left at ambient temperatures for 24 to 48 hours prior to salting. "This actually initiates the fermentation process."[38]

Next, add salt and stir thoroughly to evenly distribute it. Heavy salting is critical to protect the fish from rapid putrefaction and growth of potentially dangerous bacteria, including *C. botulinum*. Most contemporary styles of fish sauce incorporate salt at a proportion of no less than 25 percent (by weight); some use considerably more. Food historian Sally Grainger notes that ancient Roman recipes for fish sauce used much less salt, approximately 15 percent. She attributes the higher salt levels in modern fish sauce to "fear of dangerous bacteria such as botulism."[39] However, the *International Handbook of Foodborne Pathogens* states that 10 percent salt is enough to prevent the risk of botulism in fish in "the aqueous phase" at room temperature.[40]

Typically no water is added to fish sauce. Salted fish are placed in a crock, barrel, tank, or other vessel, and weighted down—as is sauerkraut—to expel air pockets and keep solids from floating to the top. Initially, salt pulls water from the fish cells by the process of osmosis; then enzyme and microbial processes cause hydrolysis. Depending upon temperature, salt content, and tradition, fish sauces ferment for between 6 and 18 months, with periodic stirring. The recipe I followed, for a Filipino-style fish sauce called *patis*, sent to me by my friend Julian (whose mother was from the Philippines), instructed to ferment in a warm place until a "desirable aroma has developed." The color also darkens as time passes, as more of the fish solids liquefy. I left mine to ferment for about six months. It tasted like fish sauce, though I cannot claim to be a connoisseur with a discerning palate. Keith Steinkraus reports on *patis* production that the fermentation time ranges from six months to a year.[41] In the Filipino tradition, the fish sauce is drained from the solids. The liquid sauce is *patis*; the residual solids, with remaining bones removed, are ground into a paste called *bagoong*, also used as a condiment. Fish sauce may be used raw after straining or is often pasteurized before bottling, sometimes with the addition of alcohol.

Microbiologists have debated the importance of fermentation in the production of fish sauce. "Generally, the number of bacteria steadily decreases in the fish following the addition of salt," writes Steinkraus.[42] Nonetheless, microbial analysis has established that salt-loving (*halophilic*) bacteria "are likely playing an important role in the maturation and development of typical fish sauce aroma and flavor."[43]

This is the basic process. A Roman cuisine enthusiast, Heinrich Wunderlich, suggests speeding fermentation of *garum* (classical Roman fish sauce) by using a yogurt maker that keeps the fish and salt at 104°F/40°C. With whole small fish, or just innards, 15 to 20 percent salt by weight, and stirring once a day, he writes that the fish liquefies in three to five days, leaving a bare skeleton. Flavor develops more slowly, and is fully developed, even in the yogurt maker, only after a few months have passed.[44] There are many variants on basic fish sauce, some using specific fish, mollusks, or crustaceans; others with added ingredients including sugar, tamarind fruit pulp, pineapple, and grains, either molded (such as *koji* or *qu*, see chapter 10), malted, in the form of lees (the solid residue from making *saké*, see chapter 9), or even outer husks. There are also hybrid fish-soy sauces incorporating soy *koji* into the fermenting mix.[45]

Pickled Fish

Fish may also be preserved by brine pickling. In contrast with fish sauces and pastes, in which the fish disintegrates, pickled fish retain their form. The most widely known styles of pickled fish, such as pickled herring in its many variations, do not involve significant fermentation. The fish are very heavily salted to remove water and slow bacterial and enzymatic degradation, then later desalted and pickled in spiced vinegar. Although most herring pickling involves limited microbial activity, it involves significant enzyme activity. When the fish are gutted, an enzyme-storing digestive organ called the *pyloric caecum* is left in place. The enzymes in the *pyloric caecum* "circulate and supplement the activity of both muscle and skin enzymes, breaking down proteins to create a tender, luscious texture and a wonderfully complex flavor, at once fishy, meaty, and cheesy," waxes Harold McGee.[46]

With more modest salting, herring and other fish are sometimes intentionally fermented. In late spring and early summer, when their fat content is greatest just before breeding begins, herring are harvested for a shorter and lighter-salt (8 to 10 percent) curing,[47] known in Dutch as *maatjes* herring, which involves more, though still limited, fermentation.[48] Historically these were only available as a seasonal delicacy, but as a result of legal requirements that these herring be frozen to rid them of parasites that can survive the lower-salt curing, *maatjes* are now available year-round.

Swedish *surströmming* is a more dramatic example of fermented herring, notorious for its strong odor and flavor. *Strömming* are the herring of the Baltic Sea. *Sur* means "sour." *Surströmming* are lightly brined (3 to 4 percent salt) Baltic herring, fermented in barrels for a month or two in the temperatures of mild northern summer. In contemporary practice, the *surströmming* is then transferred to a saltier environment and sealed in tin cans to continue ripening. The sign of ripe *surströmming* is a bulging can.[49] According to Harold McGee, "The unusual bacteria responsible for ripening in the can are species of *Haloanaerobium*, which produce hydrogen and carbon dioxide gases, hydrogen sulfide, and butyric, propionic, and acetic acids; in effect a combination of rotten eggs, rancid Swiss cheese, and vinegar, overlaid onto the basic fish flavor!"[50]

Is your mouth watering yet? I was at a conference at which Swedish food scholar Renée Valeri, the author of a paper on *surströmming*, brought some to share. Indeed, the can was bulging from the pressure of active fermentation inside. The tasting was located outdoors because of *surströmming's* assertive odor. Valeri's paper examined "the contradictory characteristics of offensive smell and good taste," and the fact that for any number of foods, not only *surströmming*, "if one is able to overcome the initial reaction and try them, the taste is quite different." As all accounts agree, the smell was horrible and putrid, but intrepid food adventurers, including me, lined up for tastes. As the smelly fermented fish on flatbread entered my mouth, I wondered whether I would be able to swallow it. But as I chewed I acclimated to the flavor, and the lingering aftertaste left me waiting for the line to be over so I could have another taste.

Norwegian *rakfisk* (also known as *rakefisk* and *rakorret*) is a somewhat similar ferment usually made from trout. Recipes generally specify that the fish must not come into contact with soil, for fear of exposure to *C. botulinum*. The most specific information I have come across is from Wikipedia, where the following process was described: Fish are cleaned and gutted, and their abdominal cavities are filled with salt, about 6 percent of the weight of the fish. Fish are placed in a crock, barrel, or other vessel, abdominal cavity up, with a pinch of sugar added to each layer. They're weighted, and as salt pulls juices from the cells, the fish become submerged under brine. Fish are fermented in this brine for two or three months at 40–45°F/4–8°C.[51] In the northern climes with suitable temperatures, especially where salt was not abundantly available, such relatively low-salt fish ferments have been a fact of life. "A surplus catch needed to be preserved in order to serve as a food supply during the winter months," explains Valeri.[52] The origin of these northern low-salt fish ferments is generally regarded to be the practice of burying fish in the ground. A generic name for these buried fish is *gravfisk*. In Scandinavia, pits gave way to barrels, and in the case of *surströmming*, cans. But elsewhere, fish-burying traditions persist, as explored in the following section, on burying fish.

Interestingly, after a period of waning interest in *surströmming*, it has become a very popular food throughout Sweden, well beyond the range of its historic use. Similarly, according to Norwegian ethnographer Astri Riddervold, *rakfisk* has gone "from the tables of mountain and inland farms to chic acceptance in urban society."[53] Valeri wonders "why the new adepts have adopted a dish which has such a bad reputation" and offers that "maybe one answer lies in today's desire to cross boundaries." Fermented fish can definitely force us to confront, and perhaps challenge, the slippery and elusive boundary between what is and is not fit to eat.

Fermenting Fish with Grains

One of the limitations of preserving flesh through fermentation is that the fermentation processes that create biopreservatives (acids and alcohol) as by-products require carbohydrate nutrients, which are in short supply in protein- and sometimes fat-rich flesh. In many Asian traditions, fish is fermented with cooked grains, usually rice. The grains provide a carbohydrate substrate for lactic acid fermentation, and the lactic acid in turn creates a selective environment that inhibits putrefaction. In Japan, fish pickled with rice is called *nare zushi* and is the precursor to the fresh sushi so popular internationally today.

H. T. Huang, author of the extraordinary and comprehensive volume *Fermentations and Food Science* (in the Cambridge University Press's epic Science and Civilisation in China series), documents the practice of fermenting not only fish, but also meat, with grains, going back thousands of years. The Chinese word *qu* incorporates both this tradition and fermented vegetables.

Huang translated from the *Qi Min Yao Shu*, Important Arts for the People's Welfare, written in the year 544, a detailed process for fish *zha* from carp. The fish is cleaned, sliced, washed, salted, and drained for several hours or overnight. "We call the salt, 'chasing water salt,' since it expels water as it is absorbed by the fish," notes the 6th-century author, who specifies non-glutinous rice, "on the hard side . . . not too soft." Rice and fish are layered in a jar, then covered by layers of bamboo leaves and stalks. "When a light liquid comes up and tastes sour, the product is ready." According to Huang, the same document also describes six other types of *zha* made with fish, as well as meat, both raw and cooked.[54]

Filipino *Burong Isda* and *Balao-Balao*

In the Philippines, fish fermented with rice is called *burong isda*, and shrimp fermented with rice is called *balao-balao* or *buro*. The Filipino ferments are relatively quick and quite delicious and offer the added comfort for the squeamish of cooking the fermented fish and rice before eating it. *Burong isda* is usually made with freshwater fish; I've made it with milkfish, one of the fish mentioned repeatedly in the literature, and tilapia. Scale, clean, and fillet your fish, and cut it into strips. Mix the fish strips with 15 to 20 percent salt, about 5 to 6 tablespoons per pound/500 g; mix thoroughly, so all the surfaces of the fish are coated with salt. Let this sit for several hours as salt both pulls water out of the fish and absorbs into it.

Meanwhile, cook rice. I'd recommend starting with about twice as much dry rice as fish, by weight, although recipes I've seen vary quite a lot on proportions of rice. Use any rice you like, and cook as you normally would. After the rice cools to body temperature, mix it well with the salted fish and it's juices, along with chopped garlic and ginger. Some recipes call for adding a small amount (1 to 2 percent) of *angkak* (red yeast rice), available in many Asian groceries as well as nutritional supplement stores. Pack the rice and fish mixture into a wide-mouth sealable jar, or a crock, pressing downward to force out air pockets. Press down any fish exposed at the surface so that it is covered by rice, and leave some space at the top for expansion. If using a jar, seal it; if using a crock, use an interior lid, a plate, or water-filled plastic bag (see *Crock Lids* in chapter 3) that will cover almost all if not all of the surface. Also cover the crock with a fabric secured by a string or rubber band to keep flies out. Ferment one to two weeks. To serve, sauté garlic and onion, then add fermented *burong isda* and a little water and cook until well heated, adding more water as necessary.[55] I've really enjoyed *burong isda* several times since I first tried it. It tastes like cheesy fish risotto. And I brought it to two potlucks where it was enthusiastically received.

Balao-balao is an identical process, only instead of fish it is made with shrimp (with shells but without heads). Shrimp is salted a little more heavily, at about 20 percent salt, or roughly 6 tablespoons per pound/500 g. It is fermented for not quite as long, 4 to 10 days. As fermentation proceeds and the shrimp and rice become acidic, the crunchy chitins of the shrimp shells soften. Like *burong isda*, *balao-balao* is cooked after fermentation. The *balao-balao* I made developed a very sharp smell as it fermented. It was a July heat wave, so I think it had to do with the temperature rather than some intrinsic quality of the ferment. I also fermented it for nearly 10 days, and perhaps given the temperature four (or even two or three) would have been plenty.

I was not concerned about the safety of the *balao-balao*, because the smell that it had is an edge that I have flirted with many times. It did, however, give me the idea to add more ingredients when I cooked the *balao-balao*, to dilute that strong smell (and potentially taste) with veggies abundant in my garden at that moment—tomatoes, okra, squash, and beans—into a stew. The flavor of the *balao-balao* turned out not to be as strong as the smell, but it was very ripe, in the way that cheeses often are. I loved the *balao-balao* stew, though I found the shrimp itself (frozen from Asia, I'm sad to report) tough and unappealing.

After I made the *balao-balao* stew, I stored it in the refrigerator and warmed it up and served it to friends a couple of times; they all seemed to like it. Each time I ate some, I liked it more. As I became more accustomed to the edgy flavor, it became more compelling. When potluck night came, I brought it, recalling how much people seemed to enjoy the *burong isda* a month earlier. Nobody said a word to me about the smell as the stew heated. After I got my food, I went to eat in another room. I heard several rounds of convulsive group laughter in the next room. I intuitively understood that it had to do with the *balao-balao*. After acting out his disgust with the smell of it, my friend Jimmy had moved the pot of *balao-balao* stew outdoors. Some people ate a little bit, in the spirit of challenging themselves; others passed on tasting it or composted what they tried. It surprised me because I was finding the flavor so compelling. I did notice, after about a week and several reheatings, that the shrimp (so tough earlier) began to literally dematerialize, shells and all, as did the grains of rice. The last of it I brought home and mixed with scrambled eggs and a little flour in a sort of shrimp soufflé, which was as delicious to me as the *balao-balao* was all along.

Online recipes for *burong isda* and *balao-balao* vary in many details. Filipino ethnologists R. C. Mabesa and J. S. Babaan observed differences in how rice is cooked (dry versus porridge), whether rice is salted, the type of fish, whether it is cleaned, how long it is salted prior to mixing with rice, and use of *angkak*. "It was noted, however, that there was no major difference in the final product in terms of overall quality in spite of the variations."[56] A 1992 paper by Minerva Olympia of the Philippine Institute of Fish Processing Technology makes the point that these methods

> were developed in homes and improvements were based on the observations of the practitioners. Fermentation processes are normally handed

down from generation to generation. There is little interest in knowing the role of microorganisms and the physical and chemical changes that occur in the products. What is recognized are changes in color, odor, and taste that result from modifications of the process or variations in the ingredients or conditions.[57]

A book can only take you so far. Once you try practices such as these, the experiential learning begins!

 ## Japanese *Nare Zushi*

Japanese *nare zushi*, historically made not only from fish, but also from mammals and birds,[58] is traditionally a much longer-term ferment. The most famous surviving example of this process is *funa zushi*, a special regional delicacy made from *funa*, a freshwater fish in the carp family (*Carassius auratus grandoculis*), unique to a single lake, Lake Biwa in Japan's Shiga prefecture. The fish are caught in spring, cleaned, and stuffed with salt. They cure just in salt, weighted down to keep them from floating to the top of the vessel, for a few months, or as long as two years. After the salt cure, they are rinsed and mixed with cooked rice, for the fish and rice to ferment together for six months to two years. Some *funa zushi* makers feel that "two years are needed for the bones to get tender,"[59] over which time the rice too gets so tender that it loses its form and becomes a "gluey, sloppy starch of lactic acid," in the words of Japanese-born food writer Kimiko Barber.[60]

There are many regional variations of *nare zushi*, some incorporating *koji*, rice malt, raw vegetables, or *saké* to speed fermentation. *Kabura* sushi is made by "sandwiching yellowtail between turnip slices and pickling this in rice *koji* for about 10 days," according to the Tokyo Foundation.[61] Barber describes a number of interesting regional styles:

> Hokkaido has "Ezushi," which is made with salted giant white radish or carrot and salmon, sailfin sandfish or Pacific ribbed sculpin, while rice malt is added and the whole left to ferment for three months. Aomori prefecture, meanwhile, offers sardine sushi, where the filleted and salted fish is layered with rice, infused with sake, and mixed while it is still warm and left to ferment in a wooden barrel with a weight for some forty days. Turnip sushi is made in Toyama and Ishikawa prefecture, where salted salmon or mackerel pieces are inserted in salt pickled turnips and fermented in seasoned rice for about a week. It has a delicately balanced sweetness from the turnip and a delicious, umami-packed taste. Soupy congee sushi is made in Yamagata prefecture as an important part of the New Year celebration dishes, with salmon, herring roe and spermatozoa of salmon, to which salt-pickled carrot, green beans and kelp seaweed are mixed with rice and malt; and in some households sake is added to ferment for between two to six weeks.

These diverse *nare zushi* techniques developed as strategies for preserving fish; the sushi we know—*haya-zushi*, or quick sushi—is an instant version, with rice vinegar replacing the traditional lactic acid fermentation. "Naturally fermented sushi came dangerously close to total extinction," writes Barber; "much of the skill and craft has been lost forever." Yet she reports that in recent years there has been something of a *nare zushi* revival. "Many small countryside villages have aspired to raise regional awareness and rekindled what were almost lost crafts, reviving fermented sushi in order to boost their village economies."

H. T. Huang hypothesizes that simple salted fish, such as fish sauces and pastes, were the earliest fish ferments, followed by the addition of *koji*-like molded grain (*qu*—see chapter 10) to produce *jiang* from both fish and meat by some time between the 6th and 10th centuries BC, followed later, between the 1st and 3rd centuries BC, by the addition of cooked rice, inspired by techniques in use earlier of fermenting vegetables with rice.[62] Huang translated a method for making meat *jiang* from the same document cited above, *Qi Min Yao Shu*, or "Important Arts for the People's Welfare," written in the year 544.

> Beef, lamb, roebuck, venison, and rabbit can all be used. Take good quality meat from a freshly killed animal, trim off the fat and chop it well. Old meat that has dried out should not be used. If too much fat remains, the meat paste will taste greasy. . . . Mix together approximately one tou (i.e. ten shêng) of chopped meat, five shêng of ferment powder [*qu*, see chapter 10], two and one-half shêng of white salt, and one shêng of yellow mould ferment [sporulated *Aspergillus* mold; see *Making Koji* in chapter 10].

These ingredients are mixed together, sealed (with mud) in a vessel, and fermented in the sun for about two weeks.[63] Other historic meat *jiang* recipes cited by Huang incorporate wine and age for much longer.

Fermenting Fish and Meat in Whey, Sauerkraut, and Kimchi

Even without live lactic acid bacteria, an acidic medium can be used to cure fish or meat. *Ceviche* is a light and delicious Latin American style of curing fish in lime juice. Over the course of just a few hours, you can see the appearance of fish transform as it is "cooked" by acidity. I was also once served raw beef, by the farmer who raised the cow, that was marinated overnight in vinegar, and underwent a similar transformation, having the appearance and texture of cooked meat, even though it had not been.

Whey, sauerkraut, kimchi, and other acidified products with dense populations of lactic acid bacteria can be similarly used as environments to safely ferment meat and fish. In Iceland, fermented whey (*sýra*) is frequently employed as a fermentation medium for a group of foods collectively known as *súrmatur*, meaning "soured food," mostly animal and fish parts. Icelandic food writer Nanna Rögnvaldardóttir recounted to me how whey preserving has been used historically, and how she uses it in her own kitchen:

> Fish was almost always dried rather than soured, although certain parts of it might be preserved in sýra—mostly parts that may not be considered food nowadays, like the stomach, the swim bladder, milt, roe, liver, skin, tail, fins etc. (We are talking about a cuisine of extreme poverty, where everything was utilized). Even the fish bones (along with other bones) were sometimes soured for a year or more, then boiled until they turned into a soft mass which was eaten. I'm told that most bones will go soft if kept in sýra long enough—I haven't tried.

> Meat was and is soured but the most common food to be soured is offal—heads and headcheese, trotters, blood pudding, liver sausage (rather similar to haggis), ram's testicles, intestines, udders, and seal flippers, whale blubber, seabirds, etc. Eggs were sometimes boiled, shelled and preserved in sýra; small seabird eggs were sometimes soured with the shell on and then the shell would gradually dissolve over time.

> I currently have a small plastic tub in my fridge, full of sýra with blood pudding, liver sausage, head cheese and ram's testicles.[64]

Rögnvaldardóttir reports that *sýra* can be continually refreshed and used as a perpetual medium. Referring to her mother, she writes: "I don't think she ever changes her *sýra*, just adds more whey as needed—I think her current batch has been going for 12 years or so."

Sally Fallon Morell, a major proponent of fermenting in whey, offers an excellent recipe in her book *Nourishing Traditions* for pickling salmon in whey, where she marinates chunks of salmon for 24 hours at room temperature in diluted whey (1 part whey to 8 parts water) with a little added honey, salt, onions, lemon, dill, and other spices.[65] Andreas Hauge, of Copenhagen, Denmark, wrote to me that he followed this recipe, but found that it "had a very powerful odor that will really challenge the tolerance of the people you share your kitchen with. A modification of the original water, salt and whey mixture with rather generous amounts of lemons or limes, will reduce the odor to level that is acceptable for most people!"

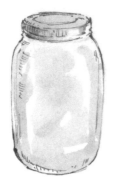

Similarly, fish or even meat can be added to kimchi. *The Kimchee Cookbook*, the most comprehensive reference on the subject that I have found in the English language, contains recipes for kimchis incorporating anchovy paste, oysters, pollack, flounder, kitefish, octopus, squid, crab, and cod. Often, but not always, the recipes call for pre-salting the fish. I've also seen kimchi recipes incorporating both raw salted meat and meat broths.

Meat and fish can be similarly incorporated into sauerkraut. In Poland I ate *bigos*, meat marinated and stewed in sauerkraut. Historically, "the dish is prepared over several days alternately heating and cooling it," according to Polish ethnologist Anna Kowalska-Lewicka.[66] Rick Headlee of Sonoma County, California, wrote to me about an old friend of his, a Swedish immigrant to Wyoming, who made vast quantities of sauerkraut "in which he often pickled pronghorn antelope loin." Fermentation enthusiast Dallin Credible of Asheville, North Carolina, wrote to report a successful experiment fermenting deer jerky in sauerkraut. "I mixed deer jerky that I cut into small pieces throughout the cabbage. It's great." I've also chopped leftover cooked sausages and added them to already mature kraut, and they preserved well, tasted delicious, and enhanced the kraut itself. In a medium like sauerkraut or kimchi that consists of salted raw plant material that will acidify in a predictable way, you can feel free to experiment with additions of small proportions of fish or meat, raw or cooked, without fear.

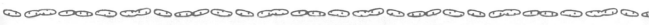

FISH FERMENTATION EXPERIMENTS IN ALASKA

Eric Haas

My most recent/exciting fish experiment is a halibut kimchi. This one has bits of mango in it. (I'm a big fan of the fruit and/or nut additions to kimchi.) I start with a strong batch of basic kimchi, being sure to use lots of ginger, which helps tenderize meat and breaks it down so that it's tastier and more fully integrated into the mix. Once the kimchi is going strong (about 10 days or so), I add the fish, mixed in as little pieces, seasoned with a bit more of my kimchi paste. I've done it with lightly steamed fish and fresh raw fish as well as frozen (thawed, of course) raw fish. The taste is basically the same. I wait about a week before starting to eat it. I've also been making really nice salmon sauerkraut, using essentially the same method as above. I do a green cabbage/grated carrot/caraway seed/salt kraut, get it going strong, then add in bits of steamed or broiled salmon, mix it up, weight it down again, and wait a week or so. The salmon becomes really tender and moist and delicious, and unlike the halibut above, retains its flavor and integrity as distinct pieces. Very nice.

Fermenting Eggs

Eggs may be fermented in a number of ways. Peeled hard-boiled eggs can simply be buried in a crock of fermenting vegetables, where they are protected by the acidification of the vegetables. Chinese cuisine has its famous century eggs, also known as thousand-year-old eggs, though they are typically preserved for just a few months. "Raw eggs are caked in a paste made from [baking] soda, quicklime, salt, and ash, often with the addition of tea leaves or grain husks, and then left in storage for about three months," writes Fuchsia Dunlop, who admits she was "revolted by their gray-black color" the first time she tried them, but "now I adore them." She describes century eggs as "something like an exaggerated egg with their rich, creamy yolks."[67] A blogger's report from a Basque confectionary museum included information on a similar technique used there in the late 19th and early 20th centuries to preserve eggs for winter, when egg production slows down. "The usual system of preservation of eggs . . . was keeping them in water with lime. The eggs were introduced in large clay pots and covered with a mixture of water and quicklime, which allowed them to keep in perfect condition for many months."[68]

H. T. Huang writes about another Chinese style of fermenting eggs, in *zao*, the residue of rice beer making, essentially the same as *saké* lees. "Lightly cracked eggs are layered between salt and wine residues and incubated for five to six months."[69] Finally, William Shurtleff and Akiko Aoyagi describe pickling soft-boiled egg yolks in miso.

> Cover the bottom of a 6-inch square container with a 1-inch deep layer of red miso. Press the large end of an egg into the miso in 4 places to make 4 depressions, then cover miso with a layer of cheesecloth and press cloth into depressions. Prepare four 3-minute eggs. Carefully remove yolks unbroken, and place one yolk in each of the 4 depressions. Cover with a layer of cheesecloth, gently top with miso, and wait for 1½ to 2 days. Serve yolks like cheese as an hors d'oeuvre or as a garnish atop hot rice.[70]

Shurtleff and Aoyagi also describe pickling hard-boiled eggs in different types of miso.

Cod Liver Oil

Cod liver oil, used as a healing supplement, particularly in some Northern European traditions, is traditionally made by fermentation. So are other fish liver oils, including shark and skate. Nebraskan David Wetzel investigated extraction processes for cod liver oil, both traditional ones and those in use in contemporary industrial production. Wetzel learned that the industrial processes used to extract cod liver oil commercially involved "alkali refining, bleaching, winterization, and deodorization. Each of these steps, especially the deodorization, removes some of the precious fat-soluble vitamins."[71] As for the traditional method, he cites an 1895 article on "Cod-Liver Oil and Chemistry" in which the author, F. Peckel Möller, describes "the primitive method." In this method, fishermen would bring home the cod livers each day after selling the day's catch and place them in barrels:

> The fishermen do not trouble to separate the gall-bladder from the liver, but simply stow away the proceeds of each day's fishing, and repeat the process every time they return from the sea, until a barrel is full, when it is headed up and a fresh one commenced. This is continued up to the end of the

season, when the men return home, taking with them the barrels that they have filled. The first of these, it may be noted, date from January, and the last from the beginning of April, and as on their arrival at their homes the fishermen have many things to arrange and settle, they seldom find time to open their liver barrels before the month of May. By this time the livers are, of course, in an advanced state of putrefaction. The process of disintegration results in the bursting of the walls of the hepatic cells and the escape of a certain proportion of the oil. This rises to the top, and is drawn off. Provided that not more than two or three weeks have elapsed from the closing of the barrel . . . to its being opened, and if during that time the weather has not been too mild, the oil is of a light yellow colour, and is termed raw medicinal oil. As may be supposed, however, very little oil of this quality is obtained. Indeed, as a rule there is so little of it that the fishermen do not take the trouble to collect it separately. Nearly all the barrels yield an oil of a more or less deep yellow to brownish colour: this is drawn off, and the livers are left to undergo further putrefaction. When a sufficient quantity of oil has again risen to the surface, the skimming is repeated, and this process is continued until the oil becomes a certain shade of brown.[72]

Wetzel writes: "After reading this passage, and foreseeing the demise of the last natural cod liver oil from Europe, I was determined to produce a light brown fermented cod liver oil according to the old methods."[73] Indeed, he has started fermenting cod liver oil and marketing it under the brand name Green Pasture.

Burying Fish and Meat

Earlier, in the section on pickling fish, I introduced the idea that the Scandinavian barrel-cured fish have their roots in a tradition of *gravfisk*, or buried fish. Along with simple sun-, air-, or smoke-drying (which, if it is effective, does not result in any significant fermentation), burying fish and meat in the ground is among the most ancient means of storing, securing, and preserving a surplus. "Originally, this might have been done to hide or protect food from insects and thieves until the hunter could return for it," speculates Sue Shephard, author of *Pickled, Potted, and Canned*. According to Shephard, in England in the Middle Ages, "venison was sometimes buried instead of being hung." She explains: "Retaining its own moisture while lying in the cool, moist ground meant the food would slowly ferment using its own yeasts and enzymes, resulting in a preserved food with a very strong flavor."[74]

The practice of burying meat or fish to preserve it has been documented widely, in varied geographic locations, though most prominently in far northern locales. Longer storage is definitely possible in cooler climates. Yet when archaeologists at the University of Capetown, in South Africa, sought to re-create the practice of burying whale meat in the sand, as recorded by early Dutch colonizers there, they found that bacterial levels did not increase beyond acceptable levels for raw consumption for about 10 days, and that if cooked the meat remained edible much longer.[75]

But it is in the far northern reaches of the Earth that burying fish is widespread and most critical to survival. Culinary historian Charles Perry cites an 18th-century account that the Itelmen people of Kamchatka, on Russia's Pacific coast, "rot fish in pits until the gristle dissolves—sometimes it rots to such a degree that it has to be removed from the pits with a sort of ladle."[76] The Scandanavian cured salmon *gravlax* (meaning "grave salmon") was historically prepared by burying salmon in the sand (although, as described previously, today its preparation involves neither burying nor significant fermentation, but rather a few days of salt- and sugar-curing, typically under refrigeration). *Kiviak* is a Greenland delicacy of whole seagulls and auks sewn into the abdominal cavity of a disemboweled seal and buried (seam up, so gases can release without rupturing the seal) under a large flat rock to ferment several months. "They bite the heads off and squeeze out the tart guts," according to a firsthand Internet account. "It tastes like a matured cheese and very pungent. There is nothing disgusting in this dish."[77]

In Alaska, Inupiat people bury king salmon heads in the ground to prepare a delicacy they call *nakaurak*, known in English as stinkheads. A collection of traditional Inupiat ways of preparing and preserving fish, collected by Anore Jones and published by the US Fish and Wildlife Service in 2006, details how to ferment *nakaurak*, as told by Mamie Beaver of Kotzebue, Alaska, near the Bering Strait. "Line a two-foot deep hole with green grass, somewhere that the sun won't shine on that ground," she instructs.

> Wash the salmon heads well, get all the blood and scum off. Leave the gills in. Put the heads in a flour sack and put the sack in the grass hole. Cover it with a few inches of grass, then cover with sand, and then with a board so people won't step on it. Let it stay until the smell is a little strong and the nose skin slips off, or can be easily broken. That skin on the nose is the best part, like soft rubber. Don't let it get too strong.[78]

Of course, "too strong" is a subjective judgment. The same document, filled with oral histories, includes the following exchange about *nakaurak* between two Inupiat elders: "I like to eat them when they are green and slimy," says one. "I can't eat them that strong," responds the other. "When they start to get green and slimy, I have to feed them to the dogs." Indeed, the dogs too are part of the overall food system and need to be fed.

Buried fish, like most fermentation, exists along a continuum, and sometimes it goes too far, at least for some people. The boundaries are typically not clear-cut. But one boundary that could not be clearer is that fish must never be wrapped in plastic for burying in the ground. Pits are lined with grass or leaves; fish may be wrapped in burlap sacks; but it is of critical importance to not use plastic in this process, because plastic can create the kind of totally anaerobic condition that encourages the growth of *Clostridium botulinum*. In North America today, Alaska accounts for a far disproportionate number of reported botulism cases, all "associated with improper preparation and storage of traditional Alaska Native foods," according to a report of the US Centers for Disease Control (CDC).[79] The CDC conducted an illuminating experiment that demonstrated the dangers of fermenting fish in plastic. The Fish and Wildlife Service report on Inupiat fish traditions included this account from a CDC official:

> We took four batches each, of the main foods where botulism was found— fish heads, seal flippers, and beaver tail. Two batches were prepared the proper traditional way, and two were prepared as some people have been doing lately, using plastic bags or buckets. One of each batch we inoculated with botulism; the other was left natural [was not inoculated]. After the fermentation process was complete, we tested them. To our surprise, those batches of foods prepared the traditional way had no trace of the botulism toxin, not even in the foods that were inoculated with botulism spores. On the other hand, both batches [the one inoculated with botulism spores and the one not inoculated] of foods prepared in plastic tested positive for botulism. The advice that came out of that experiment was—"keep on fermenting your food, but never use plastic bags or buckets, and be certain that you do it the traditional native way without any short cuts or changes."[80]

Heed that warning, please.

In Arctic temperatures, fish need not always even be buried to effectively preserve them. Another traditional fish fermentation method described in this amazing report on Inupiat fish traditions is the simple mounding of fish in piles. The mounding begins, in a shady spot, as summer wanes. Fish are not fully cleaned; only livers and bile are removed through a small incision, minimizing damage to the fish and the potential for oxidation. Each day's catch is added to the mound and covered with grass. Explains an Inupiat elder:

> As the weather cooled down they fermented more slowly, thus the top layer of fish was freshest. On these, it wasn't as important to get the liver out and we stopped doing that, just as freezing temperatures made it difficult to do with painfully numb fingers. Then we just lay the whole fish on the pile. The liver and bile ferments faster and differently than the rest of the fish and spoils more of an area around it the longer they ferment.

After the snow comes and ambient temperatures remain below freezing, the pile is rearranged, separating fish so each can freeze all the way. "If this isn't done, they keep on fermenting for weeks until the ground freezes and would become too strong."

Once frozen, fermentation stops, and fish—called *tipliaqtaaq quaq*—are removed from the pile and eaten as needed throughout the long winter. To remove a fish from the frozen pile, "take an axe and knock one loose." The pile dwindles toward the center, where the fish have more time to ferment. "The flesh of the older, earliest-caught fish changed to a cheese-like texture with no resemblance to the texture of fish flesh. . . . One analogy of the difference between fresh and *tipliaqtaaq quaq* is the difference between drinking fresh water and drinking a rich salty soup, or a strong, sweet wine. There just are so many more flavors—rich, complex, always differing, flavors—in the *tipliaqtaaq quaq*." Yet stronger is not always better: "As we eat these fish, we are continually judging what fish or part of a fish we want to eat and which parts are too strong, good only for the dogs."[81]

High Meat

In some of the literature about historical means of preserving meat and fish, flesh that has begun to putrefy is referred to as "high meat." There is a contemporary nutritional ideology, known as the Primal Diet, that advocates the consumption of high meat for health benefits. The diet's originator and promoter, a man named Aajonus Vonderplanitz, says that he came to believe in the healing power of high meat after a dramatic healing experience in Alaska, eating meat that had been buried, as described above.

The way Vonderplanitz translates the process of making high meat for people in non-Arctic climates (he himself lives in Southern California) is to age cubed meat in sealed jars in the refrigerator, airing them out periodically. A woman I've corresponded with who does this, Beverly Pedersen, of Evanston, Illinois, described the process for me:

> Just cut into bite sized pieces enough meat to loosely fill a one quart wide mouth jar half way. Put a lid on it and put it in the fridge. Every few days take it out, open the jar, and give it fresh air by swinging it around. I suggest doing this outside so it doesn't stink up your house. Put the lid back on and put it back in the fridge. Do this for a month and it is ready. It will keep a long time in the fridge.

I have encountered a number of people through the years who swear by this practice. When they have offered me high meat, however, I have not tasted it, because it always smells repulsive to me. One woman I met held her nose to eat it, and cut it into tiny pieces so she could swallow it without having to chew it. While I do not advocate this practice, and I have questions about its safety, the people I've met who eat high meat all seem to be perfectly healthy, and some of them attribute great improvements in their health to it. Despite my personal reservations, in the interest of covering the topic of meat fermentation thoroughly, I am including it here.

Meat and Fish Ethics

I cannot write a chapter about fermenting meat and fish without emphasizing that these practices evolved as strategies, each of which makes sense within its particular context. One critical aspect of this is what meat or fish may be available in abundance in a particular place at a particular time of the year. In our consumer paradise, however, most of us are woefully out of touch with this. The details of where our foods comes from and the systems that get them to us—particularly meat and fish—are usually gruesome.

There are small farmers in many places trying to raise animals with healthy, sustainable, and compassionate practices. I buy meat directly from people like this and I urge you to, too. But sustainable and compassionate practices require substantial land per animal. This not only makes meat more expensive; it also limits the amount of it there can be. If we want animals for meat to be raised in healthy and humane ways, we all have to eat less of it. I love to eat meat, and I have access to local meat from farmers I admire, and I can afford to buy it. Yet I find myself reluctant to glorify meat. I believe part of what can make meat eating sustainable is eating just a little of it.

With fish, I do not have access to anything fresh and have not (yet) taken up fishing myself. The experimentation I have done has been with frozen fish, although I don't especially want to support the global trade of frozen fish. In a coastal place with fresh fish in daily, I would be much more inclined to buy fish. Yet the drive to scale up fishing to serve global markets has led to widespread overfishing and population declines. And let's not forget how toxic water is becoming, and how fish can concentrate heavy metals and other toxins. As with meat, part of what can make fish eating sustainable is eating just a little of it.

But again, context is everything. If you do find yourself with an abundance of any resource, try to make use of it. This is how these traditions of fermenting meat and fish evolved, and how they can best be adapted to have continued relevance.

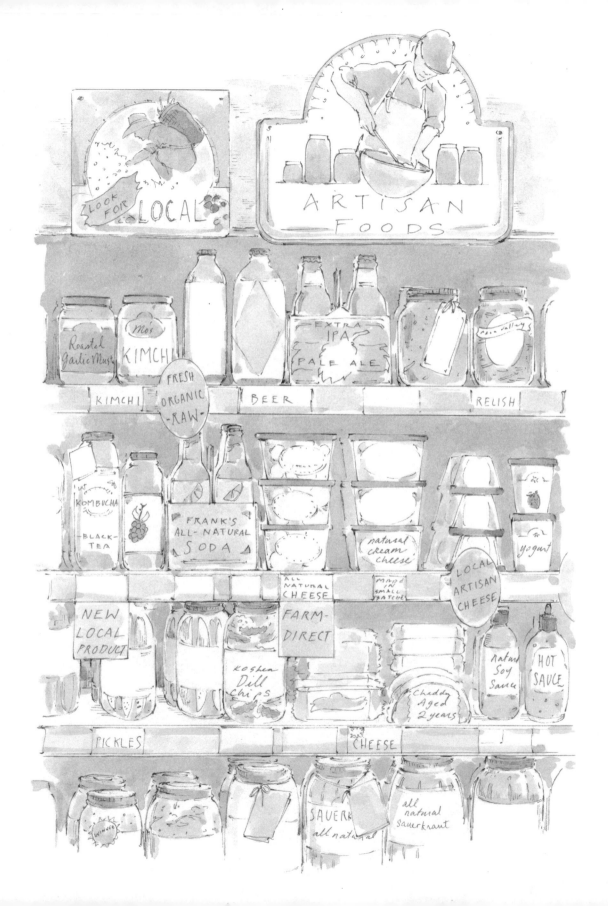

CHAPTER 13

Considerations for Commercial Enterprises

*T*he major thrust of this book is do-it-yourself fermentation, and I wholeheartedly encourage anyone with interest to experiment widely. But while I myself have done just that, I have made many ferments just one or two times; many of them not so well; and certainly I am not able to make all of them all the time. This would not be practical, nor is it desirable or necessary. Whether in the realm of informal gift exchange and barter economies, or in commercial production, some can produce beer, others bread, kraut, tempeh, kombucha, et cetera. Neither individuals nor households need (or can) be self-sufficient. Exchange can broaden everybody's possibilities.

Historically, fermentation has spawned much specialization, and through that process refinements of technique. People devote their careers and lives to each realm of fermentation that I have covered in a chapter. Though all ferments are simple enough at their core, techniques can be elaborated with great nuance. Ferments are among the original value-added products, in which the raw outputs of agriculture are transformed, via great technique and artistry, into delicacies that are stable and can be transported, and that fill our kitchens and food stores.

The revival of fermentation at the local and regional scale goes hand in hand with the revival of local agriculture in the movement toward relocalization of our food and our economics. Fermentation enterprises offer great possibilities for people who acquire the skills of fermentation to put them to use as means of economic support. This is economic development based on real production, real value, and real benefit, creating better choices for our communities by expanding the range of what is available as local food. We can revive local commercial production of ferments, as the revival of microbreweries, farmstead cheese production, and artisan bakeries demonstrate. And we do not need to wait for other people to do it. No less so than home fermentation, reviving fermentation in the form of local enterprise is a do-it-yourself venture.

In this chapter, I have collected stories and lessons conveyed to me by people who have started small fermentation enterprises. Through the work that I have been doing spreading information about fermentation, I have met many people who have started fermentation enterprises ranging from informal unlicensed underground producers to well-established businesses with sales totaling millions of dollars a year. Let me clearly state that I have never run a food manufacturing business at any scale. For me, food has been a realm of pleasure, exploration, creation, sharing, and sometimes even crusading. Ongoing commercial-scale food production has never been part of my life. Production can (but doesn't have to) be the death of pleasure, and the bottom line can (but doesn't have to) conflict with ideals. "Balancing a for-profit business with working with food as my activism has certainly been the biggest challenge," reflects Sash Sunday of OlyKraut in Olympia, Washington. "There is a certain amount of capitalism required for a sustainable business within this society and it is difficult sometimes to know what the best decision is." There are many models of production, some of which are highlighted here. The same ingenuity and creativity that people bring to fermentation itself they can bring to their efforts to use fermentation skills as a source of livelihood.

Consistency

Consistency is not necessarily important to the home experimentalist. Personally, I'm quite content for every batch of miso or kraut to be different, and that has been the source of much discovery in my experiential education. And some rare producers successfully market the utter uniqueness of each batch—for example, Enlightenment Wines in New York State, which produces and markets quirky single-batch concoctions.

However, commercial production typically requires a certain level of consistency. This can be a challenge given the vicissitudes of microbial life. The bacteria and fungi we count on exist in a much broader context. They are sensitive to temperature and humidity and other differences in environment or nutrients; their growth continually alters their population densities and creates metabolic by-products that alter their environments, giving rise to community succession. Fermentations tend to vary. "I try to educate my customers on that as much as possible," says April McGreger of Farmer's Daughter Brand in Carrboro, North Carolina, "and because I am almost completely direct sale, I can do that. I also prefer to offer tastes of new batches so people know what they are getting."

Nathan and Emily Pujol, who propagate and sell cultures as Yemoos, in Michigan, report that "generally the ferments became more consistent because we had to be more disciplined in our timing to avoid wasting ingredients and time." Nonetheless, the ferment inevitably shifts. "Cultures will go through different stages throughout the seasons . . . [we] continually adjust to get a good schedule and we are constantly finding ourselves catering to our cultures at odd hours until we make the right adjustments." Propagating cultures, more than any other fermentation practice, requires continuous attention and "would be impossible for someone who constantly enjoys being out or vacationing."

The changing of the seasons can have many implications for a fermentation enterprise. Not only do temperatures fluctuate, speeding or slowing fermentation and potentially encouraging different organisms or enzyme activity, but the availability of critical ingredients shifts as well. Cathy Smith, of Oregon, pondered these questions in an email as she considered starting a business fermenting vegetables. "I don't know how to structure a business plan based on seasonal ingredients," she wrote.

> Do I make enough of my amazing pickles to last through the year? If so, how do I refrigerate them properly? Do I run out of the cucumber pickles naturally and replace them with pickled beets in winter? These seem to appeal to different markets.

This is a huge issue for any business fermenting local vegetables. "We really like the quality of early season cabbages which we harvest June–November," says kraut maker Marko Colby of Midori Farm in Port Townsend, Washington. "The storage cabbages tend to be a little tougher and stronger in taste. We are still figuring out how to keep the product fully locally grown while meeting the demand all year long." Most producers of vegetable ferments, who are committed to using locally grown produce, ferment vegetables in their seasons, then rely on cool storage of the ferments to preserve them through the year.

Markers

Shifting temperatures through the year also impact fermentation. Some enterprises avoid fermenting in the heat of summer. "I scale back a bit on fermentation in the summer because the heat makes it harder to control yeast, as well as mold," says April McGreger. "Because summer is such a busy time for making fruit preserves, it works out for me, but I'm not sure it would work if I did strictly fermented products." Diversification can be a source of strength.

Other enterprises adapt to the seasonal highs and lows. "Luckily most seasonal variation happens gradually," observes Erin Bullock, who bakes and ferments vegetables with the Small World Collective in Rochester, New York.

> As winter approaches the loaves take a little longer to rise; we notice this and move the bulk fermentation to a warmer corner of the kitchen, turn up the proofer, increase the amount of starter, etc. More dramatic changes happen when we switch to a different crop of wheat—depending on the weather that year, the variety, the soil, the planting & harvest schedule . . . there will be big differences between them. This just takes some getting used to; hopefully those "practice" batches weren't too big or needed to fulfill an order.

In their home-based culture-propagating operation, Nathan and Emily Pujol locate shelves and cupboards "in strategic spots all over the house to avoid direct sunlight or extreme hot or cold spots throughout the seasons. When the seasons change, we have to rearrange our house to keep it optimal." Some geographic locations have more temperature stability than others. Marko Colby of Midori Farm, in Port Townsend writes: "We are fortunate that the air temperature here is regulated by the Puget Sound and Strait of San Juan, so it is really ideal most of the year for uncontrolled temperature fermentation which really helps with producing a consistent product." In contrast, Kathryn Lukas, a fermented vegetable producer located in Santa Cruz, California, reports that she was forced to install an air conditioner in her kraut-aging room to keep temperatures at 64°F/18°C after two barrels of kraut went soft in a summer heat wave. "Consistent temperatures seem to be exceptionally important in larger scale production," concludes Kathryn.

A couple of producers offered other suggestions for achieving consistent fermentation results. "Record everything," exhorts Erin Bullock, because sometimes it takes a while to gauge the significance of a small change in recipe, process, or conditions. Simon Gorman of Caldwell Bio Fermentation Canada, in St. Edwidge, Quebec, counsels a scientific approach. "Be sure you have adequate scientific back-up so that you know what is in your fermentations, in order to standardize your product, and so that you can deal with the inevitable issues that arise when you are dealing with the complexity of a 'living' process," he advises. Caldwell Bio Fermentation, which started out producing fermented vegetables, collaborated with an Agriculture Canada research station to develop a starter culture for vegetables, which it now produces and sells.

Consistency does not mean that there is no room for experimentation. A number of producers make a few primary products that are distributed widely, along with smaller batches of more experimental variations with more limited appeal. "Looking at our front fridge we currently have 10 krauts, 8 kombuchas, 15 seasonal specialty pickles, and three types of traditional Japanese pickles (nuka-zuke, kasu-zuke, miso-zuke)," reports Alex Hozven of Cultured Pickle Shop, in Berkeley, California. "The krauts are the only product we produce in volume and those are distributed around Northern CA. Everything else we retail here [at their production facility] and at farmers markets." For Cultured Pickle Shop and most other commercial manufacturers at any scale, no matter how fun and rewarding the more experimental variations are, it is the most familiar products that make up the core of the business. "We've done a pinto bean and a black bean tempeh," reports Gainesville, Florida, tempeh maker Art Guy. "Both did really well in the market. We are more just trying to get this food on the mainstream restaurants' menus rather than create oddball tempehs."

First Steps

So, you like the idea of turning your passion for fermentation into a small business. Where do you start? "Get really good at what you do first," advises Marko Colby. "Start small and focus on quality." Nathan and Emily Pujol recommend practicing your ferment through a full calendar year before going into business. "At least go through the heat of the summer and the cold of winter before trying to get into a fermenting venture."

At a small scale, it is possible to operate by word of mouth "under the radar" of regulatory agencies, but in order to establish a "legitimate" food production business you must gain the approval of regulators. "Figure out the regulations for your area first," advises April McGreger. "Every state, and sometimes county, is different." In many places, extension services, regulatory agencies, or educational institutions offer classes to help potential applicants understand licensing and certification requirements. Mark Olenick of Lititz Pickle Company in Pennsylvania suggests: "Find the closest college/university that has a food science program. Each of these schools usually has an industry-related extension program that is usually funded by grants to help support start-up businesses."

One way to minimize both start-up expenses and regulatory scrutiny is to start in a shared kitchen facility. "We spent about a year researching necessary information on how to start a small scale food production business," explains Jennifer De Marco of Fab Ferments in Cincinnati, Ohio. "We made the decision to launch our business in a shared use incubator kitchen. This was a great decision for us because the burden of maintaining and building our own kitchen was lifted." Incubator kitchens, some with extensive small business development support, exist in more and more places. If your business stays small, you can maintain it there without any big capital investment; if it flops, there are no huge losses; and if your business takes off, you may outgrow the shared facility. "After 7 years of working out of a community kitchen, we finally purchased our own building last year and turned it into our very own pickle factory, which has been working out very well," reports Dan Rosenberg of Real Pickles in Greenfield, Massachusetts.

Most of the fermentation entrepreneurs I have talked with counsel a modest start-up. "I would suggest starting small and growing organically—meaning, keep your day job at first," says April McGreger, who runs her business out of her home, which is possible in some places and not in others. "Figure out where you will source your produce. Know your market/competition—prices, demand, etc. I am a huge proponent of direct sale, and farmer's markets have been a great place to start and grow my business."

Starting small gives a new enterprise the chance to discover, before making a huge investment, whether it can sell the products that it wants to make, and whether it can make any money doing so, the ultimate questions upon which the viability of any business plan hinges, no matter what the scale of ambition. "Like any other business, a new venture must meet an unfilled need or create demand from a newly innovated product," observes Dave Ehreth of Alexander Valley Gourmet, a pickle and sauerkraut maker in Healdsburg, California. "New ventures based on fermentation should bring something exciting and new to the market."

In many places—including the rural area where I live—locally grown and fermented foods are simply not commercially available, and so the market, such as it is, is completely unserved. But how big is the market, how do you reach it, or how do you help it emerge? Brian Geier, who grows vegetables and ferments them under the label Sour Power in Frankfort, Kentucky, says "the krauts speak for themselves, and people want them, so we have our work cut out for us just trying to supply the small cities around us. . . . I have a feeling that a lot of little fermentation businesses are going to sprout in the next little while." In other places—such as, for example, the San Francisco Bay Area, or the Pioneer Valley of Western Massachusetts—there are many different types of commercial fermentation happening locally, with a multitude of available options. "Those of us who arrived early to this party were able to take advantage of the total absence from the grocer's shelves of basic live culture fermented products," reflects Dave Ehreth. "Like most markets, however, the fermented food market is becoming more competitive."

Yet there can also be a synergetic momentum when many different types of fermented products reinforce and complement one another. Will Savitri of Katalyst Kombucha and Green River Ambrosia (Meadery) in Greenfield, Massachusetts, writes: "I would like to convey to you what I feel is a very unique situation in our region of Western Massachusetts. I believe that we probably have a greater concentration of small/medium scale businesses that are based in natural fermentation than anywhere else in the country." In addition to his two ventures, within 20 miles are South River Miso Company, Real Pickles, several breweries, wineries, and bakeries, as well as West County Cider, Caveman Foods water kefir sodas, and Valley Malt, one of the nation's few small-scale malters.

Some talented and lucky producers hit the right market with the right product at the right time. Kathryn Lukas, of Farmhouse Culture, a Santa Cruz, California, kraut maker who first went commercial just three years ago, reports: "We currently sell about 8,000 lbs a month and that number is growing steadily. Californians were really ready for fresh krauts." Nathan Schomber, of Buchi, an Asheville, North Carolina, kombucha maker, says: "We can't keep up with the demand." And when Raphael Lyons, of Enlightenment Wines in the Hudson Valley near New York City, announced the debut of his "community supported alcohol" model, "I received an avalanche of interest. The blogosphere erupted and next thing I knew . . . I sold out the CSA membership over the course of a few days."

Despite the many success stories, success can never be guaranteed. "Expect to make no money and work every day all day (literally)," states Luke Regalbuto. "Do not expect to

unique ferments

make money for years." Brian Moes, founder of the year-old Viable Cultures in Asheville, North Carolina, is slightly more upbeat: "Profitability and financial success is still questionable, in my experience, but it seems very possible."

Dan Rosenberg, more than a decade and a new building into his pickle-making enterprise, cautions:

> There remain significant limitations to the markets for these foods. Natural foods- and farm-oriented markets are great venues, but it is important to be realistic about the challenges in trying to sell to more conventional markets.
>
> Wherever one is selling one's fermented products, it is important to strive for as much product consistency as possible and to be prepared to devote resources to educating one's potential customer base about the "unconventional" characteristics of the products.

The necessity of educating customers is repeated by many fermentation practitioners. "Make sure folks who buy your product know that you have to keep it refrigerated because it's not a pasteurized shelf-stable product," says Erin Bullock. "Our advice for someone starting up a fermenting venture would be to make sure that understanding and education go along with selling," offer Nathan and Emily Pujol.

Scaling Up

There is much to be learned scaling up from a home fermentation practice to commercial production. "We found that non-brined vegetable pickles (sauerkraut, shredded carrots, etc.) scaled up with no problem," recounts Dan Rosenberg:

> But, we found that brined products—particularly cucumber pickles—were exceedingly difficult to scale up, with regard to salt concentration. We never found a successful formula to guide us in choosing salt quantities as we scaled up our dill pickles recipe from quart size to 15 gallons, then 30 gallons, then finally 55 gallons. We found the optimal salt concentration only by trial-and-error. For our sauerkrauts, we actually found that our quality and consistency improved as we scaled up. It may be that a more vigorous fermentation is achieved with a bigger mass of vegetables and therefore bigger population of lactobacilli, or it may be due to a more successful airlock overall.

Alyson Ewald of northeast Missouri bakes 18 loaves of bread once a week for informal distribution within a close-knit community on a donation and barter basis. Even at her small scale, she encountered "huge hurdles" scaling up:

> I learned about temperature, humidity, the baker's percentage, and many other things I had never considered much in my home baking. I learned

that my personal connection to the dough and the bread and the fire was the most important element. That I need to stay in constant connection and keep observing and learning.

For Brian Moes, the challenges of scaling up "pertained mostly to the equipment, infrastructure, and technique" but after experimenting with different setups at different home locations, this was "just another adaptive challenge. . . . There were so many little details. . . . Not having a commercial fermented food mentor, I put to work my own creativity in making the transition points, or else, the creativity of other friends and business associates."

One of the biggest issues in scaling up is figuring out and securing appropriate vessels that are safe, legal, effective, durable, and affordable. Many small operations use ceramic crocks, even though they are expensive, fragile, and heavy. Cultured Pickle Shop in Berkeley uses stainless-steel vats, designed for the wine-making industry, with adjustable tops that can press down to the surface and vacuum-seal the contents. Be sure not to use stainless vessels that are not specifically designed to withstand acidification. "In a pinch we tried using large stainless steel brew pots," recounts Luke Regalbuto.

We found out the hard way that this can be disastrous. Often cheap stainless steel pots have handles that are fastened to the pot with aluminum. We had to throw away a large batch of product when we found that it had completely eroded the aluminum fastenings. We have also had problems with the cheap pots losing a sort of painted on stainless steel finish.

For the most part, health inspectors do not accept the use of wooden barrels. "Finding the right vessel has been super challenging," according to Kathryn Lukas:

Wood barrels are out of the question (according to the health department), ceramic too heavy and expensive and stainless steel too expensive and very hard on the earth in terms of metal extraction. We ferment in the blue plastic food safe 57 gallon barrels. It was a really hard decision. We've gone out of our way to not use plastic of any sort in our packaging (our krauts are sold in re-usable ceramic crocks at the retail level and compostable deli containers at farmers markets). Several experts have confirmed that our barrels are safe and that there is no transference but I would prefer to use wood. I'm hoping that the bio-plastics industry will soon provide an alternative.

Some producers have found it difficult to find food-grade weights to press down on their ferments. "We are currently working with a production glass manufacturer to try out using custom-made, food-grade glass discs to weigh down pickles into brine," explains Dan Rosenberg. "We have never been able to come up with any other appropriate options for food-grade weights."

Beyond vessels, the right tools can help with scaling up. "Food processors are your friends," says Erin Bullock. Marko Colby describes the continuous-feed Robot Coupe commercial shredder that Midori Farm invested in—affectionately known on their farm as "the super shredder"—as amazing: "We can shred 40 pound of cabbage in 8 minutes and control the size of shred for different products." After shredding, Erin Bullock and her fellow collective-members use a 140-quart "spiral mixer" to mix and pound the kraut.

> This works so well that after 20 minutes of mixing, lots of juice is expelled from the cabbage. We don't have to pound the kraut by hand at all. We run the mixer when it is ¼ full for 3–5 minutes to compact the cabbage that's in there and make room for more.

Brian Moes recommends getting a pH meter and learning how to calibrate and use it correctly, to monitor pH levels of your fermenting products. But don't rush out to buy a lot of expensive equipment before you start. Start small and simple, and only "upgrade your equipment as your demand increases," offers Tressa Yellig of Salt, Fire, and Time in Portland, Oregon.

THE TEMPEH SHOP

Gainesville, Florida

One fermentation enterprise I have visited in my travels really stands out in illustrating how the myriad small technical challenges of fermentation can be overcome with good systems developed over time through creative problem-solving. Jose Caraballo started making tempeh commercially in 1985. Today he operates his business, The Tempeh Shop, with his son and daughter. They sell tempeh to restaurants, at the farmer's market, and via local retail grocers.

When I toured their "factory," I was impressed by Jose's clever adaptations of readily available technology. To dry the beans, one of the most laborious parts of the process, he created a simple device in which to place the drained pot of beans. The pot sits at an angle and rotates, so the beans continually get turned over, as a fan blows air right onto them. They make the tempeh in plastic bags with holes poked in them. You can do this by hand with a pin or a fork if you are doing just a few, but hundreds? Jose created an ingenious roller with nails poking out to be a hole puncher. Jose and his family fill each bag with cooled, dried soybeans that have been inoculated with spores. Bags are flattened into 1-inch/2.5 cm slabs and placed on open shelves on a rack on rollers. (See photos in the color insert.) The rack is then taken to the incubation room, where a space heater and an air conditioner, both tied into thermostats, together function to keep the developing tempeh in the desired 85–90°F/29–32°C temperature range. It took Jose decades to refine his systems, but in doing so he exemplifies an indomitable human spirit of inventiveness. You can too!

Another consideration for any food business is packaging. Many health- and eco-conscious consumers would prefer to purchase food packaged in glass jars than in plastic tubs, although of course this drives prices higher. Some enterprises collect deposits on reusable vessels to encourage customers to return them for reuse. Some eco-friendly businesses are turning to corn-derived plastics for containers. For operations that ship food or cultures, there are more packaging decisions to make. Nathan and Emily Pujol ship cultures all across the United States. "It is a challenge to keep the cultures in their most fresh and vibrant state, since they will not be under the same conditions as they're used to. And it results in us constantly testing and tweaking our methods each season. We must also be aware of where they are shipping to, how long it will take, and the general temperature along the way."

Codes, Regulations, and Licensing

One of the biggest challenges in moving from fermentation for personal use to commercial production is the complex regulatory framework in which commercial food enterprises operate. Some people with small operations manage to avoid this by operating outside of this legal framework, "under the radar" of enforcement. This is the situation for Alyson Ewald, baking 18 loaves of bread each week in her earth oven. "I am a speck that doesn't register on any radar," she says. Jean Kowacki is a single mom in Florida who sells about 100 bottles of kombucha each week, along with fermented vegetables ("no two batches alike"), to other parents at her kids' school and people she has met through her local health food store and local nutritional advocacy groups, all through word of mouth. "I am trying to stay out of the commercial eye for now, for it would be expensive for me to legitimize my business," she says. "The amount of bureaucracy and overhead associated with a legitimate food business is overwhelming and debilitating," report Luke Regalbuto and Maggie Levinger of Wild West Ferments. Michael Thompson of the Chicago Honey Cooperative minces no words: "Fly under the radar as long as possible!"

For a small enough venture, informal and under-the-radar can be perfect, especially given ever-growing registration and reporting requirements on food production businesses from agencies at every level of government. But there are severe limitations to an under-the-radar enterprise; it is hard to develop your business if you can't freely promote it. All over the world, people are managing to ferment foods and beverages, at all different scales, successfully negotiating the terms of established regulatory frameworks.

These frameworks are evolving, and in general they seem more appropriately suited to large operations than small ones. The 2011 Food Safety Modernization Act gave the US Food and Drug Administration (FDA) "a legislative mandate to require comprehensive, science-based preventive controls across the food supply."[1] All but the very smallest food manufacturers must develop and implement a Hazard Analysis and Critical Control Point plan, better known as an HACCP plan. According to the FDA:

> HACCP is a systematic approach to the identification, evaluation, and control of food safety hazards based on the following seven principles:
>
> Principle 1: Conduct a hazard analysis.
>
> Principle 2: Determine the critical control points (CCPs).
>
> Principle 3: Establish critical limits.
>
> Principle 4: Establish monitoring procedures.
>
> Principle 5: Establish corrective actions.
>
> Principle 6: Establish verification procedures.
>
> Principle 7: Establish record-keeping and documentation procedures.[2]

This is a fine methodology for a large or possibly even mid-size organization to use. But for small, individual, partnership, family, one-or-two-part-time-employee-type enterprises, being forced to formalize so much can amount to an onerous requirement, taking time and resources that are not feasible at that scale of production. The looming specter of HACCP drove Pascal and Eric, California goat-farming and cheesemaking partners I visited a few years ago, to abandon their dream. "It would take us between 25 and 30 hours a week to perform and document all the testing that would be required," explains Pascal:

> For us that would mean a part time employee for whom we'll need an ADA compliant bathroom, a changing room and a break room plus a fully equipped laboratory. Between salary, workers comp, testing in-house and microbiological testing by a contract lab, we'll need to budget $50,000/year. We produce 5,000 lbs of cheese per year. This is why I think that to stay in business a cheese maker must produce at least 50,000 to 100,000 lbs per year.

The 2011 food safety law specifically exempted from HACCP requirements operations with gross sales below $500,000 and mostly direct sales. But some areas, notably meat and milk, face special scrutiny.

The FDA has repeatedly reviewed its policy on raw-milk cheeses, which allows cheeses from raw milk so long as they have been aged more than 60 days, a reasonable if somewhat arbitrary standard that has been in place since the 1940s. Many producers and aficionados fear that raw-milk cheeses may be banned altogether. An FDA review a decade ago was shelved after it "caused a wave of concern over imported raw-milk cheeses that many cheese fanciers feared would be banned," according to *The New York Times*.

"Today, with the artisan cheese industry booming, the focus is on homegrown cheesemakers."[3]

The American Raw Milk Cheese Presidium is a collaboration between Slow Food and members of the Raw Milk Cheesemakers' Association. To be part of the Presidium, members must adhere to strict voluntary requirements, including HACCP plans and bacterial testing to standards far stricter than the FDA's.[4] Many larger operations welcome clear science-based regulations; for some smaller operations, it may be impossible or burdensome, though others with deeper pockets persevere. I am not suggesting that healthy animals, hygienic practices, and food safety are any less important for a small-scale dairy than for a large-scale one. But the same limited scale that makes the requirements burdensome for small farmstead operators also limits the potential for and scale of danger. It is not desirable to make small farmstead production impractical.

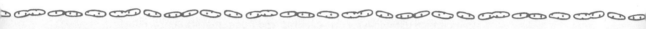

FARMSTEAD CREAMERY CHALLENGES

Nathan Arnold simultaneously started up a dairy farm and a cheesemaking operation at Sequatchie Cove Creamery in Sequatchie, Tennessee. He was mortified when the very first cheese sample he sent to the state Department of Agriculture tested positive for *Listeria monocytogenes*, and subsequent batches tested positive for *Staphylococcus aureus*. Levels were not so high that the state prohibited their sale as cheese, and no bacterially produced enterotoxins were found; whether to sell or discard the cheese was "a management decision," he was told. Nathan chose to play it safe and discarded them.

In the end, the farm culled its herd of the cows that tested positive for *S. aureus*, because as a certified organic farm they cannot treat animals with antibiotics. Nathan's advice to fledgling farmstead cheesemakers is to test cows for *S. aureus*. Test each teat when you get the cows and every month thereafter. Also test every batch of cheese at three days and at maturity for both *S. aureus* and *L. monocytogenes*. Test a sample from the bulk tank monthly. With culling and frequent testing, Nathan was able to solve the creamery's contamination problems, with the help of a French cheesemaking technical consultant and a voluntary HACCP plan, which he regards as a "proactive stance that demonstrates responsibility."

Now that Nathan and his team have the cheesemaking down, they are finding it difficult to sell all the cheese they are making, so they must increase their cave-conditions storage capacity and further develop their marketing. "The learning curve is huge!" he reflects. The dairy has spent many thousands of dollars on bacteriological testing and now routinely spends more than 4 percent of its gross income on testing. Nathan takes the long view. One season into year two, he points toward year five as his goal for achieving "consistency, marketing success, and profitability."

People's experiences of code enforcement vary widely. "It didn't seem to make any difference what product we were making; the requirements were the same regardless," explains Erin Bullock. "Actually it was easier to get our products licensed *because* they are fermented and live (not canned)," insists Marko Colby. "The doors were slammed in my face repeatedly, and I was discouraged all the way," reports Patricia Grunau, who sought to produce kombucha commercially in Virginia. "Sometimes it seems the entire industry/government is against your business," reflects Florida tempeh maker Art Guy.

Some fledgling businesses encounter outright hostility from enforcement agencies. "We had an unsettling event recently," reports Luke Regalbuto of Wild West Ferment in Marin County, California:

> I had a man in plain clothing flash a police badge and pull me aside for questioning. Right away he started out with threats and intimidation tactics, that he cleverly combined with offers of help from the trouble I might be facing. . . . He said things like, "I know where you live, don't make me get a warrant" and "there are several enforcement departments that don't like what you guys are doing and want to shut you down." When I tried to find out what exactly the problem was, he was very vague. It sounds like there was some sort of complaint/concern and there are fears that our products might contain botulism. Therefore, he wanted me to meet him first thing after the weekend to collect some samples of our product so he can drive them directly to a lab several hours away for testing. When I responded to his concern of botulism by informing him that our product is fermented, he gave me a blank stare. I met with him the following morning despite my suspicion that he might not be the special investigator that he claimed to be. After I gave him the samples I again explained that our products are live-fermented foods that are not canned and should be kept refrigerated. A light went off this time and after calling his boss, they decided it was indeed a misunderstanding, and called off the investigation. The event did sound alarms and so the county health department has proceeded to take particular interest in our obscure food processing. They now consistently go out of their way to give us an especially hard time.

He offers this general advice: "Generally it is best to have as little communication with the health department as possible."

Many people seeking to license fermentation businesses encounter officials with little knowledge or understanding of the fermentation process. "Many in the regulatory agencies are not so familiar with this type of food manufacturing," observes Brian Moes. "Same goes with insurance companies." April McGreger found that "the lack of clearly defined rules is maddening." She recalls: "The North Carolina Department of Agriculture did not know what to do with me."

> The county office had never had to deal with fermented foods before so they were learning as they went with me. I went ahead and got my licensing to sell acidified foods, but it turned out that I didn't technically need it to sell fermented foods since they fall under the 'naturally-acidified' classification. In the end, they decided that I should buy a pH meter and test the pH of each batch of product that I sell and record that in a ledger.

Others have had similar experiences, educating regulators, and finding ways to document the quality and safety of each batch. "We have generally found that the local, state, and federal regulators we interact with have little prior knowledge of lactic acid fermentation," reports a producer who asked not to be identified:

> But, we learned early on that this challenge can generally be overcome by communicating what we know about the process in a confident tone that makes the regulators trust that we know what we are doing. Our regulators have required us to document pH of each batch, but have not subjected us to any strict regimens (like HAACP, FDA acidified food rules, etc.).

The burden may be on you to present documentation of the safety of the ferments you wish to produce. "Have a list of commercially available and well known products to compare your product with," advises Luke Regalbuto. Some producers enlisted the support of research experts. "The state of California was very concerned about my 'low salt' krauts, which of course are not low salt at all (1.5 percent)," explains Kathryn Lukas:

> So they asked me to run my recipes by a microbiologist at UC Davis who in turn introduced me to Dr. Fred Breidt, a microbiologist who is also a kraut expert (North Carolina State University). Dr. Breidt has become a trusted ally, and gives me advice when I push the limits of lacto-fermentation with my sometimes strange recipes. Other than that, the public officials have been pretty cool, especially after Dr. Breidt told them that there has never been a case of food poisoning involving sauerkraut and that lacto-fermentation is considered one of the safest food preservation methods.

It is usually easy to document the effectiveness and safety of fermentation, because historical and biological facts back it up. Do the research and present the facts. Maybe you'll have an experience like Jennifer De Marco: "We feel like our inspector's main goal is to help us succeed by producing the safest food possible for others to enjoy. This is how it should be! We feel like they actually enjoy learning about fermentation and even recall stories of making kraut back in the day with their family."

There are many more specialized regulations covering alcoholic beverages, milk and meat products, and organic certification. The manufacture of alcoholic beverages (along with ethanol biofuels) is strictly controlled, regulated, and taxed in the United States by several different agencies, including the Bureau of Alcohol, Tobacco and Firearms (ATF), and the Alcohol and Tobacco Tax and Trade Bureau (TTB), both in the Treasury Department, as well as analogous state agencies. The government definitely wants its piece of the action!

Among the interests of these agencies is exactly who owns and controls the production of alcohol. Raphael Lyons promoted his Enlightenment Wines enterprise as "community-supported alcohol" and offered subscriptions as "shares" in the winery. After his unusual business model was written up in some popular blogs, he received a stern message from the New York State Liquor Authority "about the limits of my license." He was told that "owning 'shares' of my winery with a 'dividend' of three mixed cases a year is a big no-go. You can't own any part of a winery without being on the license."

Several fermentation entrepreneurs mentioned that the biggest regulatory challenge was organic certification. "For a processed food to be certified organic it takes an amazing amount of tracking paperwork," says Marko Colby. "You would think it would be easy because most of our ingredients are coming from the farm, but we need to generate invoices for each ingredient we transfer from the farm to the processing kitchen. Ahh!" Beyond the ingredients themselves, processing equipment must all be certified organic. So if a small producer of, say, apple cider brings organic apples to a larger facility for pressing, the cider cannot be labeled as organic unless that facility is certified as organic, which is typically not the case.

Different Business Models: Farm-Based Operations, Diversification, and Specialization

People start fermentation businesses with a wide range of different visions. Some want a small, personal enterprise that will provide them with some income but have no grander ambitions. Some are thrilled at the prospect of growth. Some enterprises start on farms as a complement to farming, adding value to the farm's raw agricultural products. Some businesses develop in ways that fill very specific niches. Some incorporate fermentation into broader food businesses, such as restaurants or caterers. There is no single business model for fermentation enterprises.

Many realms of fermentation have historically occurred on farms. Wine making has always been an extension of grape growing (or maybe vice versa), as cheesemaking has always gone hand in hand with keeping and milking animals. In our post-agrarian and post-industrial age, of course, wine and cheese, like any other foods, get mass-produced far from the farm. But with both these products, as well as apple cider, fermented vegetables, and probably other types of ferments, many small revivalist producers are doing so right on their farms.

Mark Shepard and his family in Viola, Wisconsin, have an unconventional farm, using permaculture ideas and diverse forest crops, with a focus on hazelnuts, chestnuts, and apples. Prime apples they can sell, but the ones that fall to the ground or are badly blemished they ferment into cider. "After 4 years, we're finally legal to sell our value-added farm product . . . Hard Cider!" announced Mark in 2010. Flack Family Farm, in Vermont, is a diversified farm offering vegetables, milk, and meat. Every fall, the Flacks host a series of workdays, inviting friends and neighbors to come join them in cleaning and shredding vegetables and pounding them into barrels. Everyone takes home a bucket of shredded veggies to ferment at home, and the Flacks get help transforming their fields of vegetables into a stable product that they can sell for the rest of the year. Nancy and Pat Curley, of Traverse City, Michigan, practice what they have termed *FARM-entation*: "from seed to plant to harvest to finished, fermented product right here on our own farm."

"Grow your own produce!" exclaims Marko Colby, whose Midori Farm grows all the veggies they ferment, except for ginger and other spices. "Fresh produce makes a superior ferment every time." My friend Brian Geier, who grows and ferments vegetables under the brand name Sour Power in Frankfort, Kentucky, envisions expanding his enterprise into a larger farmer-producer cooperative:

> My dream is to grow this business to a point where it can process and sell more than we can grow, and bring on other organic farmers as owners and producers . . . that would outgrow the kitchen we currently use [a shared incubator kitchen], and to build a completely off-grid, commercial kitchen with a root cellar for storage of fermenting vessels and finished jars. I really think it is possible, even with regs, although it will take a lot of work to get there. Good work!

Like most entrepreneurs who start small enterprises, Brian has an expansive vision. Some fermentation businesses do take off and grow fast. "Our company began about 5 years ago as a one-man garage operation," reports Dave Ehreth of Alexander Valley Gourmet in Healdsburg, California. "We now have a couple of employees and will probably double our production this year." Kathryn Lukas's Farmhouse Culture has grown in just two years to selling at nine farmer's markets and 58 retail locations in Northern California, as she explores markets in Southern California. Rather than national distribution of her products, Lukas's vision for growth is to "expand by building fermentoriums in various locations, developing recipes with ingredients that are locally abundant, and selling those krauts just in those regions."

Not every fermentation entrepreneur is eager for their business to grow. "My business is still very small, and I wrestle every day with how and whether or not I should grow it," reflects April McGreger.

> Keeping it as small as it is means that I personally make and test every batch of product that leaves my kitchen. This is how I maintain consistency at present. Currently, I am bursting at the seams in my kitchen so scaling up would mean finding a new location and new licensing (likely no longer the Department of Agriculture but Health Department instead).

Some small fermentation entrepreneurs are emphatic that they do not wish to grow. "Staying small is more than a technical or business decision," declares Raphael Lyons. "For me, it's what allows me to be revolutionary—in a permanent state of radical experimentation."

Often businesses go to the opposite extreme; rather than functioning in a permanent state of experimentation, they find a specialized niche and fill it. One interesting niche serving the DIY fermentation movement is propagating and selling fermentation cultures. For at least one culture producer, the fact that what they are selling is not itself a food has meant that they have avoided dealing with regulators. "We haven't pursued licensing because it's not technically a food product."

One fermentation business I know, the Ceres Community Project in Sebastopol, California, grew out of a non-profit agency operating "through an integrated model that gives teens experiences of growing and preparing healthy food, provides those facing cancer and other life-threatening illnesses with nourishing meals, and educates the larger community about the connection between food, healing and wellness." The sauerkraut business is an offshoot of these broader objectives. One of the foods their teen workers were preparing for the cancer patients was sauerkraut. In response to the popularity of their sauerkraut, they started packaging it and selling it through local retailers, including Whole Foods. Now sauerkraut sales are helping to support the organization's service activities.

Another model for people who enjoy variety is the "community supported kitchen" (CSK) inspired by community supported agriculture (CSA), but instead of raw vegetables it provides prepared foods, including a rotating selection of ferments. This business model was pioneered by Three Stone Hearth in Berkeley, California, but it is rapidly spreading. A related idea is a more traditional prepared meal catering service. My friend Lagusta Yearwood has a vegan meal service in New Paltz, New York, for which she makes her own tempeh, krauts, miso, and vinegar. Many restaurants have also incorporated ferments they make themselves into their menus.

This is but a cursory overview of ways in which people have transformed their passion for fermentation into their livelihood. My advice to anyone wishing to embark upon a fermentation-based enterprise is to learn as much as you can about how other people have set up such businesses. If you can, try to apprentice yourself with an experienced artisan producer whose products you admire. Reach out to other producers—just to talk to them, visit their operations, and have them to use as resources as you chart your own path. If local enterprises are reluctant to share information because they perceive you as a competitor, try reaching out to people farther away. Many people love to share their techniques and systems if someone seems genuinely interested.

Above all, I want to offer encouragement to fermentation lovers trying to figure out ways to support themselves. Fermentation may offer a viable and honorable path. The relocalization of our food demands that we create and support, beyond local agriculture, an array of local processors, fermenters prime among them.

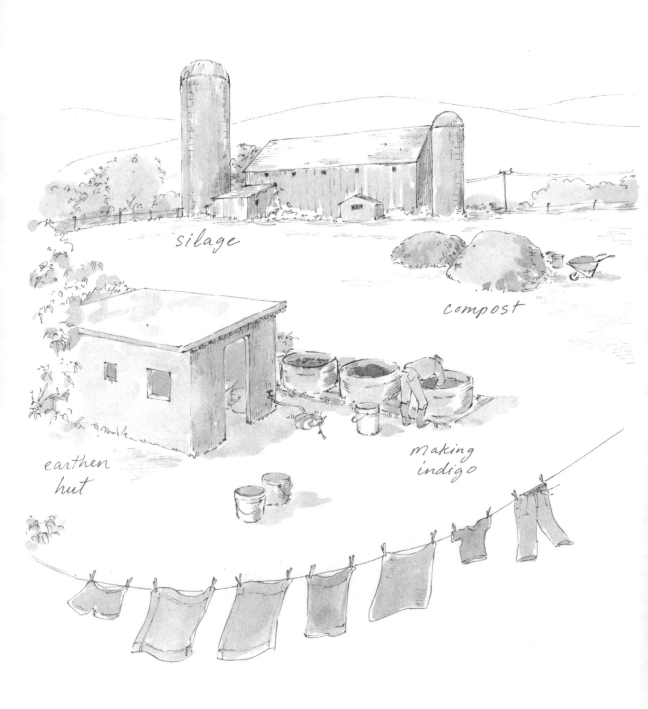

silage

compost

earthen
hut

making
indigo

CHAPTER 14

Non-Food Applications of Fermentation

$\mathcal{P}$eople have harnessed the transformative power of microorganisms for many purposes other than producing foods and beverages for our own consumption. This chapter surveys non-food applications of fermentation (defined broadly to encompass both aerobic and anaerobic microbial processes), which fall into a few broad (often overlapping) categories: agriculture; land and water reclamation (bioremediation); waste stream management; fiber and building arts; energy production; and medicine, drugs, and body care.

 ## Agriculture

Fermentation has many applications in agriculture, as fundamental as building soil fertility, saving seeds, preserving forage for livestock, and controlling pests.

Compost

In composting, bacteria and fungi transform a mix of kitchen and garden scraps, leaves, wood, manure, straw, grass—really, any organic matter—into humus that renews the fertility of the earth itself. There are many different methods of composting. Even without any method, piles of scraps of organic materials will break down. But depending upon your method, that pile can smell foul or fine, generate significant heat or none, break down faster or slower, and favor aerobic organisms or anaerobes.

The sources of both microbial inoculation and nutrients are the compost "feedstocks." In general, the more varied the feedstocks, the better. People talk about compost feedstocks in terms of balancing carbon and nitrogen. Carbon is the primary element of which all living cells are composed. Nitrogen is also essential. But the carbon-to-nitrogen ratio varies in different types of organic substances. Wood tends to have relatively little nitrogen compared with green leafy matter, or manure. It takes a mixture of higher-nitrogen feedstocks with lower-nitrogen feedstocks to create conditions for diverse and rapid microbial growth. Food scraps tend to be relatively rich in nitrogen, which is why it's best to mix them with other drier, lower-nitrogen materials, such as sawdust, wood chips, straw, or even paper. The USDA organic regulations define *compost* as a process in which the starting materials together constitute an initial C:N ratio of between 25:1 and 40:1. Commercial operations, meticulous individuals, and certified organic farms calculate how much of each feedstock will bring the average C:N ratios into that range. Many charts of the C:N ratios of different materials can be found online.

In a small backyard composting operation, there is really no reason to get too fixated on C:N ratios. Just layer a variety of green and brown organic materials. In my home practice, I use a pretty passive, effortless composting method. I just mix kitchen scraps with straw, wood chips, sawdust, and/or leaves, along with occasional bark, animal manure, or other extras. I start a new pile every so often, and turn the old one. Over time (a year or more) it breaks down, worms come, and it becomes light and beautiful humus. This process is slow and easy and suits me fine. But over at my friend Billy's farm, Little Short Mountain Farm, I've been helping him develop and implement strategies for improving fertility on many acres of pastures and fields. To restore the fertility of this land, which was farmed for years with chemicals, we're making compost (and brewing tea from it) in a much more methodical way, according to principles I learned from microbiologist Dr. Elaine Ingham.

lacto bacilli

For building soil fertility, Dr. Ingham (along with many others) recommends composting methods that encourage aerobic microbial growth, which technically makes composting not a fermentation process at all, according to the definition of fermentation as anaerobic metabolism. Dr. Ingham explains that nitrogen and other essential nutrients are most available to plants under aerobic soil conditions. Which makes sense, since the best soils have a loamy structure that allows for the diffusion of air through the topsoil. She also points out that aerobic bacteria and fungi stick to everything "like glue," binding soil together and giving it an "ultrastructure" that helps to hold water and resist runoff and erosion. Beyond these advantages of aerobic organisms, Dr. Ingham argues that certain by-products of anaerobic (fermentation) organisms can be toxic to plants, including not only our beloved alcohol (which in enough concentration can be quite toxic to us as well), but also formaldehyde, volatile acids, and phenols. Aerobic compost has a mild, earthy aroma. Anaerobic compost can (but doesn't have to) smell like a fetid swamp.

An aerobic compost pile at least a cubic yard in size, moist like a sponge but not waterlogged, will inevitably produce considerable heat. This is generally regarded as beneficial, because sustained heat above 131°F/55°C kills weed seeds, pathogenic bacteria, and pests in the composting materials and makes the process go quickly. The heat is generated by frenetic metabolic activity by microbes given ideal conditions for growth. The only problem is that if the heat in the center becomes excessive, above about 158°F/70°C, then there in the center, farthest from the free flow of oxygen, oxidative (aerobic) metabolism will no longer be able to be sustained, and the center of the pile will "go anaerobic."

A heat-generating aerobic compost pile is a miraculous thing to behold. The heat is a product of an alchemical mixing of the elements, and fills me with awe. I've even heard stories of people cooking food by burying it in the compost, or using the heat from a compost pile to heat a greenhouse. But a pile that is steaming must be monitored closely, and when the temperature in the center rises above 150°F/66°C, you have to make time to turn the pile. This releases accumulating heat in the center, aerates the pile, and remixes the elements for a more even distribution of materials and microbial activity. At my friend's farm, we use a tractor to turn the huge piles. We bought a 4-foot/1.3 m thermometer to monitor the temperature at the center of the pile, and each time the heat spikes, we turn the pile. With the tractor front loader, it takes about half an hour; with a shovel or pitchfork, it would take most of a day. After a few weeks, with four or five turns, the activity mellows and we can leave the compost to mature a few months.

The compost thus produced is gorgeous rich humus, and microscopic inspection confirms that it is a hotbed of biodiversity. We take some of the compost, place it in a mesh bag that looks like a giant tea bag, hang it in a water tank with a powerful air pump attached, add kelp powder, humic acid, and a bit of molasses, and blow a huge amount of air into the mix for 24 hours to brew it into aerobic compost tea. This tea enables us to spray beneficial microbes around the fields much farther and much more easily than we can spread compost.

On a big farm with lots of organic materials, and machinery and people to process them, an exacting process like this is not a big deal. But turning a big pile by hand, even once, is an ambitious project. Turning every few days as temperatures repeatedly spike is impossible for most busy people with backyard gardens. So as a practical matter, most people use more casual, slower, less labor-intensive composting methods. Some people (like me) just pile materials as they accumulate, turn the pile once in a while, and let time slowly decompose them. Some people use cleverly designed devices for turning. Some people use vermiculture (worms) to rapidly and efficiently transform kitchen waste, and some feed scraps directly to chickens, converting residuals to manure with hardly any work.

And some people take an approach similar to food fermentation techniques, practical for micro-scale, indoor application, using a starter culture. E. Shig Matsukawa, a composting activist who is teaching people this apartment-friendly technique in New York City, uses a vocabulary I can relate to for this, calling it "pickling food waste." Shig uses an inoculant called Efficient

Microorganisms (EM), developed in Japan and used worldwide, which is a community of organisms that includes lactic acid bacteria, yeasts, and phototrophic bacteria. "The direct utilization of the microbes gives us control of the exact species of microorganisms we know will help us with our process, as well as having enough of them ('quorum sensing') to do the job," explains Shig. "This is in contrast to creating the conditions and adding the ingredients to attract and/or bring out the desired microbes," as in the composting methods described earlier. Using many of the same organisms that are commonly used in food fermentations (and others), nutrients are broken down into forms more available to plants, acidity prevents pathogens, and waste is preserved without noxious odors, so it can be left sealed in an airtight container for many months. "The resulting odors range from vinegary to alcohol (beer-like)," says Shig.

Shig's process is actually in three steps. A preliminary process uses a liquid starter culture—EM-1—to ferment a dry, flaky medium, such as bran from wheat, rice, or oats, or sawdust, or finely shredded autumn leaves. That is fermented in an airtight container for about two weeks, then dried and stored for ongoing use as a starter. As food wastes are generated, they are placed in an airtight container and sprinkled with starter. When a container is filled, it is sealed and left to ferment at ambient temperatures about two weeks. After fermentation, the fermented food wastes can remain in the sealed fermentation containers for as long as necessary without noxious odor. As convenient, they are buried in earth (even in a pot indoors) to further cure before applying to plants. (For specifics of the process and proportions, see the sidebar.)

I was curious about the apparent contradiction between Elaine Ingham's ideas about composting—that it must be aerobic—and the EM fermentation method. Shig reflected on the question and made several excellent points. First of all, he said, "not all aerobic bacteria are beneficial and not all anaerobic bacteria are non-beneficial." He also cited a compost study done comparing piles with and without EM-1 added. The EM pile had significantly higher counts of aerobic microorganisms than the control.[1] "That trial showed that the application of EM-1 microbes in the soil encouraged the growth of other good microbes, including heterotrophs, pseudomonads, actinomycetes, and filamentous fungi such as mychorrizae, none of which are in the EM-1." Bacteria are mysterious shape-shifters! The known microbes in the starter are not the same ones that end up in the soil; the genetically fluid bacteria adapt. "What seems to be happening," Shig speculates, "is that the dominant microbes in EM-1 are influencing other microbes in the environment, and in combination with the added organic matter, these other beneficial organisms multiply more than usual, and multiply in diversity, as well." As with any ferments, any gardening technique, and almost anything in life, there is no single best method. Whatever method you find works best for you. I agree with Shig, who says, "The most important evidence is the plants themselves."

HOW TO MAKE YOUR OWN FERMENTED BRAN FOR PICKLING FOOD WASTE

E. Shig Matsukawa, recyclefoodwaste.org

Use any kind of organic material: wheat bran, rice bran, saw dust, shredded fall leaves, chipped yard waste, etc. Material has to be dry and in granular form. We use wheat bran because it is easy to use, and relatively inexpensive. For 2.5 lbs/1 kilogram wheat bran (unprocessed), use 1 fl oz/30 ml blackstrap molasses, 1 fl oz/30 ml EM-1 Microbial Inoculant, about 20 oz/600 ml water. The liquid ratio is 1:1:20, that is, 1 part molasses: 1 part EM-1: 20 parts water. Mix the liquids in a bowl, until the molasses has fully dissolved. Place the wheat bran, which should be very dry and flaky, in a mixing bin. Slowly add the liquid mixture to the wheat bran until it's about 30 percent moist (by hand, it should form into a ball but break apart when touched). Mix the liquid into the wheat bran thoroughly (no dry spots and no too-wet spots). After thoroughly mixing, put into an airtight container. Press down to squeeze out air. Put a plastic bag or sheet on top of it. Close lid tight. Let it sit at room temperature, out of direct sunlight. White mold is good if it appears. After 2 weeks, air-dry by spreading it out thinly or sun-dry it. When dry (crunchy feel to it), keep in a container or ziplock away from moisture (keeps for over 1 year), and it's ready to use.

To make fermented food waste (FFW), add a handful of fermented bran to an empty container. Sprinkle fermented bran every time you add food waste. (The ideal ratio is 1:33.) Keep container closed and airtight. White mold is good if it appears. When container is full, let it sit for 2 weeks or longer at room temperature, in an airtight container. Keep out of direct sunlight. For burying:

◎ If in a trench, bury with 6–12 inches of soil on top; can plant seeds or seedlings after 2 weeks.

◎ If in a pit, at least 1 foot away from existing plants and 3 feet away from trees; bury 1–2 feet deep and cover with at least 6 inches of soil on top; can plant after 2 weeks, or let it be the nutrients for surrounding plants.

◎ In pots or planters, you can sandwich FFW between soil in a pot or planter. First, add pebbles, small rocks, and/or sand to the bottom of the pot or planter (about 1 inch). Then add about 1–2 inches/3–5 cm of soil (or ¼ of the pot/planter). Add 2–3 inches/5–8 cm of FFW (or ⅓ of the pot/planter) And fill to the top with soil. Let it sit for 2 weeks away from rain before planting.

Or you can feed the fermented food waste to earthworms. Follow the general rules for a worm bin, except earthworms can go through FFW much faster, so you can feed them more often.

EM is a modern-day manifestation of an ancient Japanese farming tradition called *bokashi*, which involved fermenting whatever organic matter was available, including rice bran, fish meal, and the dry cake left over from oil pressing. Historically this must have begun as a spontaneous fermentation, like any other, and over time been consciously perpetuated by backslopping, adding a remnant of the previous generation into each new batch. EM has a very devoted following. I am sure it is very effective for all the varied things I've heard about people doing with it, including not only fermenting food waste but also fermenting food, probiotic supplementation, household and industrial cleaning, inoculating septic tanks and other sewage treatment, and many other applications. But *bokashi* can also be practiced as a wild fermentation; Bruno Vernier wrote to me that it "can be as simple and cheap as combining whey, molasses, water and shredded paper." Another intriguing *bokashi* practice I've heard about is known as "indigenous microorganisms" (IMO).

"Indigenous microorganisms are beneficial members of the soil biota (including filamentous fungi, yeasts and bacteria) collected from non-cultivated soil near the area where they will be applied," explains a *Bokashi Nature Farming Manual* from the Philippines. Rice or rice bran is used as a medium on which to grow existing soil organisms. I've read about two different methods. One involves mixing soil from one or more locations with rice bran and a little water to form a ball, then suspending the ball to spontaneously ferment.[2] The other involves actually burying a wooden box, with a layer of cooked rice spread in it, in the forest for four days to a week. The box is loosely covered by a paper towel, then with wire mesh to protect against rodents, then a layer of plastic to keep water out, and finally leaves.[3] In either case, the resulting grain with mold growing on it is then used as a starter for other preparations, including *bokashi* fermentation of food wastes. Much more detail on the specifics of the process is available on the Internet.

One final method of using fermentation as part of a strategy to build soil fertility is the biodynamic method. Biodynamic growers use an array of preparations (often referred to as "preps"), each of which involves fermenting an alchemical mixture of ingredients. For instance, cow horns are stuffed with fresh manure from lactating cows and buried from fall to spring. For another prep, a stag's bladder is stuffed with yarrow flowers and hung up in a tree over the summer. After its fermentation, a small amount of the prep is added to water and stirred for a full hour. Even the stirring method is prescribed: Stir in a circular motion to create a vortex; then reverse direction and create a vortex in that direction; then reverse again, and again, and again, for a full hour. These preps are intended to harness and harmonize earthly and cosmic forces. The stirring "activates" the prep energetically, or oxygenates it to encourage a rapid proliferation of aerobic organisms—whichever way you prefer to conceptualize it. The preps are then spread onto gardens and fields, directly sprayed on plants, or in some cases incorporated into compost piles.

Fermenting Urine

Another fermentation process used to improve soil fertility is the fermentation of urine. The process is simple: Collect urine and do nothing, just let it sit a few weeks. Lots of gardeners collect their own pee, and that of those around them willing to share it, to fertilize nitrogen-loving plants. Collect it in outdoor containers via pee jars or buckets. PEE HERE NOW read signs at pee stations at Short Mountain for a while. Usually pee accumulates slowly and sits around; sometimes people intentionally age it. There is even a word in English for fermented urine—*lant*—usually used to describe aged urine used for cleaning. A microscopic investigation into "The Ammoniacal Fermentation of Urine" was published as early as 1890 in the Proceedings of the American Society of Microscopists.[4] It is an alkaline fermentation that increases pH and produces ammonia.

Exactly as the acidifying fermentations destroy many pathogens, so does this alkalinizing ferment. A blogging aquaponic gardener, who uses fermented human urine as a nutrient in her system, sent urine samples to a lab for analysis, some deliberately contaminated with fecal matter. Some of each was sent to the lab fresh, and the rest was fermented until the pH rose to 9, then it was sent to the lab. Both fresh batches tested positive for fecal coliforms; both fermented batches tested negative. "This convinced me that my own urine when aged is not going to make me sick if I use it as fertilizer for a pee-ponic system."[5]

Aging urine and using it as a soil-fertilizing strategy has long been done in various places, making use of a nitrogen resource universally available. My friend Hector Black, 86 years old with beautiful gardens and orchards, swears by urine as a soil amendment, fresh and aged. "My urine is already aged," he quips. Hector applies fresh urine to his orchard, diluted 1:1 with water in dry weather, full strength when the ground is saturated with water. "I think some good stuff happens when you age it," says Hector. "I use the aged stuff on the vegetable garden. Especially nitrogen-loving plants like greens and corn. Does wonders!"

rye plant

The use of fermented urine is spreading in Uganda. "We no longer waste urine in our homes," reports farmer Mary Batwaweela. "Each member of the family is allocated a tin every night where she/he urinates then in the morning we pour it into a big container and ferment it for 28 days."[6] The aged pee is then diluted with an equal quantity of water and then applied to soil. On the Internet I found documentation of practices in China,[7] India,[8] and elsewhere.

Feeding Animals with Fermentation

Just as humans have harnessed the power of fermentation to preserve and enhance food from periods of abundance to sustain us through seasons of scarcity, we have also used fermentation to preserve and pre-digest forage crops to feed our farm animals through forage-scarce winters.

Silage is the practice of harvesting grasses, including the post-harvest stalks of corn and other grain-producing plants, and/or other green forage crops, and packing them in silos, mounds, pits, or large bales to ferment.

The fermentation is primarily a lactic acid fermentation, breaking down cellulose and lowering pH. "Efficient fermentation ensures a more palatable and digestible feed," states an extension publication of North Dakota State University.[9] If forage material is very moist, it must be dried somewhat prior to ensilage. Material must also be chopped into small pieces and packed tightly in order to minimize trapped air and thus limit aerobic activity. Typically silage is fermented spontaneously by organisms present on the plant material.

Silage is an application of the principles of vegetable fermentation to cellulose-rich grasses and stalks that humans cannot digest. In some regions, the leaves and stalks of other food crops were also fermented for animal fodder. A historical investigation into vegetable pickling in Poland states: "Until the middle of this century [20th], leaves of turnips, beet, cabbage and others were fermented in huge tubs, and used as winter fodder."[10]

Some people wishing to improve the health of their livestock soak grains in order to reduce phytic acid content and improve nutrient availability. Monique Trahan wrote telling me about the practice of her farmer grandfather: "He fed his pigs by filling pails with oats and water and letting them sit until fizzy." Many dairy operations soak grains for livestock in whey from cheese production.

Some people even make sauerkraut for their animals! My dog Kitty will sometimes eat sauerkraut, but not always. She seems to like it finely shredded rather than in bigger chunks, and she seems to prefer it only mildly sour. Rather than feeding her prime kraut to her animals, Barb Schuetz ferments the scraps for them. "All the pieces of produce that don't make it into our kraut goes in a 5 gallon bucket to ferment for them."

Seed Saving

Certain seeds are typically fermented in the pulp that holds them, prior to drying for storage. I have been watching my friend Daz'l, a master gardener in our community, save tomato seeds in this way for years. He harvests fruits at the peak of the season from the healthiest plants and scoops seeds out of the fruits in their pulp. (You can eat the fleshy remains of the seeded tomatoes.) Dazl places the seeds and pulp of each variety into a glass half full of water, and ferments about three days. Then he rinses the seeds of pulp. "The better you rinse them, the less sticky they will be," he emphasizes, therefore easier to separate as they dry. Daz'l dries them on newspaper (seeds stick less than with paper towels) and stores them in a cool, dry spot until next year's planting time.

In seed saving, as in everything having to do with cultivating plants, people use a variety of techniques. Michel and Jude Fanton, founders of

sunflower head

Australia's Seed Savers' Network and the authors of *The Seed Savers' Handbook*, use a slightly different method:

> Allow the fruits to ripen just beyond the eating stage. Cut them open, squeeze out the jelly and seeds, putting the seeds of one variety in a jar or bowl. If you are saving the seeds of a dry, meaty tomato such as the excellent Italian Plum you may have to add a tiny amount of water. Label the jars and leave in a warm spot for two to three days. If it is not stirred, a foam will form on top and a beneficial fermentation will take place, caused by a microbe, *Geotrichum candidum*, acting on the sticky gel that surrounds the seeds. Antibiotic activity deals with diseases such as bacterial spot, speck, and canker. The only danger is in leaving the fermentation process for too long, leading to premature germination. As soon as the foam forms, scoop it off the top, add water and pour the lot through a sieve. Wash and rub until clean. The jelly around the seeds will have been washed off and the seeds will appear somewhat hairy. Spread them on sheets of shiny paper in a single layer and dry somewhere safe, out of the sun. After a few hours of drying, rub the seeds between your palms to stop them from sticking.[11]

The Fantons also recommend the same procedure for saving cucumber seeds to dissolve the jelly around the seeds and "kill off any seed-borne diseases."[12] In fact, one extension officer for the University of Illinois Extension suggests fermenting the seeds of any vegetables in which the seeds are enclosed in fleshy fruits.

> Seed contained in fleshy fruits should be cleaned using the wet method. Tomatoes, melons, squash, cucumber and roses are prepared this way. Scoop the seed masses out of the fruit or lightly crush fruits. Put the seed mass and a small amount of warm water in a bucket or jar. Let the mix ferment for two to four days. Stir daily. The fermentation process kills viruses and separates the good seed from the bad seed and fruit pulp. After two to four days, the good viable seeds will sink to the bottom of the container while the pulp and bad seed float. Pour off the pulp, water, bad seed and mold. Spread the good seed on a screen or paper towel to dry.[13]

Pest Control

Another agricultural application of fermentation is in pest control. A simple old-time method is to take some specimens of pests you wish to deter, crush them into water, ferment a few days, strain, and spray on plants to protect them from those pests. One specific bacterium (*Bacillus thuringiensis* or Bt) has long been applied to crops as an insecticide against leaf-feeding caterpillars. The bacteria produce a protein that reacts with the cells lining the guts of caterpillars and other susceptible insects, causing them to stop feeding and die. Newer proprietary microbial insecticides are being developed. Spinosad comes from the fermentation of soil bacteria *Saccharopolyspora spinosa*; Abamectin from another soil microorganism, *Streptomycetes avermitilis*.

California vintner Lou Preston sprayed live-culture whey from raw-milk cheesemaking "straight from the cheese draining table (no aging)" as a foliar spray on his grape vineyards. The first year, he sprayed pure whey directly on the plants in a test patch and experienced no mildew on those vines. The next year, he mixed the whey with an aerated compost tea and spread it on more of his vineyard, with some mildew but little, and limited to the most mildew-prone varieties. Lou also noted "much better development of beneficial insect populations since they had not been disturbed by sulfur application." Sadly, the dairy that was producing the whey closed, so Lou has no large supply of whey this year. But he is fermenting grass, silage-style, and plans to experiment spraying an extract of the juices.

Bioremediation

In the emerging field of bioremediation, biological processes of nutrient cycling, involving bacteria and fungi, are encouraged in various ways, in order to decompose contaminants and clean up contaminated soils and waters. "Bioremediation has successfully cleaned up many polluted sites," according to the US Environmental Protection Agency.[14] As I was writing this book in 2010, oil was pumping at high pressure into the Gulf of Mexico from an accident at a drilling rig, the *Deepwater Horizon*. The news was filled with horrific images of oil-slicked environmental devastation. As repeated attempts to plug the well were failing, *Scientific American* declared: "Bacteria and other microbes are the only thing that will ultimately clean up the ongoing oil spill."[15]

In fact, at much lower concentrations, hydrocarbons, the chemical building blocks of fossil fuels, are part of the environment everywhere, and bacteria capable of digesting them are ubiquitous. "No single organism can break down all the components of crude oil or refined fuels spilled into the environment," explains an American Academy of Microbiology (AAM) report:

> The tens of thousands of different compounds that make up oil can only be biodegraded by communities of microorganisms acting in concert. Some bacteria can degrade several hydrocarbons or a class of hydrocarbons. The combined action of the community can degrade almost all of the components.[16]

The limitation on the ability of this to happen in an oil spill is time and speed. In the years it could take for bacteria to clean up a big spill, incalculable damage can be done.

Rates of oil degradation vary widely, depending on a variety of factors. First, there is a lag period, as the relatively small populations of hydrocarbon-digesting bacteria respond to the sudden abundance of nutrients. Then, "generally degradation rates slow as the oil concentration decreases, making it difficult to calculate a certain end-point," explains the American Academy of Microbiology. "They also slow as the more readily degradable components are used up, leaving behind the more recalcitrant components."[17] Also, when oil sinks to the ocean's depths, where temperatures are much colder and oxygen is not present, metabolism slows way down. Chemical dispersants can facilitate improved bacterial access to oil floating in water, by creating greater surface area. Fertilizers can be added to stimulate bacteria growth. Genetic engineers have attempted to create bacteria that can digest hydrocarbons more efficiently or faster. But microbiologist Ronald Atlas, who evaluated genetically engineered bacteria and other post-*Exxon Valdez* cleanup strategies, reflects, "A superbug fails because it competes with this community that is adapted to the environment."[18]

While seeding microbes into the ocean has not been effective, seeding them on land can be. Mycologist Paul Stamets has been a pioneer in mycoremediation, the use of fungi to clean up contaminated soils. "Fungi are adept as molecular disassemblers, breaking down many recalcitrant, long-chained toxins into simpler, less toxic chemicals," explains Stamets.[19] He advocates mixing fungal mycelia directly into contaminated soils, or into wood chips spread over contaminated soil, as a first step in remediation:

> The introduction of a single fungus, for instance oyster mycelium, into a nearly lifeless landscape triggers a cascade of activity by other organisms. A synergy between at least 4 kingdoms—fungus, plant, bacterium, and animal—denatures toxins into derivatives useful to myriad species and fatal to few. . . . Ultimately, nature fosters complex partnerships of interdependence, with fungi blazing the path to ecological recovery.[20]

Rather than introducing pure mycelia, Stamets emphasizes using "acclimated spawn" that have been exposed to wild bacteria:

> Bacteria proliferate alongside the mycelium and produce their own toxin-digesting enzymes. This form of mycelium is far better equipped for handling toxic waste sites than mycelium not pre-exposed to wild microbes. For this reason, using pure culture spawn for mycoremediation may not be the best choice. . . . Aged mycelium from a mushroom farm has better mycoremediation properties.[21]

One US city that has been something of a laboratory for bioremediation activists is New Orleans. Common Ground, a grassroots group formed after the 2005 Hurricane Katrina flooding disaster in the city, has published *The New Orleans Residents' Guide to Do It Yourself Soil Clean Up Using Natural Processes*. In it, they note that "every city in the United States is contaminated by chemicals that are potentially deadly."

The greater New Orleans area also has a history of oil and chemical industries that generate and store thousands of tons of toxic chemicals. When hit by the floodwaters and hurricane winds of both Katrina and Rita, many of these chemicals floated out of their storage locations and into peoples' homes in adjacent neighborhoods. . . . The sediment deposited by floodwaters contains unsafe levels of certain contaminants: arsenic, diesel fuel and other petrochemicals, heavy metals, phthalates (chemicals used to soften plastics), polycyclic aromatic hydrocarbons (PAHs), and pesticides.[22]

To clean up toxic soil, they recommend using multiple bioremediation strategies. For removing heavy metals, they suggest *phytoremediation* with "hyper-accumulator" plants, including sunflowers, Indian mustard, peas, Asiatic dayflower, brake fern, lamb's-quarters, radishes, corn, spinach, and carrots. For removing petrochemicals and pesticides they suggest mycoremediation with oyster mushroom spawn. And for everyone they recommend aerated compost tea, which the organization helps people make.

The Common Ground activists also recommend using EM, not for soil remediation but rather for removing mold from damaged interiors of flooded houses. "When EM is sprayed in an untouched moldy house and left for a day the house becomes much safer and cleaner for crews to enter," states the *DIY Clean Up Guide*. My friend Free, who went to New Orleans after Katrina to volunteer in the restoration efforts, emailed me at the time: "Mold was in the walls, the floors, the ceiling—EVERYWHERE. I couldn't help but feel like gutting was a futile act—how could this moldy environment ever be clean enough for the family to return to it?" Working with Common Ground, she learned that "EM presents a solution." As the *DIY Clean Up Guide* explains, "This group of bacteria kills and prevents further mold growth. While bleach also kills mold it has been shown to be less effective at keeping the mold from growing back over time."

 ## Waste Management

Humans create waste at a vast scale. We use excessive packaging designed to resist biodegradation. We embrace up-to-the-minute gadgetry and dispose of the outdated models. We create dangerous radioactive waste that we do not have any idea what to do with. In our insatiable collective hunger to exploit and consume resources, accidents occur, spilling oil, releasing radiation, and leaving toxic contaminants.

But our *biological* by-products do not have to be considered as waste. Waste is not inevitable. In natural systems, there is no waste. Each creature's by-products are fodder for some other creature. This is the reason the Earth is not piled with feces and dead bodies. "Feces and urine are examples of natural, beneficial, organic materials excreted by the bodies of animals after completing their digestive processes," observes Joseph Jenkins, author of the cult classic *The Humanure Handbook*. "They are only 'waste' when we discard them. When recycled, they are resources."[23]

Early human settlements did not have to worry much about disposing of their poop. In many places, traditions emerged in which human feces were recycled into nutrients for intensive agriculture. Elsewhere, dispersal was generally adequate, and as it washed into rivers, along with all the other creatures' by-products, human excrement nourished microbes and they cycled the nutrients, making them available to other life-forms and maintaining the cleanliness of the water. The problems begin when large concentrations of excrement accumulate in waterways, triggering rapid microbial growth that exhausts the oxygen in the water. Like an overheating compost pile, an "overnourished" stream can "go anaerobic." This in turn suffocates fish and other aquatic life. "Soon such a stream would be black, slimy, stinky, and dead to all but those creatures who could live without oxygen," writes Jeanette Farrell.[24]

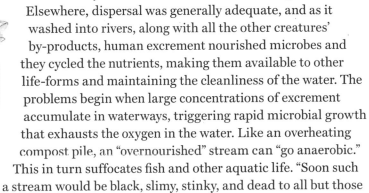

jars

Jenkins lays out simple methods for aerobic composting of humanure, along with sawdust and kitchen and garden scraps, not much different from the composting techniques described earlier, other than the inclusion of human feces as a feedstock. Jenkins addresses concerns about fecal pathogens, pointing out a hot compost pile can destroy pathogens in mere minutes:

> Lower temperatures require longer periods of time, possibly hours, days, weeks, or months, to effectively destroy pathogens. One need not strive for extremely hot temperatures such as 65°C (150°F) in a compost pile to feel confident about the destruction of pathogens. It may be more realistic to maintain lower temperatures in a compost pile for longer periods of time, such as 50°C (122°F) for 24 hours, or 46°C (115°F) for a week. . . . A sound approach to pathogen destruction when composting humanure is to thermophilically compost the toilet material, then allow the compost to sit, undisturbed, for a lengthy period of time after the thermophilic heating stage has ended. The biodiversity of the compost will aid in the destruction of pathogens as the compost ages.[25]

The techniques can be very simple and laidback, but any humanure composting takes a bit of active management.

When people live in dense settlements, such as New York, the city of eight million in which I grew up, our biological by-products require very active management. The way most municipal systems are conceptualized, the excrement is treated as a waste product rather than a resource. The waste is multiplied by the use of precious water to flush it away. We further turn our excrement from a resource into a liability by mixing into the potty water all the chemicals people pour down drains, the pharmaceuticals we take, industrial waste, hospital waste, storm sewers carrying whatever leaks onto the streets from cars, chemical tanks, or who knows where. Our nutritious shit, embodying future fertility, becomes a cesspool of chemical waste.

Sewage treatment is designed "merely to do the work of a stream, but on a grand scale," explains Jeanette Farrell. After we flush, whether it goes through an elaborate civic infrastructure into a municipal "wastewater" treatment facility, or a backyard "septic tank" system, it is bacteria that break down our feces and recycle the nutrients embedded in them.

Septic tank systems rely upon swamp-like anaerobic digestion, less efficient than oxidative metabolism, with many by-products. "Methane, hydrogen sulfide, and sulfur dioxide gases are produced, as well as a sludge of high molecular weight hydrocarbons," explains a Northern Arizona University website on the microbiology of sewage. "This sludge will readily decompose further when exposed to oxygen and aerobic bacteria."[26] Septic tanks periodically need to have sludge removed and sent to sewage treatment plants (or sometimes landfills). At any hardware store you can buy "septic treatment" products that are bacteria and enzyme mixes intended to improve or speed digestion in the tank. (My plumber friend Joe Prince says to flush a piece of bacteria-rich raw chicken skin down the toilet if your septic system is sluggish.)

In contrast with a septic tank, most large-scale sewage treatment relies upon aerobic organisms and their faster oxidative metabolism to digest massive accumulations of excrement in quite literally a river of water. "Primary" treatment filters large solids from wastewater and separates matter that sinks to the bottom or floats to the top. In "secondary treatment," the water is usually heavily aerated to promote oxidative metabolism of nutrients in the water. Like a huge compost pile, this is a closely monitored and highly managed environment, in which it is crucial to maintain adequate levels of oxygenation. Sewage treatment plants are often described as bacteria farms, in which the flows of nutrients and oxygen must be regulated in order to maintain the health of the bacterial population.

The big challenge in wastewater treatment is not removing "nutrients," as fecal matter and other organics are collectively known, but rather removing all the toxic chemicals that are also present. These unseparated toxins are what prevents the "sludge" that is a by-product of wastewater treatment from being safe to use in agricultural composts. Even at mass scale, if we could somehow collect our excrement separately from toxic chemicals, it would be easy to compost the sludge into biological fertilizers. Perhaps more intelligent designs will emerge over time. But for now, the toxic sludge remaining after sewage treatment mostly ends up in landfills. "By burying sludge, we're burying a source of food," argues Joseph Jenkins. "That's a cultural practice that should be challenged."[27] While fermentation has been effectively applied to the problems of waste management, we would do better to work toward totally eliminating the concept of waste and the problems of waste management and reframe the objective as resource recovery.

Disposal of Human Bodies

Like the feces we continually produce while we are alive, the bodies we leave behind after we die can be viewed as waste in need of disposal, or as nutritive resources to be recycled. Coffins slow down the microbial decomposition of dead bodies, as does embalming, which involves chemicals such as formaldehyde and alcohol that limit microbial growth and temporarily preserve flesh. The Egyptian techniques of mummification "bear remarkable similarity to the Egyptian practice of preserving birds and fish through disembowelment and salting," notes Mark Kurlansky in his *Salt: A World History*.[28] As discussed in chapter 12, salting preserves flesh by inhibiting bacterial growth, primarily by limiting water activity. But the fact that billions of bodies are not piling up on the Earth is clear evidence that microbes generally fully decompose corpses, undeterred by efforts to preserve them.

Where it is possible—this is legal in some places and prohibited in others—bury your dead in a hole in the ground, as simply as you can. Do you really even need a coffin? How about wrapping the body in a quickly biodegrading natural fabric or paper shroud instead? Even where you cannot just dig a hole in the ground, a growing "green burial" movement is seeking to bury dead bodies without embalming, in caskets made of biodegradable materials, and without the use of other synthetic impediments to rapid microbial decomposition. The Green Burial Council has formed "to encourage environmentally sustainable deathcare and the use of burial as a new means of protecting natural areas. Through a mix of evangelism, economic incentives, and solid science, our mostly volunteer organization has become the standard-bearer in this nascent field and the conduit for conservation at an intersection that's never been crossed."[29] Our legacy can be nutrients for trees rather than embalming fluids and garish caskets made of materials that resist decomposition.

Fiber and Building Arts

Fermentation, as a fundamental mode of processing organic materials, has been used widely in various techniques of fiber arts, construction, and decorative finishing.

Bioplastics

Most of the biodegradable plant-based plastics—being used as "green" alternatives for packaging and disposable cups, plates, and cutlery—are products of fermentation. One corn-based plastic is polylactic acid, or PLA. Corn sugars are fermented into lactic acid, which is then purified and subjected to a series of chemical manipulations to transform it into PLA. Similar processes are being applied to potato starch, cassava, sugarcane, and soybeans; they could potentially be applied to any carbohydrate fermentable into lactic acid.

Retting

The word *ret* is used to describe soaking or moistening flax, hemp, or other stalky fiber plants, as well as "coir" fibers from coconut shells, cassava tubers, and other fibrous plant materials. *Ret* comes from the same linguistic roots as *rot*. The retting initiates a spontaneous fermentation that digests pectins and other compounds, thereby releasing the fibers and making them available for use in rope, yarn, paper, and so on. (In the case of cassava and other fibrous starchy tubers, the fibers are removed, and the dissolved starch that settles in the liquid is the primary food product.)

Dyeing

Fermentation is also used in certain fiber-dyeing processes. I visited Artisan Natural Dyeworks in Nashville, Tennessee (www.ecodyeit.com), where indigo dyes were fermenting in big vats, as well as iron for another dye. Sarah and Alesandra Bellos, the sisters who operate the small-batch dyeworks, grow their own indigo, and in fact were drawn to dyeing by their desire to fuse their interests in farming with their creative pursuits. The indigo they grow (and ferment and dye with) in Nashville's temperate climate is technically of the knotweed family, *Persicaria tinctoria*—called Japanese indigo, Chinese indigo, dyer's knotweed, and undoubtedly other names—rather than the *Indigofera tinctoria* used in India. *Indigo* can describe dye made from a number of different plants, including *Persicaria tinctoria*, other plants in the *Indigofera* genus, woad (*Isatis tinctoria*), and others, all processed by fermentation, at least historically, until the discovery of faster chemical processes beginning near the end of the 19th century.

Like so many fermentation processes, indigo dyeing is an alchemical wonder. First, the pigment is extracted from the plants through a preliminary fermentation process, which can either proceed as a hot aerobic composting process yielding a pigment-rich paste, or as an anaerobic ferment immersed in water. As pigments infuse into the water and it ferments, the water goes from clear to brown to "lime anti-freeze" green, according to Sarah and Alesandra. This is the color of the pigment in its soluble form. It can be precipitated into an insoluble form by adding hydrated lime and actively agitating and aerating it. The acidic fermented infusion reacts with the alkaline lime and oxidizes, producing a blue foam and causing the blue pigment to precipitate into a sludge of insoluble particulate. This particulate can be stored wet but is typically dried into powdery cakes for transport and commerce. Then the pigment, in whichever form, is introduced into a vat of water with soda ash and a carbohydrate nutrient, such as madder or roasted barley, to undergo "reduction" (of oxygen) and fermentation. Urine has also been used in indigo fermentation vats.

As the pigment dissolves in an anaerobic environment, it loses its blue color. Minimize disturbance of the vat, as it can introduce oxygen and retard the dissolution of the pigment. As days and weeks pass, the

cassava root

vat develops a strong fishy odor. Once a coppery sheen develops on the surface of the vat, it's ready for dyeing. Fibers or garments dipped into the indigo vat come out yellow-green, and only after they are removed from the solution and exposed to air do they turn to blue as they oxidize. It's a dramatic shift, like watching a photographic print develop. To obtain a dark, rich blue color, you must generally dip the fibers multiple times, allowing full oxidation between dips.

Indigo is not the only fermented dye. In addition to indigo, the Bellos sisters had a vat of fermenting iron. Dr. S. Sekar of Bharathidasan University in Tamil Nadu, India, compiler of the *Database on Microbial Traditional Knowledge of India*, writes that "various types of natural dyes and adhesives for dyeing are prepared through traditional fermentation by *Meitei*, ethnic people of Manipur" in the northeast of India, including not only a form of indigo, but plants yielding colors across the spectrum—yellow, pink, red, violet, brown, and black.[30]

Natural Building

Building with natural materials is obviously the origin of all construction. "Even now in the 21st century, half the world's population continues to live in earthen dwellings, which are more thermally comfortable than the cement bunkers or house trailers that often replace them," writes Carole Crews, in *Clay Culture: Plasters, Paints, and Preservation*.[31] Although building practices have become more and more based upon synthetic materials—steel, cement, plastic, fiberglass, asphalt, vinyl, "pressure-treated" lumber, et cetera—there has been a revival in recent years of building with earthen materials. I was lucky enough to know some natural building revivalists in the 1990s, and I learned from them. With minimal guidance and much perseverance (and help), I built a beautiful luxurious living space out of mud and straw and fell in love with the process.

Compared to building with wood, building with mud is easy and much more forgiving. With barely any learning curve, children and anyone willing to get their hands dirty can be put right to work. Whereas carpentry errors generally get compounded, requiring remediation at each subsequent step, mudding errors are easily plastered over, as experience teaches you the nuance of judging appropriate mixing proportions.

In communicating to others how to find the right proportions, I always find myself resorting to food metaphors. Just as wheat and water can be combined to obtain so many distinctive forms, so too can earth, water, and straw. One technique I used, known as slip straw, involves first mixing a clay slip: clay and water in a liquid suspension thick like cream, thick enough to remain coating your hand when you remove it from stirring the solution. You lightly coat the straw with slip, then pack it forcefully into the wall space defined by boards affixed to the inside and outside, between structural posts. The benefit of this method is high straw content, which creates good insulation without the excessive bulk of straw bale walls. To coat straw with slip, you first disassemble part of a straw bale on a tarp, separating individual stalks as much as possible. Then you spread some slip around the pile of straw, a little at a time, and toss, just as you might toss a salad when you dress it. The objective is to coat all the straw, using as little slip as you can.

Earth, sand, water, and straw can be mixed thick into a dough-like "cob" mix that holds its own form for building walls. Like dough, it needs enough water for all the elements to become bound together, but not so much that it can no longer hold its form. In a plaster application, to finish an already constructed wall, these same ingredients (and often others) are used, but with more water to make a spreadable consistency, something like a batter.

A crucial step in all of these processes is soaking the clay, exactly as with wheat. Carole Crews explains the properties of clay:

> The crystalline nature of clay molecules enables them to bind together in a linear way to form very thin platelets of different lengths which slide over one another like a deck of wet playing cards, creating plasticity and malleability in the clay body as the platelets absorb water between the layers, in addition to that trapped within the molecular structure. Only one or two nanometers thick, the microscopic platelets stick to each other, to water, and to other objects because of an electrostatic charge on their edges. The cohesive force in clay particles is partially neutralized through the absorption of water, making the clay fluid and malleable, achieving that magic consistency between liquid and solid.[32]

When clay is left in water, after it becomes fully saturated, with water between all the layers of platelets, over time "they align themselves in a more uniform way, which improves the consistency and workability of the mass," explains Crews:

> In China, at least in the old days, each generation would prepare large pits of clay and cover them with straw for the next generation of potters, then use the one prepared for them years before. In India, builders pile up the wet mud and cover it for at least two weeks before using it.[33]

Crews describes the extended soaking of clay as "fermenting." Although minerals without organic material cannot ferment, the reality that all clays contain impurities including organic matter means that fermentation does occur. "Aged clay can begin to smell absolutely awful," warns Crews. In such an event, she recommends adding EM-1 (Effective Microorganisms) as remediation.[34]

For use in building, soaked clay is mixed with other substances, almost always fiber and aggregate, and in some applications additional binders and hardeners. Aggregate is typically sand. Clay without aggregate tends to shrink and crack. In many places, the earth you can dig already contains a good balance between clay and sand for building. In most of the earthen building I have done, I have had to add lots of sand to dense clayey earth. In addition, you need fiber to give structure and tensile strength. Straw is most famous, but other fibers can be substituted. For finer plaster work, I've used hair and dried grated horse manure, which is essentially individual grass fibers with a sticky coating. In contrast with the clay, best pre-soaked, the fiber generally is kept dry until ready to mix and use. In mixing and application it gets wet, but then begins to dry and ferments for only a minimum of time. Too much decomposition would compromise the strength of the fibers.

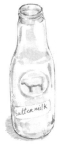

Some of the binders people use in earthen plasters and paints are foods. Wheat paste is a thin batter of flour and water cooked into a gluey paste. This mix has been popular with urban activists and street artists. I learned to mix wheat paste into earthen plasters, and it definitely contributes to the stickiness of the mix. But only mix as much as you are going to use that day, because if you leave it out overnight and the wheat ferments, the plaster loses body and cohesiveness and gets too thin to work with. Fermentation is not always the best thing!

A food-based binder that is generally fermented when used to strengthen or coat earthen plasters is casein. *Caseins* are the group of milk proteins that form curds (as opposed to whey). Casein proteins are organized as clusters floating in the milk, called *micelles*. In acid conditions, the micelles react by coming together into larger clusters. This phenomenon underlies cheesemaking and yogurt making. The same binding power that allow caseins to restructure liquid milk into solid forms can be incorporated into earthen plaster mixes via casein. I will not get into the specific plaster-making techniques, but Carole Crews's book and others have much detail. The casein itself could be yogurt hung as yogurt cheese; milk curdled with rennet or vinegar; buttermilk; or other variations. I've even used powdered milk in plaster mixes. All milk has caseins; "any milk makes good glue," summarizes Crews.

Another natural wall finish involving fermentation is lime-based paint incorporating fermented cactus, which I heard about from my friends Annie Danger and Rayna, who together used this technique to paint Annie's San Francisco apartment. The gooey fermented cactus "acts as the sticky/glossy/latexey part of the paint," explains Annie. "This was a non-toxic process to an almost disorienting degree," she says. "It felt amazing and weird to paint for a few days and never feel ill from paint fumes. What a treat!"

The first step in preparing this or any lime-based paint is hydrating or "slaking" the lime. The lime needs to soak in water for a minimum of one week (ideally longer), so mix it in a bucket that can be tied up for a while, and mix more than you think you'll need so you don't have to wait another week for more to cure if you run out. (The lime curing is not a fermentation process, but rather a chemical reaction between the lime and water.) Use "type S" lime, usually sold at building supply stores. Fill your bucket about halfway with water, then carefully sift lime into it, cup by cup, and stir. "Get out the ol'

Personal Protective Equipment, making sure to use a mask/filter to protect your lungs, and eye protection that completely wraps around," advises Annie. "You don't want the lime to hydrate using your body fluids, it's not pretty." Add lime until the water begins to thicken, something like pancake batter. A week is the minimum length of time the lime should hydrate. "The longer you slake your lime, the better it will be," says Annie. If you have extra slaked lime left over, you can store it indefinitely in a sealed container.

After your lime has slaked, it's time to prepare the cactus, *nopales*, the spiny pads of cacti of the *Opuntia* genus, available at Latin American groceries. Use another bucket for fermenting the *nopales*. Fill it no more than halfway with warm water, plus 1 cup of salt per gallon (60 ml per liter). Figure about 10 pounds of *nopales* per gallon of water (just over a kilogram per liter). Ten pounds/4 kg of *nopales* was adequate for Rayna and Annie to cover a 12-foot/4-meter-square room. There is no need to remove the spines from the *nopales*, as is typically required to cook with them. Simply slice the pads into thin (¼ to ½ inch/1 cm) slivers. Annie recommends the following method, to minimize contact between your hands and the prickly *nopales*: "Glove up on your non-dominant hand and gingerly take hold of the base of a *nopal* paddle. Using your good cuttin' hand, stand over the bucket and slash at the cactus carefully, hacking thin-as-possible slivers off the width of the cactus and letting them fall directly into the bucket." Make sure *nopales* slivers are covered with brine, stir, cover, and leave to ferment a few days, stirring daily and taking note of the changing texture as cactus goo releases into the water and ferments. "The goal is to get the cactus goo good and pickled/extracted, but not outright rotten," explains Annie. At San Francisco's moderate temperatures, it took about three days. In a warmer place, the fermentation would go faster; in a cooler spot, slower. As in any ferment, more salt would slow down the process. Rayna notes that "other kinds of cacti/succulents would work as well, if they were more abundant. For example, aloe vera has a great goo content."

Once the cactus goo has fermented, strain it through a sieve to remove cactus slivers, leaving you with what Annie calls "pure, magnificent, amber-colored, cactus goo." Then mix the goo with slaked lime. Annie and Rayna experimented with different proportions and decided to work with 3 parts cactus goo to 2 parts slaked lime. "A thinner (say 4 to 1) paint will be more like a glaze, needing many layers to build up opacity." You can work with this paint unpigmented for a "yellowish-white wash that has a bit of a luminescent sheen" or add pigments of any color(s) desired. Add pigments just a little at a time. Once you think you have achieved the color you want, test paint in an unobtrusive spot to see how the color dries, and adjust proportions and pigments as necessary. This paint dries quickly and will require a minimum of two coats, possibly more.

Yet another fermented building material, this one a new innovation rather than gleaned from clear historical tradition, is a mycelial mat, grown by fungi on agricultural by-products such as cotton burrs and buckwheat hulls, thereby binding the nutrient substrates together into a rigid board with lots of air pockets, something like Styrofoam insulation, except without glues or resins, totally natural, and totally biodegradable. Mycelial insulation is commercially available as Greensulate; the developers of the product won one of *Popular Science* magazine's Invention Awards in 2009. The magazine explained, "The mixture is placed inside a panel (or whatever shape is required) and, after 10 to 14 days, the mycelia develop a dense network—just one cubic inch of the white-and-brown-specked 'Greensulate' insulation contains eight miles of interconnected mycelia strands. The panels are dried in an oven at between 100° and 150°F to stop mycelia growth, and at the end of two weeks, they're ready for your walls."[35] The same process is also being used to create eco-friendly packaging. Unfortunately neither the *Popular Science* article nor the website of the product's manufacturer[36] specifies what species of fungus they are using, but I suppose that's the proprietary aspect of their enterprise. It would be a fun project for an experimentalist to try this DIY, experimenting with different fungal species grown in forms.

Energy Production

Alcohol, the most widely consumed product of fermentation, also known as ethanol, can be burned as fuel. Methane, another product of fermentation, can also be burned as fuel. Fermentation processes figure quite prominently in discussions of renewable energy and energy self-sufficiency.

Ethanol

Most gas stations in the United States are already pumping ethanol-gasoline blends. Government policy and industry players have been promoting this objective for years. The idea that fast-growing annual crops can be turned into fuel is very appealing, and many people believe that it is a path to energy self-sufficiency and sustainability. Most of the ethanol produced in the United States is fermented from corn, but in Brazil, the world's next biggest producer of ethanol, it is made primarily from sugarcane. After fermentation, the ethanol must be concentrated by distillation, like hard liquor, only several times over, to reach as close as possible to 200 proof, or 100 percent alcohol.

As ethanol production has risen in recent years, it has come to be blamed for rising corn prices and rising food prices more broadly. A Congressional Budget Office report explains:

> In 2008, nearly 3 billion bushels of corn were used to produce ethanol in the United States. That amount constituted an increase over the previous year of almost a billion bushels. The demand for corn for ethanol production, along with other factors, exerted upward pressure on corn prices, which rose by more than 50 percent between April 2007 and April 2008. Rising demand for corn also increased the demand for cropland and the

price of animal feed. Those effects in turn raised the price of many farm commodities (such as soybeans, meat, poultry, and dairy products) and, consequently, the retail price of food.[37]

Renewable fuel production is a laudable goal, but turning food crops into fuel has huge economic ramifications, pitting basic human needs against our insatiable desire for mobility and convenience.

Producing fuel from plant monocultures has been successfully marketed as "green," yet the push for biofuels has wrought much environmental devastation. Corn, sugarcane, and other monocultures can only be grown with heavy applications of synthetic nitrogen fertilizers. Food and agriculture writer Tom Philpott asks: "Has there ever been a 'green' technology more ecologically discredited than corn-based ethanol?"[38] In Brazil, vast expanses of the Amazon rain forest have been and continue to be cleared to make way for sugarcane fields for the burgeoning ethanol industry there. In Colombia, Argentina, and elsewhere in South America, there have been reports of people forced from land that has sustained them and their ancestors to make way for vast expanses of biofuel crops. Some of the cutting-edge research in biofuels involves finding non-food materials to turn into fuels, such as switchgrass for ethanol, or algae for biodiesel (a whole other process that does not involve fermentation). But even non-edible feedstocks require land, water, labor, and other precious resources. Biofuels are no panacea.

dried corn

The process for making ethanol from carbohydrates begins with the processes covered in chapter 9 for making alcohol from grains and starchy tubers. Usually, amylase enzymes are introduced to break down starches into simple sugars, a technological application of the molds used in Asian rice beverages. (These enzymes are also frequently used in making tuber- or grain-based distilled spirits.) Malt can be introduced rather than enzymes. After the initial carbohydrate conversion, the wort is boiled, and once it cools, yeast is introduced to initiate fermentation.

To make ethanol, the resulting fermented beverage is distilled (see *Distillation* in chapter 9) to concentrate alcohol. Ethanol of 200 proof, pure enough to be mixed with gasoline, is not generally regarded as within the reach of homebrewers without very specialized equipment. However, people have effectively run specially adapted gasoline vehicles on 180-proof (90 percent pure) ethanol, or diesel engines on even lower-proof blends.

Methane

Another combustible product of fermentation that people have developed as an energy source is methane. Methane, also known as "swamp gas" or "landfill gas," is a product of the anaerobic digestion that occurs in sewage treatment and some composting. Methane is also the primary component of "natural gas" extracted from the earth that is widely used to heat homes and water and cook food. "Biogas" produced as a by-product from anaerobic digestion of sewage can be similarly used and has also been used to power vehicles, sewage treatment, or potentially anything.

The idea of capturing methane from anaerobic decomposition processes is not new. Nearly 1,000 years ago, in the 13th century, Marco Polo reported on the practice as he observed it in China.[39] And 3,000 years ago the Assyrians were using it to heat water for bathing.[40] In recent decades, technologies have improved for capturing and refining biogas; the apparatus is usually referred to as a "digester." The Internet is full of do-it-yourself designs for building an anaerobic digester for harnessing methane biogas.

Biogas production and use accomplishes many useful things simultaneously. It turns what would otherwise be polluting waste streams of animal and human excrement into a fuel resource. Its use as fuel also prevents methane—a major contributor to global warming—from being released into the atmosphere. And by providing primarily rural people with fuel for heating and cooking, biogas also saves trees from being cut.

China is the world leader in biogas usage, with 17 million digesters and an annual biogas production of 6.5 billion cubic meters as of 2005, with ambitious plans for more. "Biogas is at the centre of a burgeoning eco-economy in China," reports the UK-based Institute of Science in Society.[41]

Medicinal Applications of Fermentation

Many traditional healing systems have prepared medications by fermentation. Chapter 4 discusses herbal elixir meads and how fermenting alcohol has been long used as a means of preserving and using plant medicine. The Indian Ayurveda tradition uses fermented forms of herbs called *arishtas* and *asavas*. "These are regarded as valuable therapeutics due to their efficacy and desirable features," according to Dr. S. Sekar of Bharathidasan University in Tamil Nadu, India, whose online *Database on Microbial Traditional Knowledge of India* describes dozens of such preparations.[42] Chinese Confucianism regarded fermented condiments as a means of regulating health by balancing individuals with the food they eat, the seasons, their individual constitutions, and so forth. Medicine derived from fermentation is not a new idea.

Every organism and microbial community secretes compounds that inhibit some of its potential competitors. This is the observation behind antibiotic drugs. Scottish biologist Alexander Fleming was studying *Staphylococci* bacteria in 1928 when he observed that an accidental mold growth in a few petri dishes destroyed those cultures. He identified the mold as being of the *Penicillium* genus and began investigating its antibacterial properties, ushering in a new era in medicine.

Mushrooms as well as molds have been found to possess antibacterial as well as antiviral properties. "Diseases of plants typically do not afflict humans whereas diseases of fungi do," points out Paul Stamets. "Since humans (animals) and fungi share common microbial antagonists . . . humans can benefit from the natural defensive strategies of fungi that produce antibiotics to fight infection from microorganisms. Hence, it is not surprising our most significant antibacterial antibiotics have been derived from fungi."[43] While most antibiotics in use are derived from molds, Stamets has been demonstrating antimicrobial action in various mushrooms, most notably the woody polypore varieties. "The pharmaceutical industry has been slow to explore mushrooms for antibiotic activity, in part because basidiomycetous fungi [mushrooms] are slower growing in fermentation and less yielding compared to the mold fungi," explains Stamets. "The mushroom genome stands out as a virtually untapped resource for novel antimicrobials . . . and may be society's greatest protection against microbial diseases."

Bacteria have come to play a very important role in pharmaceutical production. With the emergence of recombinant DNA technology, genes for producing specific compounds began being inserted into bacterial cells. Many common pharmaceutical products are now produced by genetically engineered bacteria, including insulin, interferon, tumor necrosis factor, and others. A bacteriology textbook enthusiastically summarizes: "The possibilities of biotechnology are endless considering the gene reservoirs and genetic capabilities within the bacteria."[44] In addition to bacteria, geneticists have been able to insert genes to produce pharmaceutical compounds into plants, raising the possibility that if pollen from the genetically modified plants were to escape, it could contaminate other plant populations with powerful pharmaceutical chemicals.

mortar & pestle

Like nutrients in food, nutritional supplements can also be enhanced and made more bioavailable by fermentation. The supplement company New Chapter makes food-based supplements "cultured in probiotics to deliver the full spectrum of Nature's benefits."

Very different in its nature, yet related because it is a drug, tobacco is sometimes fermented, especially for cigars. Cigarmaker Altadis explains on its website how cigar tobacco is fermented:

Tobacco fermentation means laying the leaves into huge "bulks," the centers of which develop heat. The heat in the center of a bulk should not be allowed to exceed about 115°–130° F [46–54° C], depending on the type of tobacco, otherwise it will be ruined, burned out so to speak. When it gets up to that temperature, and it will do so in its own time depending on the leaf and its condition, the bulk gets turned inside out and the heat build up (fermentation) begins again. When the heat levels off, the fermentation is complete. This could occur after four turns or eight turns, referred to as "sweats" in the Trade. Over-fermentation will ruin the leaf, cause it to become "spent" and lose its flavor and aroma. During "sweating", the fermentation process causes the emission of nitrogen compounds and other chemical compounds and reduces somewhat the nicotine content. After fermentation, further aging in bales helps to settle the leaf and enhances flavor and burning quality.[45]

That sounds exactly like a compost pile!

Fermentation for Skin Care and Aromatherapy

Another way of using fermentation is skin care. Osmosis Spa in Freestone, California, offers a Japanese tradition (since the 1940s, anyway) of bathing in a fermenting mix of sawdust and rice bran. Osmosis uses a starter from Japan to culture the mixture and ferments it for a while, turning the pile periodically, as it generates heat and slowly breaks down the plant fibers. Once the fermenting sawdust and rice bran is in the "tubs" (huge wooden crates), it is continually remixed, and the high level of microbial activity keeps it safe and clean. According to the Osmosis website:

> The heat in the Cedar Enzyme Bath differs from other heat treatments in that it is produced biologically by a fermentation process. This process requires over 600 active enzymes. The largest organ of the body, the skin, comes in direct contact with intense enzyme activity in the Cedar Enzyme Bath, which, in addition to heat, produces its own electro-chemical environment. This combination of heat and energy influences body chemistry and natural cleansing processes, and breaks down body wastes in the subcutaneous layer of the skin. The surface of your skin, your pores, and even the cells themselves are thoroughly cleansed.[46]

I had the pleasure of visiting Osmosis as the guest of its founder, Michael Stusser, who invited me to participate in the spectacular Freestone Fermentation Festival, which he organized. When I arrived at the tub, a cavity had been dug out of it, roughly my size, contoured to suggest a position halfway between lying and sitting, reclining, with head sticking out, and knees raised. I got in and adjusted my position. Then Kristen, my guide for the experience, buried me in it, reminding me of being buried in sand at the beach as a child.

It was very cozy, soft, and moist but also very hot in there! (As hot as 140°F/60°C according to Michael, though "the material in contact with your skin forms an insulation barrier.") Kristen encouraged me to uncover limbs as necessary to be comfortable. And she kept offering me cold water, with a bent straw, and swabbing my face with a cool water-soaked towel. Lying there in the sweaty heat of frenzied microbial activity, while simultaneously being pampered, it was easy to imagine the dead tissue on my skin being digested by billions of bacteria. I stayed in the tub for about 20 minutes, followed by a brush-down to remove sawdust and rice bran, a long shower and misting, and finally a deep, wonderful massage. After the whole experience I felt like jelly, reborn and deeply relaxed.

Through the years people have emailed me describing their practices and experiments with fermented skin care products. Many common ingredients in skin care products—including honey, cream, milk, coconut, botanical herbs—readily ferment. Fermenting them may alter them in some positive ways, though I have come across no research in this area and have not experimented myself beyond kombucha mother and sauerkraut facials (both wonderful).

A Canadian company, Kefiplant, with a proprietary process called Kefiech, using organisms derived from kefir grains, manufactures a starter for fermented herbal skin care products. "When botanicals are fermented by Kefiplant, the naturally occurring phytocompounds in the plant are liberated," explains the company's website.[47] "These liberated molecules can now be readily absorbed and efficiently utilized by the body."

Another related application of fermentation is the aromatherapy of potpourri. The French word *potpourri* translates to "rotten pot," and originally potpourri was not a dry mix as we find today, but rather a pot of rose petals and other aromatic herbs, fermented and moist. Fermentation was an essential part of the processing, enabling the petals and their aroma to be preserved. The process is straightforward: Layer fresh rose petals with salt at a ratio of roughly 3 parts rose petals to 1 part salt. Weigh down as for sauerkraut to keep rose petals submerged; ferment for at least two weeks or as long as six weeks. The mass of roses should dry out into a crumby moist cake. Crumble, add other aromatic flowers and spices, store in a jar, and open as scenting is desired.[48]

Fermentation Art

One final non-food application of fermentation is in the realm of art. I include in the color insert a small collection of fermentation-inspired artworks. Surely fermentation has inspired art, song, and poetry from the earliest emergence of each of these forms of expression. Some artists are using fermentation itself as a mode of expression. One example is the kombucha garments produced by Suzanne Lee, a research fellow at the School of Fashion and Textiles in London (see *Making Kombucha* in chapter 6 and a photo in the color insert). Mike Cuil writes that he and a friend performed their electronic music while they also made sauerkraut onstage. "A microphone picked up all the chopping and stomping noises and incorporated it into the mix. At the end we sang a German *schlager* about sauerkraut. It was a huge success." Jenifer Wightman is a biologist-artist who created installations of mud and water enclosed in frames, fermenting, called *Winogradsky Rothko: Bacterial Ecosystem as Pastoral Landscape*. In the artist's own words:

Made in the dimensions of a Mark Rothko painting . . . applying a micro-biology technique developed by a 19th-century soil scientist, Sergei Winogradsky, pigmented bacteria that existed in the mud and water composed a landscape. As bacteria colonize their optimal zones, they change their environments by depleting their resources and releasing by-products. As a bacterial species reaches its carrying capacity, the environment no longer hospitable to the original colonizer may now be the optimal environment for a potential successor to that zone resulting in an evolving color-field of living pigments. The appearance/disappearance of color indicates both procurement and loss of finite material resources; the agents that act out upon the landscape and synthesize change become acted upon by their consequentially changed world.

The artist explains that for her, "De/composition represents beginnings, change, contingencies of cause and effect, interconnectedness, possibility. . . . Perhaps decomposition is where my hope for the world lies."[49]

EPILOGUE:
A Cultural Revivalist Manifesto

*W*e must reclaim our food. Food is much more than simply nourishment. It embodies a complex web of relationships. It is a huge part of the context in which we exist. Reclaiming our food means actively involving ourselves in this web.

The foods that fill our contemporary supermarket shelves are products of a globalized infrastructure of proprietary genetic material, synthetic and often dangerous chemicals, monocultures, long-distance transportation, factory-scale processing, wasteful packaging, and energy-sucking refrigeration. The food being produced by this system is destroying the earth, destroying our health, destroying economic vitality, and robbing us of our dignity by breeding dependency and reducing us to the subservient role of consumer.

We need to cultivate a different set of relationships:

Relationships with Plants and Animals

This is where our food comes from, plants and animals (with microbial assistance). We cannot continue to distance ourselves from the sources of our food, relegating it to highly specialized, mostly faraway, mass-production monocultures, cut off from our lives. Historically, by necessity, we related to the plants and animals we ate. We knew them, relied upon them, and through their pursuit and cultivation, we were intimately connected to our environment. We need to become reconnected to the sources of our sustenance. Get to know the plants around you. Grow some herbs or vegetables. Glean and use unharvested fruit. Plant a tree, or care for one, or many. Forage weeds from your yard. If you enjoy eggs, milk, or meat, consider exploring the path of raising chickens or other livestock on a small scale. Find a way to observe and participate in slaughtering and butchering. Respect, honor, and appreciate the life that goes into our food. We have coevolved with these other beings, and our fates are intertwined.

Relationships with Farmers and Producers

Buy local food! Support local agriculture! Get to know farmers, and buy directly from them. Agricultural revitalization is real economic stimulus and real economic security. Beyond the raw products of agriculture, most people enjoy foods and beverages that have been processed, whether it's cheese, salami, or tempeh. Many of these "value-added" processes involve fermentation. Support small-scale local processing and production. It means fresher food, local jobs, decentralization, and greater resilience in the face of change. Local production includes not only commercial manufacturers but small informal production shared through alternative economies such as gift exchange, barter, voluntary donations, herd-shares, community supported models, or illicit underground sales. Find a niche you can fill in the reemergent web of food creators.

Relationships with Ancestors

Our ancestors paid much more attention to their ancestors than people in our time typically do. We have our God, and canonize various historical or mythological heroes into icons, but in our time we have very little appreciation for the general continuous lineage itself. However mixed our heritage may be, we are, each of us, the spawn of ancient lineages, which have bestowed upon us incredible cultural legacies. We must remember, rediscover, and reclaim our ancestors, however we can, and honor, protect, and perpetuate their gifts, including tangible ones such as seeds and fermentation processes. Cultural revival is necessary in order to maintain their great legacy to us. Keeping it alive is the ultimate in ancestor worship.

Relationships with Mysteries

Mysteries endure. Despite all the impressive advances in microscopic imaging, genetic analysis, and other forms of scientific investigation, the realm of the microscopic is still very little understood. For that matter, so is much about our own bodies and minds. Let us honor the mysteries and revel in the fact that we will never understand everything.

Relationships with Community

Self-sufficiency is a dangerous myth. We need each other. Love your circle, cultivate it, and enlarge it. Share food you grow or make with your community, and encourage others in their food production activities. Community is never perfect and takes hard work, because people have such varied visions, ideas, and values. But do the hard work of finding common ground, and build community with the people around you.

Relationships with Movements of Resistance

Our growing awareness as individuals creating change in our own lives, and communities can (and must) build into galvanizing social movements.

While reviving local food systems, we can also address inequitable access to resources by becoming part of existing movements for food justice and food sovereignty. While making use of indigenous wisdom in our cultural revival efforts, we can also acknowledge and act in solidarity with indigenous peoples struggling for survival. While trying to limit our own carbon footprints and environmental impact, we can also join social movements demanding the same of corporations and government policies. Personal actions can be powerful, but nothing like the force of collective action.

Relationships to Materials

We must strive to maximize the use of whatever is abundant, easy, low-impact, and reusable. We do not need infinitely more special equipment and gadgetry. We must interrupt the disposable society. Where feasible, scavenge materials to reuse them; process fibers from plants or animals; build a house from earthen materials. DIY culture!

These are but a few strands of a densely interwoven web of relationships that can sustain and enrich us. Fermentation is one way in which we may consciously cultivate this web. This is the daily practice of cultural revival. By engaging life forces, we rediscover and reconnect with our context.

RESOURCES

Chapter 3

Artisan Crock Makers

ADAM FIELD
Traditional Korean *onggi* crocks
www.adamfieldpottery.com

ROBBIE HEIDINGER
www.robbieheidinger.com/products-page/pickling-crocks/

SARAH KERSTEN
www.counterculturepottery.com

JEREMY OGUSKY
www.etsy.com/people/oguskyceramics

AMY POTTER
http://amypotter.com/Amy_Kraut_Crocks.htm

Chapter 4

Books

Bruman, Henry J. *Alcohol in Ancient Mexico.* Salt Lake City: University of Utah Press, 2000.

Garey, Terry A. *The Joy of Home Winemaking.* New York: Avon, 1996.

Kania, Leon. *Alaskan Bootlegger's Bible.* Wasilla, AK: Happy Mountain Publications, 2000.

Mansfield, Scott. *Strong Waters: A Simple Guide to Making Beer, Wine, Cider and Other Spirited Beverages at Home.* New York: The Experiment, 2010.

McGovern, Patrick. *Uncorking the Past: The Quest for Wine, Beer, and Other Alcoholic Beverages.* Berkeley, CA: University of California Press, 2009.

Spence, Pamela. *Mad About Mead! Nectar of the Gods.* St. Paul , MN: Llewellyn Publications, 1997.

Vargas, Pattie, and Rich Gulling. *Making Wild Wines and Meads: 125 Unusual Recipes Using Herbs, Fruits, Flowers, and More*. Pownal, VT: Storey Books, 1999.

Watson, Ben. *Cider Hard and Sweet: History, Traditions, and Making Your Own*. Woodstock, VT: Countryman, 1999.

Internet

HOME WINEMAKERS MANUAL
Free downloadable book by Lum Eisenman.
www.winebook.webs.com

THE JOY OF HOME WINEMAKING
Website of Terry Garey, author of the book *The Joy of Home Winemaking*.
www.joyofwine.net

WINEMAKING BLOG
FAQ, articles, and information provided by E. C. Kraus, a Missouri-based retailer of home wine- and beer-making supplies.
www.winemakingblog.com

WINEMAKING HOME PAGE
Basics, glossary, Q and A, recipes, and more, posted by enthusiast Jack Keller.
www.winemaking.jackkeller.net

WINEMAKING TALK
Discussion forum.
www.winemakingtalk.com

WINE PRESS
Discussion forum.
www.winepress.us

Chapter 5

Books

Andoh, Elizabeth. *Kansha: Celebrating Japan's Vegan and Vegetarian Traditions*. Berkeley, CA: Ten Speed Press, 2010.

Hisamatsu, Ikuko. *Quick and Easy Tsukemono: Japanese Pickling Recipes*. Tokyo: Japan Publications, 2005.

Kaufmann, Klaus, and Annelies Schöneck. *Making Sauerkraut and Pickled Vegetables at Home*. Summertown, TN: Books Alive, 2008.

Man-Jo, Kim, Lee Kyou-Tae, and Lee O-Young. *The Kimchee Cookbook: Fiery Flavors and Cultural History of Korea's National Dish*. Singapore: Periplus Editions, 1999.

Shimizu, Kay. *Tsukemono: Japanese Pickled Vegetables*. Tokyo: Shufunotomo, 1993.

United Nations Food and Agriculture Organization. *Fermented Fruits and Vegetables: A Global Perspective*. Online at www.fao.org/docrep/x0560E/x0560E00.htm.

Chapter 6

Culture Exchanges

CÓMO CONSEGUIR KÉFIR
A Spanish site with international listings of sources for water kefir grains, milk kefir grains, and kombucha mothers.
www.lanaturaleza.es/bdkefir.htm

INTERNATIONAL KEFIR COMMUNITY
"Real Live Kefir Grains shared by members worldwide": Users post the availability of both water and dairy kefir grains via geographic location. Some are free if you can pick them up; most entail some fee.
www.torontoadvisors.com/Kefir/kefir-list.php

KOMBUCHA EXCHANGE
An international directory organized by Günther W. Frank, in English and German.
www.kombu.de/suche2.htm

PROJECT KEFIR
An international directory "of FREE & Sometimes Not So Free Real Kefir Grains & Kombucha Tea."
www.rejoiceinlife.com/kefir/kefirlist.php

Online Sources of Mauby Bark

ANGEL BRAND SPICES, HERBS, & TEAS
www.angelbrand.com

SAM'S CARIBBEAN MARKETPLACE (NEW YORK)
www.sams247.com

WEST INDIAN SHOP (NEW YORK)
www.westindianshop.com

XNIC STORE (CONNECTICUT)
stores.xnicstore.com

Water Kefir and Ginger Beer Plant Sources

The *Culture Exchanges* listing (above) contains sources in dozens of countries of the world, mostly by individual enthusiasts. The following listings are small commercial enterprises dedicated to propagating cultures. For each listing, I have indicated which cultures they sell (WK or GBP) and the country in which they operate. I have ordered cultures from and communicated with the three in the United States. I also listed a few that I have not done business with, in Australia and the UK. In our Internet age, a quick search will yield many more options, some of which probably do not yet exist as I write.

CULTURES ALIVE (AUS) (WK & GBP)
www.culturesalive.com.au

CULTURES FOR HEALTH (US) (WK)
www.culturesforhealth.com

GEM CULTURES (US) (WK)
www.gemcultures.com

THE GINGER BEER PLANT (UK) (GBP)
www.gingerbeerplant.net

THE KEFIR SHOP (UK) (WK & GBP)
www.kefirshop.co.uk

YEMOOS NOURISHING CULTURES (US) (WK & GBP)
www.yemoos.com

Sources for Kombucha Mothers

The *Culture Exchanges* listing (above) contains sources in dozens of countries of the world, mostly by individual enthusiasts. The following listings are small commercial enterprises dedicated to propagating cultures. I have ordered cultures or otherwise interacted with all the US sources listed. In our Internet age, a quick search will yield many more options, some of which probably do not yet exist as I write.

CULTURES ALIVE (AUS)
www.culturesalive.com.au

CULTURES FOR HEALTH (US)
www.culturesforhealth.com

GEM CULTURES (US)
www.gemcultures.com

THE KEFIR SHOP (UK)
www.kefirshop.co.uk

KOMBUCHA BROOKLYN (US)
kombuchabrooklyn.com

KOMBUCHA KAMP (US)
www.kombuchakamp.com

YEMOOS NOURISHING CULTURES (US)
www.yemoos.com

Kombucha Resources

KOMBUCHA JOURNAL (BY GÜNTHER W. FRANK)
Detailed information on making kombucha and more, in 30 languages!
www.kombu.de

KOMBUCHA UNVEILED (BY COLLEEN ALLEN)
Kombucha FAQ, research, and links.
http://users.bestweb.net/~om/~kombu/FAQ/homeFAQ.html

ONLINE KOMBUCHA BREWING MANUAL (BY FRANTISEK APFELBECK)
www.noisebridge.net/wiki/Kombucha_Brewing_Manual

Vinegar Resources

Books

Diggs, Lawrence J. *Vinegar: The User-Friendly Standard Text Reference and Guide to Appreciating, Making, and Enjoying Vinegar.* Lincoln, NE: Authors Choice Press, 2000.

Internet

APPLE CIDER VINEGAR BENEFITS
Posted by a Canadian vinegar enthusiast named Wayne. Includes vinegar-making information.
www.apple-cider-vinegar-benefits.com

HOW TO MAKE VINEGAR
howtomakevinegar.com

VINEGAR CONNOISSEURS INTERNATIONAL
"The Grand Central Station for Vinegar Information," posted and maintained by Lawrence Diggs, author of the book above.
www.vinegarman.com

Chapter 7

Raw-Milk Resources

Books

Gumpert, David E. *The Raw Milk Revolution: Behind America's Emerging Battle Over Food Rights.* White River Junction, VT: Chelsea Green, 2009.

Schmid, Ron. *The Untold Story of Milk: The History, Politics and Science of Nature's Perfect Food.* Warsaw, IN: New Trends Publishing, 2009.

Internet

A Campaign for Raw Milk
The Weston A. Price Foundation's milk project website features much nutritional and legal information, as well as sources for raw milk in the United States and around the world. www.realmilk.com

Farm-to-Consumer Legal Defense Fund
Legal advocacy and legal defense for raw-milk producers and consumers. www.farmtoconsumer.org

Raw Milk Institute
"Mentors and assists farmers in the production of safe raw milk." www.rawmilkinstitute.org

Sources of Heirloom Yogurt Cultures

Cultures Alive (AUS)
www.culturesalive.com.au

Cultures for Health (US)
www.culturesforhealth.com

New England Cheesemaking Supply Company (US)
www.cheesemaking.com

Yogurt Resources

How to Make Yogurt, A Step-by-Step Tutorial
www.makeyourownyogurt.com

Yogurt Everyday
How to make yogurt, recipes, links, and more from a yogurt lover named Jenna. www.yogurt-everyday.com

Yogurt Forever
The Yogurt Encyclopaedia by Roberto Flora, translated by Fiammetta Cestaro. www.yogurtforever.org

Sources of Kefir Grains

The *Culture Exchanges* listing (see chapter 6 Resources listings) contains sources in dozens of countries of the world, mostly by individual enthusiasts. The following listings are small commercial enterprises dedicated to propagating cultures, including kefir. I have ordered cultures from and communicated with the three in the United States. I also listed a few that I have not done business with, in Australia and the UK. In our Internet age, a quick search will yield many more options, some of which probably do not yet exist as I write.

Cultures Alive (AUS)
www.culturesalive.com.au

Cultures for Health (US)
www.culturesforhealth.com

GEM Cultures (US)
www.gemcultures.com

The Kefir Shop (UK)
www.kefirshop.co.uk

Yemoos Nourishing Cultures (US)
www.yemoos.com

Cheesemaking Resources

Books

Amrein-Boyes, Debra. *200 Easy Homemade Cheese Recipes: From Cheddar and Brie to Butter and Yogurt.* Toronto: Robert Rose, 2009.

Carroll, Ricki. *Home Cheese Making.* North Adams, MA: Storey Publishing, 2002.

Emery, Carla. *Encyclopedia of Country Living.* Seattle: Sasquatch Books, 1994. A general resource that I highly recommend, which includes a very thorough section on cheesemaking, as well as milk more broadly.

Farnham, Jody, and Marc Druart, *The Joy of Cheesemaking.* New York: Skyhorse Publishing, 2011.

Hurst, Hurst. *Homemade Cheese: Recipes for 50 Cheeses from Artisan Cheesemakers.* Minneapolis: Voyageur Press, 2011.

Karlin, Mary. *Artisan Cheese Making at Home: Techniques & Recipes for Mastering World-Class Cheeses.* Berkeley, CA: Ten Speed Press, 2011.

Kindstedt, Paul. *American Farmstead Cheese.* White River Junction, VT: Chelsea Green, 2005.

Kosikowski, Frank V., and Vikram V. Mistry. *Cheese and Fermented Milk Foods.* South Deerfield, MA: New England Cheesemaking Supply Company, 1999.

Le Jaouen, Jean Claude. *The Fabrication of Farmstead Goat Cheese.* Ashfield, MA: Cheesemaker's Journal, 1990.

Morris, Margaret. *The Cheesemaker's Manual.* Lancaster, Ontario: Glengarry Cheesemaking, 2003.

Peacock, Paul. *Making Your Own Cheese: How to Make All Kinds of Cheeses in Your Own Home.* Begbroke, UK: How To Books, 2011.

Smith, Tim. *Making Artisan Cheese: Fifty Fine Cheeses That You Can Make in Your Own Kitchen*. Minneapolis: Quarry Books, 2005.

Twamley, Josiah. *Dairying Exemplified*. London: J. Sharp, 1784. Available online via Google Books. The basic techniques have not changed much.

Magazines

CULTURE: THE WORD ON CHEESE
www.culturecheesemag.com

Internet

CHEESE FORUM
"Global & Independent (Non-retailer aligned)."
www.cheeseforum.org

FANKHAUSER'S CHEESE PAGE
Posted by University of Cincinnati biology professor David B. Fankhauser.
www.biology.clc.uc.edu/fankhauser/cheese/cheese.html

GLENGARRY CHEESEMAKING AND DAIRY SUPPLY
A Canadian source of cheesemaking equipment, cultures, and supplies.
www.glengarrycheesemaking.on.ca

NEW ENGLAND CHEESEMAKING SUPPLY COMPANY
A US source of cheesemaking equipment, cultures, and supplies.
www.cheesemaking.com

Finding Raw-Milk Cheese Producers

Books

Roberts, Jeffrey. *Atlas of American Artisan Cheese*. White River Junction, VT: Chelsea Green, 2007.

Internet

SLOW FOOD USA AMERICAN RAW MILK CHEESES PRESIDIUM
www.slowfoodusa.org/index.php/programs/presidia_product_detail/
american_raw_milk_cheeses/

Chapter 8

Sourdough-Bread-Baking Resources

Books

Alford, Jeffrey, and Naomi Duguid. *Flatbreads and Flavors: A Baker's Atlas*. New York: William Morrow, 1995.

Brown, Edward Espe. *The Tassajara Bread Book*. Boston: Shambhala, 1971.

Buehler, Emily. *Bread Science: The Chemistry and Craft of Making Bread*. Hillsborough, NC: Two Blue Books, 2006.

Denzer, Kiko, and Hannah Field. *Build Your Own Earth Oven: A Low-Cost Wood-Fired Mud Oven; Simple Sourdough Bread; Perfect Loaves*, 3rd Edition. Blodgett, OR: Hand Print Press, 2007.

Hamelman, Jeffrey. *Bread: A Baker's Book of Techniques and Recipes*. Hoboken, NJ: Wiley, 2004.

Leonard, Thom. *The Bread Book: A Natural, Whole Grain Seed-to-Loaf Approach to Real Bread*. Brookline, MA: East West Health Books, 1990.

Rayner, Lisa. *Wild Bread: Handbaked Sourdough Artisan Breads in Your Own Kitchen*. Flagstaff, AZ: Lifeweaver, 2009.

Reinhart, Peter. *The Bread Baker's Apprentice: Mastering the Art of Extraordinary Bread*. Berkeley, CA: Ten Speed Press, 2001.

Robertson, Chad. *Tartine Bread*. San Francisco: Chronicle Books, 2010.

Wing, Daniel, and Alan Scott, *The Bread Builders: Hearth Loaves and Masonry Ovens*. White River Junction, VT: Chelsea Green, 1999.

Internet

THE FRESH LOAF
www.thefreshloaf.com

GOOGLE SOURDOUGH GROUP
www.groups.google.com/group/rec.food.sourdough
FAQs from this group at www.nyx.net/~dgreenw/sourdoughqa.html

DAN LEPARD'S BREADBAKING FORUM
An interactive feature on the website of the baking columnist for the UK's *Guardian*.
www.danlepard.com/forum

SOURDOUGH DAILY
www.sourdough.typepad.com/my-blog

SOURDOUGH FAQ
Posted by fermentation enthusiast Brian Dixon.
www.stason.org/TULARC/food/sourdough-starter/

SOURDOUGH HOME
www.sourdoughhome.com

Chapter 9

Further Resources for Rice Beers

Two online resources that I have found broadly survey varieties of rice beers in their respective geographic areas:

DATABASE ON MICROBIAL TRADITIONAL KNOWLEDGE OF INDIA
Dr. S. Sekar, Bharathidasan University, Tamil Nadu, India
www.bdu.ac.in/schools/life_sciences/biotechnology/sekardb.htm

GRANDIOSE SURVEY OF CHINESE ALCOHOLIC DRINKS AND BEVERAGES
Xu Gan Rong and Bao Tong Fa, Jiangnan University, Jiangsu Province, China
www.sytu.edu.cn/zhgjiu/umain.htm

Saké Resources

Books

Eckhardt, Fred. *Sake (USA): The Complete Guide to American Sake, Sake Breweries and Homebrewed Sake*. Portland, OR: Fred Eckhardt Communications, 1992.

Internet

HOME BREW SAKE
http://homebrewsake.com
This website publishes Fred Eckhardt's recipe, updated, as well as others, sells *saké*-making supplies, and contains links to other online sources of *saké* information.

SAKE WORLD
This is the *saké* information website of John Gauntner, an American expatriate living in Japan, who has written five books about *saké* and is widely recognized as the leading non-Japanese *saké* expert. The site does not contain recipes, but it does contain good information describing the process, as well as the qualities of different types of *saké*.
http://sake-world.com

TAYLOR-MADE AK—BREWING SAKE
Bob Taylor's "information resource for homebrewing sake" includes several different free recipes, including Fred Eckhardt's, and even checklists and spreadsheets for keeping track of the long process.
www.taylor-madeak.org

Small Maltsters

REBEL MALTING COMPANY
Reno, Nevada
www.rebelmalting.com

Valley Malt
Hadley, Massachusetts
www.valleymalt.com

Beer-Brewing Resources

Here are some good books and online resources to guide you through brewing classic malted barley and hops beers.

Books

Bamforth, Charles W. *Scientific Principles of Malting and Brewing*. St. Paul, MN: American Society of Brewing Chemists, 2006.

Fisher, Joe, and Dennis Fisher. *The Homebrewer's Garden*. North Adams, MA: Storey Publishing, 1998.

Janson, Lee W. *Brew Chem 101: The Basics of Homebrewing Chemistry*. North Adams, MA: Storey Publishing, 1996.

Kania, Leon W. *The Alaskan Bootlegger's Bible*. Wasilla, AK: Happy Mountain Publications, 2000.

Mosher, Randy. *Radical Brewing*. Boulder, CO: Brewers Publications, 2004.

Palmer, John. *How to Brew: Everything You Need to Know to Brew Beer Right the First Time*. Boulder, CO: Brewers Publications, 2006; available free online at www.howtobrew.com.

Papazian, Charlie. *The Complete Joy of Homebrewing*. New York: HarperCollins, 2003.

———. *The Home Brewer's Companion*. New York: William Morrow, 1994.

Sparrow, Jeff. *Wild Brews: Beer Beyond the Influence of Brewer's Yeast*. Boulder, CO: Brewers Publications, 2005.

Internet

BIOHAZARD LAMBIC BREWERS PAGE
Info on making lambic-style beers and yeast culturing.
www.liddil.com/beer/index.html

BREWERS ROUNDTABLE
Discussion forum.
www.brewersroundtable.com

HOMEBREW DIGEST
Listserv for brewing Q&A and discussions, with a searchable archive of years of postings. The same folks also run the site The Brewery, www.brewery.org.
www.hbd.org

HOMEBREW TALK
A large, well-organized discussion forum.
www.homebrewtalk.com

MAD FERMENTATIONIST
Michael Tonsmeire's brewing blog with lots of articles and links.
www.themadfermentationist.com

REALBEER.COM LIBRARY
A portal site with links to many excellent brewing resources.
www.realbeer.com/library

Chapter 10

Sources of Tempeh Starter

CULTURES FOR HEALTH (US)
www.culturesforhealth.com

GEM CULTURES (US)
www.gemcultures.com

TEMPEH.INFO (BELGIUM)
www.tempeh.info

TEMPEH LAB
PO Box 208
Summertown, TN 38483
(931) 964-4540
tempehlab@gmail.com

Tempeh Resources

Books

Shurtleff, William, and Akiko Aoyagi. *The Book of Tempeh*. New York: Harper and Row, 1979. Available full-text at www.books.google.com.

——. *Tempeh Production: A Craft and Technical Manual*. Lafayette, CA: Soyinfo Center, 1986. Available full-text at www.books.google.com.

Internet

BETSY'S TEMPEH FOUNDATION
www.makethebesttempeh.org

TEMPEH.INFO
A Belgian site selling tempeh starter with lots of information and recipes, as well as great microscopy images of the tempeh mold.
www.tempeh.info

MANFRED WARMUTH
http://users.soe.ucsc.edu/~manfred/tempeh/tempehold.html

Sources for Buying *Koji*

Commercial Koji Makers

COLD MOUNTAIN KOJI
This is a commercial brand of prepared *koji*, made in California, which I have encountered in Japanese groceries, a few homebrew supply shops, and many mail-order suppliers.
www.coldmountainmiso.com

SOUTH RIVER MISO COMPANY
This Massachusetts-based miso producer makes and sells brown rice *koji*.
www.southrivermiso.com
If you know of any nearby commercial miso makers or *saké* makers, contact them to inquire whether they sell *koji*.

Koji Retailers

CULTURES FOR HEALTH
www.culturesforhealth.com

GEM CULTURES
www.gemcultures.com

Chapter 11

Sources of *Natto* Starter

All the *natto* starter I have encountered is the same brand, Mitoku Traditional Natto Spores. It is available from:

CULTURES FOR HEALTH
www.culturesforhealth.com

GEM CULTURES
www.gemcultures.com

NATURAL IMPORT COMPANY
www.naturalimport.com
A great resource for information on all things *natto* is the website Natto King at www.nattoking.com.

Chapter 12

Sausage-Making Resources

Supplies

SAUSAGE MAKER
www.sausagemaker.com

Books

Bertolli, Paul. *Cooking by Hand*. New York: Clarkson Potter, 2003.

Fearnley-Whittingstall, Hugh. *River Cottage Meat Book*. Berkeley, CA: Ten Speed Press, 2007.

Jarvis, Norman. *Curing of Fishery Products*. Kingston, MA: Teaparty Books, 1987; originally published in 1950 by the US Fish and Wildlife Service.

Kutas, Rytek. *Great Sausage Recipes and Meat Curing*, 3rd edition. Buffalo, NY: The Sausage Maker, 1999.

Lee, Cherl-Ho, et al., eds. *Fish Fermentation Technology*. Tokyo: United Nations University Press, 1993. Out of print but available on Google books.

Livingston, A. D. *Cold-Smoking and Salt-Curing Meat, Fish, and Game*. Guilford, CT: Lyons Press, 1995.

Marianski, Stanel, and Adam Marianski. *The Art of Making Fermented Sausages*. Denver, CO: Outskirts Press, 2008.

Riddervold, Astri. *Lutefisk, Rakefisk and Herring in Norwegian Tradition*. Oslo: Novus Press, 1990.

Ruhlman, Michael, and Brian Polcyn. *Charcuterie: The Craft of Salting, Smoking, and Curing*. New York: W. W. Norton, 2005.

Toldrá, Fidel, ed. *Handbook of Fermented Meat and Poultry*. Ames, IA: Blackwell, 2007.

Chapter 13

Books

Caldwell, Gianaclis. *The Farmstead Creamery Advisor: The Complete Guide to Building and Running a Small, Farm-Based Cheese Business*. White River Junction, VT: Chelsea Green, 2010.

Fix, Mimi. *Start & Run a Home-Based Food Business*. North Vancouver, British Columbia: Self Counsel Press, 2009.

Hall, Stephen. *Sell Your Specialty Food: Market, Distribute, and Profit from Your Kitchen Creation*. New York: Kaplan, 2008.

Lewis, Jennifer. *Starting a Part-Time Food Business: Everything You Need to Know to Turn Your Love for Food into a Successful Business Without Necessarily Quitting Your Day Job*. Rabbit Ranch Publishing, 2011.

Weinzweig, Ari. *A Lapsed Anarchist's Approach to Building a Great Business.* Ann Arbor, MI: Zingerman's Press, 2010.

Chapter 14

Books

Ingham, Elaine. *The Compost Tea Brewing Manual.* Corvallis, OR: Soil Foodweb, 2005.

Kellogg, Scott, and Stacy Pettigrew. *Toolbox for Sustainable City Living.* Cambridge, MA: South End Press, 2008.

Lowenfels, Jeff, and Wayne Lewis. *Teaming with Microbes: A Gardener's Guide to the Soil Food Web.* Portland, OR: Timber Press, 2006.

Park, Hoon, and Michael W. DuPonte. *How to Cultivate Indigenous Microorganisms.* Published by the Cooperative Extension Service of the College of Tropical Agriculture and Human Resources, University of Hawai'i at Mānoa, August 2008, online at www.ctahr.hawaii.edu/oc/freepubs/pdf/BIO-9.pdf.

Wistinghausen, Christian von, et al. *Biodynamic Sprays and Compost Preparations: Directions for Use.* Biodynamic Agricultural Association, 2003; and *Biodynamic Sprays and Compost Preparations: Production Methods.* Biodynamic Agricultural Association, 2000.

Internet

RECYCLE FOOD WASTE
www.recyclefoodwaste.org

SOIL BIOLOGY PRIMER
soils.usda.gov/sqi/concepts/soil_biology/biology.html

Bioremediation Resources

Books

Common Ground Collective Meg Perry Health Soil Project. *The New Orleans Residents' Guide to Do It Yourself Soil Clean Up Using Natural Processes.* March 2006, online at https://we.riseup.net/assets/6683.

Stamets, Paul. *Mycelium Running: How Mushrooms Can Help Save the World.* Berkeley, CA: Ten Speed Press, 2005.

Internet

CANADIAN GOVERNMENT BIOREMEDIATION INFORMATION PORTAL
www.biobasics.gc.ca/english/View.asp?x=741

FUNGI PERFECTI
www.fungi.com/

US ENVIRONMENTAL PROTECTION AGENCY BIOREMEDIATION PORTAL
www.clu-in.org/remediation

Green Burial Resources

GREEN BURIAL COUNCIL
www.greenburialcouncil.org

Indigo Fermentation and Natural Dyeing Resources

Balfour-Paul, Jenny. *Indigo*. London: British Museum Press, 1998.

Buchanan, Rita. *A Weaver's Garden: Growing Plants for Natural Dyes and Fibers*. Mineola, NY: Dover Publications, 1999.

Liles, J. N. *The Art and Craft of Natural Dyeing: Traditional Recipes for Modern Use*. Knoxville: University of Tennessee Press, 1990.

Natural Building Resources

Crews, Carole. *Clay Culture: Plasters, Paints, and Preservation*. Rancho de Taos, NM: Gourmet Adobe Press, 2009.

Evans, Ianto, et al. *The Hand-Sculpted House: A Practical and Philosophical Guide to Building a Cob Cottage*. White River Junction, VT: Chelsea Green, 2002.

Guelberth, Cedar Rose, and Dan Chiras. *The Natural Plaster Book: Earth, Lime, and Gypsum Plasters for Natural Homes*. Gabriola Island, British Columbia: New Society, 2002.

Ethanol Resources

JOURNEY TO FOREVER
http://journeytoforever.org/ethanol_link.html

ROBERT WARREN'S MAKE YOUR OWN FUEL WEBSITE
http://running_on_alcohol.tripod.com/index.html

Biogas Resources

Cook, Michael. *Biogas Volume 3: A Chinese Biogas Manual*. Warren, MI: Knowledge Publications, 2009.

House, David. *The Biogas Handbook*. Aurora, OR: House Press, 2006.

People of Africa Biogas. *Biogas: Volumes 1 and 2*. Warren, MI: Knowledge Publications, 2009.

GLOSSARY

ACETOBACTER: Bacteria that, in the presence of oxygen, metabolize alcohol into acetic acid (vinegar).

ACIDIFICATION: The process of producing acidity. This is frequently the result of fermentation, and it is a critical aspect of how fermentation safely preserves food.

AEROBIC BACTERIA: Bacteria that require oxygen.

ALKALINE: Base; with a pH measuring above 7, whereas below 7 is acid.

AMYLASE ENZYMES: Enzymes that break down starches (complex carbohydrates) into sugars (simple carbohydrates).

ANAEROBIC BACTERIA: Bacteria that do not require oxygen. They may be "obligate" anaerobes, which can only function in the absence of oxygen; or "facultative," which can function with or without oxygen.

ASPERGILLUS: A genus of mold used frequently in the Asian traditions of fermenting grains and legumes.

AYURVEDIC: Describing a traditional healing system of India.

BACKSLOPPING: Introducing a small bit of a previous batch into the new batch in any fermentation process.

BIOAVAILABILITY: The degree to which a nutrient or other substance is absorbed and utilized.

BIODYNAMICS: A holistic theory and method of organic agriculture, first put forth by Rudolf Steiner.

BOTULISM: A rare but often deadly illness caused by a toxin produced by the bacterium *Clostridium botulinum*, associated primarily with improperly canned foods, but also possible in improperly fermented fish and meat.

BRINE: Salt water used as medium for pickling and preservation.

CARBONATION: Trapped carbon dioxide, resulting in bubbling once it is released.

CHLORAMINES: New forms of chlorine that are not volatile and therefore cannot be boiled off.

COAGULANTS: Substances that react with a liquid (such as milk) to transform it into a solid or semi-solid state.

CULTURE: A many-layered word; in the context of fermentation, it generally refers to starters comprising either isolated organisms ("pure cultures") or perpetuated communities of organisms ("mixed cultures").

CURDLE: The coagulation of milk, resulting in a separation of milk fats and solids from the liquid whey.

CURDS: The solid products of coagulation/curdling.

CURING: A broad expression encompassing varied forms of post-harvest maturation;

in the context of aging meat and fish, it often means the addition of nitrite and/or nitrate, known as "curing salts."

DECOCTION: A botanical extract prepared by boiling plant material, frequently roots, barks, or other dense, woody tissue.

DEXTROSE: Another name for the sugar glucose.

DISTILLATION: A process that concentrates alcohol (or other volatile substances) through evaporation and condensation.

DRY-SALTING: Salting a solid food without the addition of water.

EUKARYOTIC: Life-forms composed of cells in which DNA is contained in a nucleus and other structures are contained in membranes. Animals, plants, and fungi are all eukaryotic, while bacteria are prokaryotic.

FACULTATIVE: Organisms that can function in either the presence or the absence of oxygen.

FLORA: The indigenous microbial population found in a given substrate or environment.

GERMINATION: The sprouting of a seed.

GLUCOSE: A simple sugar that is a primary source of cellular energy.

HULL/HULLED/DEHULLED/ UNHULLED: Hulls are the outer layers of seeds (including grains, legumes, and nuts), typically hard and indigestible. Hulled or dehulled seeds have had the hulls removed. Unhulled seeds have the hulls still intact, important for certain processes, such as sprouting or malting.

INCUBATE: To maintain an environment in a specific temperature range; used in fermentation in order to encourage optimal microbial growth.

INFUSION: A botanical extract prepared by steeping plant material in hot water, rather than boiling it; generally used for extractions from leaves and flowers.

INOCULATE: To introduce a starter culture.

LACTIC ACID BACTERIA (LAB): A broad category of bacteria, encompassing several different genera, united by their production of lactic acid as their primary metabolic by-product.

LACTOBACILLI: A genus of lactic acid bacteria.

LACTO-FERMENTATION: Any fermentation performed primarily by lactic acid bacteria.

LACTOSE: The sugar present in milk.

LEAVEN: Sourdough bread culture.

LEES: The residual solids from wines and alcoholic rice fermentations.

LIQUEFACTION: The physical process of solids liquefying, which occurs in some fermentation processes.

LIVE-CULTURE: Lacto-fermented foods not heated after fermentation, so that living bacteria remain alive and intact.

MALT: Germinated barley or other grains. Germination activates enzymes that break down complex carbohydrates (starch) into simple carbohydrates that can ferment into alcohol.

METABOLISM: The chemical reactions that occur within living cells that enable them to use available nutrients. The processes specific to each nutrient and its end products are called metabolic pathways.

MYCELIUM (PLURAL MYCELIA): The network of fine filaments that fungi generate as they grow.

NIXTAMALIZATION: The process of cooking corn in an alkaline solution of wood ash or lime, which loosens and disintegrates the hard hulls of the kernels and improves the corn's nutritional value.

OXIDATION: A chemical reaction with oxygen.

PASTEURIZATION: A process of partial sterilization, most commonly applied to milk, but also wine, sauerkraut, and many other foods and beverages. Traditionally, pasteurization of milk involves heating it to 161°F/72°C for at least 15 seconds. "Ultra-pasteurization" involves higher temperatures, while "cold pasteurization" refers to irradiation.

PECTINS: Compounds found in the cell walls of non-woody plant tissue.

PHOTOSYNTHESIS: The production of energy from sunlight by plants, algae, and some bacteria.

PHYTATES: Compounds present in the outer layers of grains, legumes, seeds, and nuts, which bind minerals and render them unavailable for our absorption.

PHYTOCHEMICALS: Plant compounds.

PICKLING: Preserving in an acidic medium.

PROBIOTICS: Bacteria that confer some benefit to the organism that ingests them.

PROKARYOTIC: Unicellular life-forms, in which DNA is free-floating and not contained in a nucleus, and without specialized organelles. Bacteria are prokaryotic, while animals, plants, and fungi are eukaryotic.

RACKING: Siphoning a partially fermented alcoholic beverage into another fermentation vessel, in order to separate it from yeast sediment, and also aerate it to restart "stuck" fermentation.

RHIZOME: An underground stem, present in some plants, such as ginger, that typically grows horizontally, generating shoots and roots at periodic intervals.

RHIZOPUS: A genus of mold used in tempeh and other Asian traditions of fermenting legumes and grains.

RIND: Outer edge or skin, generally tough and hard.

SACCHARIFICATION: An enzymatic digestive process in which complex carbohydrates (starches) are broken down into simple carbohydrates (sugars), which is an essential step in all beer making.

SACCHAROMYCES CEREVISIAE: The yeast most commonly found in wine making, brewing, and baking.

SALINITY: Level of saltiness.

SCOBY: Symbiotic community of bacteria and yeast; a starter culture that has taken on a physical form, which is transferred from batch to batch as a means of perpetuation.

SIPHON: To transfer liquid from one vessel to another situated in a lower position, using a tube and the force of gravity.

SPORULATION: The reproductive phase of mold growth, typically marked by a change in color.

STARTER: Bacterial and/or fungal cultures introduced in order to initiate fermentation.

SUBSTRATE: The food or beverage we are fermenting, simultaneously food for our microbial friends and the medium upon which they grow.

TANNINS: Bitter and astringent chemical compounds present in many plants.

THERMOPHILIC: A classification of bacteria that are most active at temperatures higher than 110°F/43°C.

ULTRA-PASTEURIZED: A higher-temperature variation of pasteurization, frequently used to produce milk with a long shelf life.

WILD FERMENTATION: Fermentation that relies on organisms spontaneously present on the substrate or in the air, rather than introduced; also, the title of the author's earlier book on fermentation

WORT: Malted grain extraction, brewed, filtered, and ready to ferment.

YEAST: A broad grouping of fungi that includes *Saccharomyces cerevisiae* and others that metabolize sugars into alcohol.

A NOTE ON REFERENCES

*T*here is much excellent information available documenting fermentation practices around the world. Here I will describe some of the books and other resources that cover the topic of fermentation broadly, as well as a few notable sources that cover the ferments of specific regions of the world in especially comprehensive ways. A list of books cited follows. In addition, the endnotes and Resources section point readers to articles, additional books, Internet resources, and further sources of information.

The first book that I encountered addressing the topic of fermentation broadly was Bill Mollison's *Ferment and Human Nutrition* (Tagari, 1993). By then I had already learned several different ferments, understood that fermentation was widespread around the world, and was hungry for more information. Mollison's book really opened my eyes to the diversity of fermentation practices. His notes, observations, and investigations in the realm of fermentation from his travels and reading are extensive. This book offers a sweeping perspective, examining patterns of human fermentation practices and variations on themes, more than a usable guide to techniques for fermentation. Mollison is best known as one of the originators of the word and concept *permaculture*.

Keith Steinkraus's *Handbook of Indigenous Fermented Foods* (Marcel Dekker, 1996) is the most comprehensive book on fermentation that exists in the English language. The first edition (1983) grew out of two international events. First, a 1974 UNESCO training in Indonesia brought together microbiologists from five continents with research interests in indigenous fermentation, who realized how useful a compilation of information on these processes could be. Out of that 1974 training grew another international event, the Symposium on Indigenous Fermented Foods, held in 1977 in Thailand. Keith Steinkraus then condensed 2,500 pages of papers presented there into this book, which he updated and revised in 1996.

International conferences have generated some other excellent fermentation resources. The Sixth International Fermentation Symposium, held in 1980 in Canada, produced the book *Indigenous Fermented Food of Non-Western Origin* (J. Cramer, 1986), edited by C. W. Hesseltine and Hwa L. Wang. The Seventh International Ethnological Food Research Conference, held in Norway in 1987, resulted in the volume *Food Conservation Ethnological Studies* (Prospect Books, 1988), edited by Astri Riddervold and Andreas

Ropeid, with excellent papers mostly, but not exclusively, focused on European traditions of food preservation. Finally, the 2010 Oxford Symposium on Food and Cookery, in which I participated, was devoted to cured, fermented, and smoked foods, with many fascinating presentations that informed this book. A compilation of the papers presented at this conference has been published as the *Proceedings of the Oxford Symposium on Food and Cookery 2010: Cured, Fermented and Smoked Foods* (Prospect Books, 2011).

The Food and Agriculture Organization of the United Nations (FAO) has published a series of information-packed Agricultural Services Bulletins devoted to fermented foods, including *Fermented Fruits and Vegetables: A Global Perspective* (1998), *Fermented Cereals: A Global Perspective* (1999), and *Fermented Grain Legumes, Seeds, and Nuts: A Global Perspective* (2000). Each of these compilations is the work of a geographically diverse team of scholars, providing flow charts and detailed descriptions to facilitate the preservation and spread of fermentation knowledge.

Several books and web-based databases stand out as authoritative sources on the ferments of their respective geographic areas of China, the Sudan, and India. H. T. Huang's epic volume *Fermentations and Food Science* (Cambridge University Press, 2000), part of the Science and Civilisation in China series, presents a sweeping historical overview of the development of China's elaborate and distinctive fermentation practices, with process descriptions, from historical documents, detailed enough to follow. Hamid Dirar's *The Indigenous Fermented Foods of the Sudan* (CAB International, 1993) is an anthropological exploration of the Sudan's rich fermentation traditions, also with plenty of detail for those who wish to experiment based on descriptions in the book. S. Sekar, a professor of biotechnology at Bharathidasan University in Tiruchirappalli, India, has published online a very detailed *Database on Microbial Traditional Knowledge of India*, at www.bdu.ac.in/schools/life_sciences /biotechnology/sekardb.htm. Finally, Xu Gan Rong and Bao Tong Fa of Jiangnan University in Jiangsu Province, China, have published their *Grandiose Survey of Chinese Alcoholic Drinks and Beverages* online at www .sytu.edu.cn/zhgjiu/umain.htm.

I must also acknowledge the epic work of William Shurtleff and Akiko Aoyagi, the authors of *The Book of Miso* and *The Book of Tempeh*, as well as an ongoing project documenting the history of soybeans and soy ferments, and archiving historical references. I visited Shurtleff while I was writing this book, and when I asked whether they would be publishing the archive in book form, he launched into a passionate argument for free Internet publishing. All of Shurtleff and Aoyagi's recent books have been self-published digitally, free of charge, on both on Google Books and on their website, www.soyinfocenter .com, which is an indispensable resource.

Finally, for those seeking to reconstruct fermentation traditions, information is scattered in thousands of cookbooks, and in the practices and memories of millions of people. The realm of fermentation is too vast and non-standardized to be comprehensively contained in any single volume. Be creative in your pursuit of information on traditional ferments, and then find ways to share what you learn, so the fermentation revival can grow to incorporate ever more diverse traditions.

BOOKS CITED

Aasved, Mikal John. *Alcohol, Drinking, and Intoxication in Preindustrial Society: Theoretical, Nutritional, and Religious Considerations*. PhD dissertation, University of California–Santa Barbara, 1988.

Albala, Ken. *Beans: A History*. Oxford: Berg, 2007.

———. *Pancake: A Global History*. London: Reaktion Books, 2008.

Albala, Ken, and Rosanna Nafzifer. *The Lost Art of Real Cooking*. New York: Perigee, 2010.

Andoh, Elizabeth. *Kansha: Celebrating Japan's Vegan and Vegetarian Traditions*. Berkeley, CA: Ten Speed Press, 2010.

Awiakta, Marilou. *SELU: Seeking the Corn-Mother's Wisdom*. Golden, CO: Fulcrum Publishers, 1993.

Bamforth, Charles W. *Grape vs. Grain*. New York: Cambridge University Press, 2008.

———. *Scientific Principles of Malting and Brewing*. St. Paul, MN: American Society of Brewing Chemists, 2006.

Barlow, Connie. *The Ghosts of Evolution: Nonsensical Fruit, Missing Partners, and Other Ecological Anachronisms*. New York: Basic Books, 2000.

Baron, Stanley. *Brewed in America: A History of Beer and Ale in the United States*. Boston: Little Brown, 1962.

Battcock, Mike, and Sue Azam-Ali. *Fermented Fruits and Vegetables: A Global Perspective*. FAO Agricultural Services Bulletin Number 134. Rome: Food and Agriculture Organization of the United Nations, 1998.

Belasco, Warren. *Appetite for Change*. New York: Pantheon, 1989.

Belitz, Hans-Dieter, et al. *Food Chemistry*, 3rd revised edition. New York: Springer, 2004.

Bennett, W. C., and R. M. Zing. *The Tarahumara: An Indian Tribe of Northern Mexico*. Chicago: University of Chicago Press, 1935.

Bokanga, Mpoko. *Microbiology and Biochemistry of Cassava Fermentation*. PhD dissertation, Cornell University, 1989.

Bruman, Henry J. *Alcohol in Ancient Mexico*. Salt Lake City: University of Utah Press, 2000.

Buhner, Stephen Harrod. *Sacred and Herbal Healing Beers: The Secrets of Ancient Fermentation*. Boulder, CO: Siris Books, 1998.

Coe, Sophie D. *America's First Cuisines*. Austin: University of Texas Press, 1994.

Cushing, Frank Hamilton. *Zuni Breadstuff*. New York: Museum of the American Indian, 1974.

Dabney, Joseph. *Smokehouse Ham, Spoon Bread, & Scuppernong Wine*. Nashville, TN: Cumberland House, 1998.

Daniel, Kaayla. *The Whole Soy Story: The Dark Side of America's Favorite Health Food*. Washington, DC: New Trends Publishing, 2005.

Deshpande, S. S., et al. *Fermented Grain Legumes, Seeds, and Nuts: A Global Perspective*. FAO Agricultural Services Bulletin Number 142. Rome: Food and Agriculture Organization of the United Nations, 2000.

Diggs, Lawrence J. *Vinegar: The User-Friendly Standard Text Reference and Guide to Appreciating, Making, and Enjoying Vinegar*. Lincoln, NE: Authors Choice Press, 2000.

Dirar, Hamid A. *The Indigenous Fermented Foods of the Sudan*. Oxon, UK: CAB International, 1993.

Doyle, M. P., and L. R. Beuchat (editors). *Food Microbiology: Fundamentals and Frontiers*. Washington, DC: ASM Press, 2007.

Du Bois, Christine M., et al. (editors). *The World of Soy*. Urbana: University of Illinois Press, 2008.

Dunlop, Fuchsia. *Land of Plenty: Authentic Sichuan Recipes Personally Gathered in the Chinese Province of Sichuan*. New York: W. W. Norton, 2003.

Eames, Alan D. *Secret Life of Beer: Legends, Lore & Little-Known Facts*. Pownal, VT: Storey Books, 1995.

Fallon, Sally, with Mary Enig. *Nourishing Traditions: The Cookbook That Challenges Politically Correct Nutrition and the Diet Dictocrats*, revised 2nd edition. Washington, DC: New Trends Publishing, 2001.

Farrell, Jeanette. *Invisible Allies: Microbes That Shape Our Lives*. New York: Farrar Straus Giroux, 2005.

Farrer, Keith. *To Feed a Nation: A History of Australian Food Science and Technology*. Collingwood, Victoria, Australia: CSIRO Publishing, 2005.

Fearnley-Whittingstall, Hugh. *River Cottage Cookbook*. London: Collins, 2001.

———. *River Cottage Meat Book*. Berkeley, CA: Ten Speed Press, 2007.

Gaden, Elmer L., et al. (editors). *Applications of Biotechnology to Traditional Fermented Foods*. Washington, DC: National Academy Press, 1992.

Grahn, Judy. *Blood, Bread, and Roses: How Menstruation Created the World*. Boston: Beacon Press, 1993.

Grieve, Maud. *A Modern Herbal*. New York: Dover, 1931.

Haard, Norman, et al. *Fermented Cereals: A Global Perspective*. FAO Agricultural Services Bulletin No. 138. Rome: Food and Agriculture Organization of the United Nations, 1999.

Haggblade, Steven J. *The Shebeen Queen; or Sorghum Beer in Botswana: The Impact of Factory Brews on a Cottage Industry*. PhD dissertation, Michigan State University, 1984.

Hepinstall, Hi Soo Shin. *Growing Up in a Korean Kitchen*. Berkeley, CA: Ten Speed Press, 2001.

Hesseltine, C. W., and H. L. Wang (editors). *Indigenous Fermented Food of Non-Western Origin*. Mycological Memoir No. 11. Berlin: J. Cramer, 1986.

Hobbs, Christopher. *Kombucha: The Essential Guide*. Santa Cruz, CA: Botanica Press, 1995.

Huang, H. T. *Science and Civilisation in China*, Volume 6, *Biology and Biological Technology*, Part V: *Fermentations and Food Science*. Cambridge, UK: Cambridge University Press, 2000.

Hui, Y. H. (editor). *Handbook of Food Science, Technology, and Engineering*. Boca Raton, FL: CRC Press, 2006.

Hui, Y. H., et al. (editors). *Handbook of Food and Beverage Fermentation Technology*. New York: Marcel Dekker, 2004.

Hunter, Beatrice Trum. *Probiotic Foods for Good Health: Yogurt, Sauerkraut, and Other Beneficial Fermented Foods*. Laguna Beach, CA: Basic Health Publications, 2008.

Jacobs, Jane. *The Economy of Cities*. New York: Vintage, 1970.

Janson, Lee W. *Brew Chem 101: The Basics of Homebrewing Chemistry*. North Adams, MA: Storey Publishing, 1996.

Jay, James Monroe, et al. *Modern Food Microbiology*, 7th edition. New York: Springer, 2005.

Jenkins, Joseph. *The Humanure Handbook: A Guide to Composting Human Manure*, 3rd edition. Grove City, PA: Joseph Jenkins, Inc., 2005.

Jones, Anore. *Iqaluich Nigiñaqtuat, Fish That We Eat*. Final Report No. FIS02-023. US Fish and Wildlife Service Office of Subsistence Management, Fisheries Resource Monitoring Program, 2006.

Katz, Sandor Ellix. *The Revolution Will Not Be Microwaved: Inside America's Underground Food Movements*. White River Junction, VT: Chelsea Green, 2006.

———. *Wild Fermentation: The Flavor, Nutrition, and Craft of Live-Culture Foods*. White River Junction, VT: Chelsea Green, 2003.

Katz, Solomon (editor). *Encyclopedia of Food and Culture*. New York: Scribner, 2003.

Kaufmann, Klaus, and Annelies Schöneck. *Making Sauerkraut and Pickled Vegetables at Home*. Summertown, TN: Books Alive, 2008.

Kennedy, Diana. *The Essential Cuisines of Mexico*. New York: Clarkson Potter, 2000.

——. *Oaxaca al Gusto: An Infinite Gastronomy*. Austin: University of Texas Press, 2010.

Khardori, Nancy (editor). *Bioterrorism Preparedness*. Weinheim, Germany: Wiley Inter-Science, 2006.

Kindstedt, Paul. *American Farmstead Cheese: The Complete Guide to Making and Selling Artisan Cheeses*. White River Junction, VT: Chelsea Green, 2005.

Klieger, P. Christian. *The Fleischmann Yeast Family*. Mount Pleasant, SC: Arcadia Publishing, 2004.

Konlee, Mark. *How to Reverse Immune Dysfunction: A Nutrition Manual for HIV, Chronic Fatigue Syndrome, Candidiasis, and Other Immune Related Disorders*. West Allis, WI: Keep Hope Alive, 1995.

Kosikowski, Frank V., and Vikram V. Mistry. *Cheese and Fermented Milk Foods*. Volume I: *Origins and Principles*, 3rd edition. Ashfield, MA: New England Cheesemaking Supply Company, 1999.

Kurlansky, Mark. *Salt: A World History*. New York: Walker, 2002.

Kushi, Aveline. *Complete Guide to Macrobiotic Cooking*. New York: Warner Books, 1985.

Leader, Daniel. *Local Breads: Sourdough and Whole-Grain Recipes from Europe's Best Artisan Bakers*. New York: W. W. Norton, 2007.

Lee, Cherl-Ho, et al. (editors). *Fish Fermentation Technology*. Tokyo: United Nations University Press, 1993.

Levi-Strauss, Claude. *The Raw and the Cooked*. Translated by John and Doreen Weightman. New York: Harper & Row, 1969.

Litzinger, William Joseph. *The Ethnobiology of Alcoholic Beverage Production by the Lacandon, Tarahumara, and Other Aboriginal Mesoamerican Peoples*. PhD dissertation, University of Colorado–Boulder, 1983.

Man-Jo, Kim, et al. *The Kimchee Cookbook: Fiery Flavors and Cultural History of Korea's National Dish*. North Clarendon, VT: Periplus, 1999.

Marcellino, R. M. Noella. *Biodiversity of* Geotrichum candidum *Strains Isolated from Traditional French Cheese*. PhD dissertation, University of Connecticut, 2003.

Margulis, Lynn, and Dorion Sagan. *Dazzle Gradually: Reflections on the Nature of Nature*. White River Junction, VT: Chelsea Green Publishing, 2007.

——. *Microcosmos: Four Billion Years of Evolution from Our Microbial Ancestors*. New York: Summit Books, 1986.

——. *Slanted Truths*. New York: Springer Verlag, 1997.

Marianski, Stanley, and Adam Marianski. *The Art of Making Fermented Sausages*. Denver, CO: Outskirts Press, 2008.

McGovern, Patrick E. *Uncorking the Past: The Quest for Wine, Beer, and Other Alcoholic Beverages*. Berkeley: University of California Press, 2009.

McNeill, F. Marian. *The Scots Kitchen: Its Traditions and Lore with Old-Time Recipes*. London and Glasgow: Blackie & Son, 1929.

Miliotis, Marianne D., and Jeffrey W. Bier (editors). *International Handbook of Foodborne Pathogens*. New York: Marcel Dekker, 2001.

Mollison, Bill. *The Permaculture Book of Ferment and Human Nutrition*. Tyalgum, Australia: Tagari Publications, 1993.

Pagden, A. R. (editor and translator). *The Maya: Diego de Landa's Account of the Affairs of the Yucatan*. Chicago: J. Philip O'Hara, 1975.

Papazian, Charlie. *Microbrewed Adventures*. New York: HarperCollins, 2005.

Pederson, Carl S. *Microbiology of Food Fermentations*, 2nd edition. Westport, CT: AVI Publishing, 1979.

Pendell, Dale. *Pharmako/poeia: Plant Powers, Poisons, and Herbcraft*. San Francisco: Mercury House, 1995.

Phaff, H. J., et al. *The Life of Yeasts*. Cambridge, MA: Harvard University Press, 1978.

Piccetti, John, and Francois Vecchio with Joyce Goldstein. *Salumi: Savory Recipes and Serving Ideas for Salame, Prosciutto, and More*. San Francisco: Chronicle Books, 2009.

Pitchford, Paul. *Healing with Whole Foods*, 3rd edition. Berkeley, CA: North Atlantic Books, 2002.

Pollan, Michael. *The Botany of Desire: A Plant's-Eye View of the World*. New York: Random House, 2001.

Rehbein, Hartmut, and Jörg Oehlenschläger (editors). *Fishery Products: Quality, Safety and Authenticity*. Oxford, UK: Blackwell, 2009.

Rhoades, Robert E., and Pedro Bidegaray. *The Farmers of Yurimaguas: Land Use and Cropping Strategies in the Peruvian Jungle*. Lima, Peru: CIP, 1987.

Riddervold, Astri. *Lutfisk, Rakefisk and Herring in Norwegian Tradition*. Oslo: Novus Press, 1990.

Riddervold, Astri, and Andreas Ropeid (editors). *Food Conservation Ethnological Studies*. London: Prospect Books, 1988.

Rindos, David. *The Origins of Agriculture: An Evolutionary Perspective*. Orlando, FL: Academic Press, 1984.

Rombauer, Irma S., and Marion Rombauer Becker. *Joy of Cooking*. Indianapolis: Bobbs-Merrill, 1975.

———. *Joy of Cooking*. Indianapolis: Bobbs-Merrill, 1953.

Ruhlman, Michael. *Ratio: The Simple Codes Behind the Craft of Everyday Cooking.* New York: Scribner, 2009.

Ruhlman, Michael, and Brian Polcyn. *Charcuterie: The Craft of Salting, Smoking, and Curing.* New York: W. W. Norton, 2005.

Saberi, Helen (editor). *Cured, Fermented and Smoked Foods.* Proceedings of the Oxford Symposium on Food and Cookery 2010. Totnes, UK: Prospect Books, 2011.

Sanchez, Priscilla C. *Philippine Fermented Foods: Principles and Technology.* Quezon City: University of the Philippines Press, 2008.

Sapers, Gerald M., et al. (editors). *Microbiology of Fruits and Vegetables.* Boca Raton, FL: CRC Press, 2006.

Shephard, Sue. *Pickled, Potted, and Canned.* New York: Simon & Schuster, 2001.

Shurtleff, William, and Akiko Aoyagi. *The Book of Miso.* Brookline, MA: Autumn Press, 1976.

——. *The Book of Tempeh.* New York: Harper & Row, 1979a.

——. *The Book of Tempeh,* professional edition. New York: Harper & Row, 1979b.

——. *The Book of Tofu.* Berkeley, CA: Ten Speed Press, 1998.

——. *History of Miso, Soybean Jiang (China), Jang (Korea) and Tauco/Taotjo (Indonesia) (200 BC–2009): Extensively Annotated Bibliography and Sourcebook.* Lafayette, CA: Soyinfo Center, 2009.

——. *History of Soybeans and Soyfoods: 1100 BC to the 1980s.* Lafayette, CA: Soyinfo Center, 2007.

——. *Miso Production: The Book of Miso,* Volume II. Lafayette, CA: Soyfoods Center, 1980.

——. *Tempeh Production: A Craft and Technical Manual.* Lafayette, CA: Soyfoods Center, 1986.

Siegel, Ronald K. *Intoxication: Life in Pursuit of Artificial Paradise.* New York: Pocket Books, 1989.

Smith, Andrew F. *Pure Ketchup: A History of America's National Condiment.* Washington, DC: Smithsonian Institution Press, 2001.

Spargo, John. *The Bitter Cry of the Children.* New York: MacMillan, 1906.

Sparrow, Jeff. *Wild Brews: Beer Beyond the Influence of Brewer's Yeast.* Boulder, CO: Brewers Publications, 2005.

Stamets, Paul. *Mycelium Running: How Mushrooms Can Help Save the World.* Berkeley, CA: Ten Speed Press, 2005.

Standage, Tom. *A History of the World in Six Glasses.* New York: Walker, 2005.

Steinkraus, Keith (editor). *Handbook of Indigenous Fermented Foods,* 2nd edition. New York: Marcel Dekker, 1996.

Stoytcheva, Margarita (editor). *Pesticides: Formulations, Effects, Fate*. Rijeka, Croatia: Intech, 2011.

Tamang, Jyoti Prakash. *Himalayan Fermented Foods: Microbiology, Nutrition, and Ethnic Values*. Boca Raton, FL: CRC Press, 2010.

Tietze, Harald W. *Living Food for Longer Life*. Bermagui, Australia: Harald W. Tietze Publishing, 1999.

Toldrá, Fidel. *Dry-Cured Meat Products*. Trumbull, CT: Food and Nutrition Press, 2002.

Toldrá, Fidel (editor). *Handbook of Fermented Meat and Poultry*. Ames, IA: Blackwell, 2007.

Toomre, Joyce. *Classic Russian Cooking: Elena Molokhovets' A Gift to Young Housewives*. Bloomington: Indiana University Press, 1992.

Tsimako, Bonnake. *The Socio-Economic Significance of Home Brewing in Rural Botswana: A Descriptive Profile*. Master's thesis, Michigan State University, 1983.

Volokh, Anne. *The Art of Russian Cuisine*. New York: MacMillan, 1983.

Weed, Susun S. *New Menopausal Years: The Wise Woman Way*. Woodstock, NY: Ash Tree Publishing, 2002.

Weinert, Diana. *An Entrepreneurial Perspective on Regulatory Change in Germany's Medieval Brewing Industry*. PhD dissertation, George Mason University, 2009.

Wilson, Edward O. *Biophilia*. Cambridge, MA: Harvard University Press, 1984.

Wilson, Michael. *Microbial Inhabitants of Humans: Their Ecology and Role in Health and Disease*. Cambridge: Cambridge University Press, 2005.

Wood, Bertha M. *Foods of the Foreign-Born in Relation to Health*. Boston: Whitcomb & Barrows, 1922.

Wood, Brian J. B. *Microbiology of Fermented Foods*. London: Thomson Science, 1998.

ENDNOTES

Introduction

1. Jacobs, 3.
2. Ibid., 31.
3. C. W. Hesseltine and H. L. Wang, "Contributions of the Western World to Knowledge of Indigenous Fermented Foods of the Orient," in Steinkraus, 712.

Chapter 1

1. Geoffrey Campbell-Platt, "Fermentation," in Solomon Katz, Volume 1, 630–631, cited in Du Bois (2008), 58.
2. Deshpande (2000), 7.
3. Lynn Margulis, "Power to the Protoctists," in Margulis and Sagan (2007), 30–31.
4. Lynn Margulis, "Serial Endosymbiotic Theory (SET) and Composite Individuality: Transition from Bacterial to Eukaryotic Genomes," *Microbiology Today* 31:172 (2004); E. G. Nisbet and N. H. Sleep, "The Habitat and Nature of Early Life," *Nature* 409:1089 (2001).
5. Margulis and Sagan (1986), 131–132.
6. Sorin Sonea and Léo G. Mathieu, "Evolution of the Genomic Systems of Prokaryotes and Its Momentous Consequences," *International Microbiology* 4:67–71 (2001).
7. Jian Xu and Jeffrey I. Gordon, "Honor Thy Symbionts," *Proceedings of the National Academy of Sciences* 100(18):10452 (2003).
8. Fredrik Bäckhed et al., "Host-Bacterial Mutualism in the Human Intestine," *Science* 307:1915 (2005).
9. D. C. Savage, "Microbial Ecology of the Gastrointestinal Tract," *Annual Review of Microbiology* 31:107–133 (1977).
10. Ruth E. Ley, Daniel A. Peterson, and Jeffrey I. Gordon, "Ecological and Evolutionary Forces Shaping Microbial Diversity in the Human Intestine," *Cell* 124:837 (2006).
11. Steven R. Gill et al., "Metagenomic Analysis of the Human Distal Gut Microbiome," *Science* 312:1357 (2006).
12. Bäckhed et al. (2005)
13. M. J. Hill, "Intestinal Flora and Endogenous Vitamin Synthesis," *European Journal of Cancer Prevention* 6(Suppl. 1):S43 (1997).
14. S. C. Leahy et al., "Getting Better with Bifidobacteria," *Journal of Applied Microbiology* 98:1303 (2005).
15. Lora V. Hooper et al., "Molecular Analysis of Commensal Host–Microbial Relationships in the Intestine," *Science* 291:881 (2001).

16. Denise Kelly et al., "Commensal Gut Bacteria: Mechanisms of Immune Modulation," *Trends in Immunology* 26:326 (2005).

17. Elizabeth Grice et al., "Topographical and Temporal Diversity of the Human Skin Microbiome," *Science* 324:1190 (2009).

18. Jørn A. Aas et al., "Defining the Normal Bacterial Flora of the Oral Cavity," *Journal of Clinical Microbiology* 43:5721 (2005).

19. E. R. Boskey et al., "Origins of Vaginal Acidity: High D/L Lactate Ratio Is Consistent with Bacteria Being the Primary Source," *Human Reproduction* 16(9):1809 (2001).

20. Bäckhed et al. (2005)

21. Wilson (2005), 375.

22. Joel Schroeter and Todd Klaenhammer, "Genomics of Lactic Acid Bacteria," *FEMS Microbiology Letters* 292(1):1 (2008).

23. J. A. Shapiro, "Bacteria Are Small But Not Stupid: Cognition, Natural Genetic Engineering, and Socio-Bacteriology," *Studies in the History and Philosophy of Biological and Biomedical Sciences* 38:807 (2007).

24. Sorin Sonea and Léo G. Mathieu, "Evolution of the Genomic Systems of Prokaryotes and Its Momentous Consequences," *International Microbiology* 4:67 (2001).

25. "Interview with Lynn Margulis," *Astrobiology Magazine* (October 9, 2006), online at http://astrobio.net/news/modules.php?op=modload&name=News&file=article&sid=2108, accessed December 5, 2009.

26. Léo G. Mathieu and Sorin Sonea, "A Powerful Bacterial World," *Endeavour* 19(3):112 (1995).

27. Margulis and Sagan (1986), 16.

28. Shapiro, 807.

29. Jan-Hendrik Hehemann, "Transfer of Carbohydrate-Active Enzymes from Marine Bacteria to Japanese Gut Microbiota," *Nature* 464:908 (2010).

30. Justin L. Sonnenburg, "Genetic Pot Luck," *Nature* 464:837 (2010).

31. Margulis and Sagan (1986), 133–136.

32. Dr. Ingham made this remark September 14, 2009, at a "Soil Foodweb" workshop the author attended.

33. Buhner, 150.

34. Ibid., 151.

35. *American Heritage Dictionary of the English Language*, 4th edition, 2000.

36. McGovern, xi–xii and 281.

37. Patrick E. McGovern et al., "Fermented Beverages of Pre- and Proto-Historic China," *Proceedings of the National Academy of Sciences* 101(51):17593 (2004).

38. Aasved, 4.

39. Frank Wiens et al., "Chronic Intake of Fermented Floral Nectar by Wild Treeshrews," *Proceedings of the National Academy of Sciences* 105:10426 (2008).

40. Ibid.

41. Robert Dudley, "Fermenting Fruit and the Historical Ecology of Ethanol Ingestion: Is Alcoholism in Modern Humans an Evolutionary Hangover?" *Addiction* 97:384 (2002).

42. Siegel, 118.

43. McGovern, 266.

44. Abigail Tucker, "The Beer Archaeologist," *Smithsonian* (2011), online at www.smithsonianmag.com/history-archaeology/The-Beer-Archaeologist.html, accessed July 7, 2011.

45. Sidney W. Mintz, "The Absent Third: The Place of Fermentation in a Thinkable World Food System," in Saberi, 14.

46. Rindos, 137.

47. See Claude Levi-Strauss, *The Raw and the Cooked*.

48. D. H. Janzen, "When Is It Coevolution?," *Evolution* 34:611 (1980).

49. For a discussion of this theory, see Barlow, *The Ghosts of Evolution*.

50. Pollan, xvi.

51. Charles R. Clement, "1942 and the Loss of Amazonian Crop Genetic Resources. I. The Relation Between Domestication and Human Population Decline," *Economic Botany* 53(2):188 (1999).

52. Rindos, 159.

53. Pederson (1979), 40.

54. Erika A. Pfeiler and Todd R. Klaenhammer, "The Genomics of Lactic Acid Bacteria," *Trends in Microbiology* 15(12):546 (2007).

55. Joel Schroeter and Todd Klaenhammer, "Genomics of Lactic Acid Bacteria," FEMS Microbiology Letters 292(1):1 (2008).

56. Huang, 593.

57. Dirar, 30.

58. The laboratory, long maintained at the Northern Regional Research Laboratory in Peoria, Illinois, has become the NRRL Culture Collection, online at http://nrrl.ncaur.usda.gov.

59. C. W. Hesseltine and Hwa L. Wang, "The Importance of Traditional Fermented Foods," *BioScience* 30(6):402 (1980).

60. American Medical Association Council on Scientific Affairs, "Use of Antimicrobials in Consumer Products (CSA Rep. 2, A-00)," in Summaries and Recommendations of Council on Scientific Affairs Reports, 2000 AMA Annual Meeting, 4, online at www.ama-assn.org/ama1/pub/upload/mm/443/csaa-00.pdf, accessed December 18, 2009.

61. Lynn Margulis, "Prejudice and Bacteria Consciousness," in Margulis and Sagan (2007), 37.

62. Martin J. Blaser, "Who Are We? Indigenous Microbes and the Ecology of Human Diseases," *European Molecular Biology Organization Reports* 7(10):956 (2006).

63. "The Twists and Turns of Fate," *Economist* 388(8594):68 (August 23, 2008).

64. Volker Mai, "Dietary Modification of the Intestinal Microbiota," *Nutrition Reviews* 62(6):235 (2004).

65. Blaser.

66. Edward O. Wilson, *Biophilia* (Cambridge, MA: Harvard University Press, 1984).

67. Akio Tsuchii et al., "Degradation of the Rubber in Truck Tires by a Strain of Nocardia," *Biodegradation* 7:405 (1997).

68. Brajesh K. Singh and Allan Walker, "Microbial Degradation of Organophosphorus Compounds," *FEMS Microbiology Reviews* 30(3):428 (2006).

69. S. Y. Yuan et al., "Occurrence and Microbial Degradation of Phthalate Esters in Taiwan River Sediments," *Chemosphere* 49(10):1295 (2002).

70. Terry C. Hazen et al., "Deep-Sea Oil Plume Enriches Indigenous Oil-Degrading Bacteria," *Science* 330:204 (2010).

71. See Paul Stamets, *Mycelium Running: How Mushrooms Can Help Save the World* (Berkeley, CA: Ten Speed Press, 2005).

Chapter 2

1. Steinkraus, 113.

2. Janak Koirala, "Botulism: Toxicology, Clinical Presentations and Management," in Khardori, 163.

3. US Centers for Disease Control and Prevention, *Botulism in the United States, 1899–1996: Handbook for Epidemiologists, Clinicians, and Laboratory Workers* (Atlanta: Centers for Disease Control and Prevention, 1998), 11; online at www.cdc.gov/ncidod/DBMD/diseaseinfo/files/botulism_manual.htm, accessed December 23, 2009.

4. US Department of Agriculture, *Complete Guide to Home Canning, Guide 1: Principles of Home Canning* (Agriculture Information Bulletin No. 539, December 2009), 1–8; online at www.uga.edu/nchfp/publications/publications_usda.html, accessed December 23, 2009.

5. Michael W. Peck, "Clostridia and Food-Borne Disease," *Microbiology Today* 29:10 (2002).

6. Naomi Guttman and Max Wall, "Sausage in Oil: Preserving Italian Culture in Utica, NY," paper delivered at 2010 Oxford Symposium on Food and Cookery.

7. Akiko Iwasaki et al., "Microbiota Regulates Immune Defense Against Respiratory Tract Influenza A Virus Infection," *Proceedings of the National Academy of Sciences* 108(13): 5354 (2011).

8. US Federal Trade Commission, "Complaint in the Matter of the Dannon Company, Inc.," docket number 082 3158, December 15, 2010, online at www.ftc.gov/os/caselist/0823158/101215dannonscmpt.pdf, accessed June 5, 2011.

9. US Federal Trade Commission, "Dannon Agrees to Drop Exaggerated Health Claims for Activia Yogurt and DanActive Dairy Drink," press release December 15, 2010 (FTC File No. 0823158), online at www.ftc.gov/opa/2010/12/dannon.shtm, accessed June 5, 2010.

10. Lívia Trois, "Use of Probiotics in HIV-Infected Children: A Randomized Double-Blind Controlled Study," *Journal of Tropical Pediatrics* 54(1):19 (2007).

11. Lun Yu, Book 10, chapter 8, verse 3, cited in Huang, 334.

12. Huang, 402.

13. According to Shiming by Liu Xi, as cited in Shurtleff and Aoyagi (2009), 55.

14. Dirar, 434–443.

15. Victor Herbert, "Vitamin B_{12}: Plant Sources, Requirements, and Assay," *American Journal of Clinical Nutrition* 48:852 (1988).

16. Fumio Watanabe, "Vitamin B_{12} Sources and Bioavailability," *Experimental Biology and Medicine* 232:1266 (2007).

17. Irene T. H. Liem et al., "Production of Vitamin B_{12} in Tempeh, a Fermented Soybean Food," *Applied and Environmental Microbiology* 34(6):773 (1977).

18. Haard, 19.

19. Martin Milner and Kouhei Makise, "Natto and Its Active Ingredient Nattokinase: A Potent and Safe Thrombolytic Agent," *Alternative and Complementary Therapies* 8(3):157 (2002).

20. Rita P.-Y. Chen et al., "Amyloid-Degrading Ability of Nattokinase from Bacillus subtilis Natto," *Journal of Agricultural and Food Chemistry* 57:503 (2009).

21. Eeva-Liisa Ryhänen et al., "Plant-Derived Biomolecules in Fermented Cabbage," *Journal of Agricultural and Food Chemistry* 50:6798 (2002).

22. Farrer, 6.

23. G. Famularo, "Probiotic Lactobacilli: An Innovative Tool to Correct the Malabsorption Syndrome of Vegetarians?" *Medical Hypotheses* 65(6):1132 (2005); see also N. R. Reddy and M. D. Pierson, "Reduction in Antinutritional and Toxic Components in Plant Foods by Fermentation," *Food Research International* 27:281 (1994).

24. S. Hemalatha et al., "Influence of Germination and Fermentation on Bioaccessibility of Zinc and Iron from Food Grains," *European Journal of Clinical Nutrition* 61:342 (2007).

25. T. Heród-Leszczyńska and A. Miedzobrodzka, "Effect of the Fermentation Process on Levels of Nitrates and Nitrites in Selected Vegetables," *Roczniki Państwowego Zakładu Higieny* 43(3–4):253 (1992).

26. U. Preiss et al., "Einfluss der Gemüsefermentation auf Inhaltsstoffe (Effect of Fermentation on Components of Vegetable)," *Deutsche Lebensmittel-Rundschau* 98(11):400 (2002).

27. Aslan Azizi, "Bacterial-Degradation of Pesticides Residue in Vegetables During Fermentation" in Stoytcheva, 658, online at www.intechopen.com/articles/show/title/bacterial-degradation-of-pesticides-residue-in-vegetables-during-fermentation, accessed March 12, 2011.

28. Cecilia Jernberg et al., "Long-Term Ecological Impacts of Antibiotic Administration on the Human Intestinal Microbiota," *International Society for Microbial Ecology Journal* 1:56 (2007).

29. Michael J. Sadowsky et al., "Changes in the Composition of the Human Fecal Microbiome After Bacteriotherapy for Recurrent *Clostridium difficile*–associated Diarrhea," *Journal of Clinical Gastroenterology* 44(5):354 (2010).

30. Karen Madsen, "Probiotics and the Immune Response," *Journal of Clinical Gastroenterology* 40:232 (2006).

31. Edward L. Robinson and Walter L. Thompson, "Effect on Weight Gain of the Addition of Lactobacillus Acidophilus to the Formula of Newborn Infants," *Journal of Pediatrics* 41(4):395 (1952).

32. Irene Lenoir-Wijnkoop et al., "Probiotic and Prebiotic Influence Beyond the Intestinal Tract," *Nutrition Reviews* 65(11):469 (2007).

33. Michael de Vrese et al., "Effect of Lactobacillus gasseri PA 16/8, Bifidobacterium longum SP 07/3, B. bifidum MF 20/5 on Common Cold Episodes: A Double Blind, Randomized, Controlled Trial," *Clinical Nutrition* 24:481 (2005).

34. Heiser, C. R. et al. "Probiotics, Soluble Fiber, and L-Glutamine (GLN) Reduce Nelfinavir (NFV) or Lopinavir/Ritonavir (LPV/r)-related Diarrhea," *Journal of the International Association of Physicians in AIDS Care* 3:121 (2004).

35. Eamonn P. Culligan et al., "Probiotics and Gastrointestinal Disease: Successes, Problems and Future Prospects," *Gut Pathogens* 1:19 (2009).

36. Eamonn M. M. Quigley, "The Efficacy of Probiotics in IBS," *Journal of Clinical Gastroenterology* 42:S85 (2008).

37. Yue-Xin Yang et al., "Effect of a Fermented Milk Containing Bifidobacterium lactis DN-173010 on Chinese Constipated Women," *World Journal of Gastroenterology* 14(40):6237 (2008).

38. Joumana Saikali et al., "Fermented Milks, Probiotic Cultures, and Colon Cancer," *Nutrition and Cancer* 49(1):14 (2004).

39. Lenoir-Wijnkoop.

40. Michael de Vrese et al., "Effect of Lactobacillus gasseri PA 16/8, Bifidobacterium longum SP 07/3, B. bifidum MF 20/5 on common cold episodes," *Clinical Nutrition* 24:481 (2005); Gregory J. Leyer et al., "Probiotic Effects on Cold and Influenza-Like Symptom Incidence and Duration in Children," *Pediatrics* 124(2):e177 (2009).

41. Iva Hojsak et al., "Lactobacillus GG in the Prevention of Gastrointestinal and Respiratory Tract Infections in Children Who Attend Day Care Centers: A Randomized, Double-Blind, Placebo-Controlled Trial," *Clinical Nutrition* 29(3):312 (2010).

42. Py Tubelius et al., "Increasing Work-Place Healthiness with the Probiotic Lactobacillus reuteri: A Randomised, Double-Blind Placebo-Controlled Study," *Environmental Health: A Global Access Science Source* 4:25 (2005).

43. Stig Bengmark, "Use of Some Pre-, Pro- and Synbiotics in Critically Ill Patients," *Best Practice and Research Clinical Gastroenterology* 17(5):833 (2003); editorial, "Synbiotics to Strengthen Gut Barrier Function and Reduce Morbidity in Critically Ill Patients," Clinical Nutrition 23:441 (2004).

44. Lenoir-Wijnkoop.

45. Huey-Shi Lye et al., "The Improvement of Hypertension by Probiotics: Effects on Cholesterol, Diabetes, Renin, and Phytoestrogens," *International Journal of Molecular Science* 10:3755 (2009).

46. A. Venket Rao et al., "A Randomized, Double-Blind, Placebo-Controlled Pilot Study of a Probiotic in Emotional Symptoms of Chronic Fatigue Syndrome," *Gut Pathogens* 1:6 (2009).

47. Lívia Trois, "Use of Probiotics in HIV-Infected Children: A Randomized Double-Blind Controlled Study," *Journal of Tropical Pediatrics* 54(1):19 (2007).

48. L. Näse et al., "Effect of Long-Term Consumption of a Probiotic Bacterium, *Lactobacillus rhamnosus* GG, in Milk on Dental Caries and Caries Risks in Children," *Caries Research* 35:412 (2001).

49. Sonia Michail, "The Role of Probiotics in Allergic Diseases," *Allergy, Asthma and Clinical Immunology* 5:5 (2009).

50. D. Borchert et al., "Prevention and Treatment of Urinary Tract Infection with Probiotics: Review and Research Perspective," *Indian Journal of Urology* 24(2):139 (2008).

51. Lenoir-Wijnkoop.

52. Iva Stamatova and Jukka H. Meurman, "Probiotics and Periodontal Disease," *Periodontology 2000* 51:141 (2009).

53. Kazuhiro Hirayama and Joseph Rafter, "The Role of Probiotic Bacteria in Cancer Prevention," *Microbes and Infection* 2:681 (2000).

54. Martha I. Alvarez-Olmos and Richard A. Oberhelman, "Probiotic Agents and Infectious Diseases: A Modern Perspective on a Traditional Therapy," *Clinical Infectious Diseases* 32:1567 (2001).

55. Blaise Corthésy et al., "Cross-Talk Between Probiotic Bacteria and the Host Immune System," *Journal of Nutrition* 137:781S (2007).

56. Gerald W. Tannock, "A Special Fondness for Lactobacilli," *Applied and Environmental Microbiology* 70(6):3189 (2004).

57. Michael Wilson, 375.

58. B. M. Corcoran et al., "Survival of Probiotic Lactobacilli in Acidic Environments Is Enhanced in the Presence of Metabolizable Sugars," *Applied and Environmental Microbiology* 71(6):3060 (2005); R. D. C. S. Ranadheera et al., "Importance of Food in Probiotic Efficacy," *Food Research International* 43:1 (2010).

59. Lenoir-Wijnkoop.

60. Karen Madsen, "Probiotics and the Immune Response," *Journal of Clinical Gastroenterology* 40(3):233 (2006).

61. Michael Wilson, 398–399.

62. Mary Ellen Sanders, "Use of Probiotics and Yogurts in Maintenance of Health," *Journal of Clinical Gastroenterology* 42:S71 (2008).

63. Oskar Adolfsson et al., "Yogurt and Gut Function," *American Journal of Clinical Nutrition* 80:245 (2004).

64. Mónica Olivares, "Dietary Deprivation of Fermented Foods Causes a Fall in Innate Immune Response. Lactic Acid Bacteria Can Counteract the Immunological Effect of This Deprivation," *Journal of Dairy Research* 73:492 (2006).

65. Sorin Sonea and Léo G. Mathieu, "Evolution of the Genomic Systems of Prokaryotes and Its Momentous Consequences," *International Microbiology* 4:67 (2001).

66. Mary Ellen Sanders, "Considerations for Use of Probiotic Bacteria to Modulate Human Health," *Journal of Nutrition* 130: 384S (2000).

67. H. C. Hung et al., "Association Between Diet and Esophageal Cancer in Taiwan," *Journal of Gastroenterology and Hepatology* 19(6):632 (2004); J. M. Yuan, "Preserved Foods in Relation to Risk of Nasopharyngeal Carcinoma in Shanghai, China," *International Journal of Cancer* 85(3):358 (2000).

68. Mark A. Brudnak, "Probiotics as an Adjuvant to Detoxification Protocols," *Medical Hypotheses* 58(5):382 (2002).

69. Natasha Campbell-McBride, *Gut and Psychology Syndrome* (Cambridge, UK: Medinform Publishing, 2004).

70. Dirar, 36.

71. Andrew F. Smith, 12.

72. McGee, 58.

73. Ibid.

74. Sidney W. Mintz, "Fermented Beans and Western Taste," in Du Bois, 56.

Chapter 3

1. Clifford W. Hesseltine, "Mixed Culture Fermentations," in Gaden, 52.

2. Margulis and Sagan (1986), 91.

3. Lynn Margulis, "From Kefir to Death," in Margulis and Sagan (1997), 83–90.

4. Hesseltine, 53.

5. Pederson, 300.

6. Shurtleff and Aoyagi (1986), 143.

7. Fallon, 48.

8. www.perfectpickler.com; www.pickl-it.com.

9. S. Sabouraud et al., "Environmental Lead Poisoning from Lead-Glazed Earthenware Used for Storing Drinks," *La Revue de médecine interne* 30(12):1038 (2009).

10. www.acehardware.com.

11. Litzinger, 111.

12. Leonard Sax, "Polyethylene Terephthalate May Yield Endocrine Disruptors," *Environmental Health Perspectives* 118(4):445 (2010).

13. US Department of Health and Human Services, National Toxicology Program, Center for the Evaluation of Risks to Human Reproduction, "NTP-CERHR EXPERT PANEL UPDATE on the REPRODUCTIVE and DEVELOPMENTAL TOXICITY of DI(2-ETHYLHEXYL) PHTHALATE," NTP-CERHR-DEHP-05 (2005), online at http://ntp.niehs.nih.gov/ntp/ohat/phthalates/dehp/DEHP__Report_final.pdf, accessed June 28, 2011.

14. Christine Dell'Amore and Eliza Barclay, "Why Tap Water Is Better than Bottled Water," *National Geographic's Green Guide*, online at http://environment.nationalgeographic.com/environment/green-guide/bottled-water, accessed June 28, 2011.

15. www.lehmans.com.

16. Litzinger, 119.

17. James B. Richardson III, "The Pre-Columbian Distribution of the Bottle Gourd (*Lagenaria siceraria*): A Re-Evaluation," *Economic Botany* 26(3):265 (1972).

18. Bruman, 49.

19. Tamang, 28–29.

20. Slow Food Foundation for Biodiversity, "Pit Cabbage," online at http://www.slowfoodfoundation.com/pagine/eng/presidi/dettaglio_presidi.lasso?-id=420, accessed June 12, 2011.

21. Anna Kowalska-Lewicka, "The Pickling of Vegetables in Traditional Polish Peasant Culture," in Riddervold and Ropeid, 34.

22. Battcock and Azam-Ali, 53.

23. Steinkraus, 309.

24. www.krautpounder.com.

25. World Wildlife Federation, "Cork Screwed? Environmental and Economic Impacts of the Cork Stoppers Market," May 2006, online at http://assets.panda.org/downloads/cork_rev12_print.pdf, accessed January 1, 2011.

26. The "Yet Another Temperature Controller" (YATC) costs $80 assembled or $60 as a kit at http://store.holyscraphotsprings.com.

Chapter 4

1. McGovern, xi.

2. Kari Poikolainen, "Alcohol and Mortality: A Review," *Journal of Clinical Epidemiology* 48(4):455 (1995).

3. Buhner, 71n.

4. Cited in McGovern, 110.

5. Phaff, 136.

6. Ibid., 178–179.

7. Ibid., 84.

8. Erlend Aa et al., "Population Structure and Gene Evolution in Saccharomyces cerevisiae," FEMS Yeast Research 6:702 (2006).

9. Phaff, 200–202.

10. Ibid., 211.

11. Ann Vaughan-Martini and Alessandro Martini, "Facts, Myths and Legends on the Prime Industrial Microorganism," *Journal of Industrial Microbiology* 14:514 (1995).

12. Stephanie Diezmann and Fred S. Dietrich, "*Saccharomyces cerevisiae*: Population Divergence and Resistance to Oxidative Stress in Clinical, Domesticated, and Wild Isolates," *PLoS ONE* 4(4):e5317 (2009), online at www.plosone.org/article/info%3Adoi%2F10.1371%2Fjournal.pone.0005317, accessed July 5, 2011.

13. Sung-Oui Suh et al., "The Beetle Gut: A Hyperdiverse Source of Novel Yeasts," *Mycological Research* 109(3):261 (2005).

14. Justin C. Fay and Joseph A. Benavides, "Evidence for Domesticated and Wild Populations of *Saccharomyces cerevisiae*," *PLoS Genetics* 1(1):e5 (2005), online at www.plosgenetics.org/article/info%3Adoi%2F10.1371%2Fjournal.pgen.0010005, accessed July 5, 2011.

15. Phaff, 144.

16. J. W. White Jr. and Landis W. Doner, "Honey Composition and Properties," in *Beekeeping in the United States* (USDA Agriculture Handbook Number 335, 1980), online at www.beesource.com/resources/usda/honey-composition-and-properties, accessed December 7, 2009.

17. Steinkraus, 366.

18. Ibid., 367.

19. Litzinger, 44.

20. S. Sekar and S. Mariappan, "Traditionally Fermented Biomedicines, *Arishtas* and *Asavas* from Ayurveda," *Indian Journal of Traditional Knowledge* 7(4):548 (2008).

21. Ibid.

22. McGovern, 82.

23. Ibid., 182.

24. Standage, 75.

25. Nicholas Wade, "Lack of Sex Among Grapes Tangles a Family Vine," *New York Times* (January 24, 2011), online at www.nytimes.com/2011/01/25/science/25wine.html, accessed January 25, 2011.

26. Bruman, 33.

27. Baron, 16.

28. "Whizky, World's First Bio Whisky Aged with Granny Whiz," *Independent* (September 4, 2010), online at www.independent.co.uk/life-style/food-and-drink/whizky-worlds-first-bio-whisky-aged-with-granny-whiz-2070491.html, accessed September 6, 2010.

29. Steinkraus, 376.

30. McGovern, 260.

31. Battcock and Azam-Ali, 37.

32. Bruman, 90.

33. Battcock and Azam-Ali, 38–39.

34. Ibid., 40.

35. Bennett and Zing, 47.

36. Bruman, 69.

37. Litzinger, 32

38. Kennedy (2000), 448.

39. Bruman, 12–30; Litzinger, 28.

40. Anna Kowalska-Lewicka, "The Pickling of Vegetables in Traditional Polish Peasant Culture," in Riddervold and Ropeid, 36.

41. Bruman, 8.

42. McGovern et al. (2004).

Chapter 5

1. Personal correspondence, February 19, 2010.

2. M. A. Daeschel, R. E. Andersson, and H. P. Fleming, "Microbial Ecology of Fermenting Plant Materials," *FEMS Microbiology Reviews* 46:358 (1987).

3. Gerald W. Tannock, "A Special Fondness for Lactobacilli," *Applied and Environmental Microbiology* 70(6):3189 (2004).

4. Fred Breidt Jr., "Safety of Minimally Processed, Acidified, and Fermented Vegetable Products," in Sapers, 314–319.

5. J. R. Stamer et al., "Fermentation Patterns of Poorly Fermenting Cabbage Hybrids," *Applied Microbiology* 18(3):325 (1969).

6. Battcock and Azam-Ali, 43.

7. Erika A. Pfeiler and Todd R. Klaenhammer, "The Genomics of Lactic Acid Bacteria," *Trends in Microbiology* 15(12):546 (2007).

8. Cited by H. L. Wang and S. F. Fang, "History of Chinese Fermented Foods," in Hesseltine and Wang, 34.

9. C. S. Pederson et al., "Vitamin C Content of Sauerkraut," *Journal of Food Science* 4(1):44 (1939).

10. Fred Breidt Jr., "Processed, Acidified, and Fermented Vegetable Products," in Sapers, 318.

11. C. S. Pederson and M. N. Albury, "Control of Fermentation," in Steinkraus, 118–119.

12. Phaff, 229.

13. Nancy Russell, "Many Kitchen Tools No Longer Needed," *Columbia (MO) Daily Tribune* (July 14, 2011), online at www.columbiatribune.com/news/2011/jul/14/many-kitchen-tools-no-longer-needed, accessed August 10, 2011.

14. Mei Chin, "The Art of Kimchi," *Saveur* 124:76 (2009).

15. Mark McDonald, "Rising Cost of Kimchi Alarms Koreans," *New York Times* (October 14, 2010), online at www.nytimes.com/2010/10/15/world/asia/15kimchi.html, accessed October 16, 2010.

16. Choe Sang-Hun "Starship Kimchi: A Bold Taste Goes Where It Has Never Gone Before," *New York Times* (February 24, 2008), online at www.nytimes.com/2008/02/24/world/asia/24kimchi.html, accessed April 25, 2010.

17. David Chazan, "Korean Dish 'May Cure Bird Flu,'" BBC News (March 14, 2005), online at http://news.bbc
.co.uk/2/hi/asia-pacific/4347443.stm, accessed April 25, 2010.

18. Hepinstall, 95.

19. Mei Chin, "The Art of Kimchi," *Saveur* 124:76 (2009).

20. T. I. Mheen et al., "Korean Kimchi and Related Vegetable Fermentations," in Steinkraus, 131.

21. Man-Jo et al., 36.

22. T. I. Mheen et al., "Traditional Fermented Food Products in Korea," in Hesseltine and Wang, 112.

23. P. P. W. Wong and H. Jackson, "Chinese Hum Choy" in Steinkraus, 135.

24. Dunlop (2003), 64–65.

25. Fuchsia Dunlop, "Rotten Vegetable Stalks, Stinking Beancurd and Other Shaoxing Delicacies," paper delivered at 2010 Oxford Symposium on Food and Cookery.

26. "Indian Cooking with Mustard Oil," IndianCurry.com, online at www.indiacurry.com/spice
/mustardoilcooking.htm, accessed July 24, 2011.

27. www.friedsig.wordpress.com.

28. Tamang, 25–31.

29. Volokh, 421.

30. P. Kendall and C. Schultz, "Making Pickles," Colorado State University Extension website, online at www.ext.colostate.edu/pubs/foodnut/09304.html, accessed June 30, 2010.

31. Lilija Radeva, "Traditional Methods of Food Preserving Among the Bulgarians," in Riddervold and Ropeid, 40–41.

32. Ivan D. Jones, "Salting of Cucumbers: Influence of Brine Salinity on Acid Formation," *Industrial and Engineering Chemistry* 32:858 (1940).

33. Anna Kowalska-Lewicka, "The Pickling of Vegetables in Traditional Polish Peasant Culture," in Riddervold and Ropeid, 37.

34. Wood, 90.

35. Spargo, 90.

36. McGee, 293.

37. Frederick Breidt Jr. et al., "Fermented Vegetables," in Doyle and Beuchat, 784.

38. Ibid.

39. Kowalska-Lewicka, 36.

40. Volokh, 429–430.

41. "Personal Explanation About Fermenting Wild Foods" by Ossi Kakko (aka Orava Ituparta), summer 2006.

42. Personal correspondence, September 29, 2009.

43. Hyun-Soo Kim et al., "Characterization of a Chitinolytic Enzyme from Serratia sp. KCK Isolated from Kimchi Juice," *Applied Microbiology and Biotechnology* 75:1275 (2007).

44. Hank Shaw, "How to Cure Green Olives," October 11, 2009, posting on his blog *Hunter Angler Gardener Cook: Finding the Forgotten Feast*, online at www.honest-food.net/blog1/2009/10/11/how-to-cure-green-olives/#more-2593, accessed October 28, 2009.

45. Kaufmann and Schöneck, 16–17.

46. Irvin E. Liener, "Toxic Factors in Edible Legumes and Their Elimination," *American Journal of Clinical Nutrition* 11:281 (1962).

47. James A. Duke, *Handbook of Energy Crops* (1983), citing M. Haidvogl et al., "Poisoning by Raw Garden Beans (*Phaseolus vulgaris* and *Phaseolus coccineus*) in Children," *Padiatrie and Padologi* 14:293 (1979), published online by Purdue University, online at www.hort.purdue.edu/newcrop/duke_energy/Phaseolus_vulgaris.html, accessed June 12, 2011.

48. For a more detailed discussion of fruit kimchi, see *Wild Fermentation*, 50.

49. Madhur Jaffrey, *World Vegetarian* (New York: Clarkson Potter, 1999), 689.

50. Fallon, 109.

51. Kushi, 37.

52. Radeva, 39.

53. Volokh, 433.

54. Dirar, 412–413.

55. Ibid., 417.

56. Ibid., 433.

57. H. P. Fleming and R. F. McFeeters, "Use of Microbial Cultures: Vegetable Products," *Food Technology* 35(1):84 (1981).

58. Suzanne Johanningsmeier et al., "Effects of *Leuconostoc mesenteroides* Starter Culture on Fermentation of Cabbage with Reduced Salt Concentrations," *Journal of Food Science* 72(5):M166 (2007).

59. Battcock and Azam-Ali, 50.

60. http://users.sa.chariot.net.au/~dna/kefirkraut.html, accessed May 10, 2010.

61. http://www.caldwellbiofermentation.com, accessed February 13, 2010.

62. Arnaud Schreyer et al., "Culture Starters: Study and Comparison," Caldwell Bio-Fermentation Canada, Inc., and Agriculture and Agri-Food Canada, 2009.

63. Rombauer and Becker (1975), 43.

64. Fallon, 610.

65. Alexandra Grigorieva, "Pickled Lettuce: A Forgotten Chapter of East European Jewish Food History," unpublished paper, 2010.

66. Alexandra Grigorieva and Gail Singer, "A Pickletime Memoir: Salt and Vinegar from the Jews of Eastern Europe to the Prairies of Canada," paper delivered at 2010 Oxford Symposium on Food and Cookery.

67. Konlee, 40.

68. Andoh, 220–221.

69. Ibid., 214.

70. Ibid., 216.

71. Ibid., 217–218.

72. Dragonlife, "Takuan/Japanese Pickled Daikon: Basic Recipe," *Shizuoka Gourmet* blog, online at http://shizuokagourmet.wordpress.com/2010/01/27/takuanjapanese-pickled-daikon-basic-recipe, accessed December 2, 2010.

73. "Lephet, A Unique Myanmar Delicacy," www.myanmar.com, accessed May 22, 2010, no longer posted online as of June 14, 2011.

74. "Laphet, a Burmese Tea Snack," *In Pursuit of Tea, Travel Diary* (2002), online at www.inpursuitoftea.com/category_s/91.htm, accessed May 22, 2010.

75. Brian J. B. Wood, 54.

76. Jay, 180.

77. E. B. Fred and W. H. Peterson, "The Production of Pink Sauerkraut by Yeasts," *Journal of Bacteriology* 7(2):258 (1921).

78. Steinkraus, 125.

Chapter 6

1. A. M. Morad et al., "Gas-Liquid Chromatographic Determination of Ethanol in 'Alcohol-Free' Beverages and Fruit Juices," *Chromatographia* 13(3):161 (1980); Bruce A. Goldberger et al., "Unsuspected Ethanol Ingestion Through Soft Drinks and Flavored Beverages," *Journal of Analytical Toxicology* 20:332 (1996); Barry K. Logan and Sandra Distefano, "Ethanol Content of Various Foods and Soft Drinks and Their Potential for Interference with a Breath-Alcohol Test," *Journal of Analytical Toxicology* 22:181 (1998).

2. Toomre, 468.

3. Online at http://riowang.blogspot.com/2008/07/great-patriotic-war.html, accessed June 15, 2010.

4. See *Wild Fermentation*, 121.

5. Battcock and Azam-Ali, 35.

6. Gabriele Volpato and Daimy Godínez, "Ethnobotany of Pru, a Traditional Cuban Refreshment," *Economic Botany* 58(3):387 (2004).

7. "Making Mauby," *Tastes Like Home* blog (January 26, 2007), online at www.tasteslikehome.org/2007/01/making-mauby.html, accessed November 16, 2010.

8. M. Pidoux, "The Microbial Flora of Sugary Kefir Grain (the Gingerbeer Plant): Biosynthesis of the Grain from *Lactobacillus hilgardii* Producing a Polysaccharide Gel," *World Journal of Microbiology and Biotechnology* 5(2):223 (1989).

9. http://users.sa.chariot.net.au/~dna/kefirpage.html.

10. Litzinger, 4.

11. A. W. Bennett, ed., *Journal of the Royal Microscopical Society* (1900), p. 373, online at http://books.google.com/books?id=0ewBAAAAYAAJ, accessed May 2010.

12. Phaff, 244–245.

13. H. Marshall Ward, "The Ginger-Beer Plant, and the Organisms Composing It: A Contribution to the Study of Fermentation Yeasts and Bacteria," *Philosophical Transactions of the Royal Society of London* 83:125–197 (1892).

14. Dirar, 292.

15. Ibid., 296.

16. Ibid., 293.

17. Volpato and Godínez, 386.

18. Ibid., 390.

19. Luke Regalbuto and Maggie Levinger, "Smreka! A Fermented Juniper Berry Drink from Bosnia," online at www.regalbuto.net/Travels/?p=51, accessed May 19, 2010.

20. Anna R. Dixon et al., "Ferment This: The Transformation of Noni, a Traditional Polynesian Medicine," *Economic Botany* 53(1):56 (1999).

21. Dixon et al., 51; Will McClatchey, "From Polynesian Healers to Health Food Stores: Changing Perspectives of *Morinda citrifolia*," *Integrative Cancer Therapies* 1(2):110 (2002).

22. Dixon et al., 57.

23. www.ctahr.hawaii.edu/noni, accessed April 7, 2011.

24. Dixon et al., 58.

25. Hobbs, 15.

26. Malia Wollan, "A Strange Brew May Be a New Thing," *New York Times* (March 24, 2010), online at: http://www.nytimes.com/2010/03/25/fashion/25Tea.html, accessed June 28, 2010.

27. Meredith Melnick, "Fermentation Frenzy," *Newsweek* (July 13, 2010), online at http://www.thedailybeast .com/newsweek/2010/07/13/fermentation-frenzy.html, accessed July 14, 2010.

28. Tietze, 40.

29. Hobbs, 3.

30. Ibid., 10.

31. Günther W. Frank, "Kombucha Tea: What's All the Hoopla?" online at www.kombu.de, accessed July 14, 2010.

32. Michael R. Roussin, "Analyses of Kombucha Ferments" (Information Resources: 1996-2003), 1, online at www.kombucha-research.com, accessed July 13, 2010.

33. Roussin, 80.

34. Centers for Disease Control and Prevention, "Unexplained Severe Illness Possibly Associated with Consumption of Kombucha Tea—Iowa, 1995," *Morbidity and Mortality Weekly Report* 44(48):892 (1995).

35. Alison S. Kole et al., "A Case of Kombucha Tea Toxicity," *Chest* 134(4):c9001 (2008); A. D. Perron et al., "Kombucha 'Mushroom' Hepatotoxicity [letter]," *Annals of Emergency Medicine* 26:660 (1995); Chris T. Derk et al., "A Case of Anti-Jo1 Myositis with Pleural Effusions and Pericardial Tamponade Developing After Exposure to a Fermented Kombucha Beverage," *Clinical Rheumatology* 23:355 (2004); J. Sadjadi, "Cutaneous Anthrax Associated with the Kombucha 'Mushroom' in Iran," *Journal of the American Medical Association* 280:1567 (1998).

36. "FDA Cautions Consumers on 'Kombucha Mushroom Tea,'" US Food and Drug Administration Press Release T95-15 (March 23, 1995).

37. Paul Stamets, "My Adventures with 'The Blob,'" *Mushroom, The Journal* (winter 1994–1995), online at www.fungi.com/info/articles/blob.html, accessed July 15, 2010.

38. Jasmin Malik Chua, "BioCouture: UK Designer 'Grows' an Entire Wardrobe from Bacteria," online at www.ecouterre.com/20103/u-k-designer-grows-an-entire-wardrobe-from-tea-fermenting-bacteria, accessed July 22, 2010.

39. Hobbs, 27.

40. Roussin, 22.

41. See note 1 in this chapter.

42. US Alcohol and Tobacco Tax and Trade Bureau, "TTB Guidance: Kombucha Products Containing at Least 0.5 Percent Alcohol by Volume Are Alcohol Beverages," TTB G 2010–3 (June 23, 2010), online at www.ttb.gov/pdf/kombucha.pdf, accessed July 22, 2010.

43. Stamets (1994–1995).

44. Diggs, 92.

45. Ibid., 111-112.

46. Ibid., 118.

47. Ibid., 113.

48. See *Wild Fermentation*, 154.

Chapter 7

1. John Kariuki, "On the Hunt for Traditional Foods in Kenya," Terra Madre website, online at www
   .terramadre.org/pagine/leggi.lasso?id=3E6E345B0ca612CDC5mJT14C3621&ln=en, accessed August 17,
   2010.

2. "Ash Yogurt in Gourds . . . From a Kenyan Community of Herders and Producers," *Slow Food Newslet-
   ter* (September 2009), online at http://newsletter.slowfood.com/slowfood_time/12/eng.html#itemD,
   accessed August 17, 2010.

3. M. Kroger et al., "Fermented Milks—Past, Present, and Future," in Gaden, 62–63.

4. Sara Feresu, "Fermented Milk Products in Zimbabwe," in ibid., 80.

5. Ibid., 82.

6. Ibid., 84.

7. Ibid.

8. Joel Schroeter and Todd Klaenhammer, "Genomics of Lactic Acid Bacteria," *Federation of European
   Microbiological Societies [FEMS] Microbiology Letters* 292(1):1 (2008).

9. McGee, 45.

10. Albala and Nafzifer, 157.

11. Miloslav Kaláb, "Foods Under the Microscope," online at www.magma.ca/~pavel/science/Yogurt.htm,
    accessed August 3, 2010.

12. Kosikowski and Mistry, 92.

13. Excerpted with permission from Aylin Öney Tan, "From Soup to Dessert: Yoghurt—Not Only Fer-
    mented, But Cured, Preserved, Dried, Smoked—An Ingredient of Vast Variety Indispensible in the
    Turkish Kitchen," paper presented at the Oxford Symposium on Food and Cookery (2010).

14. For recipes, see *Wild Fermentation*, 77.

15. See ibid.

16. Tan.

17. "Our Heritage," Dannon Company website, online at www.dannon.com/pages/rt_aboutdannon
    _oheritage.html, accessed August 1, 2010.

18. William Grimes, "Daniel Carasso, a Pioneer of Yogurt, Dies at 103," *New York Times* (May 20,
    2009), online at www.nytimes.com/2009/05/21/business/21carasso.html?scp=1&sq=Daniel%20
    Carasso&st=cse, accessed August 1, 2010.

19. I purchased my heirloom yogurt cultures from www.culturesforhealth.com.

20. www.culturalfermentation.wordpress.com.

21. Personal correspondence, September 3, 2010.

22. Personal correspondence with Jim Wallace, September 9, 2010.

23. T.-H. Chen et al., "Microbiological and Chemical Properties of Kefir Manufactured by Entrapped Micro-
    organisms Isolated from Kefir Grains," *Journal of Dairy Science* 92:3002 (2009).

24. Lynn Margulis, "From Kefir to Death," in Margulis and Sagan (1997), 73-74.

25. Ibid., 73.

26. A group of Argentine investigators experimented with different kefir grain:milk ratios and found pronounced differences in resulting kefir. One percent inoculation resulted in a "viscous and not very acid" product while 10 percent "gave an acid beverage with low viscosity and a more effervescent taste." Graciela L. Garrote et al., "Characteristics of Kefir Prepared with Different Grain:Milk Ratios," *Journal of Dairy Research* 65:149 (1998).

27. http://users.sa.chariot.net.au/~dna/kefirpage.html, accessed March 3, 2010.

28. You can find detailed descriptions of methods for this on Dominic Anfiteatro's comprehensive kefir website, cited directly above.

29. Taketsugu Saita et al., "Production Process for Kefir-Like Fermented Milk," US Patent 5,055,309 (1991).

30. Chen, 3003.

31. Ibid.

32. Edward R. Farnworth, "Kefir—A Complex Probiotic," *Food Science and Technology Bulletin: Functional Foods* 2(1):1 (2005).

33. www.gemcultures.com.

34. McGovern, 123.

35. William de Rubriquis, 1253, cited in Huang, 249.

36. Rombauer and Becker (1953), 818.

37. See *Wild Fermentation*, 79.

38. Dirar, 304.

39. Ibid., 319.

40. Ibid., 319.

41. http://live2cook.wordpress.com/2008/08/22/the-secret-of-making-soy-yogurt-without-store-bought-culture, accessed August 4, 2010.

42. Tan, 3.

43. Lilija Radeva, "Traditional Methods of Food Preserving Among the Bulgarians," in Riddervold and Ropeid, 42.

44. Kjell Furuset, "The Role of Butterwort (*Pinguicula vulgaris*) in 'Tettemelk,'" *Blyttia* (Journal of the Norwegian Botanical Society) 66:55 (2008).

45. Maria Salomé S. Pais, "The Cheese Those Romans Already Used to Eat: From Tradition to Molecular Biology and Plant Biotechnology," Memórias da Academia das Ciências de Lisboa, Classe de Ciências (2002), online at www.acad-ciencias.pt/files/Memórias/Salomé%20Pa%C3%ADs/cheese.pdf, accessed August 20, 2010.

46. Grieve, 579.

47. Trudy Eden, "The Art of Preserving: How Cooks in Colonial Virginia Imitated Nature to Control It," *Eighteenth-Century Life* 23(2):19.

48. United Nations Food and Agriculture Organization, *The Technology of Traditional Milk Products in Developing Countries* (FAO Animal Production and Health Paper 85, 1990), online at www.fao.org/docrep/003/t0251e/T0251E00.htm, accessed August 20, 2010.

49. See *Wild Fermentation*, 83.

50. Kindstedt, 37.

51. Bronwen Percival and Randolph Hodgson, "Artisanship and Control: Farmhouse Cheddar Comes of Age," paper delivered at 2010 Oxford Symposium on Food and Cookery.

52. Kindstedt, 29–30.

53. Ibid., 32.

54. Ken Albala, "Bacterial Fermentation and the Missing Terroir Factor in Historic Cookery," paper delivered at 2010 Oxford Symposium on Food and Cookery.

55. Heather Paxson, "Post-Pasteurian Cultures: The Microbiopolitics of Raw-Milk Cheese in the United States," *Current Anthropology* 23(1):15 (2008).

56. Marcellino, 21.

Chapter 8

1. FAOSTAT 2008 data, accessed August 12, 2010.

2. Standage, 39.

3. Joseph A. Maga, "Phytate: Its Chemistry, Occurrence, Food Interactions, Nutritional Significance, and Methods of Analysis," *Journal of Agricultural and Food Chemistry* 30(1):1 (1982).

4. Fallon, 452.

5. N. R. Reddy and M. D. Pierson, "Reduction in Antinutritional and Toxic Components in Plant Foods by Fermentation," *Food Research International* 27(3):217 (1994).

6. Haard, 19–20.

7. Solomon H. Katz, M. L. Hediger, and L. A. Valleroy, "Traditional Maize Processing Techniques in the New World," *Science* 184 (1974).

8. Coe, 136.

9. L. Nuraida et al., "Microbiology of Pozol, a Mexican Fermented Maize Dough," *World Journal of Microbiology and Biotechnology* 11:567 (1995).

10. Rodolfo Quintero-Ramirez et al., "Cereal Fermentation in Latin American Countries," in Haard, 105.

11. Pagden, 66.

12. Coe, 118.

13. Ibid., 138.

14. Ulloa and Herrera, 164; Bruman, 43.

15. "Recipe—Aluá," *Flavors of Brazil* blog (October 14, 2010), online at http://flavorsofbrazil.blogspot.com /2010/10/recipe-alua.html, accessed March 5, 2011.

16. See *Wild Fermentation*, 112.

17. Cushing, 294.

18. Dabney, 335.

19. Mollison, 52

20. From his website www.tallyrand.info.

21. Steinkraus, 212–213.

22. S. A. Odunfa, "Cereal Fermentation in African Countries," in Haard, 37–39.

23. Ibid., 40.

24. Awiakta, 18–19.

25. Excerpted from *Simply Seeking Sustenance*, online at www.sacred-threads.com/wp-content/uploads /2008/12/simply-seeking.pdf.

26. Pitchford, 458.

27. Editorial, "Energy Content of Weaning Foods," *Journal of Tropical Pediatrics* 29(4):194 (1983).

28. Ulf Svanberg, "Lactic Acid Fermented Foods for Feeding Infants," in Steinkraus, 311–347; Patience Mensah et al., "Fermented Cereal Gruels: Towards a Solution of the Weanling's Dilemma," *Food and Nutrition Bulletin* 13(1) (March 1991), online at archive.unu.edu/Unupress/food/8F131e/8F131E08 .htm, accessed August 26, 2010.

29. Claude Aubert, *Les Aliments Fermentés Traditionnels*, cited in Fallon, 457.

30. McNeill, 202.

31. Kennedy (2010), 428.

32. Ibid., 337.

33. Dirar, 117.

34. Ibid., 169.

35. Pitchford, 478.

36. Ibid., 477.

37. In Swedish, http://porridgehunters.wordpress.com.

38. Cited in O. N. Allen and Ethel K. Allen, *The Manufacture of Poi from Taro in Hawaii: With Special Emphasis upon Its Fermentation* (Honolulu: University of Hawaii, 1933) (Bulletin; B-070), 5; online at http://scholarspace.manoa.hawaii.edu/handle/10125/13437, accessed September 30, 2010.

39. Allen and Allen, 3.

40. Sky Barnhart, "Powered by Poi: Kalo, a Legendary Plant, Has Deep Roots in Hawaiian Culture," *Maui Magazine* (July–August-2007), online at www.mauimagazine.net/Maui-Magazine/July-August-2007 /Powered-by-Poi, accessed September 29, 2010.

41. Allen and Allen, 29.

42. Amy C. Brown and Ana Valiere, "The Medicinal Uses of Poi," *Nutrition in Clinical Care* 7(2):69 (2004).

43. Amy C. Brown et al., "The Anti-Cancer Effects of Poi (*Colocasia esculenta*) on Colonic Adenocarcinoma Cells in Vitro," *Phytotherapy* 19(9):767–771 (September 2005).

44. Ramesh C. Ray and Paramasivan S. Sivakumar, "Traditional and Novel Fermented Foods and Beverages from Tropical Root and Tuber Crops," *International Journal of Food Science and Technology* 44:1075 (2009).

45. Kofi E. Aidoo, "Lesser-Known Fermented Plant Foods," in Gaden, 38.

46. Ray and Sivakumar, 1079.

47. Bokanga, 179.

48. Fran Osseo-Asare, "Chart of African Carbohydrates/Starches" (September 2007), online at http:// betumiblog.blogspot.com/2007/09/chart-of-african-carbohydratesstarches.html, accessed October 3, 2010; "Table 3. Fermented Foods from Tropical Root and Tuber Crops, Microorganisms Associated and Advantages Arising Out of Fermentation," Ray and Sivakumar, 1080.

49. O. B. Oyewole and S. L. Ogundele, "Effect of Length of Fermentation on the Functional Characteristics of Fermented Cassava 'Fufu,'" *Journal of Food Technology in Africa* 6(2):38 (2001).

50. Ray and Sivakumar, 1078–1079.

51. "Slow Food Presidia in Peru," online at www.slowfood.com/sloweb/eng/dettaglio.lasso?cod=3E6E345B1 dcfb174DBotN395D956, accessed January 2, 2011.

52. Mollison, 81.

53. www.nourishedkitchen.com.

54. P. Christian Klieger, *The Fleischmann Yeast Family* (Mount Pleasant, SC: Arcadia Publishing, 2004), 13.

55. A. M. Hamad and M. L. Fields, "Evaluation of the Protein Quality and Available Lysine of Germinated and Fermented Cereals," *Journal of Food Science* 44:456 (1979).

56. Carlo G. Rizzello et al., "Highly Efficient Gluten Degradation by Lactobacilli and Fungal Proteases During Food Processing: New Perspectives for Celiac Disease," *Applied and Environmental Microbiology* 73(14): 4499 (2007); Maria De Angelis et al., "Mechanism of Degradation of Immunogenic Gluten Epitopes from Triticum turgidum L. var. durum by Sourdough Lactobacilli and Fungal Proteases," *Applied and Environmental Microbiology* 76(2): 508 (2010).

57. Pederson, 242–243.

58. Jessica A. Lee, "Yeast Are People Too: Sourdough Fermentation from the Microbe's Point of View," paper delivered at 2010 Oxford Symposium on Food and Cookery.

59. www.sourdo.com.

60. Leader, 44–45.

61. Ibid., 45.

62. Ilse Scheirlinck et al., "Influence of Geographical Origin and Flour Type on Diversity of Lactic Acid Bacteria in Traditional Belgian Sourdoughs," *Applied and Environmental Microbiology* 73(19):6268 (2007).

63. Ilse Scheirlinck et al., "Taxonomic Structure and Stability of the Bacterial Community in Belgian Sourdough Ecosystems as Assessed by Culture and Population Fingerprinting," *Applied and Environmental Microbiology* 74(8):2414 (2008).

64. Lee, 3.

65. Steinkraus, 202.

66. *Gastronomica: The Journal of Food and Culture* 3(3):76–79 (summer 2003).

67. See *Wild Fermentation*, 105.

68. Albala (2008), 78.

69. Dirar, 173.

70. Anna Kowalska-Lewicka, "The Pickling of Vegetables in Traditional Polish Peasant Culture," in Riddervold and Ropeid, 35.

71. Ibid., 36.

72. Ibid., 35.

73. Andre G. van Veen and Keith Steinkraus, "Nutritive Value and Wholesomeness of Fermented Foods," *Journal of Agricultural and Food Chemistry* 18(4):576 (1970).

74. Herbert C. Herzfeld, "Rice Fermentation in Ecuador," *Economic Botany* 11(3):269 (1957).

75. Hunter, 234.

76. Herzfeld.

77. Ibid.

78. See *Wild Fermentation*, 78, for the recipe.

79. www.slowfoodfoundation.com/eng/presidi/dettaglio.lasso?cod=320, accessed November 6, 2009.

Chapter 9

1. McGee, 743.

2. McGovern, 255.

3. McGee, 739.

4. Sparrow, 37.

5. Buhner, 76–77.

6. Sparrow, 45.

7. Ibid., 155.

8. "Our Story: Brewing with Mystic Intentions," online at www.mystic-brewery.com/story, accessed December 12, 2010.

9. Sparrow, 4.

10. theperfectpint.com.

11. Michael Agnew, *Wild Beers* blog (February 11, 2010), online at www.aperfectpint.net/blog.php/?p=914, accessed February 16, 2010.

12. Peter Bouckaert, foreword, Sparrow, x.

13. Sparrow, 99.

14. John G. Kennedy, "Tesguino Complex: The Role of Beer in Tarahumara Culture," *American Anthropologist*, New Series 65(3), Part 1:620 (1963)

15. Litzinger, 103.

16. Ibid., 111.

17. Bennett and Zingg, cited in Bruman, 42.

18. Bruman, 41.

19. Steinkraus, 417.

20. Bennett and Zing, 46.

21. John Smalley and Michael Blake, "Sweet Beginnings: Stalk Sugar and the Domestication of Maize," *Current Anthropology* 44(5):675 (2003).

22. United Nations Food and Agriculture Organization, "Sorghum and Millets in Human Nutrition" (Rome: Food and Nutrition Series No. 27, 1995), online at www.fao.org/docrep/T0818E/T0818E00.htm, accessed November 30, 2010.

23. McGovern, 256.

24. Papazian, 202.

25. L. Novellie, "Sorghum Beer and Related Fermentations of Southern Africa," in Hesseltine and Wang, 220.

26. Steinkraus, 409.

27. Papazian, 202.

28. Haggblade, 28.

29. Haggblade, 20; citing International Labour Office, "Employment, Incomes, and Equality: A Strategy for Increasing Productive Employment in Kenya" (Geneva: 1972), 69.

30. Cited in Tsimako, 4.

31. Haggblade, 77.

32. Ibid., 34.

33. Trout Montague, "Chibuku—'Shake Shake,'" BBC (April 15, 2003), online at www.bbc.co.uk/dna/h2g2/A965036, accessed October 24, 2009.

34. Haggblade, 264.

35. Dirar, 224.

36. Ibid., 233.

37. Ibid., 225.

38. Ibid., 227.

39. Ibid., 251.

40. Ibid., 251.

41. Ibid., 228.

42. Ibid., 264.

43. Ibid., 228.

44. Ibid., 264.

45. Ibid., 229.

46. Ibid., 228.

47. Haard, 67.

48. McGovern, 70.

49. Xu Gan Rong and Bao Tong Fa, *Grandiose Survey of Chinese Alcoholic Drinks and Beverages*, online at www.sytu.edu.cn/zhgjiu/umain.htm, accessed July 12, 2011.

50. Dr. S. Sekar, "Rice and Other Cereal-Based Beverages," in *Database on Microbial Traditional Knowledge of India*, online at http://www.bdu.ac.in/schools/life_sciences/biotechnology/sekardb.htm, accessed December 5, 2010.

51. yclept, "Homemade Chinese Rice Wine" (March 8, 1004), online at http://everything2.com/title/rice+wine, accessed December 18, 2010.

52. "Jiu Niang (Sweet Rice Wine Soup)," *Lau Lau's Recipes: A Memorial to Grandma Chou* blog (February 18, 2008), online at http://laulausrecipes.com/?p=8, accessed July 12, 2011.

53. www.hmart.com.

54. http://seoulkitchen.wordpress.com/2010/02/04/homemade-sweet-potato-makgeolli, accessed February 17, 1011.

55. Tamang, 203.

56. John Gauntner, "History of Yeast in Japan," online at www.sake-world.com/html/yeast.html, accessed July 13, 2011.

57. Gaunter.

58. David Buschena et al., *Changing Structures in the Barley Production and Malting Industries of the United States and Canada* (Bozeman: Montana State University Trade Research Center, Policy Issues Paper No. 8, 1998), 7, online at http://ageconsearch.umn.edu/bitstream/29168/1/pip08.pdf, accessed December 4, 2010.

59. Janson, 41.

60. Bamforth (2006), 33.

61. Ibid., 32.

62. Ibid., 36.

63. William Starr Moake, "Make Your Own Malt," *Brew Your Own* (1997), online at http://byo.com/stories/article/indices/44-malt/1097-make-your-own-malt, accessed October 19, 2009.

64. Bamforth (2008), 86.

65. Dirar, 224.

66. Priscilla Mary Işin, "Boza, Innocuous and Less So," paper delivered at 2010 Oxford Symposium on Food and Cookery.

67. Rhoades and Bidegaray, 58–59.

68. Terry W. Henkel, "Parakari, an Indigenous Fermented Beverage Using Amylolytic Rhizopus in Guyana," *Mycologia* 97(1):1 (2005).

69. Eames, 2.

70. Grahn, 113.

71. Eames, 35.

72. Karl-Ernst Behre, "The History of Beer Additives in Europe—A Review," *Vegetation History and Archaeobotany* 8:35 (1999).

73. Buhner, 169.

74. Weinert, 33.

75. Ibid., 34.

76. Pendell, 54.

77. Weinert, 38–39.

78. Ibid., 43.

79. Ibid., 50.

80. Buhner, 172.

81. Ibid., 173.

82. Pendell, 66.

83. Buhner, 172.

84. Ibid., 172.

Chapter 10

1. Shurtleff and Aoyagi (2007).

2. Huang, 154–155.

3. Ibid., 280.

4. Ibid., 167.

5. Shurtleff and Aoyagi (2007).

6. Huang, 593.

7. Ibid., 608.

8. Tetsuo Kobayashi et al., "Genomics of *Aspergillus oryzae*," *Bioscience, Biotechnology, and Biochemistry* 71(3):662 (2007).

9. Steinkraus, 480.

10. C. W. Hesseltine, "A Millennium of Fungi, Food, and Fermentation," *Mycologia* 57(2):150 (1965).

11. http://users.soe.ucsc.edu/~manfred/tempeh.

12. The Agricultural Research Service Culture Collection, also known as the Northern Regional Research Laboratory (NRRL) collection, maintains samples of 95,000 bacteria, yeasts, and molds for research and development, available free to those with "institutional affiliation." Check out what they have at http://nrrl.ncaur.usda.gov.

13. Shurtleff and Aoyagi (2007).

14. Shurtleff and Aoyagi (1979a), 120.

15. Steinkraus, 18.

16. Robert K. Mulyowidarso et al., "The Microbial Ecology of Soybean Soaking for Tempe Production," *International Journal of Food Microbiology* 8:35 (1989).

17. Jutta Denter and Bernward Bisping, "Formation of B-Vitamins by Bacteria During the Soaking Process of Soybeans for Tempe Fermentation," *International Journal of Food Microbiology* 22:23 (1994).

18. Betty Stechmeyer, personal correspondence, July 31, 2010.

19. Steinkraus 25–26.

20. Ibid., 29.

21. C. W. Hesseltine and Hwa L. Wang, "The Importance of Traditional Fermented Foods," *BioScience* 30(6):402 (1980) online at www.jstor.org/stable/1308003, accessed December 21, 2009.

22. Shurtleff and Aoyagi's *Book of Tempeh* covers the topic in 7 pages (117–124), while their more specialized book *Tempeh Production* does so in considerably more depth in 22 pages (140–162). (Both are freely available on the Internet.)

23. Shurtleff and Aoyagi (1986), 143.

24. Hwa L. Wang et al., "Mass Production of *Rhizopus Oligosporus* Spores and Their Application in Tempeh Fermentation," *Journal of Food Science* 40:168 (1975).

25. Shurtleff and Aoyagi (1986), 145.

26. Ibid., 151.

28. www.makethebesttempeh.org.

27. C. W. Hesseltine, "A Millennium of Fungi, Food, and Fermentation," *Mycologia*, 57(2):190 (1965).

29. www.gemcultures.com.

30. Steinkraus, 480.

31. Shurtleff and Aoyagi (1980), 55.

32. Ibid., 53–57.

33. Shurtleff and Aoyagi (1976), 162.

34. Andoh, 280.

35. Kushi, 341.

36. Shurtleff and Aoyagi (1976), 162.

37. Mollison, 212.

38. Xu Gan Rong and Bao Tong Fa, *Grandiose Survey of Chinese Alcoholic Drinks and Beverages*, online at www.sytu.edu.cn/zhgjiu/u2-1.htm, accessed December 18, 2010.

39. Huang, 172–173. Reprinted with the permission of Cambridge University Press.

40. Ibid., 281.

41. Steinkraus, 451–452.

42. Dr. S. Sekar, "Prepared Starter for Fermented Country Beverage Production," in *Database on Microbial Traditional Knowledge of India*, online at http://www.bdu.ac.in/schools/life_sciences/biotechnology/sekardb.htm, accessed December 5, 2010.

43. T. S. Rana et al., "Soor: A Traditional Alcoholic Beverage in Tons Valley, Garhwal Himalaya," *Indian Journal of Traditional Knowledge* 3(1):61 (2004).

44. Cherl-Ho Lee, "Cereal Fermentations in Countries of the Asia-Pacific Region," in Haard, 70; Steinkraus, 448.

45. Shurtleff and Aoyagi (1979b), 163.

Chapter 11

1. Albala (2007), 1–2.

2. See my discussion of vegetable-nut pâtés in *The Revolution Will Not Be Microwaved*, 183.

3. "Make cashew milk by grinding up about 1 cup of cashew pieces into a powder. Add 3–4 dates and enough water to make 4 cups of liquid. Blend on high until completely blended."

4. Suellen Ocean, *Acorns and Eat 'Em* (Oakland: California Oak Foundation, 2006), online at www.californiaoaks.org/ExtAssets/acorns_and_eatem.pdf, accessed November 16, 2009.

5. www.billabbie.com/calath/word4day/sk7ee7.html, accessed January 5, 2010.

6. Pederson, 340.

7. Mollison, 214.

8. Farrell, 82.

9. Pederson, 342.

10. Farrell, 84–85.

11. Battcock and Azam-Ali, 79.

12. Pederson, 337–338.

13. Ibid., 343.

14. Wilfred F. M. Röling et al., "Microorganisms with a Taste for Vanilla: Microbial Ecology of Traditional Indonesian Vanilla Curing," *Applied Environmental Microbiology* 67(5):1995 (2001).

15. Pederson, 345.

16. Keith Steinkraus, "Lactic Acid Fermentation in the Production of Foods from Vegetables, Cereals and Legumes," *Antonie van Leeuwenhoek* 49:341 (1983).

17. Steinkraus (1996), 149.

18. McGee, 101–102.

19. "West African Cuisine in the New World," online at www.bahia-online.net/FoodinSalvador.htm, accessed March 20, 2011.

20. Edamame—Japanese steamed green soybeans—are an exception to this, but they are particular varieties, harvested before full maturity, and not dried for storage.

21. Albala, 221.

22. Sidney Mintz et al., "The Significance of Soy," in Du Bois, 5.

23. Christine M. Du Bois, "Social Context and Diet: Changing Soy Production and Consumption in the United States," in Du Bois, 210–213.

24. Benson Ford Research Center, "Soybean car," online at www.thehenryford.org/research/soybeancar .aspx, accessed January 11, 2011.

25. Du Bois, 5.

26. Ibid., 218.

27. John Harvey Kellogg, *New Dietetics: A Guide to Scientific Feeding in Health and Disease* (1921), cited in Albala, 225.

28. Belasco, 189.

29. Daniel.

30. Susun S. Weed, 163.

31. Shurtleff and Aoyagi (2009), 7.

32. www.soyinfocenter.com.

33. Shurtleff and Aoyagi (1976), 100.

34. Sidney Mintz, "Fermented Beans and Western Taste," in Du Bois, 60.

35. For historical perspectives on soy sauce, miso, and similar foods, I recommend two excellent sources: Huang, and Shurtleff and Aoyagi (2009).

36. D. Fukushima, "Soy Sauce and Other Fermented Foods of Japan," in Hesseltine and Wang, 122.

37. Deshpande, 83.

38. B. S. Luh, "Industrial Production of Soy Sauce," *Journal of Industrial Microbiology* 14:469 (1995).

39. Shurtleff and Aoyagi (2007).

40. A. K. Smith, US Department of Agriculture, ARS-71-1 (1958), cited in C. W. Hesseltine, "A Millennium of Fungi, Food, and Fermentation," *Mycologia* 57(2):187 (1965).

41. Hui (2006), 19-11 to 19-12.

42. Q. Wei et al., "Natto Characteristics as Affected by Steaming Time, Bacillus Strain, and Fermentation Time," *Journal of Food Science* 66(1):172 (2001).

43. Shurtleff and Aoyagi (2007).

44. Hui (2004), 616.

45. Shurtleff and Aoyagi (2007).

46. H. Sumi et al., "A Novel Fibrinolytic Enzyme (Nattokinase) in the Vegetable Cheese Natto; A Typical and Popular Soybean Food in the Japanese Diet," *Cellular and Molecular Life Sciences* 43(10):1110 (1987).

47. Martin Milner and Kouhei Makise, "Natto and Its Active Ingredient Nattokinase: A Potent and Safe Thrombolytic Agent," *Alternative and Complementary Therapies* 8(3):163 (2002).

48. Ruei-Lin Hsu et al., "Amyloid-Degrading Ability of Nattokinase from Bacillus subtilis Natto," *Journal of Agricultural and Food Chemistry* 57:503 (2009).

49. Charles Parkouda et al., "The Microbiology of Alkaline-Fermentation of Indigenous Seeds Used as Food Condiments in Africa and Asia," *Critical Reviews in Microbiology* 35(2):140 (2009); O. B. Oyewole, "Fermentation of Grain Legumes, Seeds, and Nuts in Africa" (chapter 2), in Deshpande.

50. O. K. Achi, "Traditional Fermented Protein Condiments in Nigeria," *African Journal of Biotechnology* 4(13):1614 (2005).

51. Food and Nutrition Library, "Netetou—A Typical African Condiment," online at www.greenstone.org/greenstone3/nzdl;jsessionid=2818D949147C6837BD89B5344237C2F7?a=d&d=HASHdee10c9b85605053eeb12f.8&c=fnl&sib=1&dt=&ec=&et=&p.a=b&p.s=ClassifierBrowse&p.sa=, accessed January 30, 2011.

52. Achi, 1616–1617.

53. Cornell University Plants Poisonous to Livestock Database, "Castor Bean Poisoning," online at www.ansci.cornell.edu/plants/castorbean.html, accessed August 24, 2011.

54. Parkouda, 144.

55. Achi, 1616.

56. Rama, "Okra Soup," *Okra & Cocoa* blog (June 24, 2007), online at http://okra-cocoa.blogspot.com/2007/06/okra-soup.html, accessed October 13, 2011.

57. Huang, 325.

58. Cited in Steinkraus, 633.

59. Steinkraus, 634.

60. Fuchsia Dunlop, "Rotten Vegetable Stalks, Stinking Beancurd and Other Shaoxing Delicacies," paper delivered at 2010 Oxford Symposium on Food and Cookery.

61. Huang, 326.

62. C. W. Hesseltine, "A Millennium of Fungi, Food, and Fermentation," *Mycologia* 57(2):164 (1965).

63. Shurtleff and Aoyagi (1998), 255.

64. Steinkraus, 634.

65. http://nrrl.ncaur.usda.gov.

66. Dunlop.

Chapter 12

1. Stephen S. Arnon et al., "Botulinum Toxin as a Biological Weapon," *Journal of the American Medical Association* 285(8):1059 (2001).

2. Riddervold (1990), 12.

3. Ana Andrés et al., "Principles of Drying and Smoking," in Toldrá (2007), 40.

4. McGee, 448.

5. McGee, 449; Karl O. Honikel, "Principles of Curing," in Toldrá (2007), 17

6. John N. Sofos, "Antimicrobial Effects of Sodium and Other Ions in Foods: A Review," *Journal of Food Safety* 6:54 (1984).

7. Eeva-Liisa Ryhänen, "Plant-Derived Biomolecules in Fermented Cabbage," *Journal of Agricultural and Food Chemistry* 50:6798 (2002).

8. McGee, 125.

9. Fearnley-Whittingstall (2007), 414–416.

10. Peter Zeuthen, "A Historical Perspective of Meat Fermentation," in Toldrá (2007), 3.

11. G. Giolitti et al., "Microbiology and Chemical Changes in Raw Hams of Italian Type," *Journal of Applied Microbiology* 34:51 (1971).

12. I. Vilar et al., "A Survey on the Microbiological Changes During the Manufacture of Dry-Cured Lacón, a Spanish Traditional Meat Product," *Journal of Applied Microbiology* 89:1018 (2000).

13. Lars L. Hinrichsen and Susanne B. Pedersen, "Relationship Among Flavor, Volatile Compounds, Chemical Changes, and Microflora in Italian-Type Dry-Cured Ham During Processing," *Journal of Agricultural and Food Chemistry* 43(11):2939 (1995).

14. Ruhlman, 153.

15. Máirtín Mac Con Iomaire and Pádric Óg Gallagher, "Corned Beef: An Enigmatic Irish Dish," paper delivered at 2010 Oxford Symposium on Food and Cookery.

16. Rombauer and Becker (1975), 507.

17. Toldrá (2002), 89; Marianski and Marianski, 20–25.

18. Fearnley-Whittingstall (2007), 418.

19. Toldrá (2002), 91.

20. Albala and Nafziger, 120.

21. Marianski and Marianski, 28.

22. Friedrich-Karl Lücke, "Fermented Meat Products," *Food Research International* 27:299 (1994).

23. Herbert W. Ockerman and Lopa Basu, "Production and Consumption of Fermented Meat Products," in Toldrá (2007), 12.

24. Ken Albala, "Bacterial Fermentation and the Missing Terroir Factor in Historic Cookery," paper delivered at 2010 Oxford Symposium on Food and Cookery.

25. Albala and Nafziger, 121.

26. Marc Buzzio, quoted in Sarah diGregorio, "The Salami Maker Who Fought the Law," *Gastronomica* 7(4):54 (2007).

27. diGregorio, 57.

28. Toldrá (2002), 89.

29. Ruhlman and Polcyn, 176.

30. Ibid., 175.

31. Marianski and Marianski, 77.

32. Margarita Garriga and Teresa Aymerich, "The Microbiology of Fermentation and Ripening," in Toldrá (2007), 130.

33. Toldrá (2002), 106.

34. Fearnley-Whittingstall (2001), 162.

35. Piccetti and Vecchio, 24.

36. Huang, 396.

37. Steinkraus, 590.

38. Robert C. McIver, "Flavor of Fermented Fish Sauce," *Journal of Agricultural and Food Chemistry* 30:1017 (1982).

39. Sally Grainger, "Roman Fish Sauce: Part 2, an Experiment in Archaeology," paper delivered at 2010 Oxford Symposium on Food and Cookery.

40. Giovanna Franciosa et al., "*Clostridium botulinum*," in Miliotis and Bier, 81.

41. Steinkraus, 586.

42. Ibid., 565.

43. Ibid., 573.

44. Christianne Muusers, "Roman Fish Sauce—Garum or Liquamen," *Coquinaria* (April 24, 2005), online at www.coquinaria.nl/english/recipes/garum.htm, accessed April 17, 2011.

45. Mollison, 127–159.

46. McGee, 232.

47. Belitz, 636.

48. Ulrike Lyhs, "Microbiological Methods," chapter 15 in Rehbein and Oehlenschläger, 318.

49. Renée Valeri, "A Preserve Gone Bad or Just Another Beloved Delicacy? Surströmming and Gravlax—the Good and the Bad Ways of Preserving Fish," paper delivered at 2010 Oxford Symposium on Food and Cookery.

50. McGee, 236.

51. http://en.wikipedia.org/wiki/Rakfisk, accessed March 20, 2011.

52. Valeri, 4.

53. Riddervold, 63.

54. Huang, 384–386.

55. Sanchez, 264; R. C. Mabesa and J. S. Babaan, "Fish Fermentation Technology in the Philippines," in Lee, 87–88.

56. Lee, 88.

57. Minerva S. D. Olympia, "Fermented Fish Products in the Philippines," in Gaden, 131.

58. Naomichi Ishige, "Cultural Aspects of Fermented Fish Products in Asia," in Lee, 15.

59. Chieko Fujita, "Funa Zushi," *Rediscovering the Treasures of Food* Volume 13, The Tokyo Foundation website, published February 16, 2009, online at www.tokyofoundation.org/en/topics/japanese -traditional-foods/vol.-13-funa-zushi, accessed February 5, 2011.

60. Kimiko Barber, "Hishio—Tastes of Japan in Humble Microbes," paper delivered at 2010 Oxford Symposium on Food and Cookery.

61. Chieko Fujita, "Koji, an Aspergillus," *Rediscovering the Treasures of Food* Volume 10, The Tokyo Foundation website, published December 16, 2008, online at www.tokyofoundation.org/en/topics/japanese -traditional-foods/vol.-10-koji-an-aspergillus, accessed April 1, 2010.

62. Huang, 391.

63. Huang, 381–382.

64. Personal correspondence, February 11, 2011

65. Fallon, 241.

66. Anna Kowalska-Lewicka, "The Pickling of Vegetables in Traditional Polish Peasant Culture," in Riddervold and Ropeid, 35.

67. Dunlop (2003), 153.

68. Katharine L Giery, *Basque Fishing* blog (April 30, 2011), online at http://basquefishing.tumblr.com /post/5075347526/xocolatl-or-however-you-call-it, accessed August 4, 2011.

69. Huang, 413.

70. Shurtleff and Aoyagi (1976), 159.

71. David Wetzel, "Update on Cod Liver Oil Manufacture," April 2009, online at www.westonaprice.org /cod-liver-oil/1602-update-on-cod-liver-oil-manufacture, accessed May 7, 2011.

72. David Wetzel, "Cod Liver Oil Manufacturing," *Wise Traditions* (fall 2005), online at www.westonaprice .org/cod-liver-oil/183, accessed May 7, 2011.

73. David Wetzel, "Update on Cod Liver Oil Manufacture," April 2009, online at www.westonaprice.org /cod-liver-oil/1602-update-on-cod-liver-oil-manufacture, accessed May 7, 2011.

74. Shephard, 131.

75. Andrew B. Smith et al., "Marine Mammal Storage: Analysis of Buried Seal Meat at the Cape, South Africa," *Journal of Archaeological Science* 19:171 (1992).

76. Charles Perry, "Dried, Frozen, and Rotted: Food Preservation in Central Asia and Siberia," paper delivered at 2010 Oxford Symposium on Food and Cookery.

77. Yann_Chef, *Food Lorists* blog (December 2008), online at http://foodlorists.blogspot.com/2008/12 /kiviak.html, accessed November 29, 2009.

78. Jones, 86, online at http://alaska.fws.gov/asm/fisreportdetail.cfm?fisrep=21, accessed February 8, 2011.

79. Centers for Disease Control and Prevention, *Botulism in the United States, 1899–1996: Handbook for Epidemiologists, Clinicians, and Laboratory Workers* (Atlanta: Centers for Disease Control and Prevention, 1998), 7.

80. Jones, 284.

81. Jones, 146–148.

Chapter 13

1. US Food and Drug Administration, "Questions and Answers on the Food Safety Modernization Act," March 4, 2011, online at www.fda.gov/Food/FoodSafety/FSMA/ucm238506.htm, accessed March 8, 2011.

2. US Food and Drug Administration, "Hazard Analysis and Critical Control Point Principles and Application Guidelines," adopted August 14, 1997, by the National Advisory Committee on Microbiological Criteria for Foods, online at www.fda.gov/Food/FoodSafety/HazardAnalysisCritical ControlPointsHACCP/HACCPPrinciplesApplicationGuidelines/default.htm, accessed March 8, 2011.

3. William Neuman, "Raw Milk Cheesemakers Fret Over Possible New Rules," *New York Times* (February 4, 2011), online at www.nytimes.com/2011/02/05/business/05cheese.html, accessed June 11, 2011.

4. American Raw Milk Cheese Presidium, "Presidium Mission and Protocol for Presidium Members," July 2006, appendix A, online at www.rawmilkcheese.org/index_files/PresidiumProtocol .htm#Appendix%20A, accessed June 11, 2011.

Chapter 14

1. See www.teraganix.com/EM-Solutions-for-Compost-s/90.htm, accessed June 10, 2011.

2. Helen Jensen et al., *Nature Farming Manual* (Batong Malake, Los Baños Laguna, Philippines: National Initiative on Seed and Sustainable Agriculture in the Philippines and REAP-Canada, 2006), online at www.scribd.com/doc/15940714/Bokashi-Nature-Farming-Manual-Philippines-2006, accessed February 24, 2011.

3. Hoon Park and Michael W. DuPonte, "How to Cultivate Indigenous Microorganisms," published by the Cooperative Extension Service of the College of Tropical Agriculture and Human Resources, University of Hawai'i–Mānoa (August 2008), online at www.ctahr.hawaii.edu/oc/freepubs/pdf/BIO-9.pdf, accessed June 27, 2010.

4. Veranus A. Moore, "The Ammoniacal Fermentation of Urine," *Proceedings of the American Society of Microscopists* 12:97 (1890). Published by Blackwell Publishing on behalf of American Microscopical Society, online at www.jstor.org/stable/3220677, accessed March 2, 2011.

5. "Pee Ponics," posting on Aquaponic Gardening: A Community and Forum for Aquaponic Gardeners by TCLynx (June 6, 2010), online at http://aquaponicscommunity.com/profiles/blogs/pee-ponics, accessed February 3, 2011.

6. Joseph Mazige, "Farmers Use Human Urine as Fertilizers, Pesticide," *Monitor* (Kampala) (August 19, 2007), online at http://desertification.wordpress.com/2007/08/21/uganda-farmers-use-human-urine -as-fertilizers-pesticide-monitor-allafrica, accessed February 3, 2011.

7. George Chan, "Livestock in South-Eastern China," Second FAO Electronic Conference on Tropical Feeds: Livestock Feed Resources Within Integrated Farming Systems (1996), 148, online at www.fao.org/ag /againfo/resources/documents/frg/conf96htm/chan.htm, accessed March 28, 2011.

8. Y. L. Nene, "*Kunapajala*—A Liquid Organic Manure of Antiquity," Asian Agri-History Foundation, online at www.agri-history.org/pdf/AGRI.pdf, accessed March 28, 2011.

9. J. W. Schroeder, "Silage Fermentation and Preservation," North Dakota State University Agriculture and University Extension publication AS-1254 (June 2004), online at www.ag.ndsu.edu/pubs/ansci/dairy /as1254w.htm, accessed March 27, 2011.

10. Anna Kowalska-Lewicka, "The Pickling of Vegetables in Traditional Polish Peasant Culture," in Riddervold and Ropeid, 37fn.

11. Michel and Jude Fanton, *The Seed Savers' Handbook* (Byron Bay, NSW, Australia: Seed Savers' Network, 1993), 152.

12. Ibid., 90.

13. Barbara Larson, "Saving Seed from the Garden," *Home Hort Hints* (August–September 2000), University of Illinois Extension, online at http://urbanext.illinois.edu/hortihints/0008c.html, accessed March 27, 2011.

14. US Environmental Protection Agency Office of Solid Waste and Emergency Response, "A Citizen's Guide to Bioremediation," EPA 542-F-01-001 (April 2001), online at www.epa.gov/tio/download/citizens /bioremediation.pdf, accessed March 29, 2011.

15. David Biello, "Slick Solution: How Microbes Will Clean Up the *Deepwater Horizon* Oil Spill," *Scientific American* (May 25, 2010), online at www.scientificamerican.com/article.cfm?id=how-microbes-clean -up-oil-spills, accessed March 29, 2011.

16. American Academy of Microbiology, Microbes and Oil Spills FAQ (2011), 1, online at http://academy.asm .org/images/stories/documents/Microbes_and_Oil_Spills.pdf, accessed March 29, 2011.

17. American Academy of Microbiology, 8.

18. Cited in Biello.

19. Stamets (2005), 82.

20. Ibid., 85.

21. Ibid., 86.

22. Common Ground Collective Meg Perry Health Soil Project, *The New Orleans Residents' Guide to Do It Yourself Soil Clean Up Using Natural Processes* (March 2006), online at https://we.riseup.net /blooming-in-space/the-new-orleans-residents-guide-to-do-it+22865.

23. Joseph Jenkins, *The Humanure Handbook: A Guide to Composting Human Manure*, 3rd edition (Grove City, PA: Joseph Jenkins, Inc., 2005).

24. Farrell, 126–127.

25. Jenkins, 151–152.

26. "The Fundamental Microbiology of Sewage," On-Site Wastewater Demonstration Program, Northern Arizona University, online at www.cefns.nau.edu/Projects/WDP/resources/Microbiology/index.html, accessed March 30, 2011.

27. Jenkins, 227.

28. Kurlansky, 43.

29. The Green Burial Council, "Who We Are," online at www.greenburialcouncil.org/who-we-are, accessed March 31, 2011.

30. Dr. S. Sekar, "Fermented Dyes," in *Database on Microbial Traditional Knowledge of India*, online at http://www.bdu.ac.in/schools/life_sciences/biotechnology/sekardb.htm, accessed December 5, 2010.

31. Carole Crews, *Clay Culture: Plasters, Paints, and Preservation* (Rancho de Taos, NM: Gourmet Adobe Press, 2009), 103.

32. Ibid., 98–99.

33. Ibid., 103.

34. Ibid., 104.

35. Jeremy Hsu, "Invention Awards: Eco-Friendly Insulation Made from Mushrooms," *Popular Science* (May 2009), online at www.popsci.com/environment/article/2009-05/green-styrofoam, accessed June 10, 2011.

36. www.ecovativedesign.com.

37. Congressional Budget Office, *The Impact of Ethanol Use on Food Prices and Greenhouse-Gas Emissions* (April 2009), vii, online at www.cbo.gov/ftpdocs/100xx/doc10057/04-08-Ethanol.pdf.

38. Tom Philpott, "The Trouble with Brazil's Much-Celebrated Ethanol 'Miracle,'" April 13, 2010, online at www.grist.org/article/2010-04-13-raising-cane-the-trouble-with-brazils-much-celebrated-ethanol-mi, accessed April 3, 2011.

39. Dhruti Shah, "Will We Switch to Gas Made from Human Waste?" *BBC News Magazine* (April 19, 2010), online at http://news.bbc.co.uk/2/hi/uk_news/magazine/8501236.stm, accessed April 5, 2011.

40. Greg Votava and Rich Webster, "Methane to Energy: Improving an Ancient Idea," Nebraska Department of Environmental Quality *Environmental Update* (spring 2002), online at www.deq.state.ne.us/Newslett.nsf/d62915495a28710806256bd5006a4d84/f60aa501092d797606256bd500646afa?OpenDocument, accessed April 5, 2011.

41. Li Kangmin and Mae-Wan Ho, "Biogas China," Institute of Science in Society (February 10, 2006), online at www.i-sis.org.uk/BiogasChina.php, accessed April 5, 2011.

42. Dr. S. Sekar, *Database on Microbial Traditional Knowledge of India*, online at http://www.bdu.ac.in/schools/life_sciences/biotechnology/sekardb.htm, accessed April 6, 2011.

43. Paul Stamets, "Novel Antimicrobials from Mushrooms," *Herbalgram* 54:29 (2002), online at www.fungi.com/pdf/pdfs/articles/HerbalGram.pdf, accessed April 6, 2011.

44. Kenneth Todar, *Todar's Online Textbook of Bacteriology*, online at www.textbookofbacteriology.net/bacteriology_6.html, accessed April 5, 2011.

45. http://altadisusa.com/cigar-101/judge/fermentation, accessed November 19, 2010.

46. "Principles of the Cedar Enzyme Bath Treatment," Osmosis Day Spa, online at www.osmosis.com/cedar-enzyme-bath/principles, accessed April 9, 2011.

47. www.kefiplant.com.

48. Arlene Correll, "How to Make Your Own Liquid Potpourri and Other Good Stuff!," online at www.phancypages.com/newsletter/ZNewsletter530.htm, accessed July 28, 2011.

49. Jenifer Wightman, "Winogradsky Rothko: Bacterial Ecosystem as Pastoral Landscape," *Journal of Visual Culture* 7:309 (2008), online at http://vcu.sagepub.com/cgi/content/abstract/7/3/309, accessed February 4, 2011.

INDEX

NOTE: *CI* page references can be found in the color inserts.

fungi. *See also* mushrooms
  bioremediation, 397–98
  compost, 387, 388, 390, 392
funkaso, 236–37

G

galangal, 151
gari, 229
gariss, 198, 199
garlic, 96, 112, 113, 120, 124, 125, 127
garum, 353
gene transfer, 3–5, 29–30
germination. *See* sprouting seeds and grains
ginger
  beer, 150–51, 274, 421–22, *CI:11*
  bug, 150–51, 162, 164
  in kimchi, 112, 113
  in kvass, 154
  in meads, 81
  sour tonic beverages, 162, 164
  in water kefir, 157
glucose, 73, 168, 342, 351
glucosinolates, 25
gluten-free beer, 253
gluten intolerance, 218
goat kefir, 164
goat milk, 182, 205, 208
  clabbering, 186
  kefir, 194, 199
  raw milk, 184
goitrogens, 31
Gouania polygama, 162
gourds as vessels, 55–56, *CI:18*
grain mills, 64
grains, fermenting, 46, 211–25, 231–45, 426–27. *See also* beer; porridges; sourdoughs; *specific grains*
  cultures, 218
  engrained patterns, 212–18
  fish, fermented with, 355–59
  leftover grains, 244
  with other foods, 244
  rejuvelac, 220
  silage, 393–94
  soaking grains, 123, 218–20
  sprouting, 219
  tempeh, 285, 288
  troubleshooting, 244–45
  in vegetable ferments, 108, 113–14
grains, kefir. *See* kefir
grapes
  juice fermented with water kefir, 157

leaves, 120
  in meads, 82
  presses, 63–64
  wines, 82–84, *CI:3–5*
grating vegetables, 98, 377
gravfisk/gravlax, 340, 363–65, *364*
green onions, 112
greens, 105–6, 118, 120. *See also specific greens*
grits, 216, 221–23
grubenkraut, 57
gruels. *See* porridges
gruts (gruits), 81, 274–75
gundruk, 118
gv-no-he-nv, 214

H

half-sours, 124, 125
Haloanaerobium, 354
hamanatto, 327–28
Hazardous Analysis and Critical Control Point
  (HACCP) plan, 379–80
health benefits of fermentation, 21–32
  detoxification, 25–26
  gluten intolerance, 218
  kombucha, 167–69
  lactose intolerance, 218
  live bacterial cultures, 26–32
  nattokinase, 330–31
  nutritional enhancement, 24–25
  pre-digestion, 24
  soybeans, 318
heavy metals, 26
Helicobacter pylori, 13–14
hemp, 402
hemp seed milk, 207
herbal elixir meads, 79–82
herbs, in beer, 273–75
herring, 354–55
heterofermentative, 96
hickory nuts, 207
high meat, 366
Himalayan *gundruk* and *sinki*, 118
HIV/AIDS, 21, 22, 136–37, 167–68
homofermentative, 96
honey. *See also* honey water; mead
  duma, 159
  jun, 175
  for vinegar, 177
  water kefir, fermented with, 155, 156
  yeasts in, 72–73, 80

condiments, 331–33
edamame, 108, 316
hulling (dehulling), 285–86, 292, 295, 332–33
in kimchi, 108, 113
koji, growing on, 298, *CI:23*
natto, 282, 328–31
proteins predigested into amino acids, 24
soydawadawa, 332–33
steaming, 64
tofu, fermenting, 333–35
United States, use in, 317–18
soydawadawa, 332–33
soymilk, fermenting, 155, 207
specific gravity, 63
spicing, vegetable ferments, 109–10, 112–14, 120
spontaneous (wild) fermentation, 5, 12, 51, 72, 92, 247
    Acetobacter and, 72
    beans, 313–16
    beers, 248–50, *CI:17*
    commercial starters compared, 134–35
    country wines, 87
    culturing *versus*, 38–39
    dry-curing, 347–49
    fruit and fruit juices, 72, 90
    mead, 74, 80
    milk, 134, 182, 183, 185–86
    tepache, 153
    tomato preserves, 117
    tubers, 228
sprouting seeds and grains, 219, 269–70
squash, 105, 106
squeezing vegetables, 100–101
Staphylococcus
    meat curing, role in, 345, 350
    S. aureus, 380
starchy tubers, fermenting, 211–12, 225–30, 244. *See also* cassava; potatoes
    beers, 271–73
    poi, 31, 226–27
starters, xviii, 38–39, 43. *See also* commercial starters; kefir; *koji;* SCOBYs (symbiotic communities of bacteria and yeast); starters, sour tonic beverages; tempeh; whey
    beans, 313
    cheese, 202–3
    Chinese pickling, 114
    compost, 389–90
    dry-curing, 347–50
    exchanges, 421
    feeding, 38–39
    fruit ferments, 129, 131
    fruit salad, 88

ginger bug, 150–51
grain ferments, 218
lactic acid, 129
mead continuous starter method, 79
millet beer, 265, 266
mold, for rice brews, 261
natto, 329–30, 431
potato beer, 272, 273
rice beers, 261–65
rules for, 40
seed cheeses, 122–23
soy sauce, 326
vegetable ferments, adding to, 132–35
viili, 196–97
vinegar, 175–77
yogurt, 186, 189–92, 424
starters, sour tonic beverages, 147–48, *CI:12. See also* water kefir
    ginger bug, 150–51, 162, 164
    kombucha mothers, 38, 167–74, 178, 422–23
    mauby, 154–55
    pru, 163
    roots beer, 162
    sweet potato fly, 164
    whey, 160–61
steamers, 64
sterilization, 41–43, 62
stevia, 87
stills. *See* distillation, alcohol
stinging nettles, 107, 199
storage of ferments, 59
    dry-cured meat, 352
    meads, 78–79
    soy sauce, 327
    tempeh, 18, 290
Streptococcus salivarius subsp. *thermophilus*, 189, 191, *CI:12*
stuck fermentation. *See* aeration
substrates, 37–38, 39
    fish ferments, grain substrate for, 355–56
    sterilization of, 41–43
    tempeh, 284–88, 293
succession, microbial communities, 41
sugar. *See also* saccharification; sugar water
    country wines, 86–87, *CI:5*
    for dry-curing, 351
    for fermented fruit salad, 88
    in kombucha, 170, 173
    yeasts in, 72
sugar substitutes, 87
sugar water, 77
    racking, adding during, 61

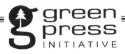

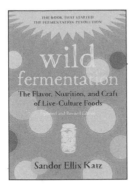
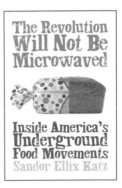
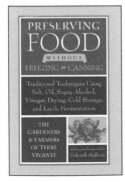
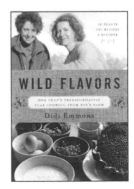
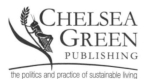

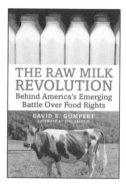
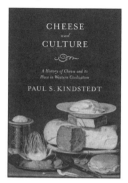
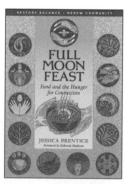
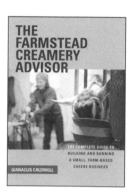
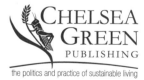